DATE DUE

APR 26 2010			
MAR 07 2011			
12/16/15 ILL			

Demco, Inc. 38-293

D1087459

A Manual Therapist's Guide to Movement

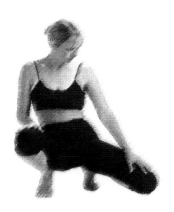

Senior Commissioning Editor: Sarena Wolfaard
Development Editor: Claire Wilson
Project Manager: Caroline Horton
Senior Designer: Sarah Russell

A Manual Therapist's Guide to Movement:
Teaching Motor Skills to the Orthopedic Patient

Gordon Browne BSC

*in Physical Therapy; Guild-Certified
Feldenkrais Practitioner;
Private Practitioner,
Bellevue, Washington, USA*

Foreword by
Darlene Hertling BS

*Senior Lecturer Emeritus, Physical Therapist,
Department of Rehabilitation Medicine,
University of Washington, Seattle, WA, USA*

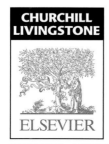

CHURCHILL
LIVINGSTONE

ELSEVIER

615.82
B882

LIBRARY
MILWAUKEE AREA TECHNICAL COLLEGE
Milwaukee Campus
WITHDRAWN

EDINBURGH LONDON NEW YORK OXFORD PHILADELPHIA ST LOUIS SYDNEY TORONTO 2006

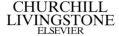

CHURCHILL
LIVINGSTONE
ELSEVIER

© 2006, Elsevier Limited. All rights reserved.

The rights of Gordon Browne to be identified as Author of this work have been asserted by him in accordance with the Copyright, Designs and Patents Act 1988

No part of this publication may be reproduced, stored in a retrieval system, or transmitted in any form or by any means, electronic, mechanical, photocopying, recording or otherwise, without the prior permission of the Publishers. Permissions may be sought directly from Elsevier's Health Sciences Rights Department, 1600 John F. Kennedy Boulevard, Suite 1800, Philadelphia, PA 19103-2899, USA: phone (+1)215 239 3804; fax: (+1)215 239 3805; or, e-mail: *healthpermissions@elsevier.com*. You may also complete your request on-line via the Elsevier homepage (http://www.elsevier.com), by selecting 'Support and contact' and then 'Copyright and Permission'.

First published 2006

ISBN 0 443 10216 3

British Library Cataloguing in Publication Data
A catalogue record for this book is available from the British Library

Library of Congress Cataloging in Publication Data
A catalog record for this book is available from the Library of Congress

Note
Neither the Publisher nor the Author assume any responsibility for any loss or injury and/or damage to persons or property arising out of or related to any use of the material contained in this book. It is the responsibility of the treating practitioner, relying on independent expertise and knowledge of the patient, to determine the best treatment and method of application for the patient.

The Publisher

Printed in China

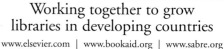

Working together to grow
libraries in developing countries

www.elsevier.com | www.bookaid.org | www.sabre.org

ELSEVIER   BOOK AID
            International   Sabre Foundation

ELSEVIER   your source for books,
journals and multimedia
in the health sciences
www.elsevierhealth.com

The
publisher's
policy is to use
**paper manufactured
from sustainable forests**

Contents

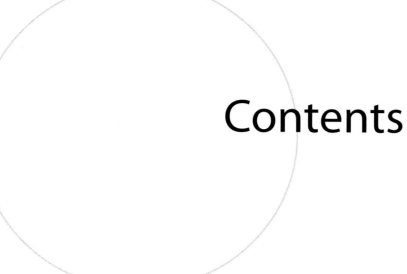

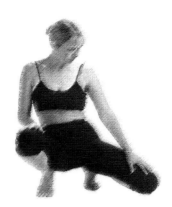

Foreword

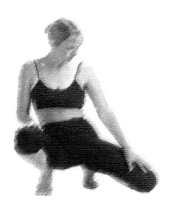

A Manual Therapist's Guide to Movement is a book for those who want to know more about human movement and how to influence it. In his analyses of postural alignment, motor control and muscle balance, Gordon Browne presents the first part of his published work on the trunk and lower limbs. A second volume is planned to cover the cervical spine, temporomandibular joint, upper limbs and autonomic balance. Written for physical therapists in clinical practice who are interested in exploring a new exercise paradigm, this excellent book is a triumph of orderly thought and presentation. It suggests that for physical therapy to continue to grow as a profession, traditional therapeutic exercise and strictly quantifiable goals need to make room for new exercise and treatment paradigms that focus on integration, self-awareness, quality and coordination of movement rather than on isolated movements and compartmentalized exercises featuring straight lines, cardinal planes and rote repetition.

Modern manual therapy has a rich and colorful heritage. As a profession, it has tenaciously held to the value of manual treatment for disorders of structure and function. Gordon Browne, with his extensive background in both manual therapy and the Feldenkrais Method, presents a unique system of therapy that has grown out of creative observation and consistent, independent development.

When the Feldenkrais Method is applied to patients in physical therapy and rehabilitation, the therapist takes on the role of teacher, facilitator and guide. The intention of the therapist is to guide the individual using verbal, visual and kinesthetic information. Rather than first evaluating the patient and then treating with soft tissue techniques and strengthening or range of motion exercises, the patient is 'invited to learn' using the discovery model. The patient is asked to explore a new focus of movement by attending to altered kinesthetic cues during a desired action. The patient is then carefully guided to compare and observe whether the new focus leads to improved adaptation during the desired function activity.

In this system, evaluation is not performed separately from the learning process. The therapist constantly observes and adapts stimuli in order for the student to maximally explore and adapt new motor patterns during a particular lesson; to experience a sense of success or the novelty of discovery. Evaluation and progress notes record the conditions that facilitate learning for this person; the key auditory, visual, kinesthetic, and/or movement cues that maximize functional performance of a desired task, illustrating in each unique case the neuroplasticity of the central nervous system.

The author of this first volume has produced a text that focuses on the functional movements that underlie every action that we participate in on a day-to-day basis. As physical therapists, we have learned to focus on the components of movement that are limited by injury – range of motion, strength and somatosensory functions. A review of physical therapy literature documents a gradual shift toward movement as its own entity. Physical measurements of joint motion and force production remain important, but new efforts address other components – motor control, balance, somatosensory awareness, movement error detection, sensory effect of somatic injury etc. – that allow us to perform our daily and recreational activities at the level we wish. This serves as the basis for determining well-organized function and success in treatment . . . achieving full range of motion or strength is no longer the final goal of treatment.

One element of functional exercise brought out in Browne's work that is worthy of consideration is the idea of 'integrated' versus 'isolated' movement patterns. Whereas most machine-based exercises isolate motion to a particular joint, effectively training a muscle in one plane, functional exercises tend to be multi-planar, since true functional movements occur in a tri-planar fashion.

After the initial background chapters covering key concepts, trunk organization and the function of the legs, the text then addresses the spinal and pelvic muscles and their potential to stabilize the spinal column. There is significant biomechanical literature describing the role of various anatomical components on stability but until recently this is not the case concerning the muscles.[1-7] Specific movement lessons focus on reactivating the deep intrinsic stabilizers such as the transverse abdominis, internal obliques, multifidus, quadratus lumborum, gluteus medius/maximus and latissimus dorsi. These functional core exercises train stability patterns in movement and positions similar those of daily life, recreation and sport or occupational demands.

Manual resistance is used to faciliate awareness of various extension, flexion and lateral stresses. Resistance is used as an evaluation tool to allow the therapist to assess the patient's global muscular responsiveness and recruitment as well as inter-segmental stability. The patient is observed and monitored through kinesthetic feedback to determine if the spine, pelvic girdle and lower limbs are well positioned and maintained in balanced alignment. Browne's text synthesizes very well the available information about dynamic stabilization of the spinal column and the role of the pelvic girdle, hip and lower limbs, which play a major part in spinal stabilization and functional movement.

The last chapter in this volume focuses on specific lessons to facilitate lower extremity function, balance and efficiency. Categories of lower extremity stressors are discussed and cor-related with needed self-awareness and movement skills. The organizing principle for this chapter is the way the foot interacts with the ground . . . and how the foot functions as an extension of and in concert with the pelvis, hips and knees.

Gordon Browne is to be congratulated for this presentation of his outstanding approach to exercise and movement therapy. He has taken the best scientific evidence available in manual therapy, integrated it with the Feldenkrais Method and applied it to clinical practice. Embracing the Feldenkrais methodology and manual therapy has finally been achieved by Mr. Browne's work.

Darlene Hertling

1. Hodges PW. Core stability exercise in chronic low back pain. Orthop Clin N Am 2003;34:245–54.
2. Hodges PW, Richardson C. Inefficient muscular stabilization of the lumbar spine associated with low back pain. A motor control evaluation of transversus abdominis function. Spine 1996;21:2640–50.
3. McGill SM. Mechanics and pathomechanics of muscles acting on the lumbar spine. In Oatis C: Kinesiology: The Mechanics and Pathomechanic of Human Movement. Philadelphia, Lippincott, Williams & Wilkins; 2004: 563–7.
4. Richardson C, Jull G, Hodges P, Hides J. Therapeutic Exercise for Spinal Segmental Stabilisaton in Low Back Pain. Scientific Basis and Clinical Approach. Edinburgh, Churchill Livingstone; 1999.
5. Richardson C, Jull G, Hides J. A new clinical model of muscle dysfunction linked to the disturbance of spinal stability: Implications for treatment of low back pain. In: Twomey LT, Taylor JR, eds. Physical Therapy of Low Back, 3rd edn. New York, Churchill Livingstone; 2000: 249–67.
6. Richardson C, Hodges P, Hides J. Therapeutic Exercise for Lumbopelvic Stabilization: A Motor Control Approach for Treatment and Prevention of Low Back Pain, 2nd edn; 2004.
7. Richardson CA, Snijders, CJ, Hides JA, et al. The relationship between transversus muscle, sacroiliac joint mechanics and LBP: Spine 2002;27:399–405.

Preface

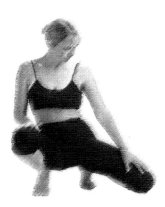

When the early anatomists first started opening up and peering inside human bodies with the intention of describing and recording what makes us tick, they made a fateful decision. They began describing things relative to cardinal planes. They divided the body into X, Y and Z axes and created the coronal, sagittal and transverse planes. They could then describe with written or verbal language exactly where a particular vein, nerve or muscle was relative to another by using the terms medial/lateral, anterior/posterior or superior/inferior. That way, they had a commonly accepted way of communicating their findings with one another.

Naturally, when they began describing human movement, they turned again to the concept of the cardinal plane. Movements of one bone relative to a stationary neighboring bone in the coronal plane became flexion/extension, movements in the sagittal plane became abduction/adduction, and movements in the transverse plane became internal/external rotation. This idea of movement in cardinal planes, and the corollary principle of fixed origin and movable insertion, has subtly but completely colored how we have viewed movement and exercise ever since.

Once movement was described in cardinal planes, the next logical step would have been to ask which muscles moved which bones in what cardinal planes. The infraspinatus externally rotates the shoulder joint in a transverse plane; the quadriceps extends the knee joint in a coronal plane; the gluteus medius abducts the hip joint in a sagittal plane. And so on it went, until over time we came to know exactly which muscles were responsible for what cardinal plane movements. Once movement was described this way and a language had been constructed that described muscular function relative to cardinal plane movement and relative to a fixed and stable point, a particular vision of human movement and exercise was destined to come into being.

Fast-forward to the early twentieth century and the advent of modern exercise principles. Armed with an accumulation of precise anatomical knowledge, modern scientific exercise was predictably designed around stretching or strengthening of individual muscles performed in cardinal planes. Destiny was fulfilled, and we have come to find ourselves under the influence of a somewhat mechanistic vision of human movement and exercise, never suspecting there could be another way of looking at things.

This vision has been one where the legs move on a stationary pelvis, instead of one in which the legs manage the pelvis from their grip on a stationary ground. This vision has been one where the arm and shoulder girdle move relative to an immobile chest and torso, instead of one in which the arms and head move synergistically with movements of the pelvis and torso. This robotic view emphasizes a fixed origin and a mobile insertion, and has the extremities moving in cardinal planes relative to an immobile pelvis and torso like a plastic Barbie doll. It localizes, isolates and compartmentalizes the body, and it has strongly influenced the way that we as physical therapists think of exercise, which is from an objective/scientific perspective.

We have based our physical therapy exercise paradigm on logic. What muscle needs to be stretched or strengthened for this particular orthopedic or movement problem? What cardinal plane movement does this muscle perform? What exercise can I prescribe that makes that muscle work in that plane and against scientifically dosed progressive resistance? With this type of circular thinking, we have constructed an entire therapeutic exercise paradigm with some unspoken but shaky assumptions.

We assume that by making the infraspinatus stronger that it will then automatically kick in at the appropriate time, with the appropriate amount of force and for an appropriate period of time to do its job of controlling arthrokinematic movement of the glenohumeral joint and reducing impingement stresses on the shoulder. We assume that making the vastus medialis stronger will make the patella track more accurately. We assume hip flexor stretches will reduce anterior pelvic tilt and relieve back pain, and that strengthening the lower trapezii makes us reach forward better.

We are making an assumption that strengthening or stretching exercises will improve a given motor skill . . . but do they really? How do we know our student is still using his new strength or flexibility appropriately? Isn't there a less circuitous route we can take to improve clinically relevant motor skills – one that teaches an integrated movement skill in a way that doesn't first disintegrate or atomize a movement? I suggest we just turn the whole equation on end and teach our students how to progressively improve a particular motor skill, then assume that the appropriate muscles will be stretched or strengthened along the way!

It is certainly simpler and cleaner to think of one muscle group controlling one direction within one joint, with one bone fixed and one bone moving. Studies based on these observations are much simpler to set up and to replicate. Exercises based on these assumptions are easier for you to teach and easier for your students to learn, but may lack the complexity or specificity required to make it stick in real life. Reality has a way of making things less tidy and increasing the degree of difficulty.

The reality is that the human body moves in incredibly complex patterns, many of which are imbalanced and inefficient and which can lead to a host of musculoskeletal miseries. These learned patterns of movement and posture are uniquely constructed by each individual and consist of the coordinated and simultaneous action of many different bones and joints, powered by the synergistic contraction of a body-wide series of muscles and controlled by some omnipotent (though not usually omniscient) wizard in the CNS.

If we acknowledge the reality of synergistic patterns of movement, we will need to start updating our exercise paradigm from isolation to integration . . . to emphasize stretching or strengthening an entire pattern of movement, and to take into account the relationship of individual parts to the integrated whole. If we acknowledge the pivotal role the CNS plays in movement and posture regulation, we will need to start finding ways to bring proprioceptive self-awareness and improved body self-image into our exercise prescription, to make it less mechanistic and more organic.

Fortunately, exercise paradigms already exist that show promise in fulfilling these requirements. Tai chi, the Feldenkrais Method® and yoga are examples of exercise systems designed not scientifically but by accumulated proprioceptive experience. These systems could be described as subjective/proprioceptive and, with modifications, have vast untapped potential for physical therapists and others who are interested in advancing their understanding of human movement and how to best influence that movement in their students.

The purpose of this book is to provide a bridge between the two visions of movement and exercise, the objective/scientific/isolationist view and the subjective/proprioceptive/integrative view. This book advocates using modifications of these proprioceptively based movement systems in therapeutic exercise, but leaves the spiritual/mystical trappings inherent to these systems for another forum and explains the science behind the movement. It analyzes the muscular components of a particular prescribed movement and relates it to clinical and functional relevance and to specific tissue strain or pathology.

Primarily, it is written for practicing physical therapists with an orthopedic clientele who are looking for new and improved ways of facilitating better movement or postural quality in their students. It is a book that challenges some of the assumptions we have always made about movement and exercise, and articulates an alternative vision of human movement and how to influence it. Rather than figuring out which muscles to exercise in order to influence a motor skill, we will be figuring out how to exercise particular motor skills and common synergistic patterns of movement that will in turn influence certain muscles.

This alternative vision of therapeutic exercise is not a quick and easy study. The subject matter is immense and intricate. On the other hand, the huge scope and complexity of these proprioceptive systems also means that there is a huge potential for use in treating a wide variety of musculoskeletal injuries or other movement-related conditions. So, if you are feeling a bit adventurous and have an inquisitive mind, dig into your *Guide* and have a safe and interesting journey.

Maple Valley   G.B.
Washington 2006

Acknowledgements

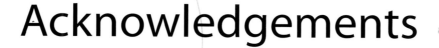

As always when advancing human knowledge, we all stand on the shoulders of others. I would like to express my gratitude and appreciation to my orthopedic/musculoskeletal instructor in physical therapy school, Darlene Hertling, who sparked an interest in orthopedics early on in my PT career.

I would like to commend the genius of Moshe Feldenkrais and thank him for his insight into the marvelous design that is the human body. My thanks go to Anat Baniel and other trainers in the Feldenkrais Method for continuing the work of Dr Feldenkrais after his death, and for making this knowledge available to me and to thousands of others.

I would like to acknowledge the incredible depth, quality and variety of movement experiences that have been developed, taught and passed on through many generations by the practitioners of Tai Chi, yoga and other eastern movement traditions. I thank those nameless masters who have kept these traditions alive through changing times.

My friend and colleague, Israel Sostrin, helped immensely with the research and was a valuable early sounding board for the content and ideas of this book, and I would like to thank him for his help. My mother put in yeoman's duty in combing through this tome three times to make editorial corrections, and I want to add a thank you for the work she did on the book to my thanks to her and my father for giving me life.

Finally, I would like to thank my family. My kids, Morgan and Derek, provided much of the inspiration for this book. Watching them grow up and develop their motor skills gave me insights into movement and learning that later became some of the main themes of this book. My wife Julie, who is a Feldenkrais Practitioner and a Physical Therapists' Assistant, has helped me every step of the way, from initial concept through outline to final changes. I want to thank her for steering me back in the right direction a number of times, for being a rock of unwavering support when I got discouraged, and for sacrificing her needs to give me the time I needed to complete this project.

SECTION ONE

Background and concepts

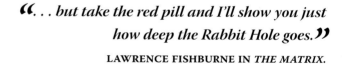

"... but take the red pill and I'll show you just how deep the Rabbit Hole goes."

LAWRENCE FISHBURNE IN *THE MATRIX*.

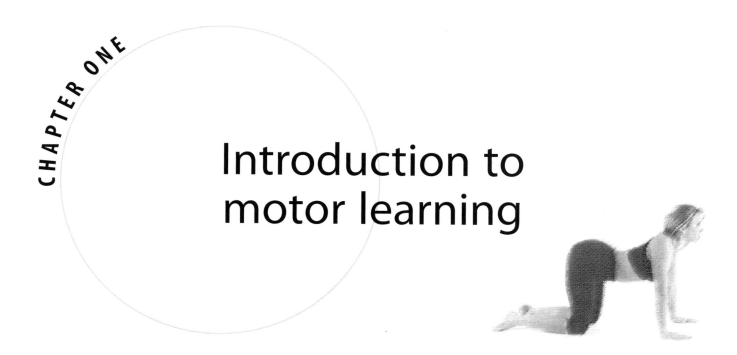

Introduction to motor learning

CHAPTER ONE

Chapter outline

1. Pathokinesiology. What happens when movement goes bad?

2. HJ Hislop coined the term pathokinesiology and called it the distinguishing clinical science of physical therapy. Pathology creates movement dysfunction, and vice versa.

3. Moshe Feldenkrais was a scientist and martial artist. Injured knee and learned to use/move again through observation and mimicking movement of others, especially children.

4. We as movement professionals need to know both objective and subjective movement . . . it is through subjective criteria that we make motor decisions.

5. Movement is behavior, learned and shaped by individual experience. We who are seeking to change the way someone moves need to be able to converse in the language of movement.

6. Proprioception is the internal body awareness sense that tells us where we are in relation to gravity, where bones are relative to each other, about the direction of movement of bones, about where the physiological end range of a joint is, and about muscular effort.

Exercise for motor control purposes

1. How can we better use exercise to improve neuromusculoskeletal function or performance?

2. We can speak broadly of three categories of motor behavior: gross motor, postural and arthrokinematic.

3. We don't want to teach mere stimulus and response behavior, but to mold our students into lean, mean and self-regulating motor planning machines.

4. Puzzle analogy – teach a process rather than imitation and repetition.

Factors influencing motor learning

1. Early childhood development

   - Developmental sequence implications. Let your students develop at their own pace. Allow progressive acquisition of motor skills instead of expecting immediate emergence of a finished product. Allowance of approximations. Start your students at a place where they can be successful, so they don't get frustrated. Progress them on as they learn, so they don't get bored.

   - The Goldilocks effect. Give your student choices, even deliberately wrong ones. By allowing them to decide between an array of choices, we are helping our students improve their proprioceptive listening skills, problem-solving abilities and decision-making, and they will become much better self-regulators. They will also be able to apply those skills to other functions and be able to modify the basic patterns you've taught to fit varied circumstances.

   - Developmental mistakes and imbalances. Early childhood learning blends into lifelong movement and postural patterns. The seeds of our destruction are sown early on. Rule of Holes: when in a hole, stop digging.

2. Injuries
   - Avoidance. Local and distal synergists: ankle sprain inhibits gluteals.
   - Compensation. Someplace else works more or moves more.
   - Tendency of avoidance and compensation patterns to habituate and perpetuate. Need to address the local and distal functional and muscular imbalances that are the unrecognized detritus of injury.
   - Self-inflicted wounds. Many injuries are insidious, created by what we habitually do. Inefficiencies, imbalances and invariance.

3. Cultural/emotional factors
   - People choose to move or hold themselves a certain way not because of either developmental reasons or injury but because of subjective factors such as communication style, chronic emotional states or acculturation.
   - We are not psychotherapists: be careful about dispensing advice outside of your scope of practice, but be aware of culture/emotion when working with movement disorders.

4. Performance enhancement
   - Another reason people move the way they do – a deliberate attempt to move in new or improved ways.
   - Important component of peak performance is neural orchestration. How accurate are the proprioceptive signals coming from your performing body, how good and how fast are performance decisions made based on that information and how accurate are the motor signals that are sent back in reply?
   - How can we get someone to practice and perform perfectly without interference or drag from inefficient or imbalanced subroutines?

Imbalances

1. Structural imbalances, muscle imbalances, functional imbalances are facets of the same gem, peas in the same pod, layers in the same onion.
   - Factors in imbalance creation. Childhood development, injuries, culture, occupation and emotion. The usual suspects.
   - Left/right imbalances normal. Asymmetrical childhood development, handedness. Advantages in bomb-proof roll or ability to throw a spear accurately.
   - Left/right imbalances contribute to asymmetrical tissue strain and musculoskeletal pain syndromes. Absolute mirror image as a clinical goal is unrealistic. Soften the asymmetry, improve efficiency and improve awareness of pattern.

Overview of motor learning

This book is for those who want to know more about human movement and how to influence it. What can we do when good movement goes bad? It is written for physical therapists in clini-cal practice who are interested in exploring a new exercise paradigm. This exercise paradigm features whole-body integrated movements rather than isolated movement of a part. It stresses the importance of being proprioceptively self-aware, and explains how to train your patients in acquiring that awareness. It makes our exercise functionally relevant by basing movements around real life or developmentally based functions. These exercises are designed to be informational, to make you a better teacher of motor skills and your patient a better kinesthetic learner.

The movements described in this book are sophisticated facilitation techniques designed to influence more efficient/less damaging movement and postural patterns. On completion of this book, you will be able to apply this material to orthopedic rehabilitation (spinal and extremity joints, tendons, muscles), to neurological rehabilitation (stroke, multiple sclerosis, cerebral palsy) and to performance enhancement (run faster, jump higher and throw farther).

Although it is not an anatomy or kinesiology book, some knowledge of anatomy on the part of the reader is assumed; keep an anatomy reference close if you are a bit hazy. Because this is a book on movement, you will need to get off your duff and out of your chair. You will be learning to move your own body to experience the techniques you will be teaching. Although you will learn a lot by reading, you will learn a lot more about human movement by feeling human movement firsthand.

We will start with an overview of movement. Why do we move or carry ourselves the way we do? Why do different people move so differently? What is the consequence of injury on normal movement? What other influences beside injury and early development affect the way we move? What are some strategies for teaching new or regaining lost movement skills?

We will discuss exercise in Chapter 2, and how we might use it as a vehicle for influencing efficient gross motor movement, postural control and intra-articular stability. How can we define ideal or efficient movement? Why do we need to make exercise look more like real life, developmental or performance activity? What makes exercise informative to the central nervous system? How do we stimulate proprioceptive self-awareness? How do we improve our students' motor planning decision-making abilities?

In Chapter 3 we will be exploring more primitive global movement patterns and focusing on the relationships among the head, spine and pelvis – trunk control. We will use this chapter and the next to introduce concepts of ideal movement and general teaching principles: what to teach and how to teach it. You will also start actively participating at this point by getting on the ground and mimicking early childhood movements. How do the pelvis and head cooperate in balance functions and in orientation from prone? How are the upper and lower extremities organized at this stage? What are the implications for influencing more mature movements? Why is it important to exercise outside of cardinal planes and in positions other than the vertical?

Chapter 4 continues with head-to-tail relationships in more mature functions: transitions and orientation from vertical. How does a baby with limited use of arms or legs roll over, or get from point A to point B? How can we use orientation or transitional movements to facilitate improved function in people with cervical strain, low back pain or hemiplegia? How can we teach the importance of coordinating head, spine and pelvis in fun and progressively challenging ways? We will introduce differentiated patterns of movement in this chapter, and will use overlapping functional necessities to create multidirectional differentiated movements.

In Chapter 5 we begin to explore the role of the legs in movement and posture. How do the biases and imbalances of the legs contribute to postural and movement dysfunction of the torso and spine? How do these biases contribute to injury or performance drag? What are strategies for teaching powerful and balanced pelvic, back and lower extremity movements?

What is the importance of hip and pelvic organization in unidirectional or bilaterally reciprocating athletic skills? This chapter is focused mainly on achieving lower torso and lower extremity musculature balance, strength and flexibility, and on facilitating a cooperative use of the opposite side hip extensors and flexors in a basic and crucial piece of the movement puzzle: the pelvic force couple.

In Chapter 6 we will focus more specifically on low back pain and lumbar stabilization. What are specific categories of movement and postural stressors for the back? How can we get our students to recognize these stressors in real life? How can we teach the physical and proprioceptive skills needed on the part of the back pain sufferer to stabilize against these stressors? How can we blend intra-articular or segmental stability with pelvic stability? What is the role of the legs in stabilizing the pelvis and lower back, or moving the pelvis adequately enough that the back doesn't have to continue to move too much? How can we facilitate low back stability without creating whole-body rigidity?

We wrap up Volume 1 in Chapter 7, with a focus on the lower extremities. What are the common movement strategies we can use for cerebrovascular accident (CVA), hip joint replacement or ankle sprain? What muscle imbalances are contributing to foot pronation, genu valgus or tibial rotation? How does hip musculature bias influence patellar tracking? How we start closed kinetic chain exercise with the person having a fresh total knee replacement short of fully bearing weight through a fully weightbearing foot?

What associative movements could we do to facilitate stronger ankle dorsiflexion and a reduction of foot drop? How can we safely and progressively teach knee stability in cutting or in changing directions? How can we use exercise designed to balance the foot on the floor for refining foot, ankle, knee and lumbar stabilization or to enhance athletic prowess?

A discussion of cervical injury and dysfunction, shoulder girdle imbalances and myofascial syndromes, neurological rehabilitation of the upper extremity and upper extremity repetitive strain or trauma-induced injuries will be covered in Volume 2. Examples include whiplash injuries, headaches, impingement syndromes, upper extremity postsurgical rehabilitation, tennis elbow and carpal tunnel syndrome. This will also include discussions of stroke rehabilitation and athletic enhancement of the upper extremities. We will also be exploring lip, tongue and jaw movements in the chapter on vegetative function, along with breathing, pelvic floor movements and strategies for facilitating autonomic balance.

Pathokinesiology

My perspective in approaching this question of how to facilitate ideal movement derives from my background in both medicine and movement. I teach movement and postural skills as a clinician working with various movement disorders. Ever since I was a kid I have been fascinated with movement and the acquisition of motor skills. Initially, this interest manifested itself in games, sports and martial arts practice. With high school graduation looming, I started looking for a job where I could use my (not good enough to be a professional athlete) movement skills.

I learned about the profession of physical therapy (PT) and decided that PT school would be able to answer the questions I had about movement: how is movement organized and regulated, what is ideal movement, and how to improve movement skills in someone else? After PT school and a couple of years in practice, I realized that my questions were still not answered. I had learned a lot about anatomy, physiology, pathology, neurology and how to work with the components of movement (muscles, joints, ligaments, bones), but my fundamental questions were left unanswered.

Whereas physical therapy/medicine/science addressed quantifiable questions about specific body parts, I was left with questions about quality of movement and the integration of those parts with the whole. I wanted to know what makes a movement *good* or *bad*, but couldn't find these answers in a purely scientific framework where the emphasis is so geared toward quantification.

I wanted to be able to do something besides tinkering with the parts: I wanted to be able to understand and influence the coordination of the whole. Knowledge about range of movement, arthrokinematics, tensile strength, collagen properties, neural pathways and force vector analysis of a muscle contraction is useful, but incomplete.

I realized that physical therapy could not be based solely on hard science, but needed to acknowledge that when working with people we are engaging in a bit of psychology: we are working with peoples' *behavior*. It is this question of motor behavior, how people come to behave the way they do, why they stick with the behavior even in the presence of negative consequences, and how to positively influence that behavior that led me to explore a discipline outside of the physical therapy field.

I am a *Feldenkrais Practitioner®* in addition to being a physical therapist, and I understand the advantages of each. This means that I can blend the countless experiential hours spent exploring complex movement patterns with my medical training and knowledge of anatomy to provide a unique perspective. I have learned to use movement for medicine, and would like to share some of what I have learned with a larger community of my peers.

Feldenkrais background

Moshe Feldenkrais was a Russian-born Israeli, trained as a physicist and a mechanical engineer, who was also one of the earliest Europeans to earn a black belt in judo. The story goes that he injured his knee playing soccer in the 1950s and that his doctors wanted to fuse it. Instead, he applied his knowledge of physics, mechanics and the balance/movement skills learned in judo to his own rehabilitation.

He began to explore movements on his own, with an emphasis on feeling and paying attention to those movements. He watched people as they moved, especially children and infants. He mimicked movements from early childhood and discovered certain principles of movement . . . among which was the realization that there are certain recurring *patterns* of movement that can be influenced most efficiently by teaching whole-body patterns of movement.

He then started working with other people who came to him with their movement problems and developed a way of manually guiding movement that he called *Functional Integration*®. As more and more people came to him for help, he needed to find a way of being able to work with many people at the same time. He then developed the movement/exercise portion of his work, called *Awareness Through Movement*®, and began teaching large group classes.

Over the next few decades he continued to develop and refine a huge body of knowledge that is both experiential and analytical, the *Feldenkrais Method*®. He led training programs in Israel and the US until his death in 1983. His early students and graduates from his training programs continued his work and are in turn running training programs in this method today. There are professional training programs, entailing 8 weeks of training a year for 4 years, throughout North America, Europe and Israel. I attended my professional training in northern California from 1990 through 1994, and was trained by Anat Baniel.

Dr Feldenkrais wrote several books and articles about his work, as have his students. I have included a sampling of these writings in the references section at the end of the chapter.[1-18] Other books and articles, as well as audio and videotapes of other Awareness Through Movement lessons, can be found by looking on the Internet. Go to www.feldenkrais.com for information about training programs, how to find a local practitioner, and general information about the Method. For articles, books and tapes, go to www.feldenkraisresources.com.

There are also some research articles in the medical literature that investigate the effectiveness of the Feldenkrais Method on various rehabilitation scenarios. Some of these articles find merit and promise in the method,[19-33] but others don't.[34,35] I'm not sure one can even gauge the effectiveness of the method itself given the relative paucity of research available to date and the subjective nature of the work itself. The work is too broad, too open to interpretation and too dependent on the skill and knowledge of the individual practitioner or practitioners doing the teaching for that particular study. What is being taught and how is it being taught?

Are we saying the Feldenkrais Method is bodywork, and do we study results from hands-on functional integration? Are we saying that it is exercise, and do we study results from randomly selected awareness through movement lessons taught in a group setting? Are we saying that the Feldenkrais Method is some exercise/coaching hybrid, and do we study results from a series of specific awareness through movement lessons taught one on one to a specific individual?

Perhaps we could ask the question another way. Instead of asking whether the Feldenkrais Method is a valid therapeutic tool, we could ask about the concepts and principles articulated and demonstrated throughout the work, and whether those concepts and principles could be applied in a clinical setting. Concepts of even distribution of movement, proportional use of synergistic muscles, conservation of energy/reduction of effort and skeletal/tensigrity weightbearing might be codified and adapted by our profession. (Tensigrity is a term coined by Buckminster Fuller. He invented the geodesic dome, a design used in some oddball buildings and in backpacking tents. Tensigrity refers to the ability of a structure to hold its shape not through the vertical compression of columns, but by the tension created by the connections between nonvertical rigid structures. It owes its integrity to the tension between the parts, hence the name. Because a skeleton has no vertical bones and contacting surfaces are not level, a true skeletal weight-bearing structure is not possible. I use the term skeletal weight-bearing as a descriptive term that matches the proprioceptive sensation of bearing weight effortlessly. In reality, the skeleton and its interconnecting ligament and fascial system is closer in kind to a tensigrity structure.)

The principles of exercising our students with whole-body patterns of movement rather than with isolated muscles or joints, linking our exercise to meaningful functional outcomes and emphasizing proprioceptive self-awareness, should not be controversial. Teaching techniques such as training the same pattern of movement in many different positions, varying speed and functional intension, applying constraints, allowing approximations, reprising developmental movements, and exercising in reciprocating patterns might be adopted by our profession and be used to greatly benefit our students.

Try taking a fresh look at this method and what it has to offer, as well as other movement disciplines such as yoga, various dance methods or martial arts. There is a wealth of knowledge in these disciplines that is wreathed in mysticism and obscured by cloudy, flowery or generalized language. What knowledge can we mine from these sources? What is there in what these methods teach or how they teach it that is consistent with what we know today through movement science?

A call to purpose

During my training I found an article, a call to arms for the physical therapy profession, which resonated with my belief that knowledge about movement is central to our work. In 1975, in the tenth Mary McMillan Lecture, HJ Hislop proposed that: 'pathokinesiology is the distinguishing clinical science of physical therapy.'[36,37] Pathokinesiology is literally the study of damaged or damaging movement. This includes the limp that follows a sprained ankle and the shoulder subluxation that follows a stroke. It includes the difficulty the child with cerebral palsy, the grandmother with a hip joint replacement and the veteran with a below-knee amputation have in standing and walking. It includes the way joint surfaces move relative to each other and the way fascial planes interact. The common denominator here is movement: what is wrong with it, what are the consequences of that movement in terms of

Box 1.1 Pathokinesiology

Injury or illness resulting in degradation of motor control
Inefficient motor control resulting in degradation of tissue
Our job is to positively influence motor behavior

pain or ability to function, and how can we as clinicians positively influence that movement?

We can think of pathology as creating alterations of movement and postural patterns. Stroke, cerebral palsy, multiple sclerosis and Parkinson's disease are examples of neurological pathology leading to movement impairment. Achilles tendon tears, anterior cruciate ligament strains and broken bones are examples of orthopedic pathology leading to movement impairments.

We can also think of alterations of movement and postural patterns creating pathology. Patellar tracking dysfunction, supraspinatus tendinitis and prolapsed discs are examples of movement impairment leading to orthopedic pathology. Sciatica and thoracic outlet syndromes are examples of movement impairment leading to neurological pathology. We can think of pathokinesiology or kinesiopathology (Box 1.1).

Anatomy is not the same as movement . . . the map is not the territory

What do we really know about movement? We have time and motion studies that tell us how various people do a particular task. We can document muscle firing sequences and graph the displacement of bones in space. We can electrically stimulate muscles and observe what bones they move. We know volumes about Golgi tendon organs, sarcomeres and neurotransmitters. We have detailed anatomical knowledge and computer-generated models that can predict obscure arthrokinematic movement.

We know that particular ways of moving our bodies have damaging consequences to our tissues. We have libraries crammed with studies and theories about motor acquisition, motor control and motor learning. These are all good things, and our *objective* knowledge about movement continues to grow exponentially. Unfortunately, for the pure scientists among us, this is not enough.

There is another perspective on movement that has not been fully appreciated: the perspective of those of us who have a *subjective* understanding of movement. Our fraternity might include Feldenkrais Practitioners, Alexander Practitioners, Laban Movement, yoga, Pilates and tai chi or other martial arts. We are concerned not just with the objective side of movement (how far, how fast, how many, how much), but also with the subjective side (how accurate, how integrated, how successful, how effortless, how comfortable, how pleasurable).

Martial art styles can be roughly divided into two schools: those that teach external styles and those that teach internal styles. External style examples include judo, aikido, karate and kung fu. In these styles, one trains ultimately to work against an opponent. Speed, power and reaction time are critical as you focus on opportunities to attack your opponent and to defend against his moves. Tai chi is a well known example of an internal martial art style. In these styles one works on improving oneself, not on defeating an external opponent. Accuracy, balance, coordination, smoothness, grace and proportionality are the goals. These are the properties of movement so sorely lacking in the typical orthopedic patient who comes to see us for low back pain, neck aches, frozen shoulders and carpal tunnel syndrome.

In modern exercise systems we have plenty of external styles. Lifting weights, sliding pulleys, running treadmills, plyometrics and progressive resistive exercise are all analogous to the external martial arts styles. Although this traditional approach to therapeutic exercise has its uses in physical therapy rehabilitation, internal styles of exercise have much to offer as well. The Feldenkrais Method and the various tai chi styles in particular have specific properties that lend themselves to translation into a physical therapy setting.

Both of these exercise styles emphasize slowing down to better control and to be more aware of your movements. They both emphasize smoothness of movement, reduction of superfluous effort and moving from the ground. They both train intentional movements of coordinated breathing and movements of the eyes and hands integrated with movements of the torso, pelvis and legs. They both contain exquisite movement combinations and clever constraints that help access some of our most obscure and neglected movement capabilities. Mostly, though, they provide an incredibly rich and diverse reservoir of subjective movement experiences.

Why would it be important for a physical therapist to have some knowledge of movement from a subjective perspective? Because it is through subjective criteria that we, and our patients, make motor decisions. We choose to posture ourselves in certain ways: to bend over, to walk, ride a bike, pet a dog, throw a ball, or to move in the million and one ways we do during our daily lives. We do this not because of what a PhD in kinesiology says is right but because of what we feel is right. The fancy word for this phenomenon is *self-affectivity*, i.e. your judgment of perceived benefit or harm from doing an action a certain way. Movement is behavior, learned and shaped by individual experience. And we who are seeking to change the way someone moves need to be fluent in the language of movement.

The language of movement is one of subjective perception. Proprioception is the internal body awareness sense that tells us where we are in relation to gravity, where bones are relative to each other, the direction of movement of bones, the physiological end range of a joint, and muscular effort. Should those of us who teach others how to move their bodies be competent in musculoskeletal organization and proprioceptive perception? Absolutely! Would you dine with a chef who can't taste? Would you hang art from a painter who can't see? Would you attend a concert of a musician who can't hear? Just as the chef needs to taste, the artist needs to see and the singer needs to hear, the physical therapist needs to have some subjective/proprioceptive understanding of movement (Box 1.2).

This book is less about scientifically observing and detailing what movement *is* and more about suggesting what movement *should be*. We will be asking not just about what is average/normal, but what is ideal. We need to know more than

Box 1.2 The subjective nature of movement and learning

Decisions about motor learning made by subjective criteria – self-affectivity

Need to develop a language consistent with subjective experience

Science not designed to decide what 'good' movement should be

Box 1.3 Motor behavior

Arthrokinematic behavior – how joint surfaces move relative to each other

Postural behavior – how bones are balanced on top of each other

Gross motor behavior – spatial relationships between bones

just how a movement creates strain, but how to get our students to recognize that strain proprioceptively, then to learn new ways of moving that are subjectively recognized as being better.

We will be introducing concepts of ideal movement and posture and the kinesthetic cues used to facilitate a change in motor behavior toward that ideal. We will be introducing principles concerning how to teach a motor skill, and will develop strategies by which our students can blend what they learn into their daily lives. Are you ready and eager to further develop your pathokinesiology skills?

Exercise for motor control purposes

This book takes a look at movement and exercise from a functional perspective. How can we better use exercise to improve neuromusculoskeletal function or performance? Is there a way to improve the qualitative results of an exercise? Although we as physical therapists use exercise for cardiovascular, collagen property or other physiological purposes, we will be focusing most of our attention on exercise performed for motor control purposes. By motor control purposes, I mean doing an exercise to affect a change in some motor behavior.

Postural and ergonomic exercises are obvious examples. Lumbar stabilization exercises, relaxation training and stretching exercises all have motor control as a primary goal. Although they are sometimes used to increase muscular bulk and torque, many strengthening exercises are performed to influence muscular coordination, so they have motor control as a primary goal. Coordination and sports-specific drills and plyometrics are other examples.

We can speak broadly of three categories of motor behavior: *gross motor, postural* and *arthrokinematic*. Gross motor behavior includes how you organize yourself to bend over, look over your shoulder, reach out with one hand, jump over a fence, throw a ball, or a billion other movements the human body is capable of. Postural behavior includes how you organize yourself to sit, stand, lie, squat or otherwise maintain a more or less static position (Box 1.3).

Arthrokinematic behavior refers to how you control the position of joint surfaces relative to each other in neutral rest and active movement contexts. Arthrokinematic, postural and gross motor behaviors are controlled by muscular effort, which in turn is controlled by the nervous system. Making some modifications to how we have traditionally taught movement skills might make exercises or drills designed to influence these behaviors more effective.

What is wrong with the way we have traditionally taught therapeutic exercise, sport activity or any motor skill? Although I am not saying that we have been dead wrong all these years in teaching what we have and the way we have, I am saying that we can do better. There is a particular framework we could use for teaching movement skills, just as there is a particular framework for putting a puzzle together.

Teaching the process of the puzzle

Imagine for a moment how you would teach a child to do a puzzle. You could send Johnny or Suzie into the next room to play while you put the puzzle together, then call them back when you have completed the puzzle. Although you could just show them the completed puzzle, give them all the pieces and then leave the room to go pay bills, success rates will probably be slim. This might work with some gifted kids, but it is not the generally accepted method for teaching a child to build a puzzle.

Putting a puzzle together is a process. First you turn all the pieces right side up and spread them out. This ensures that some pieces aren't hidden under other ones. Then you sort out all the pieces that have a straight edge, keeping a particularly sharp eye out for the four corner pieces. Then you look at colors and pictures on the edge pieces, and put together the whole outline of the puzzle. Then you start to fill in the inside by looking for matching shapes, colors or patterns from the edges in, or from one edge to another.

Our current method for teaching movement skills resembles the first strategy. We focus on the product. We have an exercise to teach and there is a particular way to do it. We describe it, we demonstrate it, we have people do it, then we correct what they are doing wrong. This is an *imitation and repetition* style of teaching. I believe a preferred way of teaching movement skills and for learning motor skills is to focus more on the process.

Our students should be active participants in finding better ways to move for themselves. They need to sort out the pieces and turn them all right side up. We should have ways of using movement and language to guide our students' problem-solving and decision-making abilities pertaining to movement. They need hints and directions for finding the edges and corners.

Our students need to recognize the advantages of doing a movement one way (good) instead of another (evil) by comparing their relative merits and drawbacks. They might have to try two or three pieces in one spot before they find the one that fits. Ultimately, we don't want to teach mere stimulus and response behavior, but to mold our students into lean, mean and self-regulating motor planning machines.

Let's go beyond teaching product and begin *teaching the process* by which we get there! This will include using specific

Box 1.4 Teaching styles

Imitation and repetition . . . show and repeat demonstrated correct form

Teaching the process – guiding self-awareness, choices and decision-making

We want to make competent self-regulators with an ability to extrapolate to daily life

Tricks of the trade: change of venue, application of constraints, allowing approximations, exercising in reciprocating patterns and reprising developmental movements

'tricks of the trade' – concepts we will use to facilitate learning on the part of our student. These tricks of the trade include changing the venue, applying constraints, allowing approximations, reprising developmental movements, and exercising in reciprocating patterns (Box 1.4).

In this book, we will be exploring fresh ways of looking at exercise. Three main themes will characterize this approach:

- That *proprioceptive self-awareness* is emphasized and taught as a co-requisite skill;
- That exercises are *pattern specific* and look something like the movement pattern you are trying to influence; and
- That exercises contain *functional context* and are designed around the basic functional categories of balance, orientation, transitional movements, locomotion, manipulation, communication or vegetation.

Factors influencing motor learning

For our purposes, motor learning can be simply defined as either the acquisition of new motor skills or the refinement or the deterioration of existing ones. This includes everything from walking to blocking to talking to frowning to looking over our shoulder to rolling out of bed and limping from a sprained ankle.

We are born with the ability to breathe, eat, digest, eliminate and circulate fluids, but not much more. We have to learn to do virtually everything else. We have to learn to coordinate our eyes to focus, and to associate the intention to look with the rolling of our head. We then roll to our bellies from our backs as an outgrowth of the intention to look overhead. We learn the beginnings of head control and the ability to bring our head to vertical from this prone position. We learn to use our arms to push ourselves higher and start precursor movements to crawling, again as an outgrowth of our intention to look around a 360° horizon. We learn to come to sit, to transfer to hands and knees and to come to stand. Creeping, crawling, walking, running and jumping follow. We learn to talk and to express ourselves through body language, learn to eat with our mouths closed, learn to throw and grasp, and learn to fall without getting hurt (mostly). Later we learn to type, to drive

a car and to use power tools and electronic toys. We learn an incredible array of motor skills in our lifetimes. Sadly, some of us lose those motor skills that we possessed earlier and some of us never learn certain motor skills very well in the first place.

Early development

Motor learning during infancy and early childhood development has a major influence on how we organize ourselves to move throughout the rest of our lives. As dynamic systems theory bigwig Esther Thelen says, '. . . new forms of behavior must arise from component abilities that are themselves continuous over time.'[38] Movement develops in patterns, and components of these patterns are put together in various ways to create new abilities. So much of how we organize ourselves to sit, bend, reach, stand, etc., is either a direct outgrowth of or is heavily influenced by what we learn in the first few years of life. It is the foundation upon which we build our movement and postural patterns. It is the time when those movement and postural patterns start becoming habitually ingrained, accruing over time almost absolute rule over our neuromusculoskeletal system. It is a time when seeds are planted that can and do eventually manifest in neuromusculoskeletal pain and dysfunction.

When working with people, there are two important concepts from early learning to keep in mind: that learning follows in a progression called the developmental sequence, and that with so much learning taking place preverbally, there is a lot of room for error.

Developmental sequence

The term 'developmental sequence' implies an order, of one thing happening before another. Alexander, Boehme and Cupps have an excellent book detailing motor development over the first year of life.[39] One would expect crawling before walking, sitting before standing, holding hands before kissing. These are a few of the major milestones in development, but there are also countless smaller ones. Interspersed throughout this book will be photographs of movements derived from the developmental sequence, movements that you will also be doing as you go through some of the described movement lessons. These steps, both large and small, blend with one another in an intricate web of interconnecting movement and postural patterns.

For instance, a baby lying on its belly will draw up a knee to look over his shoulder or to reach for a toy; this turns into a commando crawl, which is modified and turned into creeping, which leads to coming to standing, walking, etc. One step leads to another. A baby lying supine and arching his back to look above him turns into a baby lying on his belly, arching his back and lifting his head to look to the horizon. He then turns into a child sitting on the floor arching his back to look up to his father, then morphs into the incurable romantic standing on a high desert butte and arching his back to look up at the stars.

There are some basic repeating patterns here, with some important variations, which perpetuate throughout related functions and which we will explore in more depth in later chapters. These basic patterns or chunks of movement are used with either slight variations or variable synergists to assist in a number of varied functions. We'll call these chunks of recurring movement patterns 'Legos.' There are both child-rearing and clinical considerations for keeping developmental sequence in mind.

Magda Gerber is a Hungarian orphanage director who wrote books on early childhood development.[40] She advocates taking a hands-off approach in teaching children motor skills. She feels that children should be left to learn for themselves and at their own pace how to come to sit, stand, walk, etc. She observed that children developed sequentially, and that they did better if they were allowed to learn each step in that sequence fully before going on to the next. Providing a child with a safe environment, with a variety of surfaces and levels, and with a variety of objects to manipulate, stimulates motor exploration and skill acquisition.

If a caregiver sits a child up unsupported without that child having adequately learned to use his iliopsoas while lying on his belly, he may not be able to use his iliopsoas well in sitting. This might cause him to develop a strategy for sitting later that relies on rounding himself backward and holding himself up by abdominal muscle contraction. This may become a lifelong habit and contribute to a number of musculoskeletal problems.

A child who is stood up early on by a caregiver and who hangs on to fingers for support might not have learned, by crawling or by pushing himself to stand, how to fully extend his hip joints. This may predispose him to hyperlordotic postures, or rob him of a couple inches of elevation in jumping later in life. A child who is plopped in a wheeled walker may learn to associate walking with pelvic immobility. He may never learn to take a truly full stride, or to run or jump with the power inherent in integrated whole-body patterns of movement. Parents sometimes try to rush their children to the next major step in the sequence without realizing how much learning goes on underneath the radar screen that is a necessary prerequisite to that next major step (Box 1.5).

In addition to the importance of allowing sequential learning, it is also important to allow children to make motor learning mistakes. When a child is learning, it is as important for him to know what doesn't work as what does. He needs to winnow out useable movements from a number of different possibilities or choices. He needs to separate the wheat from the chaff. In that way, he knows how he arrived where he did and why he chose that particular way of doing things.

Provide safe conditions in which children can play and explore. Let them fall. Let them struggle a bit. That is how they learn. The best thing a parent can do for their children in terms of motor learning is to simply get out of the way and let them learn and develop at their own pace. Encourage activity and discourage sitting in front of a TV or computer. We don't need to teach kids to roll, to come up to sit or to stand: it will

happen, given a normal CNS (central nervous system). If the CNS is not normal (for example owing to cerebral palsy or spina bifida), we still need to provide a learning environment, but will need to get involved manually to assist the child in feeling different movement options.

Implications for teaching

It is also important to keep the developmental sequence in mind when working with your students. If you are working with someone on pivoting drills, postural retraining, spinal stabilization or ergonomics instruction, you might consider running them through a sequence of movements leading up to the finished product. Let them progressively acquire a skill over a period of time, rather than expecting perfection immediately.

If you have to teach them how to do something properly, they probably either lack the proprioceptive ability to feel what you are asking them to do or they may not have the strength or flexibility to match that ideal. If someone is not doing a movement in a biomechanically efficient way, assume he doesn't know how to do it, can't physically do it, or doesn't recognize the biomechanical advantage of doing it that way.

We might instead want to teach some basic skills leading up to that finished product: strength and flexibility skills, proprioceptive acuity and pattern recognition skills, and problem-solving and proprioceptive comparison skills. How do you do that? By incorporating these skills into motor learning lessons. If we can recognize the basic patterns involved in a particular skill and can recognize where that pattern occurred in similar functions earlier in the developmental sequence, we have a framework for progressively teaching the motor skills necessary to refine that skill. We will be introducing examples of this in later chapters.

Another implication for teaching is that we want to start teaching someone at a skill level where they can be successful and gradually progress them toward more complex, higher functions. We don't want to start them with something they are unable to do or that is painful to do. They may become frustrated. We don't want to repeat the same thing over and over again without progression. They may get bored. We might not even demand precision right away: we'll let them slowly gain in skill through successively more refined approximations of a particular movement pattern.

Think of a child learning to feed himself. Initially he'll be a messy, two-fisted eater. Later he'll learn to use a spoon, but will still spill or smear a lot. It may take him years to learn to use a steak knife and fork and follow Emily Post's Rules of Etiquette. We allow a child to perform a skill approximately right at first, then gradually expect more as he matures. We should do no less for our students. We'll call this an *allowance of approximations*.

The Goldilocks effect

As movement teachers working with students, just as with parents raising children, we want them to explore options and make mistakes. Ecological psychiatrists Turvey and Fitzpatrick hypothesize that 'nonspecific and aperiodic movements of the infant provide a rich source of random interactions with the

---

Box 1.5 Early development

Allowing for exploration and mistakes
Introduce choices in exercise
Progress at appropriate pace and in sequential manner

---

body's appendages and with the surroundings. These permit the infant to explore, in chaos-like style, various parameter spaces. Achieving fluency in intra- and inter-limb coordination is the progressive discovery of how to sculpt the force structures associated with spatiotemporal configurations of limb segments and environmental objects (e.g. gravitational, elastic and reactive forces) into the force structures that are required. The discovery is of patterns of muscular forces that are economical in time and magnitude.'[41] In other words, we move, make mistakes and learn from them.

I was working with a woman from Korea with neck pain a few years ago and she asked me about what size pillow to use when sleeping. I had her lie on her side and placed a few foam pads under her head at a neutral height where the midline of her face was parallel to the floor and her head and neck were an extension of her upper back. I asked her to focus proprioceptively on where her head was and how comfortable that height was. I then took some padding away so her head hung down more to the table and asked her to reassess her impression of her position and comfort. She could now tune into the proprioceptive sensations telling her the pillow was too low. I then put additional padding under her head to make it too high. She then was able to make an informed decision on the pillow height best for her, and had the proprioceptive reference points and sensory criteria necessary to reproduce that height at home. I then made some comment about following in the footsteps of Goldilocks . . . and got a very blank look.

Growing up in Korea, she had never heard of the story of Goldilocks and the Three Bears, so I had to tell it to her. I related how Goldilocks broke into the bears' house and sampled their breakfast, their chairs and their beds. Each item had three choices. Breakfast was too hot, too cold or just right. The chairs and beds she appropriated were too hard, too soft or just right. Goldilocks intelligently tried a number of options before choosing those that she liked the best. She knew which one she liked best because she sampled, compared and judged. When working with people teaching motor skills, the *Goldilocks effect* is an important one to keep in mind. Don't just give them the answer, let them figure it out. Give them choices, even deliberately wrong ones. By allowing them to decide among an array of choices, we are helping our students improve their proprioceptive listening skills, problem-solving abilities and decision-making, and they will become much better self-regulators. They will also be able to apply those skills to other functions and be able to modify the basic patterns to fit varied circumstances.

Developmental mistakes

In addition to the implications of the developmental sequence in motor learning, we need to be aware that early motor learning can be full of both mistakes and imbalances that have implications when working with people as teens and adults. There is no owner's manual when growing up. We are just issued this piece of equipment, this body, and have to figure out how to use it on our own. Through a Goldilocks-type process of trial and error, we gradually figure out which patterns of movement or posture work and which do not.

The problem is that there are nearly always a number of patterns that work, with some being more biomechanically efficient than others. Just go down to the local mall or airport and watch the variety of ways people choose to walk. Try mimicking them and get a sense of what they are straining as they walk! NA Bernstein first articulated this 'problem' of having too many possibilities and choices in movement in 1967.[42,43] Cleverly calling it *Bernstein's Problem*, he states that with such large numbers of degrees of freedom possible in the human body, the controlled operation of such a system requires a reduction of redundancy and a reduction in the number of degrees of freedom. We need to develop *habits*.

There is a classic book by Knight Dunlap called *Habits: Their Making and Unmaking*.[44] It is a good overview of the mechanisms of habit formation, the implications for human movement and the implications for someone seeking to change those habits.

Life would be pretty chaotic without habits. If I had to decide which of 120 ways of sequencing a motor firing pattern resulting in the movement of my hand to my mouth I wanted to use the next time I popped a grape in my mouth, lunch would take an awfully long time. We need to find a combination of firing patterns that work to accomplish a set motor task, then to reproduce that same combination the next time the motor task is performed without having to think the whole thing through again.

Think of the sequences of motor firing patterns as subroutines: chunks of ready-to-use movement of postural pattern that can be mixed and matched with other ready-made subroutines to produce variations of the same basic movement or to produce whole new movement patterns. These movement subsets are the building blocks of our organic lives and are deeply woven throughout the whole neuromusculoskeletal system.

Larry Goldfarb had a great analogy for this: imagine what it would be like if we had to control all four wheels separately as we drove down the road in our auto! Chaos would reign and carnage ensue. Instead, Mr Ford wisely chose to slave all four wheels to one control. Imagine how much more complex it would be to control the nearly infinite combinations of movements possible in the human body. Our habits serve as the steering wheels that keep our choices to a minimum.

Habits are simultaneously a blessing and a curse. On the one hand, you don't have to reinvent the wheel every time you want to go into town. On the other hand, what if you make a mistake in putting some of these subroutines together? What happens if a malfunctioning subroutine causes mechanical damage to the equipment? What happens if a neurological insult robs you of some of your subroutines? How do you weed out the faulty subroutine from the larger matrix, where it has invaded the entire CNS and has come to be associated with countless motor tasks? Worse, what if we didn't even know they were there?

Sadly but truly, most people are pretty clueless about their own biomechanical inefficiencies, imbalances and motor habits. They are invisible because they are always there and have always been there. Ask someone which shoulder is higher and they will think they are level. Ask someone whether her pelvis is vertical in sitting and she will say yes. Motor habits are like opinions: by definition, we always think we are right. In reality, all of us could use some lessons not only on how to operate the machinery, but how to listen to that machinery.

Why do we all make motor mistakes? With such an elegant design, how could there be such rampant operator error? Unlike a baby zebra, which can stand within hours of birth and run within a few days, it takes us humans a much longer time to apprentice our bodies. There are so many possibilities and so much potential that it takes a long time to learn. There is no owner's manual to guide us, but we could observe and mimic those around us. But what if our parents' motor planning is suspect too? (By taking longer to apprentice our bodies, I mean that it takes the individuals in our species much longer to attain motor proficiency. A baby zebra can stand, jump, run and feed on mama's milk without assistance within days or weeks. It takes a human a year to feed itself without assistance, come up to sit, stand and walk. It takes several more years for mature running, throwing and other higher-level motor tasks to become refined. Whereas a blacksmith apprentice learns the trade at the knee of the master, we apprentice our bodies to our environment and the school of hard knocks.)

We could assiduously apply ourselves to learning about our bodies and how they work. We could be constantly striving against our limitations and weaknesses, pushing ourselves to the limit of our endurance to achieve the pinnacle of self-awareness. But we don't. On some fundamental level, we're all pretty lazy. We like to take the path of least resistance. Once we figure out a way of doing something, we'll call it good. We may, at the first sign of success, declare victory and stop further exploration and refinement of that movement. If it works, even if it's not the easiest or most efficient way of doing things, it is often good enough . . . or the best we can do with limited exploration of choices.

We habituate our subroutines and incorporate their inefficiencies, imbalances or mistakes into subsequent steps in development.[45] The mistake may not have immediate consequences, as children are generally very resilient and can usually adequately heal any microtrauma caused by that inefficient pattern. The problem often comes later, when a lifetime of that accumulated trauma overwhelms our ability to repair the damage. This is when the chickens come home to roost.

Let's look at an example. My son, when he was 2 years old, walked with an immature and inefficient gait. He waddled. He rotated his pelvis to take a step, like ducks do. This is normal for that age. When he took a step forward with his right foot, the right side of his pelvis swung forward and his pelvis as a whole turned to the left. The mirror image was true of the opposite side. This rotational movement of the pelvis has to be accommodated somewhere, however, and that will often be at the lower back. If he swings his shoulders and chest in the same direction as his pelvis, moving his pelvis and torso like a log, his gait becomes too imbalanced.

Try it yourself. Walk with your hands glued to the front of your thighs and waddle. It is less than efficient even when performed slowly, but at the speeds at which my son zipped around it would become downright hazardous! He chose instead another option. He rotated his shoulders in the opposite direction of his pelvis and twisted around his lower back. At that age this probably caused no harm, but if this pattern were to persist into adulthood, as it does in a significant percentage of the population, it could spell trouble for him.

For some people, the locomotor function does not continue to mature: they still waddle instead of differentiating their pelvis and legs in pelvic force-coupled movements (see Section 3). They might come to us with back pain, maybe even with a history of injury, which nevertheless results largely from a lifetime of rotating too much around a few, no-longer-hardy, vertebrae in the lower back. We could surmise joint instabilities, disc shearing, articular cartilage damage and degenerative changes in either hip or back as possible outcomes of this organization.

When working with these folks, we want to apply the *Rule of Holes*: When you're in a hole, the first thing to do is stop digging. When someone is creating tissue damage by the way they are organizing their movement, we want them to stop doing that movement. How do we teach them to recognize by feeling that what they are doing is damaging? How do we get them not just to stop digging, but to organically adopt a new and more efficient pattern as a substitute for the damaging one? We will look at teaching strategies and options for stabilization in later chapters.

Other factors influencing motor behavior

In addition to the motor learning that happens naturally during the course of development, motor learning occurs at other times and is influenced by other factors. Performance enhancement and reaction to injury are examples of motor learning happening at other times. Cultural norms and emotional states are examples of common influences on musculoskeletal learning and organization. Let's look first at injuries.

Injuries

We know what happens at a tissue level following an injury. There is plentiful research on histological and physiological effects, and that information can be found through many sources. Of equal interest to those of us who work with injured people is what happens to movement quality.

When we get injured, it hurts. We want to get away from the pain, to shut it off and to make it go away. We would like to ignore it and go about our business, but we can't because if we're not careful we'll do something to hurt the injured part again. Pain is a great motivator, and we quickly learn to avoid those movements that cause us pain. The first thing to do is to self-splint, to stop movement at the site of injury.

If I sprain my ankle, for instance, I will want to stop moving my ankle. I will especially want to stop moving my ankle in the direction of injury, most likely into plantarflexion and inversion. This is just common sense, a natural reaction. This response is obvious to student and practitioner alike, but other responses to injury might more easily go unnoticed. These responses include function avoidance and compensation.[46–49]

AVOIDANCE

The term avoidance refers to not only avoiding movement at the sight of injury but also to an inhibition of certain functions that include movement of the affected part. In the case of the ankle sprain, the likely function to be inhibited is push-off in gait. By self-splinting the ankle and not letting it move into plantarflexion, we have eliminated a component of push-off in the gait cycle. The whole push-off function is then avoided to some degree, and our CNS sends inhibitory signals not only to the gastrosoleus complex but to the hamstrings and gluteals as well.[50]

The function of push off, along with related functions of standing, getting up from a chair or even rolling from supine to sitting, can be affected by this CNS inhibition of a whole-body function. The whole gait cycle can be thrown off, with crossover inhibition of the opposite iliopsoas and an alteration in synergistic torso and shoulder girdle movements.

The CNS also sends excitatory signals to certain muscles. Toe and ankle dorsiflexors and evertors will be in a heightened state of alert and, as part of the function of pulling away or withdrawing the foot from the floor, the hip flexors will probably be so as well. In motor learning terms, avoidance means both the inhibition or extinction of one group of functions and the emergence of its functional opposite in a more dominant role. These new and, by necessity imbalanced, inhibitory and excitatory signals from the CNS are appropriate and desirable for a time after injury.

We want some minimization of movement so that initial tissue healing can occur. We want to bias ourselves away from the direction of injury. What we do not want, however, is for that protective pattern to perpetuate itself indefinitely. The CNS seems to have some elements of inertia. For whatever reason, once a pattern is adopted it tends to continue and to eventually habituate unless something comes along to change its course.

We already know that as tissue healing occurs we gradually add more movement until we have full range of motion. This prevents scarring, permanent mobility loss and arthrokinematic consequences. We need to do something analogous in terms of motor learning to address the functional and muscular imbalances that are often the unrecognized detritus of injury. We need to restore both normal mobility of the part and full function of the whole.

COMPENSATION

The term compensation (or substitution) refers to the tendency for other parts of the body to make up for the loss of movement somewhere because of injury and avoidance or, as we'll see later, because of habituated disuse somewhere else. To illustrate the avoidance/compensation connection, I'll tell you about 'Nancy.'

Nancy was in her early 50s when she came to me with right-sided lower back pain. She related a history of spraining her right ankle on the first day of a 2-week vacation in Europe. She went to Europe to see and experience things, and she wasn't about to let a little swelling in her ankle interfere with her plans. She walked and walked, and near the end of the trip she began to notice that not only was her ankle not getting much better, but that her right hip and lower back were starting to hurt as well.

I saw her a couple months after she returned. Her ankle was moderately better, but the hip and back pain persisted. I noticed that she was very spasmed in her right iliopsoas and very drawn up and compressed through her right lower back. Her ankle was still stiff, and I observed incomplete hip extension in standing and incomplete push-off in walking, especially on the right side.

I then had her lie on her back with her right leg bent and right foot on the ground while the left leg was long and straight. I asked her to press her right foot into the floor to lift her right hip while I observed how she did this movement. What she tended to do, as she also did in walking and standing, was to substitute back extension for hip extension when pushing her foot into the floor. CNS inhibition of the push-off function weakened or inhibited the hip, knee and ankle extensors. That power vacuum was filled by the withdrawal or stepping function, and the iliopsoas dominated and became tight. She had little choice but to compensate for this lack of hip extension by overextending her lower back (Box 1.6).

I did not give Nancy separate exercises to strengthen the gastrocnemius, the soleus, the hamstrings, the gluteus maximus, the gluteus medius and the obturators, gemelli and other arthrokinematic hip muscles that contribute to the push-off family. I did not give her separate exercises to stretch the extensor hallucis longus, the extensor digitorum longus, the anterior tibialis, the rectus femoris, the iliacus, the iliopsoas and the lumbar extensors. What I did was to teach her basic reciprocating patterns of movement around the functions of push-off and withdrawal, and progressed her from supine to side-sit to hands and knees to Sit to Stand to walk.

I let her learn sequentially and let her make exploratory mistakes, but everything that needed to be stretched got stretched. Everything that needed to be strengthened got strengthened. We worked simultaneously on stretching, strengthening, muscle imbalances, functional imbalances and proprioceptive acuity within a framework of whole-body functional movements derived from developmental movements.

It is important to remember that motor learning happens automatically after injury but doesn't necessarily happen automatically during recovery. We need to provide the conditions in which motor learning during recovery from injury does happen. We want to help our students to re-establish normal and balanced functional movement patterns, not only to assist directly with tissue healing from trauma. We also want to re-establish those patterns to avoid secondary problems from either compensations or the habituation and perpetuation of muscular and functional imbalances.

Box 1.6 Motor control consequence of injury

Avoidance – local and distal synergist inhibition and excitation
Compensations – movement and effort increase somewhere else
Most injuries self-inflicted – repetitive stress syndromes

Self-inflicted wounds

Injuries, of course, are not always random accidents or sudden disasters. Many are insidious. There are many injuries created by our motor habits. When we move, there is tissue strain. When we move inefficiently, that strain is magnified to some degree.[51] These inefficiency-induced strains are often very small, yet are so frequent that they are able to sneak up on the unaware victim and lay him low, just as surely as a car accident or a sprained knee. It's like being devoured by ants instead of a lion.

Repetitive stress injuries are also because of invariance. Invariance is that well-worn pathway, that broken-down section of your couch you keep sinking into, the same predictable wear patterns on the soles of your shoes, or the groove in the record that the needle just keeps slipping into. This strain is like water torture: one seemingly harmless drip at a time, but always in the same exact spot. The drip lands on the same spot on the articular surface, the same part of the joint capsule, the same ligaments, the same fascial plane, the same motor units and the same combination of electrical signals in your brain.

The use of only one neuromotor pathway in any common repetitive movement is not desirable, even if that pathway is a highly efficient one. Our tissues do best when rotated on a rest/work cycle. When we move inefficiently, don't have enough variety in our movements or don't allow enough other tissues to do some of the work, we have repetitive stress syndromes. These include the noxious mix of carpal tunnel syndrome, wrist strains, various upper extremity tendinitis problems, thoracic outlet syndrome, shoulder girdle and neck tension and imbalances, headaches and the like that we associate with pecking away at a computer all day. They also include a host of other self-inflicted wounds that are the consequence, at least in part, of long-term inefficient movement patterns.

Plantar fasciitis, bunions, shin splints and anterior knee/patellar pain are some of the lower extremity examples of biomechanical faults, with walking or running being the repetitive stress. Examples of sloppy biomechanics around the pelvis and spine abound, with bending, standing and sitting being some of many possible repetitive stresses. Faulty biomechanics is a function of faulty or incomplete motor learning; it is here that we step in as teachers!

Cultural/emotional factors

Sometimes people choose to move or hold themselves a certain way not because of developmental reasons or injury but because of subjective factors, such as communication style, chronic emotional states or acculturation. Our muscular system is our means of communicating with others. The set of our lips and jaw, the use of the tongue and voice, the angle of the head, facial expression and body language are all used to communicate who we are, what we want and how we feel.

A few years ago I worked with a woman who had been in a car accident and came to me with primarily left-sided neck pain. One of the observations I made about her was that she always tipped her head (almost violently) to the left side, both as she listened and as she talked. She reminded me of how birds cock their heads to peer intently at something from a number of different angles. The expression conveyed attentiveness and had probably been adopted sometime when she was a child. After years of doing this by second nature, she was now completely unaware of what she was doing.

Did this habit cause her injury? Not entirely, but it may have been a reason why the trauma manifested itself in left-sided neck pain. It made for a weak link in the chain, or a path of least resistance. It certainly played a role in her recovery. As she became more aware of the effect that movement had on her neck, she was able to tone down its excesses and reduce that particular self-inflicted strain.

Our muscular system is also our means of expressing ourselves emotionally.[52] Facial expression and verbalizing are again part of this, but body language might be of special interest to those of us who work with people with pain. Chronic muscular holding patterns often mirror chronic emotional holding patterns. Chronic anxiety may be expressed through raised or pinched shoulders, a tight belly, a clenched jaw or other muscular means. Depression may be conveyed through slouching, slow movements, or lack of animation in speech.

Each muscle chronically held or chronically inhibited by emotional holding has consequences on tissue health, just as it did when injury was the precipitating factor. We, as practitioners, need to keep in mind the possibility of an emotional history along with that hypermobile facet or that tight iliotibial band or that elevated left shoulder. Although it may be simpler to think in terms of flesh and bone, of anatomy and pathology, of muscle bulk and elasticity, we need to remember that people who come to see us are not merely organic robots in need of repair. They are people with needs and desires, conflicting motivations and a complex emotional history.

Culture is another common influence on movement and a common detriment to rehabilitation. I can only speak having observed common American cultural influences, but I'm sure every culture has some of these influences. In American culture, a flat belly is considered an ideal of both aesthetics and health. We are acculturated to suck in our bellies by tightening our abdominal muscles. This is not the case in certain eastern traditions, where an ability to breathe into the lower belly is appreciated. Many women have been taught to sit, stand and lie with their knees close together – they are chronically contracting their adductors.

Some people have been taught not to stick their pelvis out when they bend over. Others won't move their pelvis when they walk for fear of being thought of as brazen. Men sometimes hold their shoulders up and back in a tough-guy pose. Women may cave in their chests to avoid displaying their breasts. All of these examples of accultured motor learning detract from the natural elegance of development-inspired learning and are often a hindrance to the sublimation of damaging movement patterns and the ascendance of biomechanically friendly patterns. Help your students to recognize the choice between comfort and convention!

Performance enhancement

Peak performance can be thought of as having four different components. One is metabolic: how efficiently does your body deliver and utilize oxygen and fuel? The second component is muscular: how well do your muscles apply strength and its derivatives (power, explosiveness, endurance)? The third is will: the desire to win or to achieve. The fourth component of peak performance is neural orchestration: how accurate are the proprioceptive signals coming from your performing body, how good and how fast are performance decisions made based on that information, and how accurate are the motor signals that are sent back in reply? This is a question of skill, and this is where motor learning comes in.

Motor learning for the purpose of better performance requires, as does motor learning for the purpose of pain reduction or injury prevention, more than just visually based imitation of a movement and repetitive practice of that movement to achieve excellence. Vince Lombardi, the famous football coach, had a favorite saying: 'Practice doesn't make perfect, perfect practice makes perfect.' How can we get someone to practice and perform perfectly, without interference or drag from the inbuilt and unconscious biomechanical inefficiencies and imbalances that person certainly has?

Think of upgrading the subroutines as analogous to putting premium-grade gas in your tank instead of regular. It's the difference between putting whole milk on your cereal instead of skim. It's the difference between having your car painted at the shop by professionals and painting it yourself in your garage with a brush. It's the difference between a Cuban and a Canadian cigar; it may have the same name, but there is a huge qualitative difference.

I was on vacation with my wife many years ago and we were having lunch before going out for a round of golf. Our table overlooked the tennis courts and there was a lesson in progress in the court right below us. The instructor was on one side with an inexhaustible supply of brand new tennis balls, and his hapless student was on the other side brandishing a racket and a scowl. The instructor would hit each ball to the woman's forehand, consistently and flawlessly spoonfeeding her easy shots. She, however, was anything but consistent. Some balls were captured by the net, some ended up in an adjacent court, and some escaped her swings altogether.

At first she was trying to hit the balls with her shoulders and pelvis square to the net. The instructor had her turn sideways. Then she would swing at the ball with her knees straight. The instructor had her bend her knees. He fiddled with her grip, repeatedly demonstrated good form and continued to spoonfeed her forehand, but with marginally improved results. Clearly, practice wasn't making perfect.

The woman's real problem was a fundamental biomechanical one. She didn't know how to use her legs to twist her pelvis powerfully in space or how to connect the movement of her arm and racket to her torso and pelvis. I was about to shout some instructions down to her but my wife, ever the cautious one, dissuaded me. I argued (though maybe not in these exact words) that we could have broken down her swing as a complex function into smaller chunks and taught those chunks piecemeal within a framework of an earlier developmental movement.

I thought that transitional movements from floor-sitting to side-sitting might have been a good place to start teaching her how to rotate her pelvis and to use her iliopsoas/opposite gluteal muscles in basic pelvic force-coupled patterns. We could have connected her arms to those force-coupled movements by

having her put her hands together in front and swing her arms as an extension of her turning pelvis. We could have eventually put the racket in her hand and performed the same thing in side-sitting, half-kneeling and standing.

Once she was able to learn some of the basic patterns, by moving slowly and attentively, we could have speeded it up, working on the opposite force couple with a backhand swing as the intention, and finally adding the ball. Learning would then have been through a developmentally based sequence of problem solving, pattern recognition and enhanced self-awareness, rather than the inaccurate imitation of her instructor and the continued repetition of her unsuccessful pattern.

Imbalances

Structural imbalances, muscle imbalances, functional imbalances are all pretty much the same thing. More accurately, we could say that the various imbalances are facets of the same gem. They are peas in the same pod, layers in the same onion. If you have one you probably have the other two. Have you ever heard the saying 'When you've got a hammer, everything starts to look like a nail?'

If you have been trained and are good at assessing joint glide and collagen quality you will see joint hypo- and hypermobilities and treat them with mobilization and stabilization protocols. If you test and discern muscle imbalances, you'll treat them with stretching and strengthening exercises that localize and isolate those muscles. If you see structural imbalances and feel myofascial restrictions, you will attempt to release and balance that tissue. If you see functional imbalances and biomechanical inefficiencies, you will teach movement skills.

All of us could be looking at the same person and all of us would be right. We could all benefit from taking a larger view of human function, having a number of tools in our toolbox with which to affect that function and having an inkling of how all those tools are related. Structural, functional and muscular imbalances are just three sides to the same coin! Shirley Sahrmann has a book describing muscle imbalances and their relationships to structural/fascial imbalances and to associated musculoskeletal pain syndromes.[53]

Touching the elephant

Let's say we are working with a person with anterior tilt and a hyperlordotic low back. Structurally, we might see this and reasonably surmise myofascial restrictions in the iliopsoas complex, the rectus femoris and the thoracolumbar fascia, i.e. structural imbalance. We could also look at this person and reasonably guess that not only will the iliopsoas, rectus femoris and lumbar extensors be tight and contracting, but that the hamstrings, gluteals and abdominal muscles will be weak: muscular imbalance.

Arthrokinematically, we might see joint hypermobility of the lumbar joints into extension with hypomobility into flexion, and treat with joint mobilization into flexion and with stabilization exercises: collagen imbalance. We might predict that this person will probably have difficulty with complete push-off functions such as walking or standing, with falling backward contexts, with resting comfortably supine with legs straight, or with rolling along the spine from sit to lie and back up again: functional imbalance.

The challenge from a structural perspective is to not only release the tissue that is stopping a movement, but to train weak muscles to step up and control that newly available range of movement. From a manual therapy perspective, the challenge is to achieve not only local joint release but also the release of larger fascial envelopes, and again to control that new and unfamiliar range of motion. From a muscle imbalance perspective, the trick is to functionalize that newly awakened muscle into a larger synergistic chain in a context of specific whole-body activities and to achieve accurate motor control over antagonistic pairs of muscles, both locally and distally.

The challenge from a motor learning perspective is to obtain adequate fascial movement, in terms of both local joint movement and larger fascial planes – muscle balancing and functionalization of exercise are already incorporated. The ideal clinician would be one who could mobilize specific joints to achieve collagen mobility in capsules and ligaments; who could then release myofascial elements both around those specific joints and elsewhere in distal but structurally related areas; who could then help that person to orchestrate both local and distal antagonistic muscle pairs in harmonious cooperation; and who could then help that person to recognize when to use that newly acquired and controlled movement pattern in a context of real-life or athletic function.

Think of layers of imbalances: bone, joint, fascia, muscle tissue, brain. Whenever there is a fascial or capsular restriction there is simultaneous muscle hypertonicity. This applies both to joint capsule and to interarticular ligament restriction with intrinsic muscle hypertonicity, and to myofascial restriction with extrinsic muscle hypertonicity. Specific muscles will be too tight and will need to be lengthened.

On the other side of the coin, wherever there is muscle hypertonicity there is also antagonistic hypotonicity, again applying both intrinsically and extrinsically. Specific muscles will be too weak and will need to be recruited. Recall the concept of avoidance and the example of the sprained ankle. The CNS put the evertors/dorsiflexors on alert and inhibited the ankle plantarflexors/inverters to avoid movement in the direction of injury.

A similar mechanism is at work when we have a direction of restriction caused by either collagen immobility or habitual disuse; review the gluteal weakness and iliopsoas hypertonicity of another of our hypothetical situations. Recall also another aspect of avoidance: avoidance of a particular whole-body function. The person with the sprained ankle will avoid pushing off to some extent, and not only the plantarflexors but also the hamstring and gluteal muscles are inhibited (Box 1.7).

The resultant iliopsoas domination and the functional bias toward the stepping function create muscle and functional imbalances distal to the site of injury. Resultant compensation patterns can take these imbalances even further throughout the body. These muscle and functional imbalances can, with time, lead to shortening myofascial and articular adaptations and eventual structural imbalances. Think again of layers of imbalances, like the perpetuation of a flaw in an onion through its many layers.

Factors in imbalance creation

Why do we have imbalances? Early childhood development, injury, emotional and cultural factors and occupation are the same basic list of suspects as for when motor learning occurs. They are all important, and any of them may be the predominant factor with a particular person, but early childhood development is the rough draft upon which all other factors can only edit and revise. Early development is the 800-pound gorilla of motor learning factors. And early development seems to have a soft spot for imbalances.

When a baby is struggling to learn to orient, grasp and locomote, he does not practice both sides evenly.[54] He will usually stay with movement to one side, say rolling one way from back to belly, or drawing one knee underneath first to come to sit or come to hands and knees, until he can do it well and reproduce it at will in varied circumstances and at various speeds. Whitewater kayakers, when learning to do an Eskimo Roll, will do essentially the same thing. They will practice predominantly on one side to make sure that when they are upside down going through a rapid they can rely on their dominant side roll to get them back up; they call this developing a bombproof roll.

There seems to be a developmental, and perhaps even an evolutionary, *preference for left/right imbalance*. We learn to roll to one side first and best. We learn both to come up to sit and to sit on the floor asymmetrically. When my next meal depends on the accurate cast of my spear, having a dependable side is much more important than being able to throw that spear equally well with left and right hands.

My son, when he first learned to crawl, would draw up his left knee, scoot himself forward in a half-commando crawl, and then repeat with the drawn-up left knee; only later did he make it a bilateral movement, and even then it wasn't perfectly symmetrical. Later still, when coming from hands and knees to standing, he always put his left foot standing first. When he first learned to climb stairs, he went up left knee first then right knee up to the same step. Then he learned to step up that stair with his left foot, followed by his right knee then eventually his right foot again to the same step. Coming downstairs, it's always right foot first.

This stepping function with the left lower extremity dominant was established early on and just incorporated into each successive step in the developmental sequence. You may recall that we called these movement chunks that were used with modifications throughout a number of different function 'Legos'. This developmental preference for left-to-right imbalance may be driven by a need to have a bombproof side to move.

Box 1.7 Imbalances

Functional, structural and muscular imbalances – layers of the same onion

Factors include early development, injury, emotion and occupation

Left/right imbalances a normal developmental consequence

In an emergency, or when either speed or pinpoint accuracy is critical, having the ability to just react and automatically choose the best side could be the edge we need to be successful, or to stay alive long enough to pass on our genes. Simply the fact that most of us have a dominant hand and a dominant eye guarantees lifelong muscle, structural and functional imbalances.

We could almost say that these imbalances are natural and to a certain extent desirable, and that having a goal of structural symmetry or perfect muscle and functional balance would be unrealistic. Logic dictates symmetry as the organization of choice in terms of minimizing tissue strain, but biology has other criteria. Does this mean we shouldn't treat those imbalances? No! Imbalances create tissue strain and uneven distribution of movement and effort.

Predisposition to injury

Imbalances, as Shirley Sahrmann maintains in her *movement system balance theory*, create '. . . the deviation of the PICR from the kinesiological standard, cause microtrauma that eventually leads to musculoskeletal pain syndromes (MPS) and possibly to pathology as evident neurologically or radiologically.' (PICR is the path of the instantaneous center of rotation. A state of movement system balance exists when the PICR during active motion is consistent with the standard kinesiological for the joint for each axis of motion.[53])

Imbalances predispose us to injury. They are a drag on performance when that performance is either bilaterally symmetrical (weightlifting, tumbling) or has reciprocating asymmetrical movements (running, swimming, cycling). We can work toward balance by improving the biomechanical efficiency of both sides, introducing deliberately nonhabitual directions of movement and creating some wriggle-room, so that person becomes less of a victim of his own imbalanced invariance.

In Section 2 we will direct our attention to the how-to-do part of motor learning. What do I want to teach, and how do I want to teach it? The next chapter in this section deals with exercise. Although the Feldenkrais Method has a marvelous manual technique called Functional Integration, discussion on how to teach by handling is beyond the scope or intent of this book. We will be drawing most of our Feldenkrais material from his exercise technique called Awareness Through Movement. We will first look at strengthening, stretching and coordination exercises from a motor learning perspective. We will then describe in subsequent chapters common movement and postural patterns, their clinical or performance enhancement implications, and examples of motor learning approaches to common clinical problems or sports applications.

References

1. Feldenkrais M. Body and mature behavior: a study of anxiety, sex, gravitation and learning. London: Routledge & Kegan Paul; 1949.
2. Feldenkrais M. Awareness through movement: health exercises for personal growth. New York: Harper & Row; 1972.
3. Feldenkrais M. The case of Nora: body awareness as healing therapy. New York: Harper & Row; 1977.
4. Feldenkrais M. The elusive obvious. Cupertino, CA: Meta Publications; 1984.
5. Feldenkrais M. The master moves. Cupertino, CA: Meta Publications; 1981.
6. Feldenkrais M. The potent self. San Francisco: Harper & Row; 1985.
7. Feldenkrais M. Practical unarmed combat. London: Frederick Warne & Co; 1941.
8. Feldenkrais M. Judo: the art of defense and attack. London: Frederick Warne & Co; 1944.
9. Feldenkrais M. Higher judo. London: Frederick Warne & Co; 1952.
10. Alon R. Mindful spontaneity, moving in tune with nature: lessons in the Feldenkrais Method. Australia: Interface; 1990.
11. Goldfarb L. Articulating changes: toward a theory for the Feldenkrais Method. Berkeley, CA: Feldenkrais Resources; 1990.
12. Hanna T. The body of life. New York: Knopf; 1980.
13. Heggie J. Running with the whole body. Emmaus, PA: Rodale Press; 1986.
14. Rywerant Y. The Feldenkrais Method: teaching by handling. San Francisco: Harper & Row; 1983.
15. Reese M, Zemach-Bersin K. Relaxercise. San Francisco: Harper & Row; 1990.
16. Jackson O, Gula J, Kireta A, Steeves M. Effects of Feldenkrais practitioner training program on motor ability: a videoanalysis. Platform paper, American Physical Therapy Association, Colorado, 1992.
17. Jackson O (ed) Physical therapy of the geriatric patient, 2nd edn. New York: Churchill Livingstone; 1989.
18. Jackson O (ed) Therapeutic considerations for the elderly. New York: Churchill Livingstone; 1987.
19. Narula M, Jackson O. The effects of a six-week Feldenkrais Method on selected functional parameters in a subject with rheumatoid arthritis. Platform paper, American Physical Therapy Association, Colorado, 1992.
20. Connors K, Greenough P. Redevelopment of the sense of self following stroke, using the Feldenkrais Method. Melbourne, Australia: Caulfield General Medical Center; 2004.
21. Malmgren-Olsson EB, Armelius BA, Armelius K. A comparative outcome study of body awareness therapy, Feldenkrais, and conventional physiotherapy for patients with nonspecific musculoskeletal disorders: changes in psychological symptoms, pain, and self-image. Physiotherapy Practice 2001;17:77–95.
22. Buchanan PA, Ulrich BD. The Feldenkrais Method: a dynamic approach to changing motor behavior. Research Quarterly for Exercise and Sport 2003;74:116–23; discussion 124–6.
23. Burkart S, Nair D, Burhart B, Brown V, Brantley J. Recovery of hand function following stroke using the Feldenkrais Method: the case of Norma. Palm Beach Institute of Sports Medicine Center of Complex Systems Brain Sciences. Functional Rehabilitation Associates; 2004.
24. Malmgren-Olsson EB, Branholm IB. A comparison between three physiotherapy approaches with regard to health-related factors in patients with non-specific musculoskeletal disorders. Disability Rehabilitation 2002;15:308–17.
25. Batson G. Effect of Feldenkrais Awareness Through Movement on upper extremity recovery after stroke: a case study. Provo, Utah: Rocky Mountain University; 2004.
26. Lundblad I, Eler J, Gerdle B. Randomized controlled trial of physiotherapy and Feldenkrais interventions in female workers with

neck–shoulder complaints. Journal of Occupational Rehabilitation 1999;9:179–94.

27. Hopper C, Kolt GS, McConville JC. The effect of Feldenkrais Awareness Through Movement on hamstring length, flexibility, and perceived exertion. Journal of Bodywork and Movement Therapy 1999;3:238–47.

28. James M, Kolt G, McConville J, Bate P. The effects of a Feldenkrais program and relaxation procedures on hamstring length. Australian Journal of Physiotherapy 1998;44:49–54.

29. Stephens J, DuShuttle D, Hatcher C, Shmunes J, Slaninka C. Use of Awareness Through Movement improves balance and balance confidence in people with multiple sclerosis: a randomized controlled study. Neurology Report 2001;25:39–49.

30. Gutman GM, Herbert CP, Brown SR. Feldenkrais versus conventional exercise for the elderly. Journal of Gerontology 1977;32: 562–72.

31. Nair D, Jantzen K, Fuchs A, Steinberg F, Kelso J. Assessing recovery from stroke using functional MRI: a serial case study. Boca Raton, FL: Center of Complex Systems Brain Sciences. University MRI and Treatment Centers, Florida Atlanta University; 2004.

32. Johnson SK, Frederick J, Kaufman M, Mountjoy B. A controlled investigation of bodywork in multiple sclerosis. Journal of Alternative and Complementary Medicine 1999;5:237–43.

33. Stephens J, Cates P, Fentes E et al. Awareness through movement improves quality of life in people with multiple sclerosis. Chester, PA: Physical Therapy Department at Temple University. Widener University Institute for Physical Therapy Education; 2004.

34. Ives JC, Shelley G. The Feldenkrais Method in rehabilitation: a review. Work 1998;11:75–90.

35. Ives JC. Comments on 'the Feldenkrais Method: a dynamic approach to changing motor behavior.' Research Quarterly for Exercise and Sport 2003;74:116–23; discussion 124–6.

36. Hislop HJ. Tenth Mary McMillan lecture: The not-so-impossible dream. Physical Therapy 1975;55:1066–80.

37. Purtilo R. Definitional issues in pathokinesiology: a retrospective and look ahead. Physical Therapy 1986;66:3.

38. Thelen E, Corbetta D, Kamm K, Spencer J. The transition to reaching: mapping intention and intrinsic dynamics. Child Development 1993;64:1058–98.

39. Alexander R, Boehme R, Cupps B. Normal development of functional motor skills. Tucson, AZ: Therapy Skill Builders; 1993.

40. Gerber M. RIE manual: for parents and professionals. Los Angeles, CA: Resources for Infant Educarers; 1979.

41. Turvey M, Fitzpatrick P. Commentary: Development of perception–action systems and general principles of pattern formation. Child Development 1993;64:1074–90.

42. Bernstein NA. The coordination and regulation of movements. Oxford: Pergamon Press; 1967.

43. Sporns O, Edelman G. Solving Bernsteins's Problem: a proposal for the development of coordinated movement by selection. Child Development 1993;64:960–81.

44. Dunlap K. Habits: their making and unmaking. Liveright: 1932; 3–18.

45. Juhan D. Job's body: a manual for bodywork. New York: Station Hill Press; 1987: 137–43.

46. Korr I. Collected papers of Irwin Korr. Indianapolis, IN: American Academy of Osteopathy; 1979.

47. Jayson M. Neurological aspects of low back pain. In: Jayson M, ed. The lumbar spine and back pain. New York: Grune & Stratton; 1976: 189–256.

48. Chen R, Cohen LG, Hallett M. Nervous system reorganization following injury. Neuroscience 2002;111:761–73.

49. Stokes M, Young A. The contribution of reflex inhibition to arthrogenous muscle weakness. Clinical Science 1984;67:7–14.

50. Bullock-Saxton JE. Local sensation changes and altered hip muscle function following severe ankle sprain. Physical Therapy 1994;74: 17–31.

51. Sahrmann SA. Evaluation and treatment of muscle imbalances and associated musculoskeletal pain syndromes. Level 2-UQ course manual, p 4.

52. Darwin C. Expressions of emotion in man and animals, 3rd edn. New York: Oxford University Press; 1998.

53. Sahrmann S. Diagnoses and treatment of movement impairment syndromes. St. Louis, MO: Mosby; 2002.

54. Caplan F. The first twelve months of life. New York: Grosset & Dunlap; 1971.

CHAPTER TWO

Influencing motor behavior

Chapter outline

Exercise for influencing motor control

1. Quantitative vs qualitative strengthening. Qualitative strengthening is about economy of effort – timing and coordination – it is integrative rather than isolationary, requiring a sense of purpose and an active proprioceptive awareness.

2. The main characteristics that distinguish qualitative from quantitative strengthening are proprioceptive self-awareness, pattern specificity and functional context.

   • Proprioceptive self-awareness. Importance in motor learning. Train proprioceptive self-awareness with descriptive and inquisitive language and with guiding and illuminating touch. Awareness of muscle effort, relationships to gravity, bony relationships and awareness of larger patterns key.

   • Pattern specificity. The pattern we strengthen a muscle in should look something like the pattern of movement we are trying to influence in our students – think of strengthening the pattern, not just the muscle. Studies on synergistic whole-body patterns. Movement patterns/subroutines a good thing (don't have to reinvent the wheel each time you walk) and a detriment (perpetuation of inefficient pattern and invariance of tissue strain). Global/primitive patterns (hip and back extension) less clinically relevant than differentiated patterns (hip flexion with back extension).

   • Pattern reciprocity and change of venue. Go in both directions to balance/coordinate the antagonists and

to recalibrate to a truer neutral position. Train a pattern of movement with variables. Change relationship to gravity and speed and link to functional context.

   • Functional context refers to our ability to piggyback information or skills we'd like our student to have concerning posture, strength, flexibility, gross motor skill and proprioceptive acuity on to real-life movements or developmentally inspired movements. Seven functional categories: balance, orientation, locomotion, transitions, manipulation, communication and vegetation.

3. Quantitative and qualitative stretching

   • Qualitative stretching is about changing the muscle spindle bias to a longer length: resetting the tripwire. It is about shutting off muscles that would otherwise interfere with movement in a desired direction: inhibition of antagonists. It is about general reduction of effort and muscle tone: relaxation and conservation of energy. It is integrative rather than isolationary.

   • Role of the muscle spindle. Stimulates muscle to fire to prevent joint from moving past its physiological limit. Tripwire set too short; hypomobility/stiffness. Tripwire set too long: hypermobility/instability. Hypermobility/hypomobility pairs can be local or distal: importance of addressing relationships of different parts.

   • Proprioceptive self-awareness. Effort recognition key to plastic lengthening of short muscles. Effort reduction key to relaxation and conservation of energy. Key to improving proprioceptive acuity: the Weber–Fechner Principle proposes that the ability to perceive changes in stimulus is inversely proportional to the strength of that stimulus. In relaxation training, have them do the minimal contraction they can perceive rather than the strongest contraction they can squeeze out.

- Pattern specificity makes the exercise look something like the motor behavior you are trying to influence. Differentiated patterns more clinically relevant.
- Functional context. Link to real life. Provide conditions for change; get them on the floor, squatting, kneeling, etc. SAID principle: specific adaptation to imposed demand.

4. Reciprocation of antagonists
- Come close to slapping your face with eyes closed: how do you know when to stop firing the biceps and start firing the triceps? Schematic representation of reciprocal inhibition, hypermobilities and hypomobilities as reflections of incoordination of antagonists.
- Instead of doing separate stretching and strengthening exercises, go in both directions to do both at the same time; adjust language and emphasis to encourage nonhabitual differentiated patterns.

Exercise

We might not think of exercise as being a motor learning technique, but we often use it that way. Although some exercises we do are for cardiopulmonary reasons and some for physiological reasons (blood flow change or connective tissue quality), much of our rationale for prescribing exercises is essentially a motor learning one. We want our students to move better to improve function and performance and to reduce tissue strain or damage. We already use exercise to change behavior: arthrokinematic, postural and gross motor.[1]

We strengthen the rotator cuff muscles to control glenohumeral arthokinematics and the vastus medialis to better track the patella. We stretch the pectoralis major in people who abduct their shoulder girdles, and stretch the iliopsoas in those who tilt their pelvis anteriorly. We stretch the hamstrings to make bending easier, and give balance and proprioceptive exercises to someone with a sprained ankle. These groups of exercises are designed to improve on either existing but inefficient movement and postural patterns, or injury-induced abnormal patterns. They can be broadly categorized into three groups: strengthening, stretching and coordination/balance. The purpose of this chapter is to introduce new ways of thinking about exercise and how we use it. What are the characteristics of exercise performed for motor control purposes? How does this approach differ from standard therapeutic exercise? Examples and case studies will be presented.

Qualitative and quantitative strengthening

We know how to make a muscle stronger. We can stimulate recruitment of more muscle fibers and improve their efficiency. We can increase the size of the muscle fibers and the mass of the muscle as a whole. We can measure the torque produced by a particular muscle and graph where in its range it is the strongest. This is quantitative strengthening, objective and measurable.

When quantitatively strengthening the gluteus maximus, for instance, it doesn't matter what the orientation to gravity is, whether the foot is on or off the floor, what the synergists are doing, whether the antagonists are adequately inhibited, whether the person is paying proprioceptive attention to himself, whether the contraction moves the thigh on the pelvis or pelvis on the thigh, or what his intention in moving is; it is enough to have a muscle simply produce more force. From a motor learning perspective, however, *qualitative strengthening* is a more important goal.

Qualitative strengthening is about the smooth recruitment of just enough motor units to get the job done, i.e. economy of effort. It is about firing those motor units only when needed and stopping the contraction when it's no longer needed: timing and coordination. It includes the accurate and simultaneous inhibition of antagonists and the cooperative excitation of appropriate synergists in function-specific whole-body patterns; it is integrative rather than isolationary (Box 2.1).

Qualitative strengthening requires a sense of purpose and an active proprioceptive awareness on the part of the student to make informed decisions on how and when to apply that strength. The main characteristics that distinguish qualitative from quantitative strengthening are *proprioceptive self-awareness, pattern specificity* and *functional context*.

Proprioceptive self-awareness

The need to pay attention to proprioceptive sensations when learning a motor skill seems obvious and is known intuitively. When hitting a tee shot in golf, for instance, I want to know what proprioceptive sensations are produced. If I know and can reproduce the feeling in my legs, pelvis, chest, arms, head and eyes when I hit the ball, I have a great tool for improving my game. Knowing and reproducing the proprioceptive sensations created by a ball well hit is what guides me toward refinement, and knowing the sensations created by a ball poorly hit is what helps me avoid mistakes. Studies on motor learning have confirmed what we know intuitively: that cortical involvement in learning and attending to proprioceptive perceptions are critical in learning and retaining motor skills.[2-10]

Proprioceptive sensations are our guide to comparing movement options, choosing whether to change a pattern or stay with the tried and true, and being able to reproduce that new pattern accurately and reliably. Proprioceptive receptors are

---

Box 2.1 Characteristics of qualitative exercise

Emphasizes proprioceptive self-awareness – know what you're doing to do what you want

Necessity for pattern specificity – making exercise look something like the motor behavior you are seeking to influence

Association to functional context – linking exercise to real-life movements

located in the joint capsule, ligaments, tendons, fascia and muscle, and are constantly bombarding your CNS with updated and ever-changing information from the musculoskeletal system.[11]

Proprioceptive sensations give you information about what's happening inside your body from a musculoskeletal perspective. They include an ability to discern joint position, direction and velocity of movement, relationship to gravity and muscle effort. We cannot possibly be consciously aware of every bit of proprioceptive information coming into headquarters, and most of that information is processed subcortically, but the decisions based on that information are central to motor learning.

All this proprioceptive information flooding your CNS is to aid in decision-making – decisions consciously made and abandoned, decisions unconsciously made and perpetuated. We make decisions about movement and postural patterns during childhood development, after injury and during recovery, as a manifestation of an emotional state or as influenced by cultural aesthetics and mores. We make these decisions based on internal and subjective criteria, and once a preferred pattern is selected we quickly turn it into a habit. We like that particular way of doing things and habituate our motor instructions to create the proprioceptive feeling associated with that preferred pattern.

Remember that many of these habits, along with their imbalances and errors, are formed early in development and are incorporated into all subsequent steps of the developmental sequence. It's this interweaving of motor and sensory, this blending of early learning and later function, that makes proprioceptively driven movement and postural patterns so hard to change and our work so varied and unpredictable. We have to persuade our students to change from what are often habitually ingrained arthrokinematic, postural or gross movement patterns to the new way we propose. Showing your players a film of Michael Jordan, demonstrating proper ergonomics or handing your student a packet of written home exercises is seldom enough.

Proprioceptive and neuromusculoskeletal change requires sensorimotor informative exercise. How then do we use exercise to go about changing a valgus knee or an abducted shoulder girdle, changing a hypermobile C6 or an impinging glenohumeral joint, changing a throwing motion or a swimming stroke, despite a lifetime of endless and interwoven habit selections? How can we use exercise to restore an ability to walk, climb stairs or hold a pen again for someone with a stroke or multiple sclerosis?

Learning environment

If our goal in exercise is to change muscle function to change motor behavior, we need to think about what kind of learning environment we're providing for our students. Is it reasonably quiet, or is there loud music or ongoing conversation? Are they paying proprioceptive attention while they are doing their exercises, or are they reading a magazine or worrying about work while they go through their exercises in a rote manner? Are they safely ensconced on the floor or low mat table, or are they perched on a too-high, narrow or rickety plinth? Ignoring proprioceptive cues is easy enough in the best of conditions;

Box 2.2 Training for proprioceptive acuity
Verbally guide students on search for proprioceptive clues
Guide students in decision-making process
Using descriptive and inquisitive language

unnecessary distractions or an unconscious fear of falling will make the job even more difficult.

How do we train students for proprioceptive acuity? We could ask questions about what they notice about themselves while they move or assume a posture. We could verbally guide them on their search for proprioceptive clues. How do we guide them in their decision-making process? We could ask them to feel for smoothness, ease, comfort, effortlessness and balance. We could let them use their own internal and subjective criteria, and encourage them to select new patterns from a number of deliberately introduced choices (Box 2.2).

We could use language (*descriptive and inquisitive*) and touch (*guiding and illuminating*) to help people become aware of what they are doing. What do we want them to be aware of? In addition to joint position and movement, effort sense, etc., we particularly want them to be able to recognize patterns. We want them to recognize the whole-body or integrated patterns of movement and posture that make up our real life.

Watch an infant grow through its first year and observe how basic patterns of movement (similar relationships of head to pelvis or pelvis to legs) recur throughout different, seemingly unrelated functions. This weaving of similar skeletal patterns and similar muscular synergistic relationships throughout many different functional categories makes our lives as clinicians that much more difficult. Instead of being able to simply teach our student with neck pain how to extend her thoracic spine in the context of postural support, we will have to train that same ability to extend her thoracic spine in the context of looking overhead, and will have to train that same ability to extend her thoracic spine in reaching and pushing movements, transitions and gait as well.

Instead of just teaching our student with lumbar instability how to maintain spinal neutral and core stability in symmetrical postures, with undifferentiated limb movements and in a vertical orientation, we need to provide some variety and complexity. We will need to teach those same skills in asymmetrical postures, with integrated and dynamic limb movements, in a variety of orientations relative to gravity (belly down/up, leaned forward/back, lie horizontally supine/prone/side lie) and related to many different potential stressors of the lower back (pushing, pulling, lifting, looking over one shoulder, getting out of bed, walking, washing dishes, carrying weight in front, paddling a canoe, etc.). Instead of just training your horse to walk, you'll have to train it to walk while being ridden, to walk while pulling a plow, to walk when following a lead, to walk while pulling a sleigh, and to close the barn door behind it.

We are not a huge conglomeration of discrete movement skills that can be tinkered with piecemeal, but a complex bird's nest of interwoven and interrelated intentions and patterns of movement. Recent research on how we organize ourselves to move suggests that we do so in *synergistic patterns* that help the CNS deal with Bernstein's Problem (how to select an appropriate and reproducible coordination of muscle, joint and bone in the face of the availability of practically infinite choices).[12–33]

What this means is that we are not reinventing the wheel every time we do something. We reduce degrees of freedom so we can develop a reproducible pattern of movement that we can use over and over again when a similar situation arises. These patterns or motor habits are a good thing, up to a point. With the creation of movement subroutines, we free our nervous system for other tasks. There is a potential drawback, however, with this characteristic of the CNS to create movement patterns: what happens when that habitual movement pattern is inefficient or damaging?

What this implies to the movement teacher is that teaching motor skills – attempting to modify motor behavior – is not amenable to the traditional exercise approach of localizing/isolating the muscle, repeating localized movement in selected cardinal plane an arbitrary number of times, and then increasing resistance or range to progress. We need an updated exercise approach that is consistent with what we know about how the neuromusculoskeletal system organizes itself to move in patterns. We need to bring our exercise into the Information Age.

Pattern specificity: global and differentiated patterns

Let's take a look at a couple of common clinical situations to help illustrate our second characteristic of quantitative strengthening: pattern specificity. Imagine the case of the hyperlordotic student with low back pain (Fig. 2.1). Her pain is aggravated by standing, lumbar extension and lying flat on her back, and is alleviated by lumbar flexion. We might surmise a closed-pack facet irritation and may wish to give her exercises to strengthen her abdominals and her gluteus maximus and other hip extensors to reduce excessive anterior pelvic tilt in standing.

For the hip extensors, gluteal sets, prone leg lifts or hands and knees diagonal arm and leg lifts may be prescribed and progressive resistance techniques can be applied. These would certainly quantitatively strengthen the hip extensors, but would they necessarily change the behavior contributing to her pain?

On skeletal and muscular analysis, we can see that in these exercises both the hip and the spine are in extension. Both the hip extensors and the back extensors are engaged in shortening contractions. This pattern of simultaneous hip and back extension we could call a *global extension* pattern (Fig. 2.2). Our clinical intention, however, is for the student to do a differentiated pattern of movement: hip extension along with lumbar flexion (Fig. 2.1). We want a contraction of the hip extensors with inhibition of back extensors. We want the hip extensors to work to tilt the pelvis posteriorly without the lumbar extensors kicking in to keep the low back extended in hyperlordosis.

Try the following simple experiment. Lie on your belly with your legs long and comfortably spread. Turn your head either left or right and rest it on the floor. Keep both knees on the floor as you slowly lift both feet 1–2 ft off the floor, then slowly

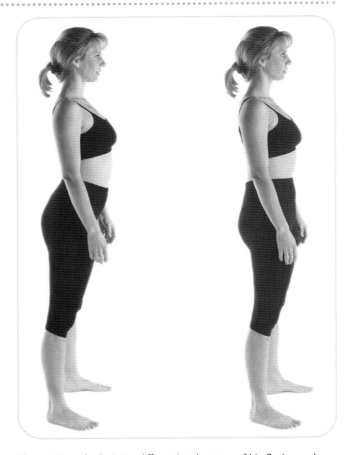

Fig. 2.1 Hyperlordosis is a differentiated pattern of hip flexion and back extension – corrected with back flexion and hip extension.

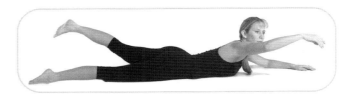

Fig. 2.2 Common hip extensor strengthening exercise is a global pattern of hip and back extension.

lower them back down. Repeat many times to feel and be aware of what happens at your pelvis and lower back as you do this. In theory, the contraction of the hamstrings should posteriorly tilt the pelvis and lengthen or flex the lumbar spine. What many of you will find, however, is that the lumbar extensors automatically kick in to counteract the posterior tilting function of the hamstrings (Box 2.3).

As you continue this movement, some of you may learn to allow the lumbar spine to flex through the inhibition of the back extensors. Some others of you will be unable to differentiate the hip and lumbar extensors and allow the pelvis to flex in this position no matter how many times you try. This

Box 2.3 Global patterns – more primitive, related to early development

Hip extension and lumbar extension
Thoracic flexion and cervical flexion
Glenohumeral external rotation and forearm supination
Hip flexion and ankle dorsiflexion

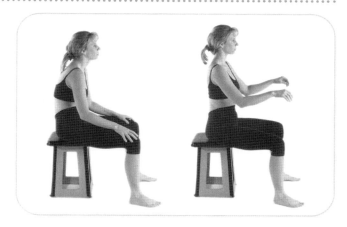

Fig. 2.4 A slumped sitting posture is a differentiated pattern of hip and cervical extension with torso flexion – corrected with hip and cervical flexion and torso extension.

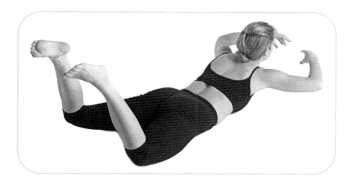

Fig. 2.3 The baby airplane – global torso and extremity extension.

becomes an even more difficult differentiation to make if we add in the gluteals by lifting the knees. Try it yourself to see if you can do it without activating the back extensors!

Developmentally, lying on our bellies and contracting our hip extensors is associated in our CNS not with standing and posteriorly rotating our pelvis, but with lifting our head to look around – to orient ourselves from prone. Children, when they are at a certain age, will spend a lot of time on their bellies with their head, arms and legs all lifted in a global extension pattern. This is the baby airplane (Fig. 2.3). Try lying on your belly and lifting your head to look forward, without pushing up with your hands.

Feel at what point your gluteals and hamstrings kick in. In this situation, the lumbar and hip extensors should be working together, as they are synergists in the intention to bring the head to vertical and look around. In our hyperlordotic student, however, we would like the hip and lumbar extensors to be antagonists in the desired action of tilting the pelvis posteriorly to better balance it over the legs, reducing hyperlordosis and its consequent tissue strain. This requires a differentiated pattern of movement, hip extension with lumbar flexion.

To strengthen the abdominals, we could have our student lie supine and do some variation of crunches, lifting the head and bringing one or both knees toward the elbows. Although this would quantitatively strengthen the abdominals, it would combine hip flexion with lumbar flexion in a global pattern of movement and make the abdominals and the hip flexors synergists. What we need in this scenario is a differentiated pattern of lumbar flexion and hip extension.

We want the abdominals and hip flexors to be antagonists. In motor learning terms, we need to be pattern specific in our exercise prescription. The pattern we strengthen a muscle in should look something like the pattern of movement we are trying to influence in our students. In other words, we can think of strengthening the pattern, not just the muscle.

Let's look at another example. Say we have someone with a habitually slumped sitting posture who works at a computer all day and complains of headaches and neck pain (Fig. 2.4). We would like to teach this student to extend her spine and come upright to better balance her head and relieve muscular strain, joint compression or shearing in the cervical spine.

We would probably prescribe exercises to strengthen the back extensors. We may even, as in our last scenario, have our student do prone (or hands and knees) arm and leg lifts, and may even add weights to make those extensors work harder. This again quantitatively strengthens the back extensors, but by combining back extension with hip extension we are again teaching a global pattern of movement, global extension.

This again would be an appropriate organization when she's lying prone and lifting her head, but our clinical intention with this person is for her to do a differentiated pattern of movement that involves back extension with hip flexion (Fig. 2.4). Here the hip flexors are synergists to the back extensors, whereas the hip extensors need to be inhibited and allowed to lengthen, as they are now antagonistic in this function. The head and neck differentiate from the extending torso by moving into relative flexion and the cervical extensors differentiate from the thoracic extensors.

The serratus anterior also now becomes a synergist to back extension rather than the rhomboids and mid to lower trapezius, differentiating the arms from the torso as well as the legs. For many people, we may even want to differentiate different parts of the torso, differentiating the lumbar extensors from the thoracic extensors. This would be especially true with students who are simultaneously excessively lordosing their low back and excessively kyphosing through their mid-back, which is another common variation of our student with neck pain and headaches. Here, the challenge is to get the thorax to extend simultaneously with lumbar flexion. Try it out in a chair (Fig. 2.5), then in standing!

With pattern specificity in exercise comes pattern recognition on the part of the student. Exercising in functionally relevant

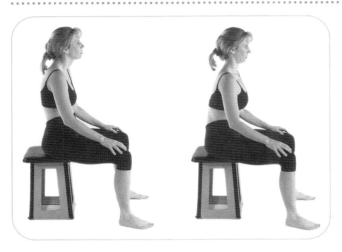

Fig. 2.5 Differentiated torso – lumbar extension with thoracic flexion – corrected with lumbar flexion and thoracic extension.

Box 2.4 Differentiated patterns – more complex, related to higher-level function

Hip extension and lumbar flexion
Thoracic extension and cervical flexion
Glenohumeral external rotation with forearm pronation
Ankle plantarflexion and toe dorsiflexion

---

patterns of movement and in a variety of positions and orientations to gravity allows our student to know what she is doing, to recognize the pattern of the movement and apply it to real-life function. With pattern recognition comes the ability to make informed decisions on movement and postural selection, and to extrapolate to real life and athletic function (Box 2.4).

With pattern specificity come whole-body integrated patterns of movement and the coordination of both local and distal synergistic muscles with the muscle we are trying to strengthen. With pattern specificity comes the ability to simultaneously inhibit the antagonists while strengthening the agonists, using reciprocal inhibition and progressive application of constraints to stretch the muscles opposing our desired function.

Although initially we might stretch and strengthen different muscles in isolation to shake those muscles from their stupor, we need to take our students further. We need to blend that newly awakened muscle into cooperative action with its neighbors. Let's use pattern specificity and whole-body movements to simultaneously do stretching and strengthening exercises, postural training, proprioceptive acuity training, spinal stabilization and body mechanics instruction. Let's look at some simple examples to illustrate what pattern-specific exercise and qualitative strengthening might look like.

Exercising qualitatively

If we want our students to change the way they are doing something (arthrokinematic, postural or gross motor behav-

ior), we first need to get them to be aware of how they are currently doing that particular movement. One of Feldenkrais' famous sayings was: 'If you know what you're doing, you can do what you want.' How do we do that? How do we get someone to recognize what he or she is doing? We may start by having our hyperlordotic student observe herself proprioceptively both in standing and in lying supine with legs long. We might ask her a series of questions about bony relationships, her perception of relationships of different bones to gravity, the degree of tension or muscle effort, and her contact pressure against supporting surfaces.

In standing, we could ask questions about the position of the pelvis in space and the shape of the lumbar spine. Can she discern the anterior spill of her pelvis and the deep hollowing in her low back? We could continue this proprioceptive scan supine with legs long (pattern specificity) and ask questions about contact against the floor. We'll use the floor as a proprioceptive mirror to help our student with pattern recognition: an anteriorly tipped pelvis will press into the floor closer to the tailbone than to the sacral base, and the lumbar spine will not have contact against the floor.

Similarly, we could have used a wall in standing as another proprioceptive mirror to clarify bony relationships. This proprioceptive awareness of what she is doing before we start a lesson provides a handy reference point that enables practitioner and student to reassess things at intervals, both during and after a lesson. Awareness of left-to-right differences is another aspect of proprioceptive awareness that enables comparisons to be made and conclusions to be drawn.

Proprioceptive awareness on the part of the student of changes in habituated muscle tone or postural and movement patterns after a lesson is the basis for the adoption of new and hopefully improved movement pathways. Try introducing some before-and-after (and left-to-right) proprioceptive reference points with your students regardless of the techniques you use!

Pattern reciprocity and change of venue

We may then have our student lie on the floor with knees bent and feet flat. We might have her alternately lift and press her tailbone, or roll her pelvis up and down on the floor by pushing and pulling with her legs (Fig. 2.6). Pressing her tailbone exaggerates her pattern and allows her to judge its familiarity and comfort. This is the differentiated pattern that causes her problems in standing: back extension with hip flexion. Lifting her tailbone is a nonhabitual differentiated pattern: hip extension with lumbar flexion. It is really the classic 'pelvic tilt' exercise, but performed for motor learning purposes with *pattern reciprocity* and *change of venue*.

Pattern reciprocity is simply going in both directions instead of in a therapeutic direction only. In the case of our hyperlordotic student, logic might dictate that we want to move in the direction of comfort only, i.e. lumbar flexion/hip extension. For pattern recognition and decision-making considerations, however, reciprocal movements are more informative, even if we can only move a small amount into that undesirable direction. Reciprocating movements help our CNS to map where we are in a movement continuum and allow us to more accu-

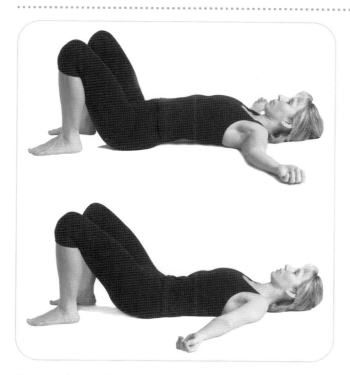

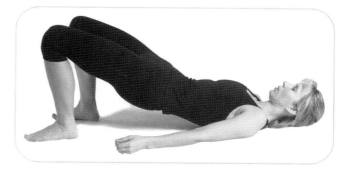

Fig. 2.7 More complete, more difficult progression of hip extension and lumbar flexion.

Fig. 2.6 Habitual and nonhabitual differentiated patterns.

Box 2.5 Reciprocating movements – going in both directions

Coordinating the antagonists – equal competence in ability to lengthen fully as to contract powerfully

Recalibrating a truer neutral – neutrality outgrowth of ability to move equally easily in both directions

Reciprocating between habitual and nonhabitual differentiated patterns is common strategy

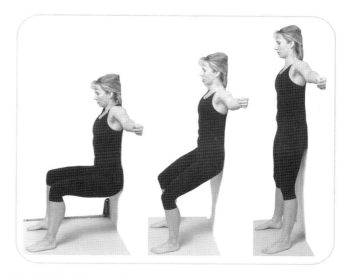

Fig. 2.8 Teach the same basic movement on the floor – roll into anterior tilt, then push into posterior tilt.

rately recalibrate neutral. Reciprocating movements also help to coordinate the antagonist pairs by having them engage in a cooperative tug-of-war (Box 2.5).

Change of venue has to do with taking the same reciprocating patterns – in this case lumbar flexion/hip extension and lumbar extension/hip flexion – and introducing an element of change. We could change speed, orientation to gravity or intention.[34,35] We might have the student enlarge the movement by lifting her pelvis off the ground and lifting and lowering the lumbar vertebrae one at a time (Fig. 2.7). This requires an even more difficult inhibition of the lumbar extensors while firing even more powerfully the hip extensors. We could introduce variations to these two movements by lying supine on a foam roller or rolled-up towel. She could lie supine with her feet on the wall instead of the floor while doing the same things and progressively move her feet closer to the floor (Fig. 2.8). We could stand her up with her butt on the wall, her feet away from the wall, and have her reciprocate patterns here and progress by standing erect and moving the feet ever closer to the wall, to achieve progressively more hip extension (Fig. 2.9).

We could take the same basic reciprocal patterns and do them supine, in side-lying, on hands and knees, hands and feet, half-kneeling, or sitting on floor or chair. We could put small rollers under her feet.

We could introduce one-sided versions of this alternating movement and do diagonal patterns in addition to cardinal plane movements. All the time we are both guiding her proprioceptive exploration and asking her questions about what she notices. These changes of venue help our student recognize pattern variations and allow her to extrapolate skills learned here to similar functions, becoming more creative and self-regulating in the process.

We could have our slouching student with the neck pain and headaches do a proprioceptive scan as well, perhaps in sitting. We can ask where her pelvis is on the seat by creating an awareness of ischial tuberosity contact. We would ask her to assess the shape of her back, the balance of her head and the

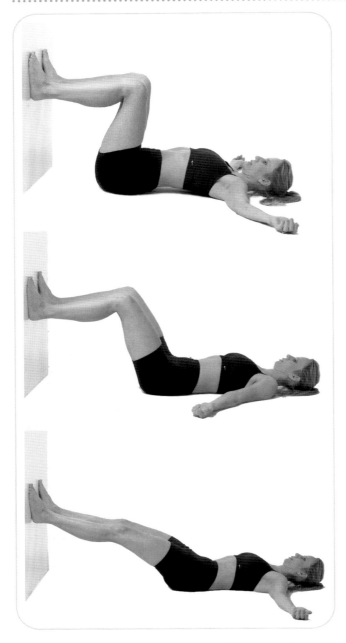

Fig. 2.9 The same pattern of movement in another position. Progress by moving feet closer to the wall.

muscular effort in her neck and shoulders. From there we could ask her to roll her pelvis deliberately forward and backward and look up and down in coordination. We could progress this to leaning back/rolling back/looking down and leaning forward/rolling forward/looking up (Fig. 2.10).

These are again reciprocating differentiated patterns, with the movement into hip flexion and back extension being of particular interest to us. Movement into this direction simultaneously strengthens the iliopsoas and back extensors while lengthening/stretching the hamstrings, piriformis, gluteals,

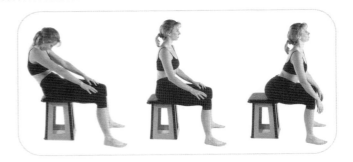

Fig. 2.10 Reciprocating differentiated movements – back flexion with hip extension to back extension with hip flexion.

Box 2.6 Change of venue – learning the same pattern in different environments

Moving slowly to learn and quickly to imprint

Adding subvariations and constraints

Repeating patterns in belly-up, belly-down and gravity-neutral orientations

Linking movements to various functional categories

---

abdominals, anterior chest wall, etc. We could progress this by rolling the pelvis forward and back while leaning on the elbows or with the hands on the floor. We could lower the seat to make it harder, or raise it to make it easier. We could progress to doing this movement while seated on the floor.

We could turn it into a transitional movement from sitting to standing, or an ergonomic movement of bending to lift. Clinically, we are asking her not just to come from slouching to erect sitting, but to go beyond vertical to gain competence in a nonhabitual direction of movement. It is this ability to move equally well in both directions that allows a more appropriate neutral and balanced posture to emerge organically. Move equally in both directions to recalibrate neutral (Box 2.6).

In the case of the student with the simultaneously lordotic low back and kyphotic mid-back, we could arrange conditions in which we can globally extend the whole spine and then constrain thoracic flexion by use of a towel roll while tilting the pelvis posteriorly and flexing the lumbar spine (Fig. 2.11). Coming from a different direction, we could constrain lumbar extension by getting to end-range hip flexion and funnel movement primarily to the thoracic spine and ribcage (Fig. 2.12). Apply principles of pattern specificity, pattern reciprocity and change of venue, and be creative!

Functional context

We will now turn our attention to the third main characteristic of qualitative strengthening. Functional context refers to our ability to piggyback information or skills we'd like our student to have concerning posture, strength, flexibility, gross motor skill and proprioceptive acuity on to real-life movements, such as coming from Sit to Stand, or from hands and knees to

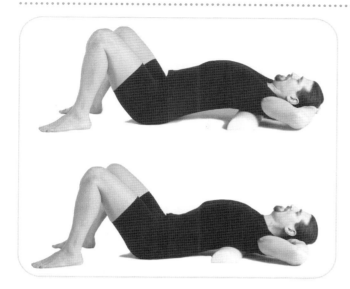

Fig. 2.11 Global extension segues into differentiated movement of lumbar flexion and thoracic extension.

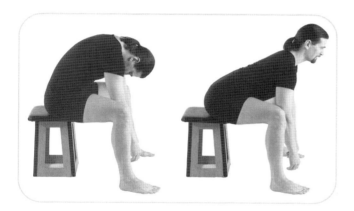

Fig. 2.12 Use lengthened hamstrings and other hip extensors to constrain pelvic anterior tilt – funnel extension movement to thoracic area.

supine. In general, it is these and similar transitional movements, other developmentally based movements and everyday movements of reaching, looking and walking, that are both our information delivery systems and our methods for stretching and strengthening individual muscles.

Consider for a moment why we move, why we tell our muscles to move our bones. We use our muscles mainly to *balance* ourselves in a gravity field, to *orient* all five exteroceptors, especially our eyes, to our surroundings, to *locomote*, to make *transitional movements*, to grasp and *manipulate*, to *communicate/express*, and for *vegetative* purposes. We rarely intend to extend our hip joints, rotate C6 to the left or move our scapula. We often, however, have the intention to stand (balance), to look to our left (orient) and to reach forward (manipulate).

We rarely intend to move our temporomandibular joint, but it often moves in coordination with moving our lips and tongue in talking (communication) and eating (vegetative). We rarely intend to weightbear through our glenohumeral joints, but may do so when getting up from the floor (transitional movements). We rarely intend to side-bend our torso, but may need to bend so as not to fall (balance). We rarely intend to move our ribs or contract our intercostals, but always have a strong desire to breathe (vegetative).

As newborn infants, we can't do much. Although there are infant reflexes present, intentional movement is not apparent very early on. As we develop, we learn to coordinate our eyes to see binocularly and to associate that desire to see with turning our heads. At some point, a baby will find itself rolling from supine to prone, not with the roll itself as the original intent but with the intention to see what is happening above her head (Fig. 2.13). With a strong curiosity about her environment she'll learn to lift her head higher, eventually learning to brace with her arms to get a better viewpoint (Fig. 2.14). Looking around 360° from here begins to trigger one leg to draw up as a precursor to a crawling movement (Fig. 2.15).

A desire to reach an object just out of her grasp might stimulate early locomotion as she straightens the leg that is cocked as a result of looking around. All this time she is learning to use her body, which muscles to contract and which to lengthen, how to listen to proprioceptive signals from her body and match them to outcome, and how to satisfy her need to negotiate a gravity field, grasp the object of her desire and bring it blissfully to her mouth. Throughout development this intimate meshing, this interweaving of intention, sensation, environment and action, is going on.[36–50]

Researchers in the field of ecological psychology study this weaving of environment, intension and action. Edward Reed has written an excellent book on the relationship of environmental affordances and motor behavior, called *Encountering the World: Toward an Ecological Psychology*.[51] Affordances are those things in the environment that have functional use: a lake to swim in, a ripe apple on a tree, a kitchen sink with nearby cup, a soft place to rest your head, a pathway through dense brush, etc.

These connections between intention, environment and action remain throughout our lives, and if we can tap into these associations of musculoskeletal organization and real-life intention, we'll have a powerful tool for helping correct many of the postural, arthrokinematic and gross motor mistakes that bring people in search of our services. Linking our exercise to functional context is what makes that exercise both informative and comprehensible to our CNS. Intentionally moving the eyes, hands, mouth and feet and linking them to whole-body patterns of movement is a common strategy in motor learning (Box 2.7).

Relearning movements first seen as part of the developmental sequence is another way of accessing forgotten skills and applying those skills to present-day and real-life activities that might have grown out of those previous steps. Breaking down a mature function such as walking, or throwing it into its constituent parts and building it back up again piece by piece, is another example of a motor learning strategy designed to qualitatively strengthen both whole-body patterns and individual

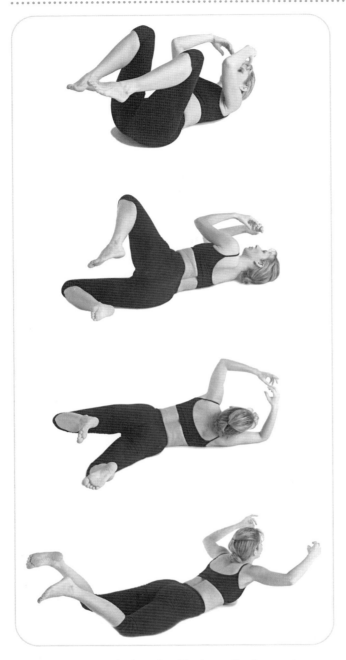

Fig. 2.13 Intension to look overhead leads to rolling from supine to prone.

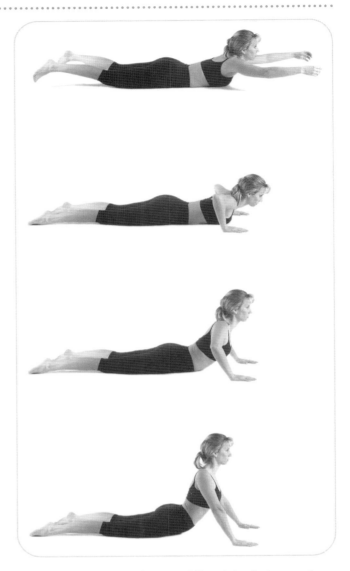

Fig. 2.14 Seeking a higher horizon – differentiating flexing arms from extending torso.

muscles. Functional context is both the information delivery system we use to help our students adopt and habituate into meaningful activity any new postural, gross motor or arthrokinematic skill, and the glue that makes it stick. Watch for examples of functional context when perusing subsequent movement lessons.

Box 2.7 Functional categories – why we use our muscles to move our bones
Balance – keeping your head off the ground
Orientation – gathering information about outside environment
Locomotion – getting from A to B
Transitions – changing positions
Manipulation – affecting your environment
Communication – speech and expression of emotion
Vegetative – breathe, eat and eliminate

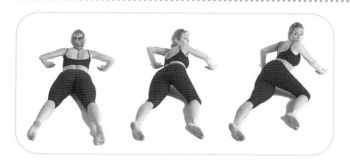

Fig. 2.15 Orientation along the horizon triggers initial stepping action of the lower extremities.

A new exercise paradigm

If, as we work with people, we acknowledge that much of our rationale for strengthening involves motor control, we need to ask ourselves about the efficacy of our strengthening exercises. What muscles do we want to strengthen, and when should those muscles be used? How do we want to teach this? Habituated motor patterns will often be unresponsive to cerebral arguments and an imitation and repetition style of teaching. Using visual information and scientific reasoning to teach proprioceptive skills and organic intelligence may be sporadically effective, but lacks subtlety, refinement and elegance.

With some modifications in how we use exercise to strengthen muscles, we can do a better job of positively influencing our students' movement. Elevating student self-awareness and enhancing proprioceptive acuity helps them become better problem-solvers, self-regulators and decision-makers. Pattern specificity helps with antagonist coordination, pattern recognition and incorporation of the affected part with the integrated whole. Functional context provides relevance, is consistent with how we learn developmentally, and is the glue that helps the CNS to functionalize exercise into real life.

Qualitative and quantitative stretching

We know a lot about connective tissue response to stretch. We know how far collagen fiber will deform, and when it will rupture if stretched too far. We know about the collagen tissue property of viscoelasticity, and know not to stretch too hard or too long to avoid microtrauma to collagen fibers. We know that most of the elasticity we see in connective tissue is due to interfiber gliding and the lubricants that makes this gliding possible, hyaluronic acid and glycoaminoglycans. We know the response of the tissue to immobilization, both with and without associated trauma. We know about the progression of scar formation, and when that scar becomes permanent. We know the effect of temperature on collagen extensibility.

This is language for describing quantitative stretching: objective and measurable. Quantitative stretching has many useful clinical implications for those who work with collagen, such as manual therapists and structural bodyworkers. This knowledge is crucial for physical therapists, athletic trainers and others working with people with injuries. But it is by no means the whole story in stretching. There are a few layers of the onion still missing.

Qualitative stretching is about changing the muscle spindle bias to a longer length: resetting the tripwire. It is about shutting off muscles that would otherwise interfere with movement in a desired direction: inhibition of antagonists. It is about general reduction of effort and muscle tone: relaxation and conservation of energy. It may include the simultaneous excitation of antagonists and the cooperative inhibition of appropriate synergists in function-specific whole-body patterns: it is integrative rather than isolationary.

Qualitative stretching requires a sense of purpose and an active proprioceptive awareness on the part of the student to make informed decisions on how and when to apply that added range of motion. Does this sound familiar? These characteristics are, in fact, eerily similar to those for qualitative strengthening. They are characteristics not of connective tissue but of neural firing patterns: brain electricity. As before, perhaps the main characteristics of qualitative stretching are proprioceptive self-awareness, pattern specificity and functional context. After a brief description of the muscle spindle, we will revisit these three characteristics within a conceptual framework of stretching.

The muscle spindle

What is it that keeps our joints from moving too far and dislocating? We could say that the ligaments and joint capsule fill that role, and we would be partially correct. Joint capsules and ligaments do check movement in certain directions, but should be the last line of defense against moving a joint too far. They provide static stability for a joint and help to guide the arthrokinematics of that joint, but shouldn't be relied on as the primary structures to stop a joint from moving too far – especially when movement forces are fast, explosive or repetitive. For example, when preparing to throw a baseball I will wind up by abducting and externally rotating my shoulder joint. This is a direction of movement that is commonly associated with glenohumeral dislocation; do I really want to trampoline my bones off my capsule and ligaments every time I throw? No!

Instead, I want to be able to decelerate and stop that movement into abduction/external rotation before banging into delicate connective tissue. I want my pectoralis major and subscapularis to catch the bone before it lands on my collagen. This is where the muscle spindle comes in. The role of the muscle spindle is to recognize the length of the muscle in which it is embedded and the physiological limit of the joint it crosses. It is a specialized type of muscle fiber that responds to stretch and then stimulates a contraction of its associated muscle group.[52–54] The classic example is the knee-jerk reflex. When the patellar tendon is tapped with a reflex hammer, a quick stretch is applied to the quadriceps muscle. Some of the various muscle spindles that are interspersed throughout the quadriceps are stretched, stimulating a reflex arc that results in a contraction of the quadriceps as a whole – the knee straightens. The CNS interprets the knee tap as a movement of the knee into flexion and as a lengthening of the quadriceps. This then stimulates the contraction of the muscle to prevent too much movement into knee flexion or too much stretch of the quadriceps.

This basic mechanism is present in slower or more controlled movements as well, with the muscle spindle responding to a stretch nearing the end range of the joint. The effect and the intention are the same as with the quick stretch, preventing the joint from moving too far and causing connective tissue strain, damage or frank dislocation. Think of the muscle spindle as a tripwire: the CNS sets the sensitivity of the spindle to respond to boundary violations of the bone.

What can go wrong with this mechanism? The CNS could set the muscle spindle too long, where the tripwire isn't triggered until the physiological limit of the joint has been violated. Knee hyperextension, either as an injury or as part of a habitual standing posture, is a classic example of this. Spinal joint instabilities, shoulder subluxations associated with strokes and foot pronation are further examples of the failure of dynamic stability. In these cases, not only do we have to strengthen the muscles that control the movement into unstable directions, we also have to train our students to recognize proprioceptively the physiological limits of the joints and to reset the muscle spindle tripwire to a shorter length.

The other mistake in relation to the muscle spindle is that of setting too short. In this situation, the tripwire is set to stimulate the stretch reflex well before the physiological limit of the joint is reached. We call this stiffness, hypomobility or muscle spasm. This is a very common occurrence in many clinical syndromes. Tight hamstrings, adductors, hip flexors, pectorals, scalenes and upper trapezius are the stuff of legend and all have short muscle spindles.

Spinal hypomobilities will have both a collagen component and a muscle spindle keeping a short leash on its muscle. The paradox comes in when we see tight muscles and try to stretch them. What we often end up doing is to stimulate a stretch reflex and stretch the muscle like a rubber band – whereupon it will quickly spring back to the length set by the muscle spindle and the CNS (Box 2.8).

In a very real sense, we can't stretch tight muscles. Muscle tissue, when separated from its various fascial envelopes, is loose and elastic. What makes a muscle tight is the fact that it is contracting (present tense, active verb). We can't stretch tight muscles, but we can reduce the level of contraction and reset the muscle spindle to a longer length that more accurately reflects the true physiological limit of the joint.

Stretching is really a motor skill that needs to be learned, and we as movement teachers need to know how to teach it better. How do we achieve a reduction of underlying muscle tone and get the CNS to recognize how to allow a muscle to lengthen past its preset length and not stimulate a stretch reflex? Stretch qualitatively: introduce elements of proprioceptive self-awareness, pattern specificity and functional context.

Proprioceptive self-awareness

Recall our need to pay attention to proprioceptive sensations when learning a motor skill. We want to be able to recognize and learn to duplicate those proprioceptive sensations that result in a desired outcome – a golf shot, a dive into a pool, or the allowance of more movement at a hypomobile joint. These proprioceptive sensations include the ability to discern joint position, direction and velocity of movement, relationship to gravity and muscle effort. It is this sense of muscle effort that is of particular interest to us in stretching.

Have you ever watched someone trying to stretch a muscle they are contracting at the same time? I see it all the time. Some people go too fast and stimulate a stretch reflex in the muscle they are trying to stretch. Some people try too hard and stretch too far, again stimulating a stretch reflex. Some people stretch into pain and stimulate an avoidance reflex. Some people anticipate pain moving into a certain direction, and will actively protect themselves. They are all contracting the muscle they are trying to stretch. What they need is an enhanced sense of effort recognition.

Effort recognition

I once had a student named John, a physician, who complained of having been stiff all his life – back, hamstrings, shoulders, you name it. The straw that finally broke this particular camel's back was the difficulty he was having swimming. His ankles were so stiff into plantarflexion that his feet didn't serve as good fins: he flailed with his legs and moved inefficiently through the water.

On observing John standing, sitting and lying, I noticed that he was always actively dorsiflexing his toes and ankles. The anterior tibialis tendon on both sides was the size and consistency of a rope, and his common toe extensor tendons bulged on the dorsum of his foot like piano wires. He was obviously working way too hard with his dorsiflexors. In standing, he habitually rocked his weight back on to his heels, creating the balance reaction of dorsiflexion.

Stand up and try it yourself right now – rock your weight back on your heels and notice the reaction in your toes and anterior tibialis tendon. His sitting organization was similar. He rolled his pelvis back on the seat, which necessitated the chronic contraction of his iliopsoas to hold him up. The synergistic relationships of the iliopsoas to the ankle and toe dorsiflexors through association with the stepping or withdrawal function was enough to create dorsiflexor hypertonus in this posture as well. Try it yourself to see if you have a similar association; sit well forward in a chair and roll your pelvis way back while rounding your spine – do your ankles or toes react by dorsiflexing? Be your own experiment for a minute!

Rather than succumb to my logical self's desire to perform myofascial release and stretch the bejeezus out of his anterior

---

Box 2.8 Muscle spindle – tripwire for the CNS

Antagonists should have well calibrated muscle spindles – allowing full physiological movement but not beyond

Muscle spindle set too short creates hypomobility

Muscle spindle set too long creates hypermobility

compartment muscles, I tried a different course of action. I started with proprioceptive awareness training of how he was standing and sitting, and had him exaggerate those backward-rocking tendencies to bring his attention to the consequences of those exaggerations. I had him deliberately increase the effort in the anterior compartment muscles to give him the opportunity to feel effort where, even though he is constantly doing it, he never felt it!

We did a few lessons on balance and orientation functions, helping him to better coordinate his pelvis, head and spine. We then did several lessons on accessing and balancing the pelvic power plant before even starting on his feet.

To have done otherwise would have run the risk that change in detail at the feet would be overwhelmed by the ponderous inertia of those more powerful systems. One day, when I thought he was ready, I taught him a lesson that made amazing changes in his feet.

I had him side-sit on the floor and play with his toes. I had him gently make circles with his toes by grasping and moving them with his fingers. I had him interlace his fingers and toes. I had him press the pad of his thumb and the pad of his big toe very gently against each other as if holding a butterfly's wing. I had him proceed by pressing his index finger and second toe, middle finger and toe and so on all gently against each other and slowly lifting away from each other. After having him do this sequence of movements on one side, I had him feel for differences throughout his two sides before going on to the other side. I finished with having him sit with the soles of his feet together and press corresponding toes into each other, before finally having him interlace his toes.

He just had a hoot with this lesson, and when he came to stand his anterior tibialis and toe dorsiflexors were relaxed and (for the first time in probably decades) his toes were on the floor with his weight naturally distributed more forward on his foot. His whole standing, sitting and walking organization had changed. He was ready, after having learned effort recognition specific to his feet and to specific functional contexts, to peel open a few more layers of the onion. It was here that we started some joint mobilization, myofascial work and functional movements into challenging plantarflexion movements, such as sitting back on his heels from hands and knees.

Language is a very powerful thing. When you define the problem in terms of muscles being tight, you define the solution to that problem as stretching. There are, however, other ways of defining the problem and other solutions. Early on, John had adopted these particular imbalanced postural (always falling backward) and movement patterns, which resulted in muscle imbalances (hyperactive anterior compartment and weak plantarflexors, as well as associative and compensatory hip and torso muscle imbalances) and structural imbalances (through selective adaptive shortening). Remember our layers – bone, joint, fascia, muscle and brain.

Beginning (appropriately enough) at the beginning, we started with the brain. In this lesson, we emphasized the sensorimotor skills of effort recognition and quality of control. He was able to use his fingers both to move his toes passively and to assess his degree of hypertonicity. He was able to contract his toe plantarflexors, and have either fingers or toes there as both a destination and a sounding board. How hard am I pressing, and how steady/controlled is that pressure? How does toe

control compare to finger control? The ankle plantarflexors were overflow stimulated by the activation of the toe flexors, and a degree of reciprocal inhibition occurred with his anterior tibialis.

Sitting and leaning forward to play with his toes allowed him to gain competence in a falling-forward direction and allowed for a more balanced standing posture afterwards. From brainwork, we made our way back through the fascial and joint layers. My question is this: if our students can't recognize inefficient effort in context-specific movement and lessen it, if they can't change the tripwire of muscle spindle bias to allow more normal osteokinematic and arthrokinematic movement, how long will the movement gains made through the release of myofascial or articular tissues by manual techniques last?

Effort reduction

Effort recognition is a necessary proprioceptive skill for learning to allow muscles to soften and lengthen when stretching and for resetting muscle spindle bias. Effort recognition is also a main ingredient in effort reduction, also known as relaxation. We have traditionally treated relaxation training separately from flexibility training or stretching, but they are really just different aspects of the same thing, a keen sense of muscle effort.

Relaxation has traditionally implied a reduction of muscle tone and a reduction in heart rate and blood pressure. Relaxation traditionally has been associated with certain breathing exercises, contract–relax techniques and associative imagery. Relaxation training is commonly taught when the student is lying supine or reclining in an overstuffed chair. The whole effect is to learn to do less while doing nothing. It runs the risk of being situation specific.

Someone can learn to relax just fine while in an easy chair listening to running water and bird sounds. They relax completely when on a beach on Maui sipping a Mai Tai. But they may have difficulty in applying those relaxation skills in the context of their daily lives. Traffic, work, deadlines, kids and spousal relations – this is when you really need these skills. Effort reduction does include this ability to completely let go, but can also be extended to include 'relaxing while doing.' Let me tell you a story to help illustrate this concept.

Dave was an endodontist who came to me with bilateral shoulder impingement syndromes, neck stiffness and tension headaches. He spent a lot of his day hunched over an open mouth with his arms held in abduction and internal rotation and his head thrust forward to peer inside his patients' orifice. This in itself is bad enough, but he also had a strong culturo-emotionally based torso flexion and upper extremity internal rotation pattern (Fig. 2.16). He held his belly in and rounded his back. He held his shoulders up and forward while sitting, standing and lying. He would breathe with his upper chest and raise his ribs using his neck muscles. He was one tense individual.

Upper trapezial bias led to lower trapezius weakness through reciprocal inhibition and habitual disuse. This resulted in poor control over upward scapular rotation and the superior orientation of the glenoid fossa. Abdominal and anterior intercostal bias robbed him of an ability to arch or extend his thoracic spine in another necessary auxiliary movement useful

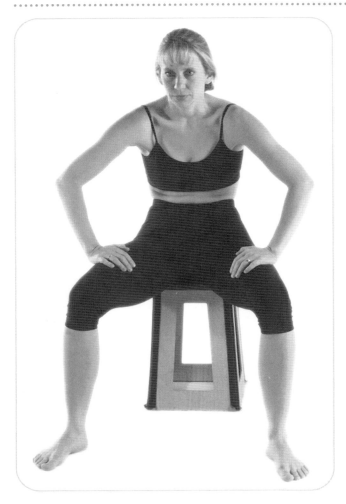

Fig. 2.16 Flexion/internal rotation combination – what is she afraid of?

in reducing glenohumeral impingement. Chronic abdominal muscle contractions disallowed full use of his diaphragm and necessitated upper chest breathing and suboccipital tension and compression.

He had tried neck, shoulder girdle and pectoralis stretches. He had tried rotator cuff strengthening with weights and rubber tubing. He had tried relaxation training and biofeedback machines, and could even relax and lower his biofeedback readings with techniques he had learned. What he could not do was to 'relax while doing.' In his work as an endodontist – and really in the context of all functions involving the use of his arms out in front of him – he had associated those upper extremity reaching functions with upper trapezius and abdominal muscle contraction. This is a fairly common pattern and will be addressed in more depth in Section 4. We'll also look at anxiety patterns in more depth in Section 5.

Let's just say for now that the hypertonicity of the upper trapezius, abdominals and anterior intercostal muscles was woven into patterns of movement associated with both emotional holding patterns/expressive functions and upper extremity reaching functions. To relax, he had to learn to move

his arms without associative belly and upper trapezius involvement. To do this, he had to learn to relax. He was in a Catch-22 situation.

As long as he was unable to recognize similar patterns of effort in different functional contexts, he was doomed to repeat them both. We went through a learning process that helped him make the necessary connections between intention and specific muscle relaxation, both in resting and while doing. He learned this not by just performing his habitual pattern, but by selecting another pattern of movement and another pattern of muscle recruitment as a clearly preferable alternative that worked better for him, both in resting and when doing. Relaxation training is part of qualitative stretching.

Implications of effort reduction

Effort reduction has implications for biomechanical efficiency not only when working with somatic symptom-producing postural and movement patterns, but also in performance enhancement situations. Effort reduction implies a conservation of energy; it reduces unnecessary or parasitic muscle effort to leave more gas in the tank in endurance events. Effort reduction implies an ability to selectively inhibit the muscles you need to move your bones in a certain direction while powerfully or even explosively using other muscles to perform that movement, a reduction of contradictory or oppositional muscle effort to produce the flexibility of the gymnast.

Effort reduction can sometimes be a hard sell in the land where hard bodies and high tone are presented as functional ideals, where the washboard stomach is considered highly aesthetic. The attempt, however, is worthwhile. When presented with the choices and asked to make a decision on preference, most people will choose comfort, biomechanical efficiency and effort reduction over artificially high tone maintained as a cultural artifact. Give them a choice and let them decide!

Finally, effort reduction is a useful skill to develop for proprioceptive self-awareness purposes. The ability to perceive changes in a sensation is proportional to the strength of that sensation. The Weber–Fechner Principle proposes: 'the principle that gradations of stimulus strength are discriminated approximately in proportion to the logarithm of stimulus strength. It emphasizes that the greater the background sensory intensity, the greater also must be the additional change in stimulus strength in order for the mind to detect the change.'[53] Visually speaking, the brighter the sun, the more difficult it is to see a firefly. The louder the orchestra, the harder it is to hear someone sniffling four rows away.

Proprioceptively, this means the harder you try the less you can feel. More muscle effort equals diminished ability to feel subtle proprioceptive signals, such as muscle effort. If you place a one-pound weight in your hand with your eyes closed and then place another one pound on top of the first, you will certainly be able to tell the difference. If you place 50 pounds in one hand and add that same extra pound, it will be unlikely that you will be able to perceive it. When working with students on stretching, go slowly and gently so they have the opportunity to recognize effort when it comes (Box 2.9).

Stop at that point and continue further into the range once successful effort reduction and muscle spindle recalibration

Box 2.9 The Weber–Fechner principle

'The greater the background sensory intensity, the greater also must
   be the additional change in stimulus strength in order for the
   mind to detect the change'

Reduce effort to enhance proprioceptive acuity – not maximum
   contractions to elicit temporary reflex relaxation

Effort recognition and pattern recognition skills taught by
   progressively finer discrimination of ever more subtle changes

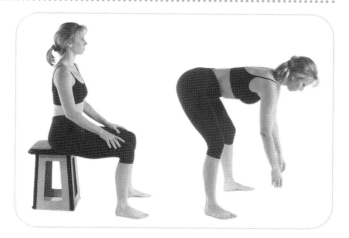

Fig. 2.18 Similar nonhabitual patterns need to be taught throughout different functions.

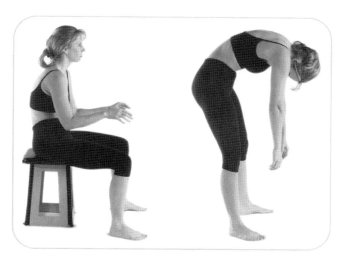

Fig. 2.17 Similar habituated patterns occur throughout different functions.

have been achieved. When working with students on relaxation using contract/relax ideas, have them do the minimal contraction that they can perceive rather than the strongest contraction they can squeeze out. Doing smaller contractions can train them to feel for subtleties and to find levels of relaxation they didn't think were possible. When teaching, go slow, go small and go gently if you want your students to have the proprioceptive acuity necessary to stretch qualitatively and relax while doing.

Pattern specificity example 1

Let's look again at global and differentiated patterns of movement, this time within a framework of stretching. We will again illustrate these differences with some examples.

Cliff was a forestry worker who went to see a colleague of mine several years back. He complained of bilateral lumbosacral pain of sudden onset soon after he had been digging holes and planting seedlings at work. The pain persisted even after taking time off work, and was particularly aggravated by bending, lifting and sitting. When I observed Cliff in standing, I noticed how posteriorly rotated his pelvis was. On sitting, he rolled his pelvis back on the seat and rounded his back (Fig. 2.17). On bending, he flexed very well through his whole back but had very little hip joint flexion (Fig. 2.17).

My colleague had picked up on the tight hamstrings, gluteals, piriformis and other hip external rotators that were preventing Cliff from moving his pelvis into anterior tilt. This lack of anterior tilting movement constrained his ability both to sit erect and to forward-bend with a neutral back (Fig. 2.18). For Cliff, the consequence of this lack of hip hinge was too much movement at the lumbosacral junction into flexion. We could reasonably surmise capsular and ligament overstretching or disc derangement as the possible outcome of this particular habitual muscle imbalance combined with this particular occupation.

My colleague applied myofascial work and exercises with Cliff. He did strengthening exercises for his back and stretching exercises for his hamstrings, hip extensors and rotators. She instructed him on proper sitting posture and correct bending ergonomics. Cliff didn't get much better. Every time I saw him in the waiting room he was sitting slumped, looking at a magazine in his lap.

Whenever I saw him bend over to pick up his shoe or to get a hand-weight when the movement wasn't part of his exercise routine, he would revert to his old habit and bend mostly at the lumbosacral junction. You can bet he was still bending the same way at home, and would have resumed that same thing when he did go back to work. For Cliff, the exercises (which he performed diligently and well) were not translating into use in the real-life functions where the damage was occurring.

Part of the problem with his exercise was lack of pattern specificity. When stretching his hamstrings, for instance, he would stand, put one heel up on something and reach toward that foot with both hands. Alternatively, he would sit on the floor with one leg bent in front and one leg long out in front, again reaching with both hands toward his foot (Fig. 2.19). He feels a stretch in his hamstrings. Why aren't they getting longer when he needs them to?

Because he was practicing a global pattern of movement – hip flexion with back flexion. By the time he felt a stretch in his hamstrings, he was already past the normal physiological range of the lumbosacral junction into flexion. With the intention of reaching his feet, his CNS selected the path of least

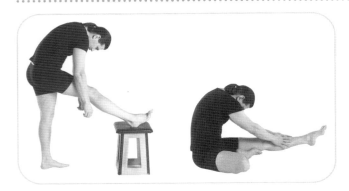

Fig. 2.19 Similar stretching mistakes in different positions – global patterns of hip and back flexion.

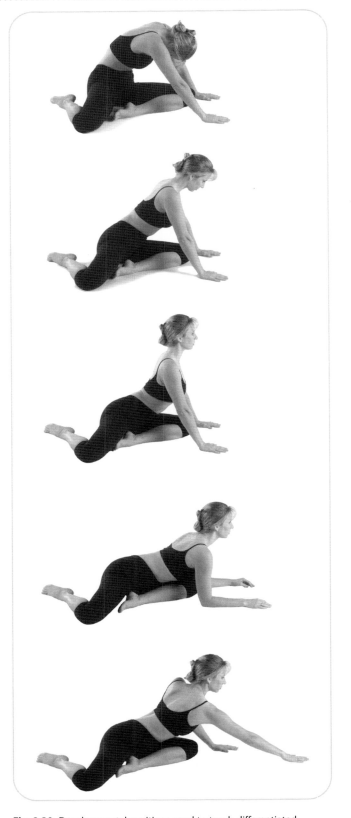

resistance, the tried and true, the old familiar – and flexed first and most at his low back. Cliff needed to learn how to do differentiated patterns of movement – hip flexion with back extension.

Cliff might have performed better by starting in a side-sitting position and simply looking up and down. Describing for him what to feel for and giving him suggestions on what to try, we could have led him to coordinate his whole body with those neck and eye movements so that his whole torso alternately arched and rounded and his pelvis rolled forward and back on the floor.

Looking up, arching his back and rolling his pelvis forward go together; this differentiated pattern features back extension with hip flexion. Looking down, rounding the back and rolling the pelvis back go together; this differentiated pattern features back flexion with hip extension (Fig. 2.20). This is another example of what we saw in the strengthening scenarios, reciprocating differentiated patterns.

We could have changed the venue by having him do the same movements in side-sitting and leaning on his elbows, or by introducing a different intention and having him slide or reach a hand forward on the floor (Fig. 2.20). We could have extended the same basic movement by turning it into a transitional movement up to hands and knees. We could have brought him up to a chair and taught him essentially the same sequence of movements, this time culminating in a transitional movement coming up to stand.

Bending to reach the ground with either one or two hands and coming to sitting erect are within the same family of differentiated patterns – hip flexion and back extension. So too are sitting movements of looking up and these described transitional movements to hands and knees and standing. They all require differentiated patterns of movement, emphasizing hip flexion and back extension. We would probably have worked initially on hip flexion with the knee bent so that Cliff could first recognize the pattern. We would then have added in a straighter knee in sitting and standing, but with continued awareness of moving within that same differentiated pattern.

For those functions where he created damage to his back (sit, bend, lift), stretching the hamstrings with a bent knee

Fig. 2.20 Developmental positions used to teach differentiated pattern specificity – progressions to get lower.

is more functionally relevant. We could have progressed Cliff roughly through a developmental sequence using reciprocal differentiated patterns of movement, proprioceptive acuity and pattern recognition training and change of venue concepts, all linked to a variety of functional contexts. This not only stretches the muscle but, more important functionally, it stretches the pattern.

Pattern specificity example 2

Take a hypothetical situation of someone who comes to us with left-sided neck and shoulder girdle tension and aching. We assess her structurally and notice that her left shoulder girdle is elevated in comparison to the right (Fig. 2.21). We assess her range of motion and notice a decrease in range in right cervical side bending, with a subjective feeling of tightness along the left neck and upper shoulder girdle.

We palpate musculature and notice tightness, elicit tenderness, and note myofascial restrictions along the left scalenes, upper trapezius and levator scapulae. We assess joint play and note cervical facet capsular restrictions into right side bending. We mobilize, we release fascia, we prescribe stretching exercises for the scalenes, trapezii and left levator. This is a very logical approach, but still misses something.

Why is her left shoulder girdle elevated? It is probably not only because of a hyperactive upper trapezius. We might want to step back to look at the forest for a moment to see if some whole-body pattern of movement may be part of the mix. It is unlikely that we will see an elevated left shoulder girdle on a perfectly symmetrical torso. We could assess the angle of the sternum relative to vertical, and will probably (though by no means always) see the bottom of the sternum angled off to the left.

The whole torso/ribcage will probably be bent in some fashion to the right. We could observe for subtle differences in weight distribution in sitting and standing, and might find her weight biased toward her left side. Take a closer look at Figure 2.21. See if you can pick out some of these details and recognize that the details reflect the big picture.

Think first of balance reactions. Hold a baby up by its pelvis in vertical, then start to tilt the baby from side to side. As you tilt to the right the baby will make a compensatory balance adjustment to side-bend in a C-curve back to the left – tilt to the left, side-bend to the right. When sitting or standing vertically, we all have some degree of weightbearing bias. If we habitually put more weight on our left ischial tuberosity in sitting, or on our left foot in standing, this unlevels the pelvic base and necessitates a compensatory side-bending movement of the spine and ribcage, in this case to the right. If we continue this C-curving movement all the way through our spine, we will end up with our head cocked to the right as in the example of the baby; this is a global pattern of movement throughout the whole spine. The head and neck are moving as an extension of the torso. However, this is not how we typically organize ourselves.

What we really do is to bring our head to vertical to orient the eyes and ears along a horizontal axis. This is a differentiated pattern of movement – the right torso side-bending with left cervical side-bending that we saw in Figure

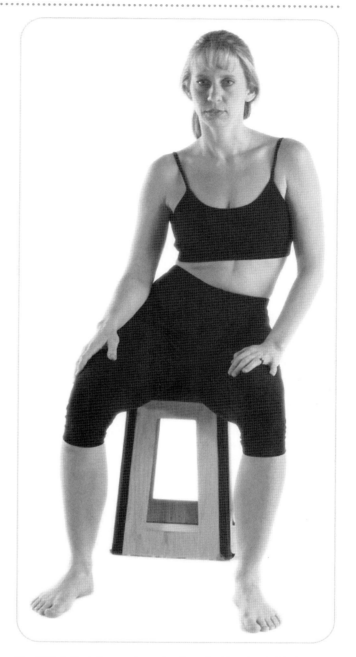

Fig. 2.21 Is the left upper trapezius the only thing that holds that shoulder up?

2.21. The pattern is driven by two functional necessities: an equilibrium or balance reaction to an unbalanced pelvis creates the torso side-bend, and the functional need to orient to the horizon creates the differentiation of the head and neck.

We could stretch the scalenes, upper trapezius and levator on the left. We could stretch the latissimus dorsi and lower trapezius on the right. We could stretch the right torso inter-

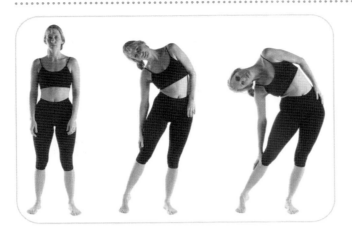

Fig. 2.22 Weight shift to the left and side bend to the right – head moves globally with torso.

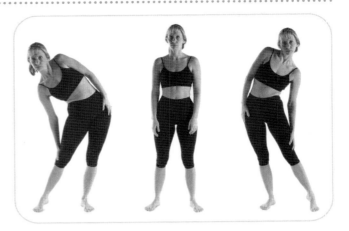

Fig. 2.23 Same movement but with differentiation of head and neck from torso.

costals, quadratus lumborum and lateral abdominals. We could stretch the right gluteus medius and the left adductor. We could strengthen the left intercostals, latissimus dorsi, lower trapezius and left-sided back and belly. We could strengthen the right adductor and iliopsoas and the left gluteus medius and maximus.

All of these muscles and their fascia are imbalanced in this scenario. They all contribute to the elevated left shoulder girdle, the local muscle tightness and the manifestation of pain for our student. We could send her home with 17 different exercises and hope her CNS can make some sense out of it, or we could do some motor learning lessons.

We might start with her standing with her feet about shoulder-width apart and have her slide her right hand down the outside of her right thigh in the direction of her foot. We might encourage a weight-shifting component by having her lift her right heel as she does this (Fig. 2.22). We would encourage a full weight-shift to the left along with a full C-curve bend to her right, including her head and neck.

We would then go to the other side to compare and contrast these two global movement patterns (we might even predict that she might have more difficulty with range or coordination of movement into left side-bending and right weight-shifting). We could continue the same global movements in both positions with a variation: we could have her head stay vertical by keeping her eyes horizontal and on the horizon (Fig. 2.23).

These are now reciprocating differentiated movement patterns built around the functions of balance, orientation and reaching/manipulation. Pay particular attention to the movement into right-side weightbearing, left torso side-bending, and differentiation of the head and neck into right-side bending. These are nonhabitual differentiated patterns and are mirror images of the habitual pattern that contributes to her problems. We could teach this movement as home exercises in standing, lying and sitting, and direct her specifically to find and use that nonhabitual differentiated pattern, not only in posture but also in some common, daily

functional context such as walking with shoulder girdle participation.

Functional context

Recall in the section on strengthening the question of why we move and why we tell our muscles to let our bones move through their whole physiological range. Again, we use our muscles mainly to *balance* ourselves in a gravity field, to *orient* especially our eyes to our surroundings, to *locomote*, to *transition*, to grasp and *manipulate*, to *communicate*, and for *vegetative* functions. Movement lessons around these functions are our information delivery systems and the glue that makes it stick in our CNS. Linking exercise to function is what makes our stretching and strengthening exercises relevant.

Motor learning lessons regarding creeping, crawling, reaching, eating, breathing, rolling, lifting the head to look from prone, transitional movements and balancing encourage dynamic, multiplanar neurological lengthening of chronically contracting muscles, rather than static, uniplanar tugging on a swathe of connective tissue.

A teaching strategy for stretching involves initial neurological lengthening or inhibition of muscles in relatively easy functional contexts to allow for success and pattern recognition. We then gradually apply constraints to place ever more demand on the CNS to inhibit the contraction of those muscles that are getting in the way. This also gradually imposes a demand on the collagen component. We then have the person use that specific pattern, applied to a specific function and used commonly in daily activities, to gradually stimulate connective tissue remodeling. In physical therapy school, we called this the SAID Principle: Specific Adaptation to Imposed Demand.

We impose a functional demand (a constraint) on the muscle spindle to lengthen and on the tight intra- and extra-articular fascia to remodel, hydrate and allow more movement. We might have someone stretch their hamstrings in the context of picking up their shoes, reaching into their refrigerators, loading their dishwasher and other bending-to-reach functions.

We might have someone stretch their iliopsoas while standing, half-kneeling, walking, balancing on one foot and other pushing-against-the-ground functions. We might have someone stretch their piriformis by getting up and down from the floor, getting up from sitting, getting out of bed and other transitional functions. We impose a new demand on muscle and connective tissue by incorporating specific patterns into daily function, as in these examples, or by teaching a 'new' function.

Get them on the floor

The 'new' function we teach to impose demand on muscle and connective tissues is really just old functions that have been forgotten. We ask them to spend more time on the floor: no chairs, no shoes and no props. We might ask someone to side-sit or tailor-sit on the floor while watching TV or having conversation. Long sitting and leaning on hands, sole-sitting or sitting on the heels could also be used.

Side-sitting or coming on to hands and knees while reading a book or newspaper might be suggested. Prone-prop side-lying with head propped on hand, or side-lying propped up on an elbow are other possibilities. We might have them kneel or half-kneel at a computer or at the breakfast table. These positions not only hold stretching possibilities in themselves, but also require transitional movements. Transitional movements include standing to kneeling, sitting to lying, hands and knees to sitting, belly to side or back to standing.

These positions and transitional movements will be familiar to anyone who has watched children at play. Young children spend a great deal more time on the floor and exhibit a great deal more variety and complexity in their everyday movements than the typical adult does. With a deferential nod to physiology as a factor in the gradual stiffening of the average person with age, I believe that it is invariance that is the main culprit in accelerating this slow slide into decrepitude. We don't spend enough time playing or otherwise functioning on the floor or on natural surfaces.

We no longer put ourselves in the position to move like we did as children. It's no wonder few of us can still move that way. We spend too much time sitting and walking on flat, homogeneous surfaces. Our conveniences are stiffening us. Cars have replaced walking. Washing machines have replaced hand-washing clothes and hanging them to dry. Oil heats our homes, so we don't have to chop wood. Water comes from taps instead of being hauled up from the river, winched up from a well and carried home by a yoke on our backs. We walk on sidewalks and stairs instead of dirt paths and variable slopes. The good old days? Hmmm – maybe not.

We already substitute working out at the gym for the volume and intensity of movement missing in our daily lives in comparison to those of our human ancestors and their animal relatives. We could also substitute relearning to be comfortable being on and moving around the floor for some of the missing variety and complexity of movement in our daily lives. We could take a yoga or a Feldenkrais class, learn tai chi or other martial arts and practice at home. We need to get off our collective duffs and use our bodies both qualitatively and quantitatively.

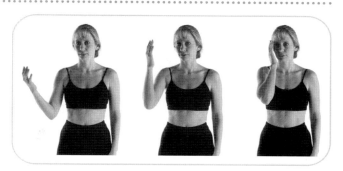

Fig. 2.24 How does your hand know when to stop?

Reciprocation of antagonists

Try the following simple experiment. Close your eyes and move the palm of your right hand toward the right side of your face as if you were going to cup it (Fig. 2.24). Don't actually touch your face but come as close as possible. Do it a few times slowly then do it quickly, still with your eyes closed. Move your hand quickly toward your face as if you were going to slap yourself, but again stop just short; how close did your hand get to your face? Repeat the movement quickly a few times and see how accurate the movement is. How close do you come to touching without actually making contact? Most of you will find that you have a very accurate ability to stop just short of contact, both when moving slowly and when moving quickly. How is this possible with your eyes closed?

Proprioception is the ability to know where one bone is in relation to another. Your hand has traveled that path to your face many times in your life and you have the route, time and distance down pat in your CNS. You know how to contract your biceps and when to stop it. You know precisely when to deploy the parachute and hit the brakes: your triceps fires to decelerate and stop elbow flexion.

If you whack yourself in the face with this movement, does that mean that your elbow is hypermobile? If your hand always ends up well away from your face, does that mean that your elbow is hypomobile? In some respects, yes! Both hyper- and hypomobilities are manifestations of an inability of the CNS to recognize where one bone is in relation to another. Both rigidity and instability can result from this incoordination of antagonists.

Schematic of antagonist relationships

Let's look at a schematic representation of antagonist coordination. Say we have a wide ring or doughnut-shaped disc suspended horizontally by strings (Fig. 2.25). A wooden post is placed vertically in the exact center of the ring. The ring represents the bone, the strings are two antagonistic muscles, and the post represents the end of the normal physiological range of motion for that joint.

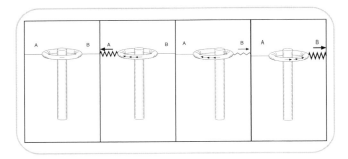

Fig. 2.25 Schematic representation of normal coordination of antagonists – reciprocal inhibition.

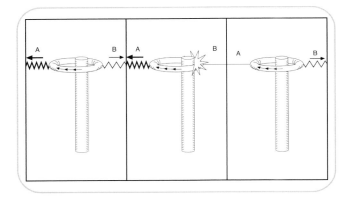

Fig. 2.26 Schematic representation of co-contractions – hypermobilities and hypomobilities.

Muscle A is the agonist that contracts to pull the disc leftward on the page and Muscle B is the antagonist that lengthens to accommodate the movement. In a well organized system excitation of Muscle A inhibits Muscle B (Fig. 2.25). This is called reciprocal inhibition. Muscle A keeps contracting until the edge of the disc approaches the post, then stops contracting as Muscle B fires to decelerate and stop the ring from striking the post (Fig. 2.25). Muscle B then becomes the agonist and contracts to pull the ring to the right on the page, while Muscle A is now antagonistic and needs to be inhibited and lengthened to accommodate the movement in this direction (Fig. 2.25). This is how things should work. The antagonists work cooperatively in this schematic to move the bone fully within its physiological limits, but not beyond it.

Let's say now that Muscle A really prefers the on-switch to the off-switch, and it doesn't stop contracting when the disc nears the post. Because Muscle A likes the on-switch, this means that Muscle B will habitually hit the off-switch (aided by reciprocal inhibition) and may be slow or completely negligent in decelerating the ring. We get a train wreck as the bone violates its physiological limit (Fig. 2.26). Ligaments stretch and are damaged. Joint capsules strain to contain the runaway bone. Joint surfaces collide and cartilage is mashed. We call this joint hypermobility or instability.

Taken to extremes, we get joint subluxation or even dislocation. Whoever is in charge of the on- and off-switches is not paying attention. If we make Muscle B lift weights to get stronger, will that stop movement past the physiological limit? Maybe – but Muscle B also needs directions on when to apply that strength, and Muscle A needs directions on when to stop pulling. For that to happen, someone needs to be cognizant of where one bone is in relation to another. Antagonists need to be coordinated by the CNS.

Say that Muscle A fires to pull the ring leftward on the page but stops firing before the ring gets to the post. At the same time, Muscle B kicks in prematurely and actively stops the movement of the ring at the same time as Muscle A stops working (Fig. 2.26). This we call hypomobility. The results of this scenario could include eventual capsular, ligamentous and myofascial remodeling as these tissues shorten to accommodate the truncated range of movement.

Joint surface lubrication through synovial fluid production and distribution might be affected, with long-term consequences on the health of the cartilage. The lack of movement at this joint may necessitate the overuse of another joint and contribute to instabilities and train wrecks both proximal to and distal to the hypomobile site. If we stretch Muscle B, will that restore full mobility of the joint? Maybe – but Muscle B also needs instructions on allowing movement past its current muscle spindle tripwire point, and Muscle A needs instructions on shortening more completely. For that to happen, someone needs to be aware of where one bone is in relation to another. Antagonists need to be coordinated by the CNS.

Let's say now that Muscle A receives instructions to pull the bone leftward on the page but that Muscle B didn't receive the order to allow that leftward movement to happen (Fig. 2.26). Muscle A not only has to drag the bone to the left on the page, but has to do it while Muscle B is trying to pull the bone back to the right. We call this a co-contraction. One muscle has to work much harder than it would normally to move the bone. Adequate reciprocal inhibition is not present. This scenario might result in a general squeeze of the tissues: joints compress, tendons are strained, fascia thickens and blood supply is compromised. Energy is expended working against yourself: you are driving with the brakes on! Again, antagonists need to be coordinated by the CNS.

Changing the schematic a little, we could now orient the ring vertically and the post horizontally. Muscle A now performs a shortening or concentric contraction to move the ring upward, then a lengthening or eccentric contraction to lower the ring back down in a controlled way. Muscle B still needs to cooperate by paying out the line (Fig. 2.27) as Muscle A shortens, and by reeling in the slack as gravity pulls the ring back down and Muscle A performs an eccentric contraction (Fig. 2.27; Box 2.10).

Just as in our horizontal orientation schematic, this new orientation can still be plagued by hypomobilities, hypermobilities and co-contraction problems. The antagonists need to be coordinated by the CNS. This scenario illustrates the need to work in both vertical and horizontal orientations when stretching, strengthening, stabilizing or otherwise coordinating the antagonists. We will now flesh out these schematics a little with some clinical examples illustrating the advantages of reciprocal movements.

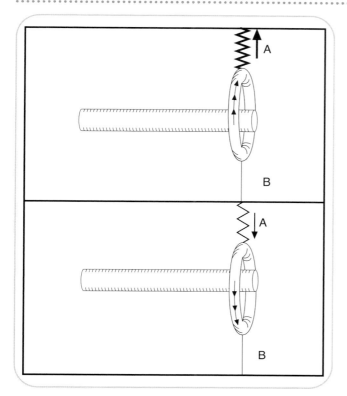

Fig. 2.27 Representation of change in relationship to gravity – muscle 'on top' does lengthening and shortening contractions to control the ring.

Box 2.10 Coordinating the antagonists
Hypermobilities – agonist doesn't stop contracting and antagonist doesn't kick in
Hypomobilities – agonist doesn't finish the job and antagonist kicks in too soon
Co-contractions – antagonist never fully inhibited when agonist working
Stretch and strengthen simultaneously – and in pattern-specific and functionally relevant ways while you are at it

Reciprocity examples

When prescribing exercises for muscle or structural imbalances, the approach most often taken is the obvious and logical one: stretch the tight muscle and strengthen the weak one. For instance, when working with someone who flexes too much in their lower back when bending, we may want to stretch the hamstrings and strengthen the back extensors. When working with someone who tends toward excessive anterior pelvic tilt in standing, we will probably give exercises to stretch the hip flexors and other exercises to strengthen the hip extensors.

The logic is sound, but a question arises: do we stretch first or strengthen first? Let's look at a couple of our clinical examples within a framework of some commonly used movement lessons: Pelvic Tilts and Half-kneel Bending. Both of these

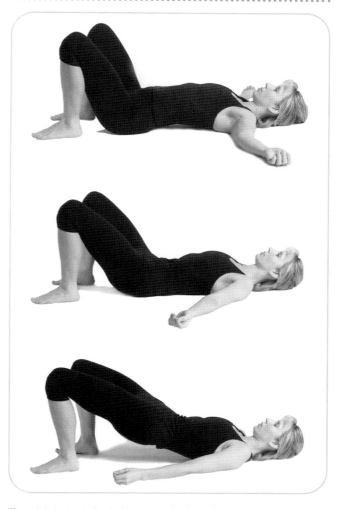

Fig. 2.28 Going in both directions of pelvic tilt – reciprocating movements train antagonist balance and cooperation.

lessons feature reciprocating movements, but in differing orientations.

With Pelvic Tilts, we will start both of our students (too much flexion on bending and too much extension on standing) on their backs with their knees bent. They will then alternately roll their pelvis up and down on the floor. This results in an alternate flexing and extending of the lower spine. We will direct them to use their legs in accomplishing this movement – pushing the feet into the floor with the gluteal group to posteriorly rotate the pelvis and flex the lower back, and lightening the feet from the floor with the iliopsoas group to anteriorly rotate the pelvis and arch the lower back (Fig. 2.28).

The supine position is a neutral one in terms of the pelvis and its relationship to gravity: the gluteals do a shortening contraction to flex the back and the iliopsoas does a shortening contraction to arch the back in an organization reminiscent of our schematic with the horizontal ring. Recall also in our schematic how, with reciprocal inhibition, we also get an inhibition or stretching of the antagonists: gluteal contraction inhibits the iliopsoas, and vice versa.

The movement into posterior pelvis tilt/hip extension and back flexion is the nonhabitual differentiated pattern needed by the person with the hyperlordotic standing posture. The movement into anterior pelvic tilt/hip flexion and back extension is the nonhabitual differentiated pattern needed by the person who over-flexes in the lumbar spine when bending or sitting.

Why not just go in the direction most needed by each of these individuals? One reason to go in both directions with both of our students is for pattern recognition purposes. We tend to focus with these students on movements of the back, but it is really the relationship of the back to the pelvis and legs that is often the primary problem in both cases. Going in both directions helps our students feel these differentiated patterns of movement and helps to enhance for them an awareness of the relationship of their legs to their back.

Your students can better recognize their direction of ease/familiarity and their direction of difficulty/unfamiliarity and make comparisons. They may even recognize that moving into their habitual direction recreates their pain, even though (or maybe because) it is the path of least resistance. This information can be invaluable to our students – most of them wouldn't have known this about themselves before starting this lesson.

With respect to postural training, when we get proprioceptive recognition of oppositional (but cooperative) movement patterns, an accurately calibrated home or neutral posture can be more easily found, recognized and reproduced volitionally. We could think of neutral posture as being that place where you could as easily fall in any direction. As an example, reciprocating movements of falling forward and back while sitting on a chair contain the sort of information needed by the CNS to find that neutral or balanced posture. It is this ability to move equally well in each direction that allows a more effortless and balanced posture to emerge organically.

Another reason for going in both directions is to assist in coordinating the antagonists. As the gluteals and iliopsoas play off against each other in this cooperative tug-of-war, the CNS learns to more accurately inhibit the antagonist to allow smoother and easier movement and learns to recognize physiological limits. Movement approaching end-range can also stimulate a stretch reflex or a spring-loading effect on the antagonist and makes the subsequent contraction more powerful. This is another way the antagonists work cooperatively. As the iliopsoas contracts to pull the pelvis into anterior tilt and as it approaches its fully shortened length, it stretches the gluteal muscle spindles and stimulates them to contract.

This results in a pushing of the pelvis back into posterior tilt. Then the hip extensors are fully shortened and the hip flexors are reflexly stimulated to contract in their turn. Going in both directions helps the CNS orchestrate the antagonists and helps to apply that newfound coordination to hypermobility, hypomobility and co-contraction problems. As this supine position is neutral in terms of gravity, the agonists are both working against gravity with shortening contractions as the antagonists are inhibited and lengthen. We will look at other positions/orientations now to get a further perspective on antagonist coordination.

As a continuation of our pelvic tilt lesson, we can bring our students up to sitting on the floor, having them place their

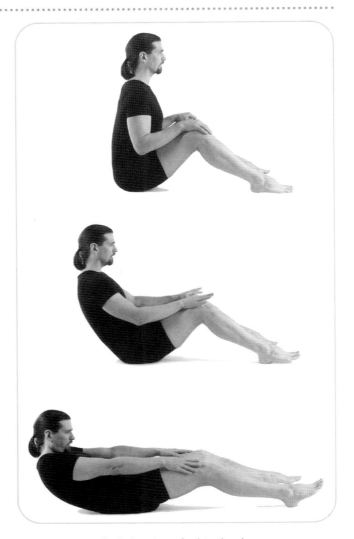

Fig. 2.29 Going in both directions of pelvic tilt – the same reciprocating movement but harder.

hands on their thighs near their knees and alternately rolling their pelvis forward and back (Fig. 2.29). Coming forward is a shortening contraction or a strengthening of the iliopsoas and back extensors, along with a simultaneous inhibition or stretching of the hamstrings, gluteals, other deep posterior hip external rotators and the abdominals. This direction could be especially beneficial for the person who flexes too much at the lumbar spine when bending and sitting.

Rather than separate exercises for stretching the hamstrings, gluteals, etc. and separate exercises for strengthening the iliopsoas and back extensors, we can do them all simultaneously and, in doing so, greatly enhance the likelihood of influencing their particular damaging motor behavior. Taken a step further to incorporate functional imbalances, we are training our students here to pull forward toward a more erect sitting posture, simulating the balancing function that gives them so much difficulty.

Coming back toward lying is a lengthening contraction of the iliopsoas, a shortening contraction of the abdominals and an inhibition of the back extensors. This direction could be especially beneficial for those who hyperlordose and anteriorly tilt their pelvis in standing. Rather than separate exercises to stretch the iliopsoas and the back extensors and strengthen the belly (but not the gluteals in this scenario), we can do them all simultaneously and in doing so greatly enhance the likelihood of influencing their particular damaging motor behavior.

Taken a step further to incorporate functional imbalances, we are training our students here to allow their pelvis to fall backward, simulating a direction of movement they have such difficulty with in standing (where they allow their pelvis to fall too far forward). This is a belly-up orientation that emphasizes the reciprocity between a shortening contraction of the iliopsoas and a lengthening of the iliopsoas. Even though it emphasizes one muscle group, it is still a coordination of antagonistic directions of movement.

This scenario is much like the schematic of the vertical ring and the horizontal post. The iliopsoas is the muscle on top and provides power to control both the fall backward and the return to a higher center of mass. The gluteals are the muscles on the bottom and serve to pay out the line and to reel in the slack. This reciprocating movement is useful for both of our students.

Our hyperlordotic person is helped by strengthening the abdominals and lengthening the iliopsoas (falling back); our hyperflexing person is helped by strengthening the iliopsoas and back extensors and stretching the hamstrings and gluteals (pulling center of mass back up). We could vary this basic movement by different placements of the hands, the introduction of diagonal directions, or by changing speed or intention – more on this later.

Changing orientation to gravity

Let's look now at our two hypothetical students in a belly-down orientation. In a variation of Half-kneel Bending, we could start both of our students in a three-and-a-half point stance and have them alternately round and arch their back, with the intention to look down and up as a functional context (Fig. 2.30). Arching requires a lengthening contraction of the gluteals and hamstrings, inhibition of the abdominals and a shortening contraction of the back extensors. This direction would be especially useful for our person who bends with too much lumbar flexion.

Again, we are simultaneously stretching and strengthening that which needs to be stretched and strengthened, rather than going about balancing these muscle groups piecemeal or sequentially. Rounding the back requires a shortening contraction of the hamstrings, gluteals and abdominals, and inhibition of the iliopsoas and back extensors. This direction would be especially useful for our hyperlordotic stander. This is again performed simultaneously and with integration, rather than sequentially and in isolation. This belly-down orientation emphasizes the shortening and lengthening contraction of the gluteals and hamstrings – and even though it emphasizes one muscle group, it is still a coordination of antagonistic directions of movement.

This is again like our vertically oriented ring schematic, but this time with the gluteals on top and the iliopsoas on the

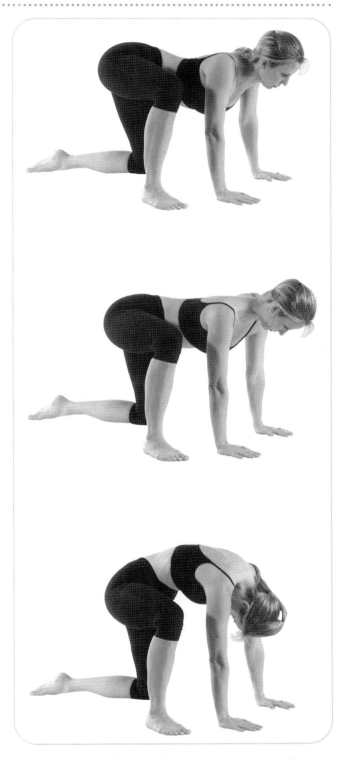

Fig. 2.30 The same differentiated reciprocating movement with a changed relationship to gravity.

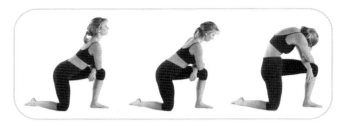

Fig. 2.31 A midway position between bending all the way over and standing all the way up – another step in the progression.

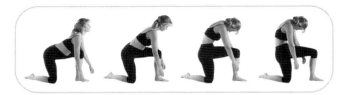

Fig. 2.33 Putting the different parts and positions together to create functional reciprocations – bending and standing.

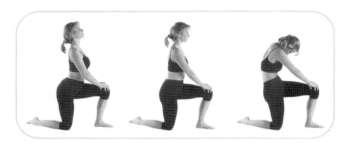

Fig. 2.32 Gaining skill in pushing the pelvis toward vertical in this position – useful for hyperlordotic students: hip flexor length and hip extensor strength.

bottom. This reciprocating movement is also useful for both of our students. Strengthening the gluteals and hamstrings and lengthening the iliopsoas when pushing the pelvis toward vertical helps our hyperlordotic student. Strengthening the back extensors and lengthening the hamstrings and gluteals when moving the pelvis to or past horizontal helps our hyperflexed students.

Let's try other variations of the same lesson. Do the same reciprocating movement when leaning on your elbows and forearms on your knees (Fig. 2.31) and up further to lean on your hands (Fig. 2.32). These progressions place increasingly more demand on the hyperlordotic student, especially coming all the way up to half-kneeling. This position is nearing (or surpassing for some people) end-range for hip extension and hip flexor length; rounding the back and posteriorly rotating the pelvis requires shortening contractions of the gluteals and hamstrings and the inhibition of the iliopsoas and back extensors.

We are again reciprocating directions of movement and simultaneously stretching and strengthening. Taken a step further to incorporate functional imbalances, we are training our student to recognize how to push the pelvis posteriorly toward vertical, simulating the balance function that is giving this person so much trouble by allowing his pelvis to fall too far forward.

Now we can combine movements of posteriorly rotating the pelvis and rounding the back to come to half-kneel and anteriorly arching the pelvis and rotating the back to bend over to the three-and-a-half point position: moving from bending to standing while in a half-kneeling position (Fig. 2.33). We already know the movement in the direction of pushing-to-

stand is particularly beneficial for our students who hyperlordose. The movement in the direction of bending, paradoxically, will be particularly useful for the person who bends from her back.

Directing this person into a specific differentiated pattern involving hip flexion and back extension strengthens the back extensors and lengthens the gluteals and hamstrings. Taken a step further to incorporate functional imbalances, we are training our student here to recognize how to allow her pelvis to fall forward more completely on the legs, simulating the bending-to-reach function that gives her so much trouble, but emphasizing bending from the hips rather than from the lumbar spine.

Notice that in all our orientations (gravity neutral, belly down and belly up) there is something valuable to be learned by both of our hypothetical students. By doing reciprocating movements to enhance pattern recognition and to coordinate the antagonists in a number of different positions, we can use the same exercises/lessons for a wide variety of people. We can simply emphasize things differently for the two opposite types. These examples are from the legs section, and we will look at each of these lessons in more depth there, but watch for this reciprocation strategy throughout the rest of the book.

Preview of section 2

On completing this first section on background and principles, we turn our attention to the nuts and bolts of motor learning: what do we want to teach and how do we want to teach it? One of the main difficulties in both writing and reading this sort of book is that the subject matter – ideal movement and how to influence it – doesn't lend itself well to written words and static pictures. Describing dynamic multiplanar movement patterns and proprioceptive sensations is hard enough, but trying to imagine the effects of movement lessons on neuromusculoskeletal organization without having experienced those movements is even more difficult.

I have used specific language, pictures, diagrams, metaphors and phrases to describe certain phenomena to help you to understand functional movement and functional exercise in a framework you have perhaps not thought of before. Your job, as you continue through this book, is to be an active participant. This is no comic book: you won't learn the whole story by just looking at the pictures, or even by reading the whole text. This is a book on human movement and exercise – get active!

You will have to digest this book slowly. Taking the time to go through the movement lessons personally will help you to get much more from the book than just reading it will. Get on the floor. Follow the directions. Think about what you are doing and feeling. Notice what you feel afterwards as a result of the lessons. Repeat the lessons again in whole or in parts, to learn in more depth and to refine your understanding of that movement.

Try the lessons out on some of your hardier students first. You will probably make mistakes initially, but with experience comes a more knowledgeable eye for movement and better judgment on what kind of person can benefit from what kind of lessons, at what kind of pace, and with the use of what sort of descriptive or inquisitive language.

Pay attention! When doing the lessons, you'll need a relatively distraction-free environment – fairly quiet and with minimal interruptions. Start each lesson by resting quietly in the described position and take the opportunity to ask yourself questions about yourself and how you are organized. What is your contact against the floor? What is your orientation to gravity? What are the relationships of different bones to one another? Can you discern left/right differences in length? Weight distribution? Comfort? Clarity of self-image? Each lesson will have a brief description of what to feel for. Do take the time to answer these questions for yourself and to the best of your ability.

Take care of yourself

As you start moving, do so gently and slowly to start with. This not only helps you to avoid injuring yourself by going either too far or in a damaging direction before you have an opportunity to become aware of that fact, but it will also help you to perceive proprioceptive sensations more accurately. As you reduce excessive chatter from your CNS by reducing muscle effort, reducing movement volume, closing your eyes, being in a quiet environment and moving slowly and gently, hitherto unnoticed proprioceptive information about muscle effort or imbalances can seep into your consciousness.

Dr Feldenkrais had a famous saying: 'If you know what you're doing, you can do what you want.' Go slow and small to know what you're doing. Go faster and larger later, after you've learned a comfortable and interesting movement. This will help solidify learning, make it more spontaneous, and do what you want with power, speed and confidence. Needless to say, this also applies when working with your students!

Take the time also to make proprioceptive comparisons during and after the lessons, and between left and right sides. Part of the game here is to puzzle things out, make discoveries and connections, and come to some sort of qualitative judgment or decision about a way of moving that you most prefer. The descriptions and breakdown of the lessons might lead you to think that there is a right way of doing the movement, but those descriptions are really of a hypothetical ideal that may or may not be right for you and your own particular skeletal organization.

Find your own path of least resistance – your own sweet spot. Use the pictures as general guides, but don't move just

---

Box 2.11 Taking care of yourself

Go slow and small to start – progress to larger and faster after proving safety

Make proprioceptive comparisons – before/after and right/left

Find the path of least resistance

Ask what other parts you can invite to participate – even distribution and proportional effort

---

like the pictures. These are photos of professionals, and many/most of you will not move as far as the pictures suggest. A general rule of thumb is to move about 75% of what you think you can do until you are certain of the safety of that movement. Figure out ways to use a newly learned movement pattern in everyday life. Start looking for recurring patterns both in the lessons, in daily life and with your students. In summary, please take the time with this book to make it as much a proprioceptive experience as an intellectual one!

In subsequent sections we will look at functional movement patterns and some common movement lessons with which to influence those patterns. Section 2 starts with primitive movements: earlier developmental movements. We can imagine a torso with a neck and head: we'll call it the worm. We will look at head-to-tail relationships in balance, orientation, early transitions and early locomotion. We will move the extremities mostly in a global way with the torso, but will explore differentiation of the head and neck from the torso (Box 2.11).

These are simpler lessons in terms of grasping intellectually, as some of the movements will be similar to what we already do in therapeutic exercise, though for some of you they may be more difficult to do physically. Some of you with sensitivity in the lower back and neck will need to be particularly self-aware when doing these global head/tail movements. You will have to be especially vigilant to move proportionally.

Section 3 explores how the legs move the pelvis and are therefore initiators of movements of the torso, head and arms. We will look especially at the gluteal and iliopsoas groups and will describe them as the four cornerstones of the skeleton. We will explore how imbalances of the leg musculature accompany imbalances of the torso. We will explore these relationships both in a front/back direction and in left/right directions. Section 3 expands on our knowledge of the worm to look at matured orientation and balance, advanced transitions and upright locomotion.

We will look especially at lower back and lower extremity dysfunction as manifestations of imbalances and insufficiencies of the four cornerstone muscle groups, and describe ways of influencing them. Lessons featured in this section will explore primarily differentiated patterns of movement with the legs moving opposite to the torso, and are mostly closed kinetic chain as befits the role of the legs.

Section 4 looks first at cervical stabilization and then at the arms and shoulder girdles and their role in higher-level functions. These include balance reactions and orientation, advanced transitions, integrating the upper extremities with locomotion, and manipulation of our external environment. After exploring ways of working with students with cervical dysfunction, we will look at shoulder girdle movement and postural patterns and relate them to pelvic and torso patterns.

We will focus on differentiating the arms from the torso and on using upper extremity closed kinetic chain exercises to facilitate shoulder girdle and upper back integration with walking, and to facilitate impingement-free reaching. We will look at elbow, forearm and wrist syndromes and discuss treatment plans incorporating the integration of the hand with the shoulder girdle and torso and incorporating nonhabitual global and differentiated movements.

Section 5 scratches the surface of a huge topic: communication, emotion and vegetation. Lessons on eye movements, lip/tongue/jaw relationships, breathing and coordination of the pelvic floor are featured. After a discussion of communication and emotion, we will look more closely at anxiety patterns, their clinical manifestations, and how to influence better autonomic balance.

Have fun! Stay focused! Good luck!

References

1. Sahrmann SA. Evaluation and treatment of muscle imbalances and associated musculoskeletal pain syndromes. Level 2-UQ course manual, p 4.
2. Singer R. Cognitive processes, learner strategies, and skilled motor behaviors. Canadian Journal of Applied Sports Science 1980;5: 25–32.
3. Keele SW. Attention and human performance. Pacific Palisades, CA: Goodyear Publishing; 1973.
4. Singer R. Motor skills and learning strategies. In O'Neil HF Jr, ed. Learning strategies. New York: Academic Press; 1978.
5. Hazeltine E, Grafton ST, Ivry R. Attention and stimulus characteristics determine the locus of motor-sequence encoding. A PET study. Brain 1997;120:123–40.
6. Sanes J. Skill learning: Motor cortex rules for learning and memory. Current Biology 2000;10:R495–7.
7. Singer R, Gaines L. Effects of prompted and problem-solving approaches on learning and transfer of motor skills. American Educational Research Journal 1975;12:395–403.
8. Keele SW, Summers JJ. The structure of motor programs. In: Stelmack GE, ed. Motor control: issues and trends. New York: Academic Press; 1976.
9. Wickens JR, Reynolds JN, Hyland BI. Neural mechanisms of reward-related motor learning. Current Opinion in Neurobiology 2003;13:685–90.
10. Singer R, Pease D. A comparison of discovery learning and guided instructional strategies on motor skill learning, retention, and transfer. Research Quarterly 1976;47:788–96.
11. Guyton A. Neuroscience: anatomy and physiology. Philadelphia, PA: WB Saunders; 1991: 122–3.
12. Whiting HTA (ed) Human motor actions. Bernstein reassessed. Amsterdam: North-Holland; 1984.
13. Arshavsky YI, Gelfand IM, Orlovsky GN. Cerebellum and rhythmical movements. Berlin: Springer Verlag; 1986.
14. Gelfand IM, Gurfinkel VS, Tsetlin ML, Shik ML. Some problems in the analysis of movements. In: Gelfand IM, Gurfinkel VS, Formin SV, Tsetlin ML, eds. Models of the structural–functional organization of certain biological systems. Cambridge, MA: MIT Press; 1971: 329–45.
15. Gelfand IM, Gurfinkel VS, Tsetlin ML, Shik ML. Certain problems in the investigation of movement. In: Tsetlin ML, ed. Automata theory and modeling of biological systems. New York: Academic Press; 1973.
16. Saltzman E. Levels of sensorimotor representation. Journal of Mathematical Biology 1978;20:91–163.
17. Turvey MT. Preliminaries to a theory of action with reference to vision. In: Shaw R, Bransford J, eds. Perceiving, acting, and knowing: Toward an ecological psychology. Hillsdale, NJ: Lawrence Erlbaum; 1977: 211–65.
18. Kots YM, Syrovegin AV. Fixed set of variants of interaction of the muscles of two joints used in the execution of simple voluntary movements. Biophysics 1966;11:1212–19.
19. Soechting JF, Laquaniti F. Invariant characteristics of a pointing movement in man. Journal of Neuroscience 1981;1:710–20.
20. Soechting JF, Laquaniti F. An assessment of the existence of muscle synergies during load perturbations and intentional movements of the human arm. Experimental Brain Research 1989;74: 535–48.
21. Bradley NS, Bekof A. Development of coordinated movement in chicks: I. Temporal analysis of hindlimb muscle synergies at embryonic days 9 and 10. Developmental Psychobiology 1990;23: 763–82.
22. Soechting JF, Laquaniti F. Coordination of arm movement in three-dimensional space. Sensorimotor mapping during drawing movement. Neuroscience 1986;17:295–311.
23. Scholz JP, Kelso JAS. A quantitative approach to understanding the formation and change of coordinated movement patterns. Journal of Motor Behavior 1989;21:122–44.
24. Buchanan TS, Almdale DPJ, Lewis JL, Rymer WZ. Characteristics of synergic relations during isometric contractions of human elbow muscles. Journal of Neurophysiology 1986;56:1225–41.
25. Ganor I, Golani I. Coordination and integration in the hindleg step cycle of the rat: Kinematic synergies. Brain Research 1980; 195:57–67.
26. Turvey MT, Fitzpatrick P. Commentary: Development of perception–action systems and general principles of pattern formation. Child Development 1993;64:1175–90.
27. Greene PH. Why is it easy to control your arms? Journal of Motor Behavior 1982;14:260–86.
28. Lee WA. Neuromotor synergies as a basis for coordinated intentional action. Journal of Motor Behavior 1984;16:135–70.
29. Nashner LM, McCollum G. The organization of human postural movements: A formal basis and experimental synthesis. Behavioral and Brain Sciences 1985;8:135–72.
30. Shik ML, Orlovsky GN. Neurophysiology of locomotor automatism. Physiological Review 1976;56:465–501.
31. Viviani P, McCollum G. The relation between linear extent and velocity in drawing movements. Neuroscience 1983;10:211–18.
32. Kelso JAS, DelColle JD, Schoner G. Action–perception as a pattern formation process. In: Jeannerod M, ed. Attention and performance XIII. Hillsdale, NJ: Lawrence Erlbaum; 1990: 1639–92.
33. Kugler PN, Kelso JAS, Turvey MT. On the control and coordination of naturally developing systems. In: Kelso JAS, Clark JE, eds. The development of movement control and coordination. New York: John Wiley; 1982: 5–78.
34. Schmidt RA. Motor control and learning. Champaign, IL: Human Kinetics Publishers, Inc.; 1988.
35. Shea CH, Kohl RM. Specificity and variability of practice. Research Quarterly Exercise and Sport 1990;61:169–77.
36. Thelen E, Corbetta D, Kamm K et al. The transition to reaching: mapping intention and intrinsic dynamics. Child Development 1993;64:1058–98.

37. Gibson JJ. The ecological approach to visual perception. Hillsdale, NJ: Lawrence Erlbaum; 1986.

38. Carello C, Turvey MT, Kugler PN, Shaw RE. Inadequacies of the computer metaphor. In: Gazzaniga M, ed. Handbook of cognitive neuroscience. New York: Plenum Press; 1984: 229–48.

39. Ashmead DH, McCarty ME, Lucas L, Belvedere MC. Visual guidance in infants' reaching toward suddenly displaced targets. Child Development 1993;64:1111–27.

40. Kugler PN, Turvey MT. Information, natural law, and the self-assembly of rhythmic movement. Hillsdale, NJ: Lawrence Erlbaum; 1987.

41. Bushnell EW, Boudreau JP. Motor development and the mind: The potential role of motor abilities as a determinant of aspects of perceptual development. Child Development 1993;64:1005–21.

42. Whitall J. A dynamical systems approach to motor development; applying new theory to practice. In: Stinson WJ, ed. Moving and learning for the young child. Presentations from the Early Childhood Conference, 'Forging the Linkage between Moving and Learning for Preschool Children', Washington DC, 1–4 December 1988.

43. Goodwin B. Developing organisms as self-organizing fields. In: Yates FE, ed. Self-organizing systems: The emergence of order. New York: Plenum Press; 1987.

44. Clancy WJ. The frame of reference problem in the design of intelligent machines. In: Lehn JV, ed. Architectures for intelligence. Proceedings of 22nd Carnegie Symposium on Cognition. Hillsdale, NJ: Lawrence Erlbaum; 1992: 357–423.

45. Turvey MT. Preliminaries to a theory of action with reference to vision. In: Shaw R, Bransfore J, eds. Perceiving, acting, and knowing: Toward an ecological psychology. Hillsdale, NJ: Lawrence Erlbaum; 1977.

46. Haken H. Information and self-organization. Berlin: Springer Verlag; 1988.

47. Edelman GM. Neural darwinism: The theory of neuronal group selection. New York: Basic; 1987.

48. Abraham R. Dynamics: a visual introduction. In: Yates FE, ed. Self-organizing systems: the emergence of order. New York: Plenum Press; 1987: 543–97.

49. Tuller B, Kelso JAS. Environmentally-specified patterns of movement coordination in normal and split-brain subjects. Experimental Brain Research 1989;75:306–16.

50. Thelen E, Kelso JAS, Fogel A. Self-organizing systems and infant motor development. Developmental Review 1987;7:39–65.

51. Reed E. Encountering the world: toward an ecological psychology. New York: Oxford University Press; 1996.

52. Oliveira FT, Goodman D. Conscious and effortful or effortless and automatic: a practice/performance paradox in motor learning. Perception and Motor Skills 2004;99:315–24.

53. Guyton A. Neuroscience: anatomy and physiology. Philadelphia, PA: WB Saunders; 1991: 122–3.

54. Juhan D. Job's body: a manual for bodywork. New York: Station Hill Press; 1987.

Movements of the worm

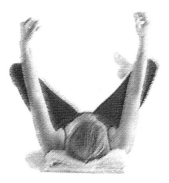

"He who controls the Worm controls the spice and he who controls the spice controls the Galaxy"

KYLE MCLAUGHLIN IN *DUNE*

CHAPTER THREE

The early worm

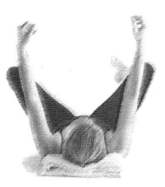

Chapter outline

Balance – falling from vertical

1. Falling back. *Global torso flexion.* Protect the head and provide a rounded surface to absorb shock.

   - Even distribution of movement as characteristic of ideal movement – the *good housekeeping rule.*

   - Head moves as an extension of torso and pelvis. Proportionality principle. Larger muscles do bulk of work while smaller muscles do fine-tuning. Another characteristic of ideal movement.

2. Falling forward. *Global torso extension.* Protect the head and provide a rounded surface to absorb shock.

   - Description of extremities moving globally with torso – primitive pattern. Sometimes desirable (arm extension with torso extension), sometimes differentiated pattern useful (arm flexion with torso extension).

   - Falling from vertical and dropped horizontally elicit same global patterns.

3. Falling sideways. *Global torso side-bending.*

4. Falling diagonally. *Global torso right flexion* (fall back and to left), *left flexion* (fall back and to right), *right extension* (fall forward and left), *left extension* (fall forward and to the right).

5. Do reciprocating movements to establish/recalibrate *neutral.* Place where antagonists balanced and weight borne skeletally/tensigrity. Another characteristic of ideal movement/posture organization.

6. Well-organized posture is really just an acute sense of balance and effort recognition.

Orientation – looking around

1. Orientation from supine. Lesson 1: *Be a Better Ball.*

   - Introduction of use of static and dynamic baselines. Use of proprioceptive reference points to check back for comparisons. Used throughout all lessons. Changes before/after and left/right opportunities for learning.

   - Torso flexion movements with side-bending and rotational variations. Head/eyes move as an extension of the torso.

   - Introduction of descriptive and inquisitive language. Used throughout all lessons.

   - Clinical applications and positional variations described for this lesson. Used throughout all lessons.

   - Application of constraints. Move this while moving that – do the same movement but in this more difficult position – put head and hand together and move them together to facilitate movement of the torso/common denominator.

2. Lesson 2: *London Bridges.*

   - Looking overhead from a supine position – beginning global extension patterns and precursor to rolling to belly.

3. Orientation from prone. Lesson 3: *Xs and Os*. Torso extension patterns with side-bending and rotational variations.
    *   Head and arms moving as an extension of the torso – global movements.
    *   Importance of raised vantage point – a high horizon. Links to skeletal weightbearing.
4. Orientation from side-lie. Lesson 4: *Be a Better Bow*.
    *   Patterns of falling from vertical and orienting from horizontal nearly identical.
    *   Global side-bending movements with flexion and extension variations.

Balance – falling from vertical

We will begin our inquiry into the nature of human movement by observing falls. Balance is the first function we will analyze. To simplify things a little conceptually, we are going to imagine how a worm with some modicum of intelligence would react if it had either dropped from a height or had lost its balance while standing on its tail and fallen over. The image of the worm is just a metaphor for the torso. This includes the pelvis, spine, ribcage and chest, with an attachment on top: the head and neck.

This worm doesn't include the extremities: no scapula, clavicle, arm bones or legs. We will use this image of a worm as representing the torso because of its multidirectional flexibility – a squirmy, wriggly, writhing tube of muscle. Worms have the advantage of being boneless, of course, but just because we have some bones embedded in our torso musculature shouldn't mean that those bones need restrict our movements unduly. This image of the torso as a flexible tube with somewhat predictable motor behaviors is an important one to keep in mind as you progress through this book.

The purpose of this chapter is to introduce examples of motor control exercise and use these relatively simpler movement lessons to introduce concepts of ideal movement and posture and to explain some of the tricks of the trade. Lessons in this chapter are conceptually fairly simple, as they pertain mainly to head/pelvis relationships and trunk control and balance. In this chapter, you will begin the experiential portion of the book. Please take the time to experience the movements you are going to be teaching – you will need some kinesthetic experience to make sense of the lesson breakdowns.

Falling backward

Let's stand our imaginary worm on his tail for a moment and see what happens. Worms aren't particularly good at standing on their tails, so he would probably topple over pretty quickly. If he falls backward, what is he going to do? How will his body move in reaction to the fall? Being a worm with a modicum of intelligence, he will probably move to protect his head. Lots of important gear is stored in there and the consequences of injury are dire. He will move his head forward, away from the uprushing floor, and will round his torso forward to assist in this. He flexes. This flexion or rounding serves the additional purpose of softening the landing by rolling along his backside like a rocking-chair runner (Fig. 3.1).

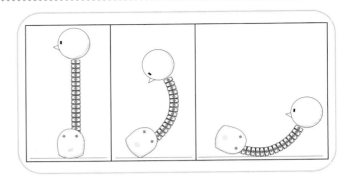

Fig. 3.1 Falling backward and protecting the head – global flexion.

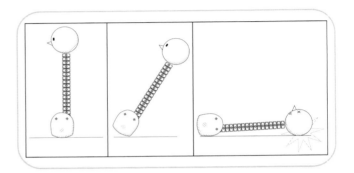

Fig. 3.2 Consequences of not adjusting to fall backward – ouch!

We will name this basic pattern of torso/pelvis/head relationships *global torso flexion*. What happens if the worm doesn't react? His body stays straight and the whole length of his body, along with his head, slams into the ground (Fig. 3.2). This strategy is to be avoided. Our evolutionary ancestors and cousins learned to avoid this outcome, and somewhere in the murky corners of our brains we have built-in mechanisms at work that help us to keep our own heads off the floor in the event of an emergency landing.

These mechanisms are partly inherited and partly learned, and that learning happens early in life. I remember an incident when my son was about 6 months old, sitting on the floor and playing with some toys. This was very soon after he had learned to come up to sit, and he was still a bit shaky way up there on his pelvis. As I walked into the room, he looked up at me and in doing so threw his head too far back and lost his balance. He was very surprised and his eyes got as big as mine did as I watched him. He didn't react quickly enough and hit the back of his head, with authority. He wasn't happy, but he did learn a valuable lesson.

A few days later the same situation arose and, as before, he looked up a little too far and a little too quickly and lost his balance again. This time, however, he reacted. He flexed his little torso and tucked his little chin and managed to ease his head down to the floor without damage. Over the course of the next couple of weeks he refined this fall back until one day he was able to catch himself in mid-fall and haul himself back upright again (Box 3.1).

Box 3.1 Falling in cardinal planes

Falling back – global torso flexion
Falling forward – global torso extension
Falling left – global torso side-bending right
Falling right – global torso side-bending left

He was very pleased with this development and practiced that movement at every opportunity over the next several weeks. How he caught himself we will discuss in the third section, when this story continues. For now, just be aware of how old and ingrained these balance reactions are and how most of us get to be so familiar with them that we are no longer even aware that we are constantly working and adjusting to maintain our balance in a gravity field.

The worm being a metaphor, let's look at what happens with a real live torso. As our pelvis starts to roll or fall backward in sitting, we would like the abdominals and anterior torso intercostal muscles to contract and shorten to round or flex the spine and assist in moving the head forward. I specifically included the intercostals in this description because we can easily lose track of their function or even their existence. They are the muscles between the ribs that squeeze those ribs together anteriorly; they are prime movers of thoracic flexion.

By extension, they are prime culprits in chronic or excessive thoracic kyphosis. Because the abdominals are also synergists in this direction of movement, they are accomplices in excessive kyphosis. Therefore, there are many times clinically where we might want to stretch both the intercostals and abdominals to reduce thoracic kyphosis and its attendant cervical strain. As the abdominals and intercostals work to flex the torso when falling back, the back extensors and posterior intercostals should be inhibited to allow the spine and back of the ribcage to flex. Falling back strengthens the abdominals and stretches the back extensors (and fascia). This is an example of accurate reciprocal inhibition.

Good housekeeping rule

Ideally, we hope both the worm and the torso would flex evenly throughout their whole lengths. With the movement distributed evenly, we get a smooth rolling back without flat spots and without one place having to move more to compensate for lack of movement somewhere else. This concept of *even distribution of movement* is a main characteristic of the Feldenkrais Method.[1] A Feldenkrais teacher named Larry Goldfarb coined a phrase for this characteristic of ideal movement: he called it the 'good housekeeping rule.'[2]

The good housekeeping rule states that just as everyone in a family has to pull his or her own weight, every joint and muscle should also contribute what they can to a movement. In that way, no one member needs to work too hard or move too far, causing tissue strain or damage. Another movement system that emphasizes whole-body participation and even distribution of movement is tai chi.[3] In these and other movement disciplines, the advantages of whole-body movement are learned experientially and then codified as a general principle. Do we ever see this in real life? Observing the torso and ribcage

of babies clearly shows an ability to move more evenly throughout their whole length than typical adults do, with the thoracic spine and ribcage being pliable and soft.

Many athletes move with this same quality of bonelessness, and it is this adherence to the good housekeeping rule that makes their performance appear so effortless. Sadly, violations of this rule are very common clinically, and we will describe many of them as we progress through the book. For example, very commonly we find that people we work with have stiffness/immobility through the thoracic spine, primarily because of the added complexity with the additional muscular and bony constraints of the ribcage.

Proportionality principle

As a corollary to the good housekeeping rule we have the *proportionality principle*. This refers to the varying strength of different muscles. In a family, the dad might chop wood and operate power-cutting tools, whereas the 5-year-old might set the table or feed the dog. In bodies, the proportionality principle means that the largest bones and the biggest muscles initiate movements and provide most of the bulk and power of that movement. In the case of the torso in particular, it means that the pelvis, as the largest bone with the biggest muscles attached to it, is the key to balance. Where the pelvis goes the torso is sure to follow. In tai chi and other martial arts, this principle of moving the pelvis first and letting the rest of the body follow is a common one. In tai chi this is called 'moving from your one point'.[3]

If the pelvis is rolled back on the chair in sitting, if the worm tucks his tail, we would like the lower spine to go along for the ride and move into flexion. As we progress farther up the spine, the rest of the back can either follow the lead of the pelvis and lower spine in a sequential movement of flexion or can differentiate somewhere along its length and move in the opposite direction. Clinically, we see the former posture fairly frequently.

Recall our hypothetical slumped sitter in Figure 2.4. We might say she has a posteriorly rotated pelvis and lumbar and thoracic kyphosis in sitting – or we might take a dynamic and functional view and say that she is allowing her pelvis to fall backward and is flexing her torso as part of an unspoken intention to keep her head from hitting the ground. Posture is an activity – and the posture of the torso is a direct outgrowth of the vertical balance of the pelvis.

Proportionally, the pelvis is a much larger bone with much stronger muscles attached to it than are, say, the upper cervical vertebrae. The spinal system is composed of two bookends, the head and pelvis, and 24 ring-shaped bones strung between the two bookends like pearls on a thread. The pelvis is by far the largest of these bones, and the vertebrae themselves get successively smaller as you go from lumbar through thoracic and cervical segments (Box 3.2).

Contrast as well the size and potential strength of the muscles that attach the ribcage to the pelvis (rectus abdominis, internal and external obliques, the back extensors and quadratus lumborum) to those that attach the head to the spine (semispinalis capitis, rectus capitis posterior minor and major, obliquus capitis superior and inferior, rectus capitis anterior longus capitis and longus colli).

Box 3.2 Characteristics of ideal movement

Even distribution of movement – good housekeeping rule

Using larger muscles to do more of the work – proportionality principle

Intention to move distally, initiating a proximal response

Bearing weight 'skeletally' – bones stacked approaching vertically and connective tissue providing tensigrity

Economy of effort – driving with your brakes off

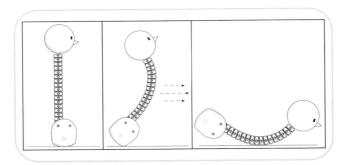

Fig. 3.3 Falling forward and protecting the head – global extension.

The larger bones and bulkier muscles of the pelvic area are clearly better suited to grosser and more powerful movements, whereas the upper cervical vertebrae and the smaller muscles of the upper neck are better suited to delicacy and fine-tuning. Unfortunately, average movement is rarely ideal movement, and clinically we find many people experiencing musculoskeletal misery owing to organizing their movement and posture with uneven distribution of movement and disproportionate distribution of effort.

Falling forward

What happens when the worm falls forward? Being a worm with a modicum of intelligence, he will move to protect his head. Being a worm with a modicum of vanity, he will also probably move to protect his comely face. He will move his head backward, away from the uprushing floor, and will arch his little worm torso backward to assist in this. He extends. This extension or arching movement of his torso serves the additional purpose of softening the landing by rolling along his front side like a reverse rocking-chair runner (Fig. 3.3). We will call this basic pattern of torso/pelvis/head relationships *global torso extension*.

With the worm as a metaphor, let's look again at what happens with a real live torso. As our pelvis starts to roll or fall forward, the back extensors, quadratus lumborum and posterior torso intercostal muscles have to contract and shorten to arch or extend the spine and assist in pulling the head backward. I specifically included the intercostals again because they are important contributors to thoracic extension. By extension, they are important muscles to recruit when dealing with someone with chronic or excessive thoracic kyphosis.

As the back extensors and posterior intercostals work to extend the torso, the abdominals and anterior intercostals should be inhibited while falling forward, allowing the spine and back of the ribcage to arch. Exercises designed around falling forward strengthen the back and stretch the front. This is another example of accurate reciprocal inhibition and coordination of the antagonists.

We have been talking so far as if we were just a tube of muscle, but in reality we do have arms and legs. What happens to the extremities in each of these scenarios? My son was about 2 years old when we went to a neighborhood park for a little playtime. It was one of those places that used a layer of small round rocks to cushion falls from the play equipment, and my son kept getting those rocks stuck between his sandals and his bare feet. I rummaged around the back of the car for a bit before I found some of his older sister's rubber boots. Foolishly, I put those oversized boots on my son.

This was a mistake. As he ran back toward the playground, he tripped and fell face forward on the cement path. The fall looked like slow motion to me and I was able to note, with that peculiar part of my brain that seems to be always analyzing and thinking about movement, that he did a perfect global extension pattern – I was so proud! His torso extended evenly and he kept his face from being rearranged by the ground.

Extremities move globally with torso

He also extended his arms and legs away from the ground as a continuation of the global extension pattern – the extremities are moving as an extension of the torso in a pattern reminiscent of the baby airplane in Figure 2.3. The posterior upper extremity muscles (rhomboids, mid and lower trapezius, posterior deltoid, infraspinatus and teres minor) all contract synergistically with the posterior torso musculature.

The posterior lower extremity muscles (gluteus maximus, hip rotators, hamstrings, and maybe even gastrosoleus) also contract synergistically with the posterior torso musculature. We can say that both the upper and lower extremities are moving globally with the torso, and that all the extensors or posterior musculature are contracting globally throughout the body. Later, he learned to catch himself with his arms as he fell forward, differentiating the upper extremities from the still-extending torso.

The organization of the arms and legs in falling backward is much the same. The arms flex forward along with the legs in a global flexion pattern. Anterior upper extremity musculature (anterior deltoid, biceps, pectoralis major and minor, serratus, and possibly the subscapularis) contract synergistically with the anterior torso musculature. The hip flexors (iliacus, iliopsoas and rectus femoris) also contract synergistically with the anterior torso musculature in this global flexion pattern. This scenario, like the fall forward of my son, is a bit primitive.

Later, we learn to extend our arms back in a differentiation of the arms from the torso to help break our fall. Whereas therapeutic exercise often tends to emphasize global patterns of movement, qualitative/informational exercise will add in the use of differentiated patterns. In therapeutic exercise, we might ask the gluteals to work to facilitate the lumbar extensors, or the lower trapezii to work to facilitate the thoracic extensors.

In motor learning there are many times when we want the gluteals to work independently of the back extensors, or the thoracic extensors to fire without having to squeeze the shoulder girdles down and back. Although global patterns can be useful initially, differentiated patterns are essential progressions from these more primitive patterns and are much more like what happens in real life with our students. We will get into differentiated movements both later in this chapter and in subsequent chapters.

If we change our scenario a little from having the worm standing on his tail and falling, to one of his being suspended horizontally and belly up then dropped to the floor, the response is much the same. The torso flexes, the arms flex, the hips and knees flex and the worm presents an entirely round structure to absorb the blow and to protect the head, throat, soft underbelly and genitals. Infants at a certain age have this as a reflex, though I wouldn't suggest trying it out as an experiment.

If the worm is dropped horizontally from a belly-down orientation, a global extension pattern is triggered. The arms, legs and torso all extend to present a bow-shaped structure to the floor to absorb the blow, and to again protect the head/face, throat and genitals. In global patterns, then, the arms and legs are moving as an extension of the torso. In some respects, we can even think of the head and neck as a fifth extremity. In both of these falling scenarios the head and neck are also moving globally as an extension of the torso. We will see this later in the discussion on orientation functions, then later still will explore differentiations of the head and neck from the torso.

Falling sideways

When our worm falls to the left from standing on this tail, he will now bend to the right. Right torso side-benders (right internal and external obliques, quadratus lumborum, intercostals and back extensors) are excited and the left torso side-benders are inhibited again to protect the head and to present a bow-shaped structure to the floor (Fig. 3.4). The top or right leg will abduct and the left will adduct, with right gluteus maximus, medius, minimus and tensor fasciae latae all engaging with the left adductor magnus, brevis and longus.

The top or right arm will adduct and depress and the bottom arm abduct and elevate. Right latissimus dorsi and

pectoralis major are strengthened, along with the left deltoid, upper trapezius and others. Recall that for each muscle that is strengthened there is a corresponding antagonist that is stretched or inhibited. This applies both to torso and extremity musculature. The legs, arms and head are again moving globally with the torso – they are neurological extensions of the activated torso pattern. Falling to the right is a mirror image. Movement lessons that simulate falling sideways can be a functional context for working with scoliosis or other lateral torso asymmetries. We will call these movements *global torso side-bending*.

Falling diagonally

Our traditional cardinal planes of flexion/extension and left/right are only four of 360 possibilities for falls. What happens if the worm falls forward and to the left? He will bend back and to the right. We will call this *right torso extension* – he is extending back and to the right. Right back extensors, quadratus lumborum and right posterolateral intercostals are strengthened. Left abdominals, anterolateral intercostals are stretched. Think of painting in the quadrants. Notice that in all our scenarios there is this relationship between front and back or between right back and left front.

The muscles described in the diagonal movements are antagonists and need to be coordinated. Clinically, we will use diagonal patterns a lot. They help with both anterior/posterior and left/right imbalances, which nearly all of our students have concurrently. They also follow asymmetrical use of the legs and arms, and are therefore relevant to many more functional daily movements than either straight anterior/posterior or straight side-bending movements are.

If our worm falls back and to the right, he will bend forward and to the left – *left torso flexion*. Falling back and to the left is *right torso flexion*. Falling forward and to the right is *left torso extension* (Fig. 3.5). We will be working a lot with eight directions of movement, four cardinal and four diagonal. Many lessons will flesh out this framework with circular movements – moving in all 360 directions. In all these falling scenarios, the head, arms and legs move globally with the torso. The same kind of organization applies when being dropped from a height with varying angles of orientation to the floor.

To summarize balancing, when we start to fall in one direction we would like to see a bend in the opposite direction. We would like to see an even distribution of movement and proportional muscle use. We can examine falls in 360 directions, in the case of both the standing worm and the dropped worm, but will focus most of our lessons with our students on eight of them. Cardinal plane movements are global torso flexion and extension and right and left global torso side-bending. Diagonal patterns are left and right torso extension and left and right torso flexion (Box 3.3).

In falling, antagonists are coordinated: one side or diagonal corner of the torso is strengthened while its opposite side or corner is stretched. The upper extremities, lower extremities and head/neck move globally or as an extension of the direction of movement of the torso in these earlier or more primitive falling reactions (the arms differentiate from the torso later to assist with breaking a fall). The descriptions so far have been of the stylized variety: few people actually move this ideally.

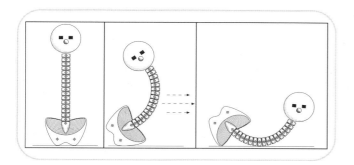

Fig. 3.4 Falling sideways and protecting the head – global side-bending.

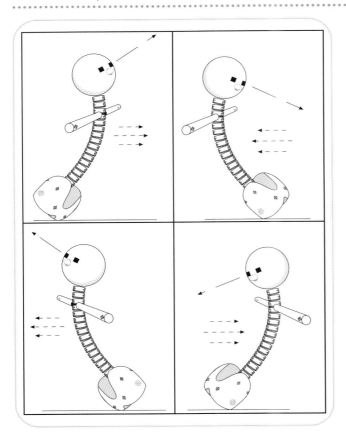

Fig. 3.5 Falling in diagonals – right extension, left flexion, left extension and right flexion.

Box 3.3 Falling in diagonal directions
Falling back and left – right torso flexion
Falling back and right – left torso flexion
Falling forward and left – right torso extension
Falling forward and right – left torso extension
Head and extremities move globally with torso

There are a few different ways of thinking about falls. We could take falling literally: in the context of the person who has had a stroke, or the child with cerebral palsy who can't sit upright. We can also think about falls metaphorically: how people organize themselves to stay upright in a gravity field – their posture.

We can say that our student who tends to slump when sitting is allowing her pelvis to fall backward (see Fig. 2.4). She is neglecting to do something to keep her pelvis vertical, and some part of her back has no choice but to follow the lead of the pelvis and flex. The worm is falling backward, but catches herself with her belly and holds herself in that falling state.

We could say that our student with excessive lordosis in standing is allowing her pelvis to fall too far forward on her legs (see Fig. 2.1). She is also neglecting to do something to keep her pelvis vertical. The worm is falling forward on her legs, but catches herself with her back and holds herself there in mid-fall. In both of these scenarios she is holding herself in a constantly falling state, which necessitates constant muscular effort from one of the two paired antagonists.

Both of these cases result in muscle imbalances, as the unused antagonist is chronically inhibited, and invariant stress on supportive connective, circulatory, nervous and articular tissues in the lower back. Both of these folks could benefit from movement lessons featuring reciprocating movements that both balance and coordinate the antagonists and allow a more accurate neutral posture to emerge as an outgrowth of an ability to move more or less equally well in both directions.

Skeletal weightbearing

A neutral postural position in this anterior/posterior plane could be defined as that place where the antagonists are balanced or almost imperceptibly reciprocating, and where neither the abdominals nor the back extensors are working harder or longer than the other. This place approximates a vertical orientation of the pelvis and a place where neither the ligaments of the spine nor the facet joints are doing the bulk of weight support. We would like to organize our vertebrae in space and in relation to one another in such a way that the subjective feeling is one of *bearing weight skeletally*, more through the vertebral bodies than through the posterior structures.

In reality, there are no flat surfaces, straight bones or vertical columns in our bodies. A truer representation of how our bag of bones organizes itself upright is described by Buckminster Fuller[4] and SM Levin.[5] Fuller described the solid pieces (bones) of the *tensigrity* structure as spacers and the connecting guy wires (connective tissue) as weight supporters. We will be using the language of vertical bones and skeletal weightbearing throughout the rest of the book because it is the subjective feeling of solidity, of being grounded, and of being balanced on top of solid bone that we will usually be teaching our students. Just keep in mind that skeletal weightbearing and tensigrity are used here interchangeably.

This principle emphasizes the central role of the floor in supporting your weight and is the antithesis of the sky-hook analogy. To a tai chi practitioner, bearing weight skeletally is described as 'keeping weight underside.'[2] The subjective feeling is one of effortlessness, of being grounded, and a sense of being able to fall equally easily in either direction. If we can train a student to fall equally easily in both directions and to feel the effort involved in arresting those falls, we have some of the proprioceptive cues the student needs to be aware of to monitor and correct her postural organization. The same framework is true for left/right and alternating diagonal falling patterns. We will be exploring this process experimentally a bit later. Try this idea for size: well-organized posture is really just an acute sense of balance and effort recognition.

Orientation from supine

Balancing, or preventing oneself from falling and hitting one's head, is learned relatively early on in the developmental sequence and gets more refined as we get older (then begins

Box 3.4 Two definitions of orientation

Relationship to gravity – prone, supine, side-lie or vertical
Gathering information from outside world – sight, touch, hearing, smell and taste
Vision is king

to deteriorate as we get older still). Another very early function, probably even preceding balance, is orientation. In motor control language orientation has two meanings. It can mean your relationship to gravity: supine, prone, side-lie, vertical, etc. It can also mean your relationship to the horizon and to the points of the compass: forward/back, left/right, up/down are all orientations. This definition of orientation is about body position in space.

The other definition of orientation refers to movements executed with the intention to orient our exteroreceptors. Exteroreceptors include hearing, smell, taste, touch and sight. All of these senses except touch reside in your head. We turn and cock our heads to listen. We move our head forward and up to lick an ice-cream cone. We may raise our nose in the air to smell. The big daddy of orientation, however, is sight.

We seem to have an insatiable curiosity about our environment when we're born. Babies get into anything they can. Because they can't walk or crawl around to feel or taste things at a distance, they develop a special fondness for looking around. There is a very early association between the intention to look and the movement of the head and, as we'll see later, the rest of the skeleton in cooperation (Box 3.4).

How does a worm orient itself to see from a horizontal position? If a worm is lying on its belly and lifts its head to look forward to the horizon, we will see a global torso extension pattern. This pattern matches the global extension pattern of falling forward. It is the same basic pattern, but with a different intention. If it's lying on its back to lift its head, we will see a global torso flexion pattern. If lifting to orient to the horizon in side-lying, we will see global torso side-bending (Fig. 3.6).

Let's now do some personal research. Our first experiential lesson will be orienting our eyes toward the horizon from supine; this will be a global flexion pattern. Next we will orient from prone, an extension pattern. Finally we'll orient from side-lying, a side-bend pattern with some exploration of flexion and extension components. They will be mostly global patterns, arms and legs moving as an extension of the torso. Please read through the general instructions for doing the movement lessons at the end of Chapter 2 before starting.

For this first lesson, pay particular attention so that you don't pull strongly on your head. Get your chest to fold and your back to lengthen, instead of pulling your neck strongly into flexion. Some of us have hypermobilities or instabilities in the lower neck due to postural or movement stresses that tend to shear one vertebra forward on the other. Move proportionally!

When starting and finishing lessons, you will be asked to pay attention to some things about yourself and to compare the before-and-after answers to those questions. Take a moment to quiet yourself in preparation for the lesson. Bring your attention internally.

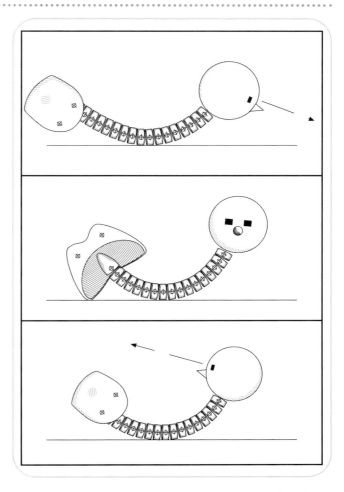

Fig. 3.6 Orientation from horizontal – global extension, global side-bending and global flexion – patterns identical to falls.

Box 3.5 Orientation from horizontal

From supine – global torso flexion
From prone – global torso extension
From supine – global torso side-bending
Head and extremities move globally with torso
Patterns identical to falling

When you begin to follow the directions and move, start your experimentation slowly and gently. Don't go fast or hard to begin with. This enhances safety and reduces proprioceptive chatter, making subtle proprioceptive sensation more easily felt.

During the breaks in the lessons, between sections designated by the capital letters, come back to your starting position (usually lying on your back) and rest for a bit. Take that time to compare your initial proprioceptive sensations to what you are experiencing after having moved (Box 3.5).

If you have any discomfort while doing the movements, stop for a moment and reassess how you are doing things. Have you gone too far? Is it a simple matter of making the movement smaller or slower? Have you tried another possibility, another trajectory of movement, another solution to the problem? Try working around discomfort – don't work through it. Pain stimulation will cause the CNS to reject what you are trying to learn.

The general structure of most lessons is to move from simpler and easier movements to more complex or demanding ones. There may be a time during the lesson in which it would be wise for you to opt out – there are some very challenging movements in this book, and I wouldn't expect most readers to be able to do all of them. I don't want to teach to the lowest common denominator, however, so I include some movements here that can challenge your fittest students or your highest-level athlete. Recognize your own limits and don't push your round peg into a square hole. Also, please extend this same courtesy to your students. Be reasonable and use your judgment about how far to take it.

Be a Better Ball

Variations

A. Lie on your back with your legs down long and comfortably spread. Have your arms and hands resting somewhere on the floor away from your sides.

- Be aware of the contact you make against the floor.

- Feel the position of your pelvis. Is your tailbone pressing into the floor or lifting away? Is it rolled left or right?

- Feel how your weight is distributed along your spine. What parts press into the floor and which parts are lifted from the floor?

- Feel the position of your head. Is it tipped nose up or chin down? Is it rolled left or right?

B. Still lying on your back, bend your knees so the soles of your feet are flat on the floor. Arms are still on the ground a bit away from your sides.

- Lift your head to look between your knees (Fig. 3.7). Is this easy or difficult? How heavy does your head feel? Can you see your feet? Try this a few times.

C. Still lying on your back, interlace your fingers and put them behind your head.

- Lift your head with the assistance of your arms and move your elbows gently toward your lower belly (Fig. 3.8).

- Try this with an exhalation. Does this help? How about an inhalation?

- Try lifting your hips a little away from the floor to reach your lower belly toward your elbows. Coordinate lifting both your head and your tail.

D. Still lying on your back, place your right hand behind your head and your left hand holding on to your right knee on the upper shin just below your kneecap.

- Lift your head with the assistance of your right hand and move your right elbow and right knee toward

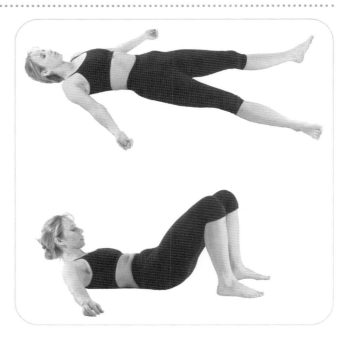

Fig. 3.7 Starting position and initial movement – lie on your back and look between your knees.

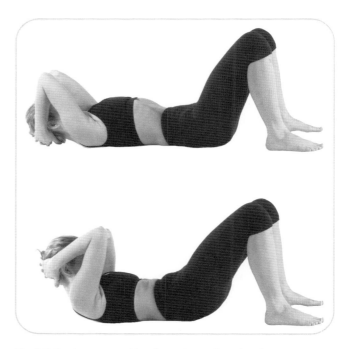

Fig. 3.8 Putting arms and head together and moving them as one – constraint to get whole torso involved.

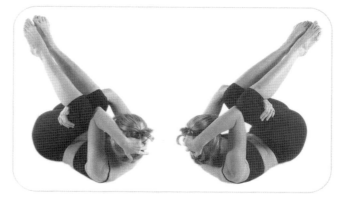

Fig. 3.10 Holding knees with forearms and moving elbows to knees on each side.

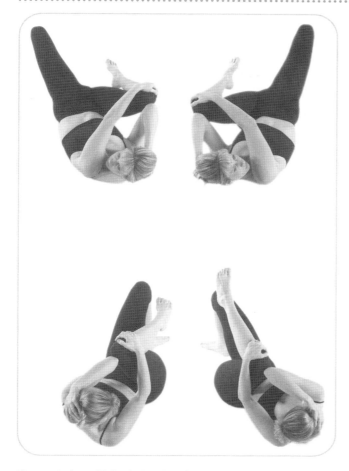

Fig. 3.9 Right and left side-bending/flexion and right and left diagonal or rotation/flexion movements.

each other as you look between your thighs toward your left foot (Fig. 3.9).

- Try it by folding your torso to the right. Bend to the right as you flex or curl up. Let your right hip open up to the right as you try this. Now try moving elbow and knee toward each other in a straight line. Which feels like the path of least resistance?

- Time the movement with your breath. Rub your elbow around your knee if easy.

E. Do a mirror image of D: left hand behind head, right hand holding left knee.

- Move left knee and left elbow toward each other. Where is the path of least resistance here? How does this side differ from the other (Fig. 3.9)?

F. Still lying on your back, place your right hand behind your head and your left hand holding on to your left knee just below your kneecap. This is a diagonal or twisting movement rather than a bending movement.

- Lift your head with the assistance of your right hand and move your right elbow and left knee toward each other (Fig. 3.9).

- Try lifting or peeling both right shoulder and left hip and lower back away from the floor.

- Time with your breath, look around your left hip toward your left foot.

G. Do a mirror image of F: left hand on head and right hand on right knee.

- Move left elbow and right knee diagonally toward each other. How does this side compare to the other (Fig. 3.9)?

H. Lie on your back with your knees bent. Lift both feet from the floor and hold on behind your knees with your right forearm. The hand reaches under both legs to hold left thigh. Left hand behind head.

- Lift head to move left elbow toward both knees. How does your chest and ribcage have to bend to do this (Fig. 3.10)?

I. Do a mirror image of H. Hold both knees with left forearm, right hand on head.

- Lift head to move right elbow toward both knees. How does this side compare (Fig. 3.10)?

J. Lie on your back with both knees bent and both arms on the floor.

- Lift your head now without the assistance of the arms to look between your thighs. How does this compare to when we began?

- Lie on your back with your legs down long and compare contact against the floor to when you began. How is your weight distributed along your spine? How are your head and pelvis resting on the floor in comparison?

- Stand up, feel the shape of your spine and the balance of your head and pelvis here. Walk around to feel mobility and coordination of your torso.

Static baselines – Be a Better Ball

A proprioceptive awareness scan is our first order of business, as is outlined in variation A. If our intention in exercise is to change postural, gross motor or arthrokinematic behavior, the first thing to do is to train your students to feel and be aware of that behavior. Those who can't learn from their history are doomed to repeat it. The first instruction in this lesson, lying on your back on the floor and being aware of contact against the floor, is here to establish a *static baseline*.

We will use this static baseline as a reference point that we can return to during and after the lesson and over a series of lessons to assess change or progress. Feeling the contact your pelvis, spine, ribcage and head make against the floor can give you clearer information about your shape, about relationships among various segments of your spine, and about differences in organization of your torso left to right.

Different people lie supine differently. Some will lift their lower back – some will lift so little an ant could crawl underneath. Some will lift it a lot and a mouse might squeeze under. Some go overboard and lift their lower backs so far off the floor that a kitten could chase that mouse right under the arch. Others will press their lower backs into the ground. This degree of spinal arch will correspond to the position of the pelvis on the floor. Roll the pelvis down toward the tailbone and the lower back will extend and lift from the floor.

Roll your pelvis up toward the sacral base and your lower back will move toward flexion and press into the floor. The position of the pelvis in space and the shape of the lumbar spine are linked. This assessment of the relationship of the lower back to the floor is an assessment of the habitual bias of this person toward either posterior pelvic tilt and lumbar flexion or anterior pelvic tilt and lumbar extension. This bias is partly a result of torso muscular imbalances between the abdominals and the back extensors. It is also partly a result of muscle imbalances in the legs. Those muscles that cross the hip have a tremendous influence over the organization of the back, as we'll see in Section 3.

How the floor supports the mid-back is also of interest to us. In many of our students the thoracic spine is often biased toward kyphosis or rounding. The floor can help them to feel and be aware of that thoracic shape, just as it helped in the assessment of the shape of the lower back. Often the thoracic spine stays rounded/flexed and there will be a short section of vertebrae that is supported by the floor.

If the thoracic spine and the dozen pairs of ribs that attach to it are resilient, that section of the torso can become flatter as gravity pulls those bones toward the floor and the weight becomes more evenly distributed. Think of those vertebrae as pearls on a thread: if you hold that string at both ends and lower the middle to the floor, the round shape will flatten as it accommodates to the shape of the floor (Box 3.6).

Awareness of the space between the back of the neck and the floor and the contact point of the back of the head against the floor also gives us important information. Infants will lie supine with their neck flat against the floor, but the only adult I've seen do this was a woman with a seriously deranged cervical spine. We wouldn't expect or want to see a completely flat neck, but one that is very extended and shortened/compressed at the back is not ideal either. If the contact of the head is closer

---

Box 3.6 Structure of a lesson

Static baselines – position changes before/after, left/right

Dynamic baselines – movement changes before/after, left/right

Application of constraints – funneling movement options toward the desired outcome

Use of descriptive and inquisitive language to match attention to intention and outcome

---

to the base of the skull than to the top of the head, the neck is flatter and longer at the back.

With the weight of the head borne more toward the top of the head, the neck becomes more arched and shortened posteriorly. Observe yourself, your colleagues and your students for this phenomenon. We can look at the angle of the face relative to the ceiling. Are the face/eyes oriented to the horizon, looking down or looking up? Angle of the face, contact point of the back of the head on the floor and space under the neck go together and are again handy reference points for both therapist and students to assess changes as a result of the lesson. Did your head/neck organization relative to the floor change afterwards?

Part of this bias toward orienting downward/flattening the neck or orienting upward/arching the neck is a reflection of anterior/posterior muscle imbalance. This is also a reflection of thoracic mobility. With a rigid kyphosis, the head has no choice but to hang back as the upper thoracic spine lifts or rounds away from the floor. The same is true in vertical orientations. The more the thoracic spine kyphoses, the more the cervical spine has to extend to orient the eyes to the horizon. If someone is markedly like this, put a pad under the head for this lesson to get the head/face more oriented to the horizon and the neck in a more neutral position.

What we are aiming for in this scan is to hone the ability of our students to discern the shape of different parts of the spine and the relationships between them. It is a handy way to start to train proprioceptive acuity – it gets students to think about and ask questions about what they habitually do. Note the *inquisitive language* in this section. We are asking questions about what your students notice about themselves, which can be a much more powerful way of honing proprioceptive clarity than telling them what they feel. Use inquisitive language with both static and dynamic reference points.

Dynamic baselines – Be a Better Ball

Our first movement is described in variation B. With legs bent up, lift head to look between knees. This is a test movement, a *dynamic reference point* with a functional intention to look. We can see around our environment best when we bring our head to vertical with our eyes on the horizon. Few people will do this initially; did you? Some people when they lift their heads to look don't have a sense of how to distribute movement evenly or distribute effort proportionally.

These folks may lift their head mostly with their neck, without a preparatory or simultaneous contraction of the abdominal muscles. What happens here is that the chest will lift as the neck muscles pull the sternum and ribs upward. There

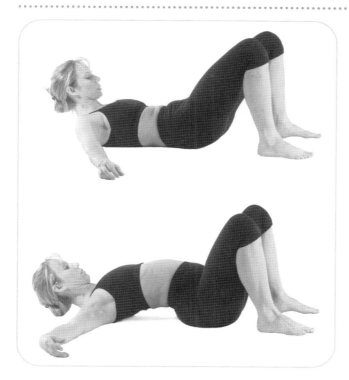

Fig. 3.11 Lifting head with and without abdominal and anterior intercostal participation – which choice looks easier and more successful?

is not a stable base for those muscles to work from or a dynamic partner for them to work with. The back may even lift slightly from the floor (Fig. 3.11).

With a well-distributed movement, the whole back will flex as the abdominals and anterior intercostals fire to move the head as an extension of the torso. Proportionally, the belly and chest muscles are stronger than the neck. Reduce neck strain by involving the stronger synergists. How did you make this test movement? What was your strategy? The rest of this lesson is designed to facilitate an improvement in this coordination of head and torso.

Our next instruction in this sequence is to interlace your fingers and place hands together behind head, as in variation C. Use your arms to assist in lifting your head to look, and time with exhalation. Both of these variations of the initial movement are auxiliary movements. Put the hands on the head so you have to move head and arms as one unit; this requires the torso to participate. This is a common motor learning strategy that we can call an *application of constraints*. Put two bones together and move them as one: 'do this while also doing that.' Constraints are designed to require a different organization from what the student habitually does, and will be a commonly used strategy throughout many of the lessons in this book.

Physical therapists are already using constraint-induced (CI) movement therapy in children and adults with acquired brain injuries and are showing promising results.[6–14] Arrange environmental conditions in such a way that the central nervous system (CNS) needs to learn/figure out how to use body parts

in certain ways. If we already use this technique for our neuro students, why not apply the same ideas to acute and repetitive musculoskeletal injuries? A brain is a brain, and it responds to puzzles in the same way.

Applying constraints

The timing of the breath is another example of a constraint. Exaggerating your exhalation with lifting your head is another auxiliary movement. In this case, it stimulates the abdominal and anterior intercostals contractions that we want to be part of this movement. This introduces the function of vegetation to the mix. The instruction to lift the hips to meet the elbows as the elbows move toward the hips is to get both ends of the spine (pelvis and head) to move simultaneously and to encourage a more even distribution of movement.

Variations D and E ask you to hold right knee with left hand and place right hand behind head – lift head to move right elbow toward right knee and to look between knees toward left foot (the foot that is still on the floor). Here again we have constraints – 'do this while also doing that.' This directs or encourages an asymmetrical movement that emphasizes a combination of torso flexion and right side-bending. This encourages more right anterior and lateral abdominal excitation and left posterior and lateral extensor inhibition. Note the diagonal relationship. As you try this movement on the other side, you have an opportunity again to ask questions about left-to-right differences.

Part of the game in training motor control is to be aware enough to make comparisons and to make good motor decisions. We started with static and dynamic baselines and will end the lesson with the same: we make before and after comparisons. We also can make comparisons of opposite directions, left and right, front and back, right and left flexion and extension diagonals. This emphasis on making comparisons, of directing the students' attention to those differences by asking specific questions, aids our students in proprioceptive acuity and pattern recognition skills (Box 3.7).

Other comparisons made in this variation of the lesson are about different ways of moving on the same side. We want our students to try a few different options of the same movement. Recall the Goldilocks effect from the first chapter. Although there are a number of ways to bring the same-side elbow and knee toward each other, this particular variation asks you to compare two versions. One version is to come straight up in more of a cardinal plane or classic global torso flexion pattern, and another version is to flex with a component of bending to the right. Most people will find that bending to the right to accommodate the asymmetrical nature of this movement is easiest. It is the path of least resistance. Some of you may even find that it is possible to do this movement and barely lift your head at all!

Box 3.7 Application of constraints
Do this while doing that
Put hands and head together and move them as one
Use of timed breath to facilitate skeletal movement
Feldenkrais, tai chi and yoga all make liberal use of constraints

In variations F and G, hold left knee with left hand and place right hand behind head. Lift head to move right elbow and left knee toward each other. This is an asymmetrical movement that emphasizes a combination of torso flexion and rotation. It is a diagonal pattern of left torso flexion. Recall our muscular analysis from the falls, as it is the same. Left abdominals and anterior intercostals are strengthened and right back extensors and posterior intercostals are stretched.

The diagonal corners lift; the left hip lifts when left knee moves diagonally upward and the right shoulder lifts as the right elbow moves diagonally downward. The opposite side (right torso flexion as you bring left elbow and right knee toward each other) will be different. Were you able to sense those differences in your own body? Can you spot differences between the two sides in your students? How do you organize your head as you add the simultaneous intention to look around the hip toward the lifted foot?

It is this ability to know what you are doing with your own body and the ability to feel differences and judge preferences between two or more ways of doing the same thing that help you to better see errors or inefficiencies in your students; help you to understand why they might be doing it that way; what some of the consequences are of doing it that way; and guide you in helping them to learn a new and better way.

Our final movement variations in H and I are to hold behind both knees with a forearm and place the opposite hand behind the head – move elbow and both knees toward each other. This variation is also an asymmetrical one that encourages a side-bending component with the flexion. It is also a more difficult progression of the previous variations. Holding the knees with the forearm requires both more flexion of the hips and more rounding and bending of the torso.

Recall from our background discussion our desire to progress our students systematically to keep interest high and avoid boredom. This is important, not just to keep people doing their home exercises but also to prevent them from going on autopilot as they are doing them. We want them to pay attention, not only when they are learning the movements, but we'd also like those movements to be challenging enough that they always have room for improvement. Generally, motor control exercises start with simpler instructions and more open-ended movements and progress to more complex, demanding or constrained movements toward the end.

Comparing baselines – what has changed from the beginning?

In K, we return to our original questions: our static and dynamic baselines. Lie on your back with knees bent and arms at sides again as in our very first movement, and lift head to look between knees. How does this movement compare to the beginning? For many people, the answer will be: 'its easier;' 'it feels lighter;' 'I notice I'm not holding my breath anymore;' 'I'm using my belly and moving my chest much differently.' This is the dynamic baseline we first explored early in the lesson. What happened during the lesson that changed the organization and ease of this test movement?

By applying constraints of moving head and arm together, requiring a specific intention to look in a specific direction and

timing the breath, we have informed the CNS of the advantages of moving the head and eyes as an extension of the torso and of using more fully the powerful abdominal muscles. We have taught our students the advantages of the good housekeeping rule and the proportionality principle. If you can demonstrate to your students proprioceptively that a different way of moving is clearly easier than, more pleasant than, hurts less than or serves them better than that which they were doing before, half the battle is won.

They will not necessarily be convinced by double-blind studies and expert advice, but by what they subjectively feel and know to be true from personal experience. Once they feel differences as a result of the exercise, especially if as part of that difference they are feeling less pain/better fluidity of movement/less muscle effort/easier posture, they will be much more likely to follow up with those exercises at home and will place more weight on what you have to tell them in subsequent appointments. You obviously know what you are talking about.

We finished this lesson by lying supine and feeling contact and left/right balance on the floor, comparing that contact and balance to the beginning of the lesson. This is our static baseline. Did you feel supported differently by the floor? Was more of your torso in contact with the ground? Were some of the left/right differences you felt at the beginning lessened?

If differences were narrowed from side to side, why? Because we all have both a preferred extension diagonal (right or left torso extension) and a preferred flexion diagonal (right or left torso flexion) in daily movement, those differences in preference will still be present when resting supine because of residual or habitual patterns of muscle recruitment and inhibition. If someone always sits with the pelvis falling back and to the left, the resultant right torso flexion pattern will create an asymmetrical or imbalanced neurological firing pattern.

The resultant right anterior intercostal and abdominal muscle excitation and left posterior intercostal and back extensor inhibition remain even at rest, and can account for some of the left/right differences in weight distribution and orientation of head, shoulders and pelvis that you may have felt at the beginning of the lesson. Try observing your students supine while asking yourself about those differences. If you observe closely, you will probably see that the ribcage is a little longer on one side, or the space in the waist is different on one side compared to the other.

The pelvis will probably be rolled on the floor one way or the other and the head offset from geometrical midline in some way. We are all asymmetrical as we lie on the floor, and that asymmetry is a result of muscle – and hence functional – imbalances that echo upright asymmetries of posture and movement. You can learn to read and anticipate those imbalances by observing your students closely while they are resting supine (or sitting, standing, walking, etc.).

If there was a reduction of left/right differences, we might reason that by asking the CNS to perform variations of the basic movement in asymmetrical ways and to both sides, we have helped to balance out the motor firing patterns that were creating the asymmetries in the first place. By directing attention to differences in the two sides and directing intention to making those mirror image movements more like each other, we get the CNS to recognize through movement the hitherto unrecognized imbalances and thereby reduce them.

If differences in your contact with the floor were noted before/after, what happened? We might anticipate a reciprocal inhibition of the lumbar extensors through repeated, intentional and varied use of the abdominal muscles. The back extensors need to lengthen to allow this movement of knee and elbow toward each other, and this may be part of the reason that in many people the lumbar spine is closer to the floor at the end of the lesson. The low back loses some of its lordosis and the extensors now allow the vertebrae to sag toward the floor more easily as gravity pulls those bones back.

This common effect of the lower back flattening toward the floor can also be a result of changes in the shape of the thoracic spine. If we thought of it logically, we might think that the repeated firing of the abdominals and anterior intercostals would result in an accentuation of any thoracic rounding or kyphosis. This is not usually the case. Although it is true that the abdominals and anterior intercostals are shortening while we are lifting the head and moving the elbow and knee toward each other, we are getting a lengthening contraction of those same muscles as we return the head slowly and gently to the floor.

Recall our muscle balance schematic in Chapter 2, where the top muscle both lifted the bone upward and lowered it back down by lengthening. This is a peculiar version of reciprocating movements (raising up and lowering back down) that balances the antagonists. Throughout this book we will find many instances of using controlled lengthening contractions to help stretch muscles.

As the abdominal and intercostal muscles alternate between flexing and allowing a flattening of the torso, there may be a change in muscle spindle bias in these muscles. They may find a new and longer resting length that allows freer extension of that often flexed mid-back. As the thorax is allowed to flatten or extend, it brings the vertebrae at the bottom of the kyphosis (the apex of the lordosis) closer to the floor and helps flatten the lower back into flexion.

Changes in those left/right differences from beginning to end may come about because of intentional and self-aware movement into both habitual and nonhabitual directions. In the case of students who allow their pelvis to fall back and to the left and have a balance reaction of right torso flexion, we might anticipate their being more easily able to do variations of right elbow to right knee and left elbow to right knee. The variations of left elbow to left knee and right elbow to left knee would be less familiar – the left abdominals would be weaker than the right and the right back extensors would be tighter than the left.

It is these *nonhabitual directions* of movement we want to emphasize as a home program. By initially doing all the variations, we assist our students in recognizing the differences in those habitual and nonhabitual patterns and motivate them to learn to move in a more balanced way. As you explore those nonhabitual directions of movement and gain some degree of competence in accessing those nonhabitual neurological firing patterns of muscle inhibition and excitation, you can get a reduction of one-sided tone bias and a change (hopefully toward better balance or symmetry) in how bones are arranged on the floor.

Using reference points with other interventions

Try teaching this lesson to a few students. Observe them lying supine and guess in which directions they are likely to move more easily. Observe them as they move. See if you can pick up what they are doing differently left and right, and what they might do to make the movements easier, more comfortable or more complete. It is this attentive observation of postural patterns and of complex, integrated, noncardinal plane movements with a variety of students with different body types that will deepen your understanding and observation skills in both evaluation and treatment.

It is difficult to exaggerate the importance of having reference points in movement and posture retraining (anything that seeks to change postural, gross motor or arthrokinematic behavior). Although it is extremely important in a motor learning approach to have before/after and left/right reference points and contrasts, this simple device can be of great benefit to both student and practitioner no matter what approach is used.

Manual therapists who are mobilizing C6 into left rotation could use a dynamic baseline before the mobilization to heighten students' awareness of differences in the ease and comfort of movement side to side and before and after. Ask them to turn to look over their left shoulder. Ask them to swing their arms to the right while still looking forward. Ask them to lie on their belly with their head turned to the left.

Ask them to do a movement and go slowly and gently enough to notice subtle differences in organization or ease side to side. Do your magic and have them reassess afterwards. Hopefully, range and ease of movement will have been improved and you will have helped to communicate to their CNS that a newly available movement has been reclaimed.

That newly available range or coordination of movement will now need to be recognized as useful and incorporated into some useful daily activity – such as looking over their shoulder while changing lanes, other orientation contexts, or walking. That new range now needs also to be controlled differently by the antagonist pairs, and muscle spindle recalibration needs to occur. Make them aware that they have now a different way of moving, and instruct them specifically on where and when they might use it – otherwise your magic may fade with time and a return to the more familiar motor habits that caused their problems in the first place becomes more likely.

Rolfers and other structural bodyworkers who work to release tight thoracolumbar fascia might use slumping while sitting or falling back from floor sitting to roll along the back as possible test movements. Muscle energy, strain/counterstrain and other techniques used to reduce muscle and structural imbalances would be enhanced by a little student self-awareness of the subjective and internal differences in musculoskeletal organization achieved as a result of that technique. If they know what they're doing, they can do what they want. If they know what they are doing differently as a result of your intervention, they will be more likely to be able to maintain or reproduce it at home, at work and at play. Make them pay attention!

This lesson, as it did in the schematic representation of falling earlier in this chapter, features the extremities moving

Box 3.8 Be a Better Ball

Global torso flexion – rotational and side bending variations

Head moves as extension of torso, linked to orientation downward from supine

Orientation from supine and falling backward contexts for torso flexion

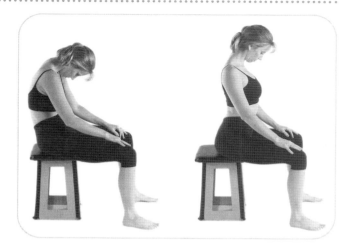

Fig. 3.12 Looking down with and without integration of pelvis and torso – disproportionate movement at lower cervicals, leading to shearing/hypermobility.

globally with the torso. It combines hip flexion with torso flexion; the iliopsoas and abdominal muscles are synergists in this movement. This lesson also combines shoulder flexion and adduction with torso flexion; the pectoralis major and its underlying intercostals, as well as the abdominals, are synergists. These global patterns of movement, with the arms and legs moving as extensions of the torso, can be very useful clinically but are primitive.

By primitive, I don't mean unrefined or outdated. I mean that these patterns emerge and are used early in life. Although babies use these global movements a lot, adults don't so much: they use mostly differentiated movements and need to be taught movement skills within a context of those more frequently used movements. Williams Flexion and McKensies Extension exercises (or informational exercise versions of them) can be useful initially but need at some point to evolve to a more mature level.

Applications

We could use this lesson with students having some types of lumbosacral dysfunction. If it hurts to extend the lumbar spine, move toward flexion. If they have a habitually lordotic lumbar spine or are unable to fully flex the lower back, use this lesson. Hyperextension in the lumbopelvic region could be associated with facet joint irritation, sacroiliac (SI) or lumbar ligamentous strain, SI or lumbar joint shearing and instability, spondylolisthesis, or disc shearing and derangement (Box 3.8).

These can all be local tissue dysfunctions resulting from gross motor movement imbalances – in this case anterior pelvic tilt and lumbar hyperlordosis. Regardless of the exact tissue under stress, we can take a motor learning approach to our exercise prescription and treat the postural or gross motor behavior that contributes to the problem.

We could use this lesson with our students who shear the lower cervical segments forward on top of the upper thoracic segments when looking down. Some people who do this have a very flat and rigid thoracic spine, and this could be a good lesson for these folks to understand how to allow the torso to participate by rounding when looking down (Fig. 3.12). Paradoxically, I could also use this lesson with people who are hyperkyphotic through the thoracic spine and ribcage.

Performing alternating shortening and lengthening contractions of the anterior intercostals and abdominals can help set the muscle spindle at a new and longer length and thereby reduce the action of kyphosing. We may even be stimulating a stretch reflex in the elongating back extensors and posterior intercostals and encouraging an increase in tonus of these muscles. This increase will be even more likely if we get a longer muscle spindle tripwire in the anterior torso muscles because of the reduction of reciprocal inhibition.

As abdominal tone decreases, the CNS reduces inhibitory signals to the back. Clinical manifestations of excessive thoracic kyphosis include lower cervical joint instabilities (as the more delicate cervical vertebrae and musculature are asked to pull heavy loads into extension without assistance from the mid-back), disc and joint degenerative changes, and postural stresses on muscle and connective tissue as the head unbalances toward falling forward. We will examine some of these scenarios in more detail when we look at lessons combining orientation and balance functions.

We could use this lesson with people who have suffered a stroke, using it to help them regain left/right balance in movement and to regain confidence in controlling falls backward by taking them all the way back to basics. Perhaps by directing the different variations of torso flexion we can help in redirecting neurological signals to wake up the affected side. By placing hand and knee together and moving both extremities in coordination with the torso, we can begin to reintegrate the extremities with the torso.

By directing orientation (look toward the foot as you lift your head) and side-bending and rotating in both directions, we can influence one-sided neglect. By engaging the abdominals and intercostals, we might get a rebound effect of doing a stretch excitation of the back extensors and improve their ability to sit or stand more erectly, or to look or reach overhead.

We could use this lesson for people who have had heart surgery, mastectomy or chronic obstructive pulmonary disease, using it to help mobilize the ribs and chest and to work the intercostals in shortening and lengthening contractions. Use this lesson for anyone in whom trunk control or mobility is an issue: multiple sclerosis, Parkinson's disease or ankylosing spondylitis. Be creative: think of these early/primitive lessons as the nuts and bolts of movement that can provide great benefit for a wide variety of conditions.

What sorts of performance could we enhance with this lesson? What activities require flexion? Gymnastics/tumbling or diving maneuvers that require a tuck might be refined. Some wrestling or grappling-style martial arts moves are performed lying supine with legs and head lifted. In falling-style martial arts such as judo or aikido, an ability to flex fully both to fall safely and to roll back up again is useful.

Variations

Here are some other variations of the same basic lesson you may wish to explore. Changing hand position on either the knee or the head adds several subvariations that you can progress your students toward and which introduces increasingly complex and refined options to the same basic movement. Holding on to your knee from the outside, holding instead behind the thigh near the knee from either the outside or the inside, holding one knee with your forearm, or holding the foot from either the outside or the inside are possibilities. Describing the complexity and subtlety of differences in these subvariations is beyond the scope of this book. You'll have to do your own research here.

Holding the back of the head, holding the same-side or the opposite-side ear, or holding the opposite side of your face with your forearm behind your head are subvariations for hand placement on the head. Subvariations are ways of applying increasingly complex constraints on movement that result in increasingly specific skeletal trajectories and antagonist coordination.

Positional variations can be performed in sitting. Sit on the floor and lean back on one hand. Place one hand behind your head and move to bring your elbow and first one knee then the other towards each other. Subvariations are as described above for hand on head. Alternatively, sit on the floor and lean back on one hand. Hold the same then the opposite knee or foot, and move knee or foot and forehead/chin/temple/cheek toward each other. Subvariations for this lesson include hand placement on knee or foot as described above and leaning back on elbow/forearm instead of hand (Fig. 3.13).

This positional variation takes advantage of a *falling backward* functional context to further facilitate torso flexion. It also introduces an upper extremity closed kinetic chain component that we will come back to in Section 4. Here is a toy variation. Do it with a rolled-up towel or hard foam roller lengthwise along your back. Add up the variables and try to guess how many different movements we have performed with just this one lesson and a few described variations – this might give you an appreciation of how vast this body of knowledge is! And it is just one lesson of thousands!

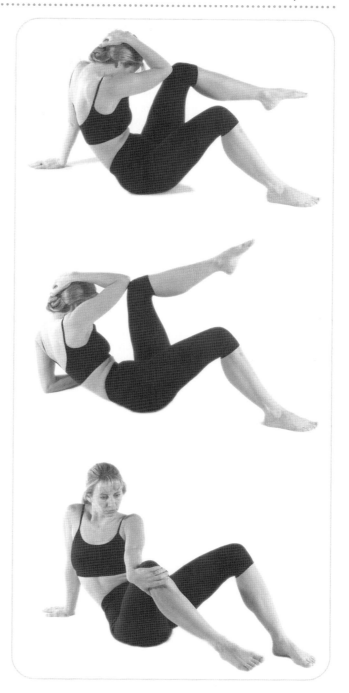

Fig. 3.13 Some positional options and subvariations for this lesson.

Next up

Logically, the next lesson should be lying on your belly and lifting your head to look forward toward the horizon in a mirror image of our last lesson. I could have done this and almost did, but decided instead to do another lesson that leads up to it. We will continue here with orientation from supine. Developmentally, we are born and spend early infancy in a torso flexion bias. Newborns generally don't like to be laid on their bellies. Their flexion bias mashes their face into the floor, and they don't have the extensor control or strength yet to lift their heads to see their environment. They eat dirt and see carpet close-up.

Newborns are best put on their backs so they can at least see the volume of the room (or the sky) and can roll their heads to look left and right. Because this is also limited orientation capability, they soon learn to slide their heads to look above them (see Fig. 2.13). By above, I mean overhead. When describing movement directions in this book, I will describe those directions from the perspective or orientation of the mover.

When lying on your back, the ceiling is forward, the floor is behind you, up is overhead on the floor and down is toward your feet. If you are on your belly, the floor is forward and the ceiling is behind you. Lying on your right side, the ceiling is to your left and the floor to your right. You will need to pay close attention to directions and be precise in how you move while experiencing the movements.

At any rate, when a baby lying supine wants to see something overhead, it will arch itself to one side or the other and slide its head backward to accomplish this. These are precursor movements to rolling to lie on its belly. Babies are learning to use their back extensors (and to reduce torso flexion tone/bias) before they get on their bellies: they don't have to be placed there by their parents to facilitate back extensor and hence head control. This next lesson mimics this early developmental movement and features homolateral global extension patterns.

Take particular care in this lesson if you have any sensitivity in either your neck or your lower back when moving into extension – a common lament. Follow the good-housekeeping rule and move proportionally. For many of us, this means focusing movement on the mid-back and ribcage and deliberately limiting movement in our necks and lower backs. The other tip to reduce extension strain in your lower back is to make sure your hip joint extends as completely as possible. Get on the floor and try it out but do move gently and slowly. Don't get too ambitious!

London Bridges

Variations

A. Lie on your back and scan your contact against the floor.
- Notice spaces between you and the floor, especially under your neck and lower back. Feel whether your mid-back is flattening toward the floor or is staying rounded and pressing into the floor along just a few vertebrae.
- Feel also your chest. How long is it top to bottom, how deep front to back, and how wide left to right?

B. Still lying on your back, spread your legs and arms out a bit and turn your head to look at your left hand.
- Slide that left hand upward on the floor as if reaching for something above your head.
- Follow that hand with your eyes as it slides upward. Keep looking at your hand as you slide it first overhead then down on the floor toward your left thigh (Fig. 3.14).
- Don't force the movement, but see both how far your hand slides up without lifting away from the floor and how well you can see above you.
- Try it a few times to the left, then switch. Look at your right hand and slide it alternately up on the floor

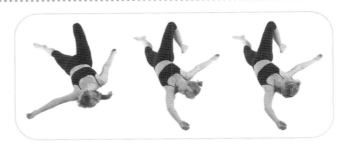

Fig. 3.14 Sliding one arm up and one arm down – looking at left hand, then right.

and down toward your right hip. Follow the movement with your eyes by sliding the back of your head on the floor. Compare the two sides for range, ease and comfort.

C. Lie on your back and bend up your right leg so your right foot is flat on the floor. Find a place where it is best balanced, where it could as easily fall inward as outward, and where weight is distributed evenly on your foot. This is at least hip width.
- Place your right hand on the floor near your right ear with your palm on the floor and your elbow pointed toward the ceiling. Point your fingers as much as possible toward your feet.
- Now place your left hand on your right elbow and move your right elbow left and right with the assistance of your left hand. Balance the weight on your palm so the weight is evenly distributed from thumb side to little finger side (Fig. 3.15). Once you have found that balance point, stay there.
- Now begin to make a small movement to bring your right elbow and right knee away from each other. You will lightly press both the palm of your right hand and the sole of your right foot into the ground as you do this (Fig. 3.15).
- Continue to do this movement of pressing hand and foot and moving elbow and knee away from each other, then gently move elbow and knee toward each other while still keeping your foot and hand on the ground. Alternate a few times.
- This time you press hand and foot and extend the movement to lift your hip, shoulder and whole right side of your torso away from the floor. You will have to arch your back and push your chest and belly out and to the left (Fig. 3.15).
- Try experimenting with the timing of your breath. Do you inhale or exhale as you do this? Rest a bit with arms and legs down and compare the two sides.
- Come back to the same position and resume the movement of right elbow and right knee away from each other. Segue into lifting your whole right side from the floor.
- Lift both shoulder and hip together, but now lower first your shoulder to the floor, then your ribs, then

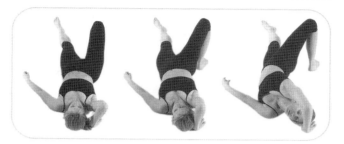

Fig. 3.16 Looking under the bridge – right torso extension.

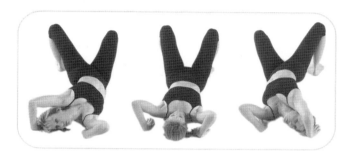

Fig. 3.17 Alternating bridges – can you keep both elbows and both knees pointed to the ceiling?

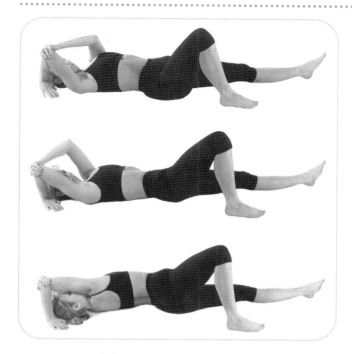

Fig. 3.15 London Bridge with knee and elbow close – separating – apart – lifting the whole right side.

your waist, then finally your hip. Lower sequentially from shoulder to hip (Fig. 3.15).

- Try lowering sequentially from hip to shoulder. Which way is easiest?

D. Do a mirror image of C. Bend up left leg and place left hand on floor with right hand on left elbow. Follow same directions as in C.

E. Come back to the position of lying on your back with your right leg bent up and your right hand standing on the floor near your right ear, still holding right elbow with left hand.

- Press hand and foot into the ground to move elbow and knee away from each other and lift right hip, shoulder and torso from the floor.
- Then slide the back of your head under your right elbow. You will be facing to the left and sliding the back of your head to the right as if you wanted to look toward your right wrist.
- Remember to move proportionally. Be careful of your neck and lower back and emphasize the movement at your mid-back and hip (Fig. 3.16).

F. Do a mirror image of E. Left leg and left hand up and slide head under left elbow as if looking toward left wrist. Compare sides.

G. Lie on your back with both legs bent and both hands standing with palms flat on floor near your head and elbows pointed forward toward the ceiling.

- Move right elbow and right knee away from each other and slide head under right elbow. Can both elbows and knees stay pointed toward the ceiling?
- Do it now with the left side and compare.
- Alternate from side to side. Rest and review contact, contrasts (Fig. 3.17).
- Simultaneously move both right elbow and right knee and left elbow and left knee away from each other. This may flatten your whole back and neck towards the floor.
- Extend this movement if you'd like to lift both hips, then both shoulders, then both hips and shoulders from the floor to hang your head backward and upside down, as if you wanted to put the top of your head on the floor. Do this only if you are very confident in your abilities (Fig. 3.18).

H. Lie on your back with your legs long and arms down on the floor somewhere out away from your sides.

- Compare and contrast the contact you make against the floor to when you started this lesson.
- Compare and contrast your impression of the dimensions of your chest/ribcage to when you started.
- Slide left hand overhead and watch it as it goes. Do the same with the right hand. How do these movements feel in comparison to the beginning?
- Stand up and feel balance of head. How tall do you feel?

are using both orientation (look at hand as it slides) and manipulation (as if reaching for something overhead) as functional contexts.

Making the hand analogous to the foot

In variations C and D you are instructed to place the ipsilateral palm of the hand and the sole of the foot on the ground and point the elbow and knee to the ceiling. Find balance of both hand and foot on the ground and move elbow and knee away from each other. This encourages a pushing of both hand and foot into the floor. I will defer discussion of the muscular breakdown of both the upper and lower extremity until later chapters, but we can say now that we are pushing the extremities backward to facilitate an extension movement through the torso.

The hip is clearly extending and the arm and shoulder girdle are moving in a version of extension that is clearly backward and clearly assisted by torso extension. This could be said to be true of any movement of the arm behind the frontal plane, whether the arm is down at the side, in 90° abduction or in full forward elevation. This is a global extension pattern, performed homolaterally. The right lower and upper extremities are extending along with the right side of the torso; this is the right torso extension we saw in the schematic of falling forward and to the left, but in an entirely different relationship to gravity and in a different functional context.

Recall from Section 1 the term Legos. This is a basic, recurring pattern or chunk of torso movement that is put together in different ways relative to the head and extremities, to gravity and to varying functional contexts. We'll keep an eye out for this particular movement in later sections and in later lessons in this section – it's a very good one to know! The muscular breakdown for this movement at the torso is the same as in the description for the schematic of falling forward and to the left movement of right torso extension.

How did you organize your breath with these movements? In the first lesson around flexion, you may have found an exhalation on the effort of lifting and flexing to be most effective. In an extension movement, we may wish to direct our students to inhale on the effort. Bringing a breath in while extending helps expand and lengthen the anterior chest and belly and inhibits the abdominals and anterior intercostals. Attention to breath also brings in that aspect of vegetative functioning, as it did in the first lesson.

Variations of lowering shoulder first or hip first require an ability to differentiate upper from mid-thorax, mid-back from lower and pelvis from lower back. They are constraints that allow the student to explore options off the same basic movement. We ask that Goldilocks question again: which way of differentiating upper from lower torso seemed easiest to you? Probably 90% (estimate out of a hat) of you will find lowering the shoulder first to be easiest.

Is this because the scapula is somewhat detachable from the torso and can touch the ground even before the back does? Is it because the leg is stronger and can better hold the weight of the body off the ground? Is it because lowering the hip first requires both more strength and more flexibility in the direction of extension from the mid to the upper thorax?

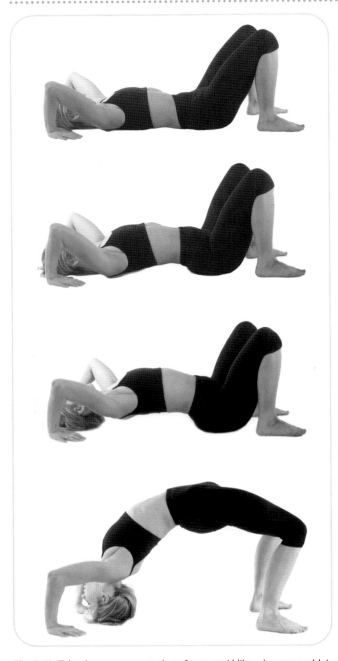

Fig. 3.18 Take the movement only as far as you'd like – be reasonable!

Static and dynamic baselines

The first two instructions in variations A and B are to again provide proprioceptive reference points. What is your contact? What are the dimensions of your ribcage? How easily did your hand slide overhead, and how did that change by the end of the lesson? How easily were you able to look over your head from lying on your back, and how did that change? How did the two sides compare? We saw this technique of getting our students to subjectively measure static and dynamic baselines in our first lesson, and we will see it throughout this book. We

Can we answer such a question with EMG (electromyographic) findings?

Regardless of how well or accurately someone does these more complex variations of the same basic movement, they are learning something that will very likely result in their feeling a positive difference in themselves (providing they followed the good housekeeping rule) in general. We might also anticipate their feeling that both our simpler variation of lifting and lowering hip and shoulder simultaneously and our original test movement became easier. How does this happen?

What I have observed is that by introducing complex variations of basic movements with my students, movement that in the beginning felt difficult or jerky becomes easier and smoother. Movement quality changes. The changes are both visible to an experienced eye and felt by the attentive participant, and are therefore more likely to be adopted and used.

What's up with the opposite hand on the elbow? That hand is there for a couple reasons. One is to help to position the standing hand. This is a somewhat difficult position for many people to get into, and especially to hold for a while. The holding hand is partly to give the standing arm some help in staying upright. The other reason is for biofeedback purposes. The hand can help us feel where the held elbow is in space and what direction it is moving in. Some of the instructions were to find a place where the elbow is vertical over the palm. Some of the instructions were to move the elbow upward away from the descending knee and downward toward the ascending knee.

Both movement and position awareness can be enhanced by monitoring the action through touch. The hand is chock-full of information being fed to the CNS. The opposite hand is also a representative from the other side of the brain. Perhaps learning is occurring already that results in easier movement to the other side. In homolateral movements we sometimes invite a witness from the other side to observe and learn from the festivities. Why move elbow and knee both toward and away from each other? As before, making reciprocating movements helps coordinate antagonists, establishes more accurately where middle is, and spring-loads the antagonists.

Slide your head to look – linking exercise to functional context

In variations E and F we have a continuation of the same movement with the additional intention to slide your head back underneath your standing elbow to look toward the standing hand. This is the movement that mimics the description of a baby's movement at the beginning of this segment. It is not exactly the same, as babies are unlikely to use the leg and arm this way, but it's close enough. Adults often have difficulty going all the way back to the primitive global torso patterns, especially global torso movements, without extremity support.

Even though something may happen earlier in the developmental sequence, it doesn't necessarily mean that this is where we will start. It has been a long time since infancy for most of our students, so movements from later in the sequence are usually more appropriate places to start. Work backward from there to more primitive if you like. In general, I will start with simpler differentiated movement lessons and decide

whether to progress or regress them from there. I like and use this lesson more than I do a lot of the other global movement lessons, not just because of how it facilitates torso movement but also because of what it teaches about control of the scapula.

How did you do with this variation? Did the intention to look make a difference for you in terms of your coordination, ease or range of movement? Orientation is an early and powerful influence on movement organization, and this movement closely approximates a very important step in our early development. The CNS is now reminded of some of those older, unused movement patterns and can dust them off and bring them back out to help with this odd riddle we have provided. When was the last time you did this movement? It is novel enough to the adult nervous system that it provides a puzzle to be solved.

We give hints and suggestions, but the solution to how to move your own body has to be arrived at personally. Presenting the CNS with a puzzle forces it to figure out how to move several different bones in such a way as to fulfill the requirement to look toward the hand. It has to figure out what muscles need to work and what muscles need to be inhibited. It has to coordinate the antagonists. It has to pay attention and learn to choose wisely from different options. It searches past experiences for clues to the riddle, and happens to find them in the early orientation-from-horizontal bin.

Come to the same basic position in variations G and H but with both legs and both arms standing. Alternate movement of sliding head under elbow and looking toward hands, both left and right. This both allows a back-to-back comparison of differences between left and right sides and provides another sneaky constraint. By alternating sides, we are helping to coordinate and balance the extensors on the two sides and helping to bring about a more accurate neutral. By asking both elbows and both knees to remain pointed toward the ceiling, we are putting an additional constraint for horizontal adduction on the opposite-side hip and shoulder, for more precise and proportional movement of the torso or both.

This position also lends itself well to the coup de grace, pushing both hands and feet into the floor to lift the whole body away from the floor in an antigravity, bilaterally symmetrical global extension pattern. The movement is beautiful but deadly; please be careful whom among your students you progress into this variation. You can nibble around the edges and feel them out by having them lift first both hips high in the air, then lifting the shoulders and upper back away from the floor as if putting the top of the head on the ground (Fig. 3.19). If they can't do both of these movements with comfort and aplomb, think twice before giving them the idea of lifting both.

Comparing baselines – what changed from the beginning?

We come back to our baseline in variation I. How are you contacting the floor? Could your lower back be closer to the floor even though you have been moving into extension? This happens fairly frequently, especially with people with thoracic kyphosis. As they learn to access their mid-back extensor

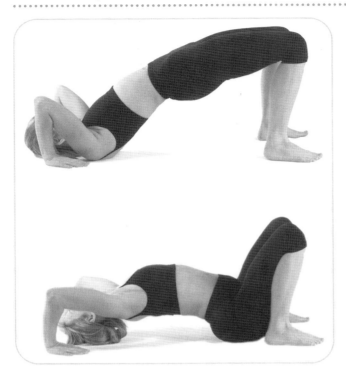

Fig. 3.19 Use these two movements as criteria to determine whether to progress to a full bridge.

muscles and posterior intercostals, they are also learning to inhibit their anterior intercostals and upper abdominals – the thoracic curve flattens and brings the very bottom of the kyphosis (the apex of the lumbar lordosis) closer to the ground.

Often the reason a person extends in the lumbar spine so much and has such hard-working lumbar extensors is because the thoracic spine is unable to move in that direction. If the thorax is unable to extend, the low back and neck have to do more (a reverse good housekeeping arrangement) and can become overworked. One thing to look for in people with lordotic postures and pain on extension is the shape and mobility into extension of the thoracic spine and attached ribcage. This is a classic example of looking past the local diagnosis to include relationships to other areas.

What were the dimensions of your chest? How long, how wide, how deep? What kind of question is this? It is a question of self-image. Many people can't accurately point to bottommost and topmost ribs – try this out with a few of your students and see how they answer. Many people don't know their ribs are attached to their spine or their sternum. Many people don't even know that ribs are supposed to move! For the majority of us, this is a place in our bodies that both moves the least and has the poorest self-image. So many problems clinically come from an inability to move through the torso proportionally. This puts strain on the lower back, neck, shoulders and arms (Box 3.9).

If our students can learn to recognize the possibility of movement in this area and incorporate that newly learned (or freshly remembered) movement into everyday activities of

---

Box 3.9 London Bridges

Global torso extension – emphasizes unilateral extension
Head moves as extension of torso, linked to orientation upward from supine
Precursor to rolling to belly and orientation from prone – early extension

walking, looking, breathing, reaching or balancing, they can reduce or eliminate much of the strain on overworked areas. If I had to zero in on the two things I most commonly do with my students, it is teaching them how to move their pelvis from their legs and how to mobilize and integrate movement through the chest/ribcage/thoracic spine.

Applications

Who could we use this lesson with? Beside shoulder and shoulder girdle movement impairments, which we will cover in Section 4, use this lesson to help someone with neck or back pain that results, in part, from excessive thoracic kyphosis and an inability to arch their mid-back. We might use it with people who posteriorly tilt their pelvis and flex too much in their lower back when sitting, or who flex too much in bending. We could also use this lesson with people with scoliosis and left/right torso imbalances. These homolateral movements can help the person feel more clearly their imbalances and give them resources for use at home. We might ask them to work more often in the nonhabitual direction to help balance out the two sides.

We might use this lesson, as we did the previous lesson, in people with strokes. Start on the unaffected side first to educate the CNS about extremity-to-torso synergistic relationships, and then progress to the affected side to encourage reintegration and discourage one-sided neglect. Use extremity movement to facilitate trunk control, and integrate trunk activity with the extremities to wake up the hip and shoulder extensors. As with the global flexion lesson, we could use this lesson for people who have had heart surgery, mastectomy or chronic obstructive pulmonary disease, helping to mobilize the ribs and chest and helping to work the posterior intercostals in shortening and lengthening contractions. Use this lesson for anyone where trunk control or mobility is an issue: multiple sclerosis, Parkinson's disease or early ankylosing spondylitis.

What sort of performance requires global extension patterns? Rebounding in basketball, serving in tennis, and spiking or serving in volleyball. Many swimming strokes have an extension phase: the crawl, breaststroke, backstroke and butterfly all have the upper extremities and torso moving synergistically in global or unilateral extension patterns. Certain movements in ballet and figure skating are examples of global extension use in artistic performance.

Variations off the main path

How about a few variations? You can do this movement with the standing hand against the wall and sliding the back of the head underneath the elbow while either sitting or standing. Try it with both hands against the wall in sitting and standing, and moving as if to put the top of the head against the wall. Some people cannot get their hands into this standing position because of sensitivity in their wrists or limitation of movement in their shoulders or mid to upper back.

We can still do the same basic movement by sliding the hands and head with just the foot standing. We could start with both arms on the floor out at shoulder height and keep the relationship between them the same, as if holding a long stick between the hands. With your right leg bent, simultaneously slide your right hand down toward your right foot and your left hand overhead while keeping a real or imaginary stick between your hands (Fig. 3.20).

Try variations of rolling your head to look at the right hand as it reaches toward your right foot. Try sliding your head and keeping your nose always pointed toward the ceiling. Try sliding your head backward on the floor to look at your left hand as it reaches overhead. This is the variation that most closely approximates our baby movement.

Subvariations to this basic sequence involve placing one or both hands on the head and sliding hand and head together. This is a commonly used constraint that we also used in our last lesson – 'move this and that together as one.' This whole variation of sliding the arms rather than standing them can be brought up to vertical and against a wall. Stand leaning with your back and pelvis against a wall and with your feet placed out away from the wall at about shoulder width. Your hips and knees should be bent at an angle that mimics your original position on the floor. Interlace your fingers and put both hands behind your head, then slide your elbows, shoulders and head from side to side on the wall. How are you going to coordinate the movement of your pelvis on the wall with this?

Be creative and come up with some of your own variations – you could easily build another three or four lessons from the above descriptions!

Orientation from prone

This next lesson features global extension patterns linked to orientation while lying prone. Those of you with sensitivity in your lower back when lying prone, or who experience discomfort on lumbar extension, will have to be particularly careful. Although this is not a lesson I use a lot in my practice, there are several therapeutic exercise variations of this type of movement. If you are familiar with and like that family of exercises of lying prone and lifting an arm, a diagonal arm and leg, or if you like doing the same basic thing up on hands and knees, this lesson will be familiar.

This lesson will have a few more variations, will be a bit more dynamic and multiplanar, and will contain elements of proprioceptive self-awareness training and functional context. Although this is a popular exercise among physical therapists, I believe that for many people it is a bit advanced. When doing global extension patterns it is very easy to extend dispropor-

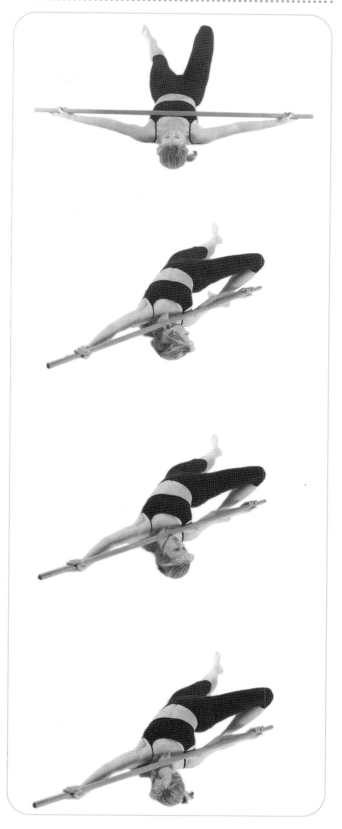

Fig. 3.20 Starting position and head variations for related lesson.

tionately, with most movement occurring at the low back and neck and less in the mid-back/chest. There are safer and more functional ways of training the back extensors, as we'll see in subsequent chapters.

Developmentally, lying prone and lifting the head is an all-important and much sought-after skill for the ambitious young-ster. Once a baby has learned to roll on to its belly (as an extension of the intention to look above its head, as in London Bridges), the first order of business (before it learns to support its weight with its hands, crawl, creep, or come to sit) is to lift its head to orient to the horizon and to learn to control the fall of its head back down to the floor.

When she was very small, my niece was a very crabby and demanding baby. She was born with the idea that she should be able to do everything that she saw adults do. She especially liked to be held upright and faced outward. She wanted to see what was going on and to be part of the action. If we put her on the floor, she cried and begged to be picked up. She was very persistent, and earplugs were standard equipment when baby-sitting.

Although she didn't like the floor all that much, we tried to get her to at least spend some time there so that she could learn to roll to her belly, lift her head, come up to sit and so on. When she was finally able to roll to her belly and lift her head to look around on her own, she became much less crabby. When she learned to crawl around to get to stuff, she was happy. When she learned to stand and walk, we were all ecstatic.

We all have a very strong desire, manifest at a very early age, to explore our environment. To do that, we need to gain some control over our bodies. Because our CNS at birth is so plastic and has so relatively few hard-wired movement patterns, we have to learn that control through experimentation. We struggle and fail and struggle again. I remember watching both my own kids and my niece when they were at that early stage of learning to lift their heads from prone. They would wriggle and squirm, lifting head, arms and legs in globally synergistic patterns, then collapse back to the ground again. Resting a moment, they would try it again. Learning to control the lowering of the head back down again is another skill; going too fast and hitting your head is a developmental no-do. I watched them bob their heads in a jerky fashion as they tried to lower down, went too fast, caught themselves but overcorrected and lifted too high, lowered back down again and so on. Sometimes they would face-plant, but we tried to keep them off the tile floor and no permanent injuries occurred.

This is where we begin to learn balance, which in essence is the need to keep our heads from hitting the ground. These children would spend several frantic minutes learning and prac-ticing this new skill, then would need to lie back down to rest. They reminded me of salmon struggling to jump a waterfall: they put everything they had into it and knew that failure was not an option. If only our students would be that motivated with their home exercises!

Get down on the floor and do what you can with this lesson. Remember the good housekeeping rule and remember that causing yourself pain as you move is highly undesirable from a motor learning perspective. Remember to stop and rest at each major break, designated by the capital letters.

Xs and Os

Variations

A. Lie flat on your back with legs down long on the floor and with arms on the floor somewhere below shoulder height.

- Be aware of how your body rests on the floor. Where are there spaces or gaps between you and the floor?

- How are your arms and legs arranged? Are your legs spread apart or close together? Are your arms held in closely or out away from your sides?

B. Still lying on your back, place both arms on the floor over-head and spread your legs fairly wide on the floor. Imagine trying to make an X, with one leg and its oppo-site arm lined up. Do the same to the other side and you have made an X.

- Gently press your right heel and the back of your left hand backward into the floor. Press along this diag-onal and feel the consequences or the contribution of your torso to this movement. How easy is it to move, and how easy is it just to be in this position (Fig. 3.21)?

- Press now the opposite diagonal – left heel and back of your right hand press back into the floor. Compare this diagonal to the first.

- Press all four extremities back into the floor at the same time. What happens in your back? Your shoul-der blades? Your neck?

- Now lift your legs and arms off the ground and move both elbows and both knees towards each other in front of you. You can slide up your feet and bend your knees before you lift your legs.

- Just bring everything together in front as you round your back and lift your head from the floor. Think of curling up into a ball, or into the shape of an 'O' in this position (Fig. 3.21).

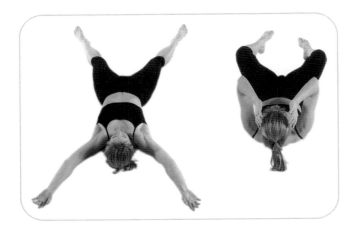

Fig. 3.21 X is the starting and open position – O is the curling movement to close.

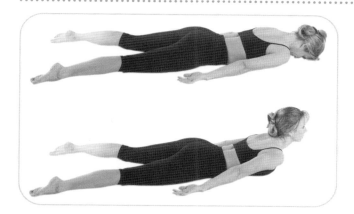

Fig. 3.22 Initial movement of lifting head to look forward.

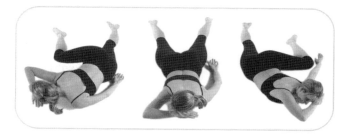

Fig. 3.23 Lift and lower a few times – slide hand and head side to side – lift and move side to side.

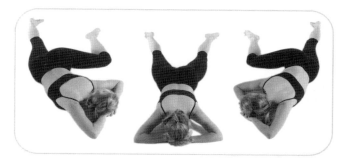

Fig. 3.24 Alternating sliding elbows – head turns as you come through the middle.

C.   Turn to lie on your belly. Lie for just a moment with your forehead on the floor and both of your arms down on the floor by your sides.

* Lift your head off the ground as if you wanted to look forward along the floor. Can you see the bottom of the wall in front of you? Don't strain your neck as you get a sense of how you do this movement. How easy is it? How far forward/up can you see (Fig. 3.22).

D.   Lie on your belly with your head turned to the right; the left side of your face will be contacting the floor. Place your left arm down on the floor by your side and your right arm up on the floor near your head, with hand and elbow resting on the floor.

* Rest the left side of your face on the back of your right hand and lift your right hand, forearm and elbow a little bit off the floor along with your attached head.

* Lift arm and head together with nose still pointed to the right. How heavy does this seem? How do you organize your back to assist? What happens down in your legs? Do one or both start working or lifting away from the floor (Fig. 3.23)?

* Keep your right hand/head together and on the floor this time as you slide your whole elbow/arm/head/shoulders/upper chest from side to side on the floor. Slide to the right as if reaching with your right elbow and looking downward toward your right hip.

* Slide to the left as if reaching with your right elbow and looking upward above you on the floor (Fig. 3.23).

* Alternate this movement a few times, then lift the whole arm/head/elbow off the floor and continue the same side-to-side movement while lifted just a fraction off the floor. Feel your back and your ribcage move and work.

E.   Do the same to the other side. This is a mirror image with your head turned to the left, your right arm by your side and your left arm up by your head.

* How does this side compare to the other? How are your legs and back contributing to this movement?

* Lie on your back and curl up in an 'O.'

F.   Lie on your belly with both arms up by your head. Rest one hand on top of the other and your forehead on top of your hands.

* Slide both elbows/forearms/hands, along with your head on your hands, alternately left and right. Turn your head in the direction you are sliding your elbows. Turn to look to the right as you slide elbows to right and turn head to left as sliding elbows left. (Fig. 3.24).

* Continue to do the same alternating movement of sliding elbows and looking right and left with elbows/forearms/hands along with head lifted off the floor.

* Are your legs or is part of your back waking up? Have they pitched in to help yet?

* Come back to resting your forehead on the floor with your arms at your sides. Lift your head to look forward along the floor, then up along the wall in front of you. How is this movement organized now in terms of range or ease?

* Lie on your back and curl into an 'O.'

G.   Lie on your belly with your head turned to the right. Place the left side of your face against the back of your right hand as before. Now place your left arm somewhere on the floor above shoulder height.

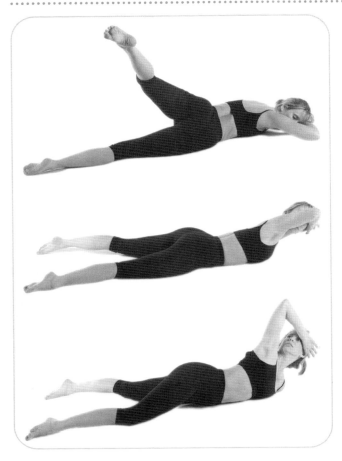

Fig. 3.25 Reaching elbow toward the ceiling – rocking along the diagonal.

- Lift your hand/arm/elbow/head together again, but this time reach with your right elbow toward the ceiling. You will also be turning your face more to the right to look behind you toward the ceiling. Do this a few times then rest. (Fig. 3.25).

- Continue the same movement, but now as you lower your right arm and head back down to the floor, lift your left leg off the ground as if reaching your left foot toward the ceiling.

- Think of rocking all along the front of your torso with your opposite arm and leg moving like a teeter-totter; as you lift your left leg to reach your foot, allow your left hip and left lower belly to also lift from the floor and your weight to roll up the front of your torso to press the right side of your chest into the floor.

- As you lower your left hip and leg back to the floor, you lift again your right elbow/arm and head to look toward the ceiling. Roll alternately along your front side like a runner on a rocking horse, making a diagonal from the front of your right shoulder and chest to the front of the left hip and lower belly (Fig. 3.25).

H. Do the movement as a mirror image to the other side. Head turned left, lifting left elbow and right leg and rolling along diagonal from left front of shoulder and chest to front of right hip and lower belly.

- Compare this diagonal to the previous one. Which is easier? How are your back and legs participating now?

- Come back to our original movement with your forehead on the floor and your arms at your sides. Lift your head to look forward and up again. How does this feel now? How much of your front side lifts away from the ground?

- Lie on your back and feel your contact – compare to the beginning. Put your arms above you on the floor and spread legs to make an X – press along diagonals and all four at the same time. Compare this to the beginning.

- Alternate between making an 'X' and making an 'O' while lying on your back.

- Stand up and feel the balance of your head and the shape of your back and neck. Look overhead – look up and to the right – up and to the left. How does your whole body move to support this intention to look up?

Static and dynamic baselines – Xs and Os

In variation A we are again lying supine and scanning for information. These are the usual questions about contact as a whole and about differences between left and right. Questions about the distance of the upper and lower extremities from the sides are interesting. Did you feel a change in how far out from the midline you placed your arms and legs compared to the beginning? Without getting metaphysical here, I have observed how some people tend to pull in more than others. They stay narrow, with arms and legs pulled in close to the core while sitting, standing and lying. The analogous movement in the torso is toward flexion or pulling together.

As some people progress through this extension lesson, they begin to pull apart and spread themselves wider. They open up their chests and bellies and allow their extremities to abduct and externally rotate as a synergistic echo of the changing torso bias. Although generally I think this is a good thing, there is a point to be clarified here. I am not saying it is bad to make a movement of pulling in the extremities and torso and getting narrow. I do not believe there are any inherently bad movements, and believe that the more options we have in movement the better.

The problem comes in when someone always does the same thing or does that thing poorly. It is the invariance or the inefficiency of the movement that is causing problems, not necessarily the movement itself – repetitive stress injuries are not only common in the arms and hands, but are epidemic in the spine and legs. If someone is holding herself consistently narrow, teach her lessons that access that oppositional direction.

Conversely, we also work with people who are markedly biased in the other direction. These folks will lie supine with legs and arms wide and externally rotated, and are very restricted in adduction, horizontal adduction and internal rotation. With these students we would also emphasize movements into unfamiliar or nonhabitual directions. Do not think in terms of good and bad movements, just imbalanced ones.

Motor control exercise is not so much about always avoiding 'the bad thing' and doing 'the good thing' as it is about balancing and coordinating antagonists (muscles and directions of movement), helping people to know more clearly what they are doing and integrating individual parts into the bigger picture of relationships and functional context.

Does primitive mean easy?

With the first movement coming in variation B, lie on your back with your arms above you on the floor and legs spread apart to make an 'X.' Press back of left hand and back of right heel back into the floor – try the same to the other side and compare. Press all four simultaneously. This is another reference point, a dynamic baseline. Does the intention to move distally (hands and feet) elicit a proximal response (did your back participate)? It should, but often doesn't initially. Some people have no idea they can move their extremities as an extension of their torso.

This test movement is likely to have changed by the end with many of you, and it is likely to with many of your students as well. The meat of the lesson was devoted to helping your CNS rediscover the advantages of using extremity and torso musculature synergistically. The 'O' part of the lesson is really just to minimize the likelihood of making your lower back sore. Many people are sensitive going in this direction, so we are balancing out the 'Xs' with 'Os' – balancing the global extension pattern with a global flexion one. You could just do some of the variations from 'Be a Better Ball', or anything that rounds out and relieves extension stress on the low back.

In variation C, lie on your belly with arms at sides and forehead on floor. Lift your head to look forward. We are lucky enough in this lesson to have two dynamic reference points. This is an approximation of the early baby movement we were describing before starting the lesson – lifting the head to orient forward to the horizon. By having your arms down at your sides, you can't cheat (or jump to a later developmental step) by using them to push yourself up. I have seen many people attempt this movement initially with the neck only.

The curse of the doll body

This is a violation of the good housekeeping rule and most people who do this movement this way don't really like the way it feels, and would have a hard time continuing it for any length of time. They are trying to do everything with just the smaller and more delicate neck vertebrae and muscles without asking for help from the larger muscles. When a person is violating the good housekeeping rule in this way, Larry Goldfarb has coined another phrase: 'the curse of the doll body'. Try putting your daughter's Barbie doll on the floor face down and play with what she has to do to lift her head to look forward.

Having a solid plastic trunk that closely approximates the mobility of some of our students, she is only able to extend her poor, overworked neck and can't really see very far. This movement is probably a microcosm for how this person habitually

organizes herself to orient overhead while upright in vertical postures as well. It is unlikely she will be moving her pelvis and back so that her head and neck can move proportionally as an extension of her torso. As we move through the lesson, we progressively require more participation from the extensors (both torso and extremities) to help address this common movement impairment.

What we would like to see is a movement that mimics the response of the worm to falling forward. We would like to see a global torso extension pattern with the upper and lower extremity extensors firing cooperatively and the movement distributed evenly throughout the whole torso. For practical purposes, this means that we would like to see thoracic extension that matches the ability of the cervical and lumbar spine. The muscular breakdown for this movement through the torso is (should be) then exactly like the breakdown for the falling worm.

Why is the involvement of the legs critical to this movement? We can imagine that a worm lying on its belly might lift its head to look forward. As the head raises and the torso extensors kick in, they will have a similar effect on the tail. As the tail lifts (as the pelvis tilts anteriorly), the whole torso bows and both ends are lifted equally off the floor. If we take the tail of that worm and push it back on to the ground, his head can rise up higher and he can see around himself from a much better vantage point (Fig. 3.26). The legs serve a similar purpose. By contracting his hip extensors, the baby is effectively making his pelvis much heavier and a base from which he can lift his head more and with greater ease.

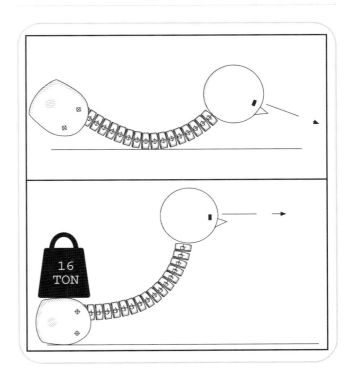

Fig. 3.26 Weighting the pelvis with the legs allows for a higher horizon.

The high horizon

This desire to see from the highest possible vantage seems to be universal across a variety of species. Snakes rear up high on their coils when danger threatens. Turtles push themselves higher with their front legs and lengthen their necks up and forward. Think of how a dog looks when excited: head high, ears lifted, chest out. When looking out for danger (don't want to be eaten) or for opportunity (food, mates, etc.), all species want to get their exteroreceptors as high as possible. Some animals, such as bears, prairie dogs or meerkats, that are officially quadrupeds have even developed an ability to rise up on two feet, all the better to see you with.

We as individuals have followed a similar path. When very young, we had to figure out how to better survey our environment from prone. This determination to see more than carpet leads to lifting the head and activating the torso extensors. By contracting the gluteals we raise the head higher, then higher yet as we discover our arms. Prone prop gets us an even higher horizon. This pushing with the arms continues in a hands and knees position, again with the intention of pushing to an ever-higher horizon. Progress to sitting and standing. This developmental imperative to get the best view or the highest possible horizon is our ally when teaching posture to our students.

We can use orientation from prone or in vertical to encourage our students to lengthen upward as much as possible. This not only enhances orientation, but also improves the balance of the head over the torso by moving the mid-back and chest forward. This brings the thoracic spine underneath the head to push it up higher, and moves the supporting bones of the upper and mid-thoracic spine into a place where they can better carry the weight of the head skeletally.

This functional imperative to get taller is emphasized by this lesson. The ability to become taller is enhanced later when we can push up higher with the assistance of the weightbearing arms (we will use this later to facilitate scapular control for reaching contexts). This ability gets better still after learning to come to sit and to stand. We will later use variations of this intention in those positions to teach the motor, proprioceptive and intentional skills needed for better posture.

Applying constraints – moving like a baby is hard work

In variations D and E you lie on your belly with one arm down at your side and the other up by your head. Place hand and head together and lift them both a little off the floor. This should be a familiar strategy by now: put head and hand together and move them as one unit. This again encourages torso participation, which we want to relink to an intention to see or reach. Now place your face on the back of your hand and slide them together alternately right and left while still on the floor.

Keeping hand and elbow on the floor initially helps to provide a reference point or sounding board for the movement, and is easier than doing it with the head and arm lifted right off the bat. This movement alternates between shortening and lengthening the two sides of the torso and ribcage. It is a version of coordinating the antagonists: in this case the left and right lateral intercostals and, depending on how you do it, the left and right quadratus lumborum and back extensors or the left and right lateral abdominals are playing a cooperative game of tug-of-war.

When we add in lifting the head and arm as a unit and sliding them right and left, we are funneling the side-bending bias toward extension. Needing to extend against gravity and side-bend to look and reach at the same time, we are especially asking the quadratus lumborum, back extensors and postero-lateral intercostals to do some heavy lifting. This is also more like how we really moved as babies. We lifted our heads to look around us 360°. This movement leads later to triggering the same-side knee to draw up in a precursor to a crawling movement (see Fig. 2.15).

Some of you may even have found that you did this drawing-up-the-leg movement in this lesson. What tangled webs we weave! Comparing the two sides, we are likely to feel differences in ourselves and notice differences in our students. None of us is balanced in our torso, and the muscles that side-bend to one side will be stronger (or conversely more flexible) than those on the other side. Because part of the game in motor learning is getting someone to recognize these differences to lessen them, this can be a nice place to make those discoveries (Box 3.10).

In variation F, alternating from side to side gives us another opportunity to make those comparisons and mimics a primitive swimming motion that later gets folded into a commando crawling motion, then a creeping (hands and knees) motion and then a walking motion. This alternating side-bending movement is linked to primitive locomotion because we want to have our students move their ribs in a combination side-bending and rotational movement while walking upright.

We are also crossing the midline with this movement and alternating orientation from left to right. This combination of bending and turning your head in the opposite direction is yet another way to help your student associate an intention to look alternately from side to side with an ability to support this with alternating movements of the pelvis and torso. An intention to move distally (eyes) should elicit a proximal (pelvis and torso) response or initiation. This is another Lego piece, another reprogramming of a subroutine.

Coming back to the original movement of lifting the head to look forward while the arms are at the sides is to again check in with how this important movement is organized. What was your ease and range of torso movement? How are the back and legs participating? Many people will already be feeling improvement in ease and range as a result of recruiting more of themselves to assist in moving. This could easily be the end of its own mini-lesson, or would be a good place to break the lesson in half if you run into student fatigue or run short of time.

Box 3.10 Xs and Os

Global torso extension – rotational and side-bending variations

Head moves as extension of torso, linked to orientation forward or backward from prone

Orientation from prone and falling forward contexts for torso extension

Looking back toward the ceiling rather than forward to the horizon

Progressing to variations G and H, lie on your belly with both arms up. One hand is glued to your head and the back arm long on the floor above your head. Lift head/hand/arm to reach your elbow toward the ceiling and look toward the ceiling at the same time. We make a bit of a switch in the lesson at this point. The direction of orientation changes from looking low along the floor downward (toward hip) and upward (along the floor above your head) to looking backward toward the ceiling. All three of these directions are variations of left or right torso extension. Lifting the head and right arm and moving to look toward the right hip is a right torso extension pattern.

Lifting head and left arm with head turned left and looking/reaching left elbow toward the ceiling is another variation of a right torso extension pattern. Lifting head and left arm with head turned left and moving to look/reach upward is yet another movement into right torso extension (get on the floor to confirm it for yourself). The same is true in mirror image for left torso extension. These asymmetrical torso extension patterns are very important, so keep the variations from this lesson and the London Bridges lesson in mind when we cover differentiation of torso and head later in this chapter.

Why is the back arm now overhead instead of down at your side? Try the diagonal rocking with both variations: arm overhead on the floor and arm down at your side. Which is easier? For many people, having the back arm overhead helps control the movement better. It also asks that the armpit on that side flatten more to the ground when lifting the opposite arm/head – it opens the upper chest and stretches the pectorals.

Lifting right elbow/hand/head Lego from the floor and reaching your right elbow toward the ceiling requires both strength and flexibility. Strength of the back extensors and posterior intercostals, especially the left side, is a prerequisite for this movement, just as it was for falling forward and to the right. Flexibility of the abdominal flexors and anterior intercostals, especially along the right side, is also a prerequisite, just as for falling forward and to the right. Why not just teach this in one position and be done with it?

Putting the same information in different folders

These global orientation and global balance patterns, though very much alike, need to be trained separately because of the tendency of the CNS to place each individual file or Lego into separate folders: a balance folder, an orientation folder, a locomotion folder, a transition folder, a manipulation folder and so on. Exercising an individual muscle, or even a whole-body pattern of movement in just one position, one orientation to gravity or one functional context, is not going to be nearly as effective an approach as one that teaches the same basic movement patterns in a wide variety of positions relative to gravity and relating to a wide variety of functional contexts.

We need to spell it out for the brain: 'use this particular pattern when you have this particular intention.' This is why you will be seeing some of the same basic patterns recurring over and over throughout the different lessons in this book.

You will see asymmetrical torso flexion and extension patterns not only in this chapter on balance and orientation, but also later when we explore transitions and locomotion, and later still when we address upper quarter coordination in gait and manipulation functions. Just remember that knowing what to teach (what needs to get stronger and what needs to get longer) is only half the job. Knowing how to teach is at least as important and is, sadly, a more difficult task.

The next instruction, to lift the opposite leg as you lower the head/arm/elbow back to the floor, is a variation designed to bring attention and intention to the lower extremity contribution to this movement. Physical therapists are no doubt already familiar with this basic movement as a therapeutic exercise performed both prone and on hands and knees. Although the idea is much the same – to facilitate the back extensors to work and the front of the torso to lengthen – there are a few important differences. The therapeutic exercise versions are more static; get into the correct position and hold for the count of ten.

Comparing therapeutic and informational exercise

The intention in quantitative exercise is to contract and strengthen muscles. The informational exercise version is more dynamic: get into the same basic position but move from there into a variation of that position. The intention in the informational exercise version is orientation (look to the ceiling), manipulation (reach elbow or opposite foot toward the ceiling) and balance (rolling along your front side like a rocking-chair runner to lower your head back in a controlled way to the floor without banging your head or mashing your face).

You may have also noticed other differences between the therapeutic exercise and the informational versions. One difference is variety. In therapeutic exercise, we look to position our students in the correct position and have them hold it there, then repeat the exact same movement several times. Depending on whether the intention of the lesson is to gain motor control or achieve muscle hypertrophy, you may have your student move gently and slowly or have them pile on some weights and go to work. In informational exercise, the intent is always motor control.

We nearly always have our students move slowly and gently at first to learn to recognize patterns and reduce extraneous effort, then progress them to faster and larger movements as they gain competence (an aspect of change of venue). This lesson is an example of this strategy. It starts off slowly with lifting, then sliding your elbow/hand/head accompanied by proprioceptive awareness questions. It finishes with a grandiose rocking/swinging movement that will get your average student huffing in no time. In between, there are a variety of movements that are really just subvariations of the same movement: torso extension.

We could say that one difference between therapeutic and informational exercise is that whereas therapeutic exercise is composed of one movement performed precisely in one direction, informational exercise is composed of many movements performed exploratively in several directions (especially reciprocating directions). Therapeutic exercise is the repetitive toot of the one-note flute, whereas informational exercise is a song with many notes and an overall theme or story. Some songs are the simple equivalent of Chopsticks and some are the complex equivalent of Beethoven's *Fifth Symphony* (this lesson is probably somewhere in the range of *The Star-Spangled Banner*).

This is not meant to denigrate therapeutic exercise in any way. It's just that the two versions have a different role to play. Therapeutic exercise is precise in its positioning and disallows compensatory or other undesirable contractions of other muscles. It is designed to activate a specific muscle that does not for some reason participate appropriately in the whole-body actions that it should. Vigilance and precision are mandatory to ensure that the lazy muscle doesn't revert to old habits and leave action to others.

Repetition is necessary to whip the recalcitrant muscle into shape and deepen the pathway in the CNS. Informational exercise encourages exploration of movement variations and invites participation of synergists, both local and distal. It is designed to integrate individual muscles into a coherent whole-body movement system. Creativity and self-awareness are mandatory to ensure that the habit-driven CNS can recognize, choose and change whole-body movement and postural patterns in beneficial ways.

Another difference between a traditional approach to exercise and the motor control approach is the language used. Informational exercise uses both descriptive and inquisitive language. 'Lift your head off the ground as if you wanted to look forward.' 'Slide to the left as if reaching with your right elbow.' 'Turn your face more to the right to look behind you toward the ceiling.' This is descriptive language. What is the action? Reach, look, press, lift, slide, rock, etc. What is the direction? Up, down, forward, backward, toward your chest, toward the ceiling, toward the wall in front of you.

What should it feel like? Pressure changes against the floor, effort, and the participation of other areas in your body. What are you supposed to pay attention to? We use language to train our students in proprioceptive listening and motor decision-making skills. 'How easy is it now?' 'How heavy does it feel?' 'What are your legs doing?' 'How much of your chest lifts from the floor?' This is inquisitive language. Describing movement to someone is difficult. When using these exercises with your students, use language that describes, language that informs, language that directs attention and language that inspires them to want to learn more about themselves to take better control of their musculoskeletal health. This is where the art of teaching comes in.

Baselines and applications

Come back to the original position with your forehead on the floor and arms at your sides. Lift your head to look forward along the floor. Dynamic baseline number one – how did you do? Did you learn anything? Are things moving more proportionally? Further? Are your legs participating?

Now roll back on your back with arms and legs in an 'X.' Press your diagonals and all four extremities at once, as we did to begin with. This is dynamic baseline number two. How goes it? Lie on your back and feel contact against the floor. This is our familiar static baseline. Our final baselines are in standing.

How are you balancing your head? Might you be holding your head higher, as a result of thoracic extensor and posterior intercostals activation, to orient from a higher vantage point? Try looking toward the ceiling, or up and over one shoulder and then the other. Do you organize these orientation movements with global torso extension or right/left torso extension patterns?

Who would we use this lesson with? This is a progression of the London Bridges lesson and would therefore be used for the same sort of clinical problems. Ditto for sport and artistic performance. See further variations of 'belly lessons' in the sections on shoulder girdles and neck.

Orientation from side-lie

The next stop on our tour of horizontal orientation is looking around from side-lying. As you might guess, orientation from side-lying is much like falling sideways. We will be looking at global side-bending patterns. Schematically, the movement lesson in this section is much like some of our previous lessons. We will be applying constraints by putting the hand and head together and having them move as one.

We will be directing and exploring the organization of the breath. Functional contexts will still be orientation (as you lift your head to approach the horizon), balance (controlling the 'fall' of your head as you lower back down), manipulation (reaching hand to foot) and vegetative (breathing). Because it is a relatively simple lesson with many of the concepts having already been developed, we will go through this one fairly quickly.

Be a Better Bow

Variations

A. Lie on your back and sense your contact against the ground.

- Feel how your weight is distributed along your torso from pelvis to head. Is it even or lumpy?

- Feel how your weight is distributed side to side on your pelvis, chest, shoulders and the back of your head.

- Notice if you perceive one side of your torso as being longer than the other. Is the space at your waist the same side to side? Are the ribs along your sides closer together on one side?

- Does your breath fill up one side of your chest or ribcage more than the other side?

B. Lie on your left side. Bend your hips and knees to about 90°. Rest your head on your left upper arm. The left elbow is straight and the arm is on the ground as far overhead as you can comfortably place it. If this position is not possible, roll up a towel or blanket to support your head.

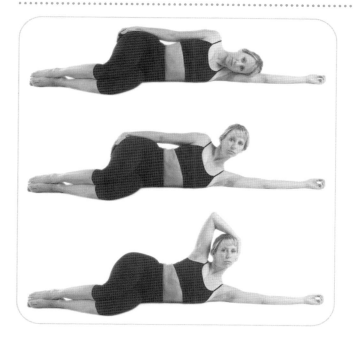

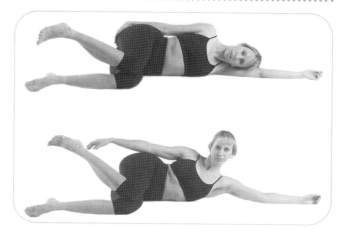

Fig. 3.28 Lift foot and slide hand to lift both ends of the torso at the same time – press the middle to the floor.

Fig. 3.27 Initial position on side – initial lift of head – combine arm and head to lift.

- Lift your head a little away from your left arm, feel the weight of your head and slowly lower back down (Fig. 3.27).

- How much of the side of your torso contributes to this? Does anything along your left side press into the floor? How high does your head lift?

- Reach your right forearm across the top of your head to hold on to your left ear. Lift your head with the assistance of your arm as if you wanted to bring your head to vertical. Don't strain your neck (Fig. 3.27).

- How do you organize your breath with this movement? Try exhaling with the intention of squeezing the air out of the right side of your chest. Try inhaling with the intention of expanding the left side of your chest.

- Making sure your hips and knees are at 90° and keeping your knees together, lift your right foot away from your left and toward the ceiling (Fig. 3.28).

- The knees stay together and the leg maintains its 90°/90° shape. This is a rotational movement at your right hip.

- Does your pelvis move, or does the space in the left side of your waist narrow? Does the left side of your waist and lower ribcage press into the floor? Try lifting both feet, keeping your knees on the floor.

- Start to add in reaching with your right hand toward your lifting right foot. You will have to lift your head to do this and will have to squeeze the whole right side together. Pelvis and shoulder blade move toward each other (Fig. 3.28). Rest after trying this a few times.

- While still lying on your left side, lift your head again. Has its perceived weight changed? Is it lifting any higher or more easily?

- Hold on to your left ear with your right hand as before. Lift your head with the help of your arm, and stay there. Look down toward your knees or feet, along your hip and waist, up along your ribs and under your right armpit. You will have to round yourself to do this. Look up overhead and beyond as if you wanted to see behind you. You will have to arch yourself to do this (Fig. 3.29).

- Alternate rounding and arching movements to look around you as much as possible. Can you see 360° around yourself?

- Lift your head again without the assistance of your hand and notice how this movement is in terms of ease or organization compared to the beginning.

- Turn to lie on your back and compare your contact against the floor to when you started. Compare especially your two sides. Does one feel longer or larger? Does your breath move more easily into one side? Is one side preferable to the other?

C. Do the mirror image of B to the other side. Lie on right side, repeat instructions as above.

- How does the movement of lifting your head feel initially? How does it feel by the end of the lesson?

- Which side of your torso feels stronger? Which one is longer?

- Compare contact and left/right differences while lying on your back once again.

- Stand up; feel left/right balance of torso. Is one side longer here? Walk around. Are there any bending movements of your ribcage or waist as you walk?

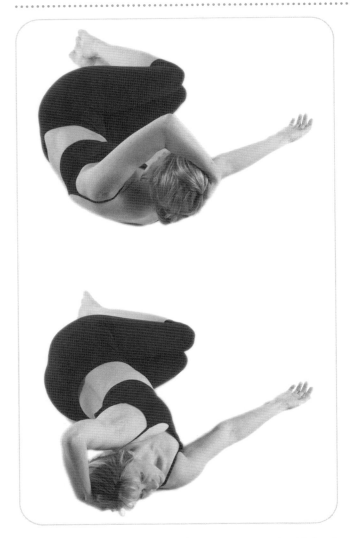

Fig. 3.29 Adding a rounding and arching component to the side bend.

Static and dynamic baselines – Be a Better Bow

This is our familiar static baseline again in variation A. Questioning directs more attention to left/right differences and an awareness of the two sides of the torso. Space in the waist and between the ribs – differences in ease and volume of breath into the two sides. This lesson is a little different from previous lessons in that we spent half the lesson on one side only, running through all the variations, before going in the other direction. We came back to our dynamic baseline (lifting head without arm) during and after the first half, but didn't alternate between sides as we have been doing.

Why might we do this? To create larger differences and more easily perceived contrasts between the two sides. Did you have noticeable or even marked differences between left and right sides at the halfway point in the lesson? Did those differences blur by the end? This strategy of doing all the variations to one side to heighten sensation from and awareness of one

side is a somewhat common one that we will be using again later. We do this especially when working with left/right differences.

The first variation in this long set of instructions in variation B is to establish a dynamic baseline by lifting your head to feel its weight, organization and range. Were you able to get your eyes horizontal? This is another good housekeeping test. Did you use your proportionally larger muscles? We would like those lateral muscles that connect the pelvis and ribcage, the lateral intercostals and the shoulder girdle depressors, to assist the cervical musculature in this movement. As with previous lessons, many people will do this movement initially without integration – they try to do everything with the neck.

The meat of the lesson is designed to help the CNS make these connections and to recognize the disadvantages of moving in a compartmentalized fashion. If you did this movement initially by using quadratus lumborum and lateral abdominals, get on the floor and try it again but doing it deliberately without the assistance of these stronger muscles. This technique of trying out your students' mistakes and experiencing what they feel like proprioceptively can give you valuable insight into what they are feeling and can make you a better teacher. Try mimicking the walk, posture, reaching and orientation habits of your students!

Constraints and subvariations

Our second instruction should be a familiar one by now – put hand and head together and lift them as a unit. By applying this constraint again, we are encouraging the more powerful torso side-benders to participate. The other auxiliary movement in this variation was directing the timing of the breath. Exhaling with the effort emphasizes the contraction of the top muscles of the torso. Inhaling with the effort emphasizes the inhibition and lengthening of the bottom muscles of the torso. Could you do either variation with equal aplomb?

Our third variation is designed to bring the lower torso musculature into the equation if it hasn't awakened yet. Lifting the top foot to internally rotate the hip can trigger a synergistic hip hike on that side and help fire the dormant muscles of the lower torso. Lifting both feet is a more difficult subvariation in terms of requiring the waist to work. Reaching the top hand towards the lifting top foot deliberately coordinates the simultaneous lifting of both head and tail. Feel how powerfully the whole top side has to contract to do this.

Our fourth variation introduces an exploration of flexion and extension bias. Lifting the head and hand together and then looking around triggers torso flexion when looking down and underneath the armpit. Looking overhead and behind you triggers torso extension. How far around yourself can you see? Is your personal bias more toward side-bending with flexion or with extension?

Observing your students as they do previous variations may enable you to guess which bias they have and to direct them to emphasize the nonhabitual direction. This is another example of the dynamic nature of informational exercise. Instead of just doing cardinal-plane side-bending, we are doing side-bending while in varying degrees of flexion or

Box 3.11 Be a Better Bow

Global torso side-bending – flexion and extension variations
Head moves as extension of torso, linked to orientation to the
    horizon from side-lie
Orientation from side-lie and falling sideways contexts for torso
    side-bending

extension. This enhances motor control over both excited and inhibited musculature, and gives our students more options to choose from in real-world situations.

Comparing baselines and applications

At the end of the first half we compared dynamic and static baselines, and then did the whole thing again to the other side. We all have side-bending bias in our torsos – what was your easiest side? Was your easiest side predictable from an awareness of differences between the two sides during our static baseline? There is a good chance that you will be able to bend most easily in the direction that you perceived to be the shortest initially, as that shortness is going to be a reflection of habitualized muscle tone imbalance. We finished the lesson with some observations in standing and walking. Did you feel some side-bending movement in your ribcage when walking? Should there be?

Clinically, we could use this lesson with people with mid- to upper-spinal and shoulder girdle impairments. This side-bending movement tends to be a good one for accessing movement of the upper chest, upper back and cervicothoracic junction. Two of the main stressors for the cervical spine are the lack of mobility of the chest and thoracic spine and the movement and postural imbalances of the upper chest/ back. The floor acts almost as a passive masseur and helps our students to be more aware of a part of their bodies that might seldom participate in functional movement (Box 3.11).

This is really just another lesson in a broader category of lessons: coordinating head and tail. As such, its primary purpose may be to mobilize and gain accurate antagonist reciprocation over the movement of the chest/ribcage/thoracic spine. It is this section of the back that most consistently lags in movement range and control. Because lack of movement in one section of an integrated system necessitates too much movement somewhere else, it is not surprising that what we see clinically are predominantly lower back and mid-lower neck movement impairments that lead to joint, disk or ligamentous breakdown.

This whole first section is filled with head/tail lessons, and most of them are to get the chest to move. Use this lesson for stroke, multiple sclerosis, Parkinson's disease, chest surgeries and other neurological and medical conditions as described in previous lessons in this section. Mobilizing the ribs/chest/thoracic spine and gaining motor control over the trunk and the globally moving extremities is beneficial for many different conditions.

What sports use global side-bending movements? Falling sports such as football and certain martial arts need to have

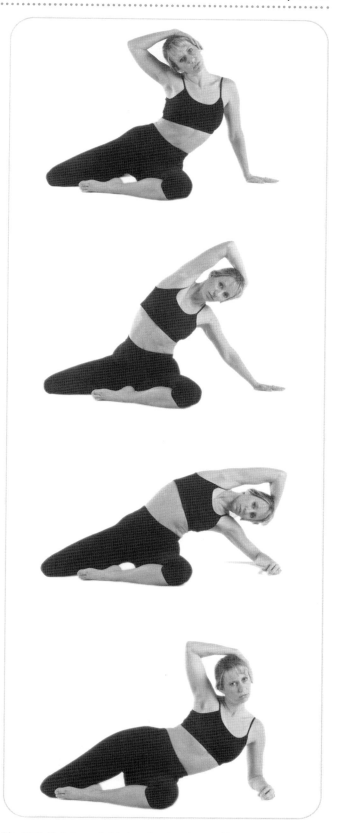

Fig. 3.30 Variations of side-bending in other positions.

flexible and strong sides to avoid players hitting their heads in sideways falls. Kayakers use side-bending movements for low braces, high braces and rolls.

Variations

Variations of this lesson might be performed in more upright positions. Come to side-sit on the floor with your right foot and leg behind you and lean on your left hand out to your side. Place your right hand either on top of your head or, as you did in the original variation, with your forearm reaching across the top of your head to hold your left ear. Alternately, move elbow and hip towards and away from each other as you alternately bend your whole torso from side to side. The key to doing this movement is to roll your pelvis from side to side on the ground – shifting weight from way to the left to nearly on to the right ischial tuberosity. If you allow the right knee to slide toward and away from yourself on the floor, it may help facilitate this rocking of the pelvis. Subvariations include hand placement on the head and leaning on elbow and forearm instead of hand (Fig. 3.30).

References

1. Feldenkrais M. Awareness through movement: health exercises for personal growth. New York: Harper & Row; 1972.
2. Goldfarb L. Articulating changes: toward a theory for the Feldenkrais Method. Berkeley, CA: Feldenkrais Resources; 1990.
3. Kotsias J. Tai-chi tao for physical therapists: applications and interventions. Caledonia, MN: American Tai-Chi Tao; 1996.
4. Fuller RB. Inventions: the patented works of R Buckminster Fuller. New York: St Martin's Press; 1985.
5. Levin SM. A different approach to the mechanics of the human pelvis: tensigrity. In: Vleeming A, Mooney V, Dorman T, eds. Movement, stability and low back pain. Edinburgh: Churchill Livingstone; 1997: 157–69.
6. Byl N, Roderick J, Mohamed O et al. Effectiveness of sensory and motor rehabilitation of the upper limb following principles of neuroplasticity: patients poststroke. Neurorehabilitation and Neural Repair 2003;17:176–91.
7. Winstein CJ, Miller JP, Blanton S et al. Methods for a multisite randomized trial to investigate the effect of constraint-induced movement therapy in improving upper extremity function among adults recovering from a cerebrovascular stroke. Neurorehabilitation and Neural Repair 2003;17:137–52.
8. Wongphaet P, Butrach W, Sangkrai S. Improved function of hemiplegic upper extremity after cognitive sensory motor training therapy in chronic stroke patients: a preliminary report of a case series. Journal of the Medical Association of Thailand 2003;86: 579–84.
9. Karman N, Maryles J, Baker RW, Simpser E, Berger-Gross P. Constraint-induced movement therapy for hemiplegic children with acquired brain injuries. Journal of Head Trauma and Rehabilitation 2003;18:259–67.
10. Stevens JA, Stoykov ME. Using motor imagery in the rehabilitation of hemiparesis. Archives of Physical and Medical Rehabilitation 2003;84:1090–2.
11. Bonifer N, Anderson KM. Application of constraint-induced movement therapy for an individual with severe chronic upper-extremity hemiplegia. Physical Therapy 2003;83:384–98.
12. Jang SH, Kim YH, Cho SH, Lee JH, Park JW, Kwon YH. Cortical reorganization induced by task-oriented training in chronic hemiplegic stroke patients. Neuroreport 2003;14:137–41.
13. Schaechter JD, Kraft E, Hilliard TS et al. Motor recovery and cortical reorganization after constraint-induced movement therapy in stroke patients: a preliminary study. Neurorehabilitation and Neural Repair 2002;16:326–38.
14. Page SJ, Sisto SA, Levine P. Modified constraint-induced therapy in chronic stroke. American Journal of Physical and Medical Rehabilitation 2002;81:870–5.

CHAPTER FOUR

The maturing worm

Chapter outline

Segue from orientation to transitions

1. Lesson 1: *Cherry Turnover.*
   - Coordinating the flexors and extensors. Using spring-loading principles.

2. Transitional movements. Changing positions for the purpose of orientation, manipulation, locomotion, etc. In motor learning approaches, we use transitional movements a lot because:
   - It's a good way to access motor pathways learned in childhood that may have been forgotten or long unused.
   - It's a discrete movement that has a clearly defined goal (functional context) and that students seem to take pride in accomplishing. They can clearly tell they are doing something.
   - Transitional movements, especially towards or within a vertical orientation, always necessitate balance reactions and most often include an orientation component. We can file a newly learned or freshly relearned movement into several functional categories at the same time.
   - Summary lessons and cumulative movements. Use movements you have been building up to as home exercise programs.

3. Why work horizontally at all?
   - Helps to reduce proprioceptive volume.

   - We can go back in history and work with some earlier, developmentally based movements that are ancestors or precursors to the current dysfunctional movements.
   - Use the floor as a passive masseur, rubbing and pressing various parts of ourselves against its untiring and inexpensive surface.
   - The unfamiliarity of the position for most adults: it requires movement out of the habitual. Can't just be on autopilot.

4. Lesson 2: *Baby Rolls.*
   - Really just Cherry Turnover with both arms and both legs off the floor. Literal revisitation of earlier developmental movement.

Orientation from vertical

1. Lesson 3: *Sitting Circles.*
   - Head to tail connections in flexion/extension and in diagonal patterns. Connect the dots into a circle. Even distribution of movement and proportional effort again emphasized in orientation context.
   - Finding anterior/posterior and left/right postural balance as an outgrowth of an ability to move equally easily in all directions. Facilitates skeletal weightbearing organization and a high horizon.
   - Balance responses and direction of orientation congruent.

- Anticipating movement imbalances and inefficiencies through observation of postural organization: posture and movement two sides of the same coin.
- Some differentiation of arms from torso.

2. Lesson 4: *Heads Will Roll*.
   - Positional variation of Sitting Circles.

3. Lesson 5: *Side-sit Spirals*.
   - Orientation left and right along the horizon.
   - Deliberate movements of the eyes – link to functional context of orientation. Disproportional representation of eyes (tongue, lips, thumb) in the CNS.
   - Disadvantages of organizing orientation movements from the top down: violation of proportionality principle. Advantages of proximal initiation and moving from the ground up.
   - Importance of spiraling movement rather than pure rotation: higher horizon and access more upper thoracic segments.
   - First foray into differentiating head/eyes from torso/pelvis. Differentiated patterns created by the juggling of multiple functional contexts. Wind up and throwing ball while looking in the same place. Swinging arms/shoulders in gait while orienting forward.
   - Cumulative movement combines balance, orientation and transitional movements.

Combining orientation and balance

1. Lesson 6: *Eskimo Roll*.
   - Combining falls left and right with intention to read vertical writing (global pattern where head/eyes move as extension of torso).
   - Combining falls with orientation to the horizon (horizontal eyes) to create differentiated patterns.
   - Connection between injury and habitual postural/movement patterns: story of spilling kayak. Impact of injury going to path of least resistance/weak link in the chain. Injury rehabilitation implications.
   - Therapeutic emphasis on nonhabitual differentiated pattern, but do work with habitual differentiated pattern as well. Need to know what not to do as well as what to do.
   - The 'Simon says' phenomenon. People tend to interpret movement instructions as moving in a compartmentalized fashion rather than integrated fashion.

2. Lesson 7: *Sitting Circles II*.
   - Differentiation of head/eyes from torso/pelvis in flexion/extension direction.
   - Fall back (posterior rotation pelvis and flexed torso) combined with orientation to the horizon (cervical extension) to make a differentiated pattern.
   - Fall forward (anterior tilt and extended torso) combined with orientation to the horizon (cervical flexion) to make a differentiated pattern.

- Diagonal differentiations. Circular differentiations if it doesn't fry your circuits.
- Supine facilitation of oh-so-desirable differentiated pattern of lumbar flexion/thoracic extension/cervical flexion. Facilitation of longus colli and rectus capitis as intersegmental stabilizers.
- Roller/toy facilitation of same.

Segue from orientation to transition

Have you ever wondered how it is that babies learn to roll to their bellies initially? Do they just wake up one day and realize that the developmental manuals say they are old enough to try a new position? No, it is the intention to look overhead, as described in Chapter 2, that triggers the roll. This chapter has a lesson and a described variation that recreates this early transitional movement. Recall that at this age the extremities are not generally able to differentiate from the torso, and so global patterns are still emphasized.

This will also be our first lesson where we are officially making reciprocating movements. We will be reciprocating torso flexion and extension movements in the Cherry Turnover, and will be describing 360° rolling in a lesson called, appropriately enough, Baby Rolls. This is a progression of the Cherry Turnover and affects both anterior/posterior and left/right muscular, structural and functional balance. Both of these lessons are integrative: they incorporate elements of all our previous lessons in that we will be doing flexion, extension and side-bending movements all in the same lesson, and will be linking them to the important new functional skill of making transitional movements.

The purpose of this chapter is to continue our exploration of head to pelvis relationships and of trunk control and balance. Horizontal transitional movements will be first, with an emphasis on more complex circular and spiraling movements, followed by balance and orientation movements in a vertical orientation. We will introduce and discuss the clinical relevance of movements that differentiate the head and neck from the pelvis and torso. Principles and concepts of ideal movement and teaching technique are reinforced.

Cherry Turnover

Variations

A. Lie on your back with your legs long on the floor and spread a comfortable distance apart. Arms are also on the floor, somewhere below shoulder height.
   - Be aware of your contact against the floor. Notice what parts along the back of you are pressing into the floor and what parts are lifting away. Where are there spaces between you and the floor?
   - Compare your perception of length along your two sides – compare the length of the two arms – legs – sides of your torso.

- Feel the volume of breath into each side. Which side moves more freely with the movement of your breath?

B. Lie on your right side with your hips and knees bent up to about 90°. Interlace your fingers, place your hands behind your head and support a portion of the weight of your head (the more the better) with your hands.

- Move both elbows and both knees towards each other. The right elbow and knee/thigh will slide on the ground and your whole torso has to round or curl up in a ball. Come back to where you started and repeat.

- Move both elbows and knees away from each other. The elbow and knee still slide on the floor, but now the back arches or straightens.

- Alternate sliding elbows and knees toward and away from each other. How do you time your breath with this? Where are you looking?

- Can you do this movement without rolling toward your front or back? How proportional is the movement of your back in each direction (Fig. 4.1).

C. Repeat instructions as for B to the opposite side. Lie on your left side with interlaced fingers supporting your head and slide elbows and knees toward and away from each other.

D. Lie on your right side with your right hand and forearm supporting the weight of your head as before, but now place your left hand on top of your head. Make sure your hips and knees are bent.

- Move your left elbow and left knee toward each other. Let your head come with the left hand and look toward your belly. Right elbow and knee stay where they are on the floor – they do not slide. Repeat many times.

- Move left elbow and left knee away from each other many times (Fig. 4.2). Right knee and elbow stay where they are, and you look up overhead.

- Alternate moving elbow and knee towards and away from each other.

- Is this movement easier or harder than moving both elbows and knees? Are you still able to be aware of the timing of your breath?

E. Continue to lie on your right side to rest, then place hands as before with left hand on top of head.

- Move left elbow and knee toward each other as before, but this time as you move them away from each other . . .

- Let your left hand separate from your head and reach along the floor overhead. As you straighten your left elbow to reach overhead, also straighten your left knee to reach your foot downward on the floor.

- Both elbow and knee straighten along with your hip, back and shoulder as you turn this movement into . . .

- Rolling back on to your back (Fig. 4.3). You are straightening your arm, leg and back as you

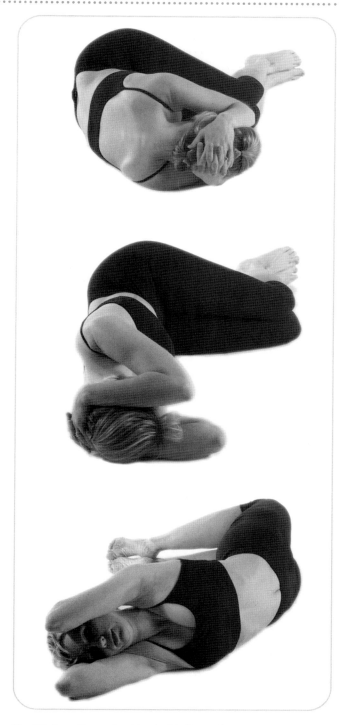

Fig. 4.1 Rounding and arching in side-lie position.

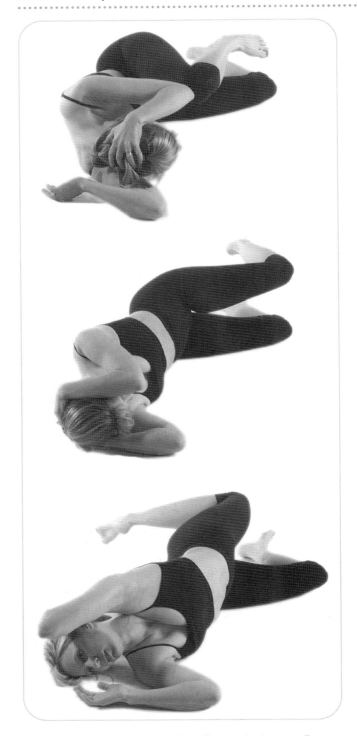

Fig. 4.2 Rounding and arching unilaterally – moving just top elbow and knee toward and away from each other.

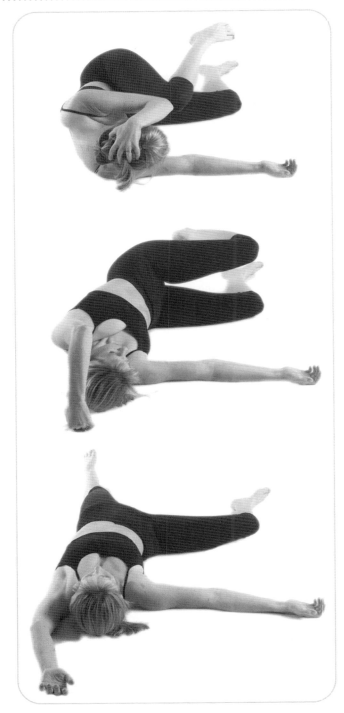

Fig. 4.3 Segue movement into rolling to your back with the arch and rolling back to your side with the round.

simultaneously use that straightening movement to roll yourself back on to your back. Left arm is overhead and left leg is straight down and long. Your head rolls a bit off your right hand, and your right elbow and knee stay in more or less the same place on the floor.

- Reverse the movement to return on to your side – curl yourself up as you slide your left elbow and knee back towards each other to roll once again on to your right side. Left hand slides on the ground above your head.

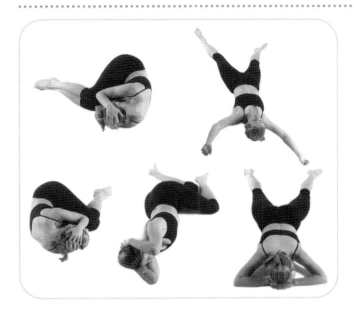

Fig. 4.4 Making transitions to roll across the floor – side-lie to back to belly.

- Alternate between arching and straightening yourself to roll on to your back, then rounding or curling yourself to roll on to your right side. Repeat many times – search for fluidity and ease – for coordination (the moment you are on your back is the moment that the arm and leg fully straighten).

- Rest on your back with legs and arms long – compare contact against the floor to when you began – compare length and breath in the right and left sides.

F. Repeat instructions as in D and E – all done rolling left side to back and return.

G. Lie on your back with legs long and spread your arms on the floor somewhere above your head if possible.

- Slide your right knee and right elbow towards each other on the floor – elbow and knee both bend and stay pretty close to the ground then:

- Follow by sliding your left arm overhead and your left leg to the right to roll yourself on to your right side with both knees and elbows bent and torso curled up into a ball.

- Reverse the movement to return to your back – left arm and leg straighten, the back straightens, which is then followed by the right arm as it slides overhead and the right leg as it slides down long.

- Repeat rolling from back to right side – leading with one side and following with the other.

- Try this movement to roll yourself on to your left side. How does this side compare?

- Alternate rolling back to right side, to back, to left side, to back, to right, to back, to left (Fig. 4.4). Pause for a moment on your back and rest.

- Continue to alternately round and straighten yourself, but now add in using the straightening movement to roll on to your belly.

- From your right side, you will slide both left and right arms overhead and simultaneously straighten your legs down long to end up lying on your belly (Fig. 4.4).

- Roll across the floor in sequence: right side to back to left side to belly to right side to back to left to belly to right. Now reverse the direction. How much room do you have on your floor?

- Lie on your right side and slide both elbows and both knees toward each other as you did at the very beginning.

- How does this movement feel now? Does it feel any easier? Are the movements any more proportional? How does the right side compare to the left now with this movement?

- Lie on your back and rest. Notice changes in contact against the floor or differences in perception of length in arms, legs or torso. Feel the ease and balance from side to side of your breath.

- Compare to the beginning. Get up on your feet and stand, then walk around. How is your head balanced? How do your shoulders move as you walk? Reach overhead with each hand. How is this movement organized?

Static and dynamic baselines – Cherry Turnover

Here again in variation A is our familiar proprioceptive scan and static baseline. With attention to contact, we are again asking questions about flexion/extension bias throughout different parts of the torso. Did any of your curves smooth out with this lesson? We also asked about left to right differences relating to both the perception of length and ease of movement of breath into each side. This is a question about side-bending bias in different parts. Which was your easiest side to lengthen? For most right-handed people, it will be the left side.

You may have noticed that each of the lessons that had a side-bending component started with having you either bend yourself to the right or lengthen your left side. All the lessons described so far in this section have followed this general pattern (go back and look!) because it is the direction of ease for the majority of people and because we would like to have people make movements to their easiest and most familiar side first. This gives them a sense of competence, the comfort of the habitual. It also serves to heighten awareness of differences between the two sides, both with the static scan and with the movements themselves.

Part of the game for the practitioner is to make observations that lead you to guess which direction will be easiest for your student: just be prepared to be wrong at least 25% of the time, and don't get too attached to your guesses.

Let's roll

Variations B and C ask you to lie on your right side with hips and knees bent and hands interlaced behind your head to support its weight. Slide both elbows and knees towards and away from each other. The hands on the head trick should be a familiar one by now – it's a common constraint. You are sliding elbows and knees toward each other to elicit a global torso flexion pattern first, simply because most people are more comfortable and less liable to damage themselves by moving into flexion.

Many people will tend to over-arch in their neck and lower back with the extension component of this movement while underutilizing the thoracic extensors and posterior intercostals. By flexing first, we also are taking advantage of the stimulation of a stretch reflex to the extensors. We are *spring-loading* the back by contracting the front. This helps to bring in the often dormant mid-back. We will use this phenomenon of spring-loading frequently in subsequent chapters, as well as describe its use in everyday and sports activity. It is one of the major benefits of doing reciprocating or alternating movements.

The movement of elbows and knees away from each other is to elicit a global torso extension pattern. How global does yours feel? How proportional is this movement in your students? Both the flexion and extension patterns at the beginning of this lesson are dynamic baselines that we return to at the end of the lesson. Did the quality of movement change for you from beginning to end (Box 4.1)?

Alternating between global torso flexion and extension is our first real foray into true alternating movements (previous versions have been mostly of the 'move in one direction then come back to home' variety). Both the flexors and extensors get to work in a gravity-neutral position and both legs and arms are moving globally as extensions of the torso. Do we ever actually use this alternating global flexion/extension movement as adults?

In variation D, lie on your right side as before but with your left hand on top of your head. Move your left elbow and left knee toward and away from each other while keeping your right elbow and knee where they were. This variation is really just a halfway step to rolling to your back. It sets up the direction and the one-sided nature of the movement as the right side extremities are now differentiated from the rest of the movement.

With the head now being less supported by the right hand (which is constrained from moving on the floor) and the left leg and thigh being slightly lifted because of the loss of support from the stationary right thigh, the lateral torso musculature has to get a bit more involved. The flexion component of the movement emphasizes contraction of the lateral abdominals and lateral and anterolateral intercostals.

The extension component emphasizes the quadratus lumborum, back extensors and lateral and posterolateral intercostals. Alternating between flexion and extension while still contracting to side-bend can help balance the torso in an anterior/posterior direction through the coordination and equalization of two of the four torso quadrant movements (left torso flexion and left torso extension).

In variation E, continue from right side-lie to make alternating movements to curl and straighten. Now you straighten your back, left leg and left arm simultaneously to roll on to your back. Reverse to come back on to your right side. This strategy of continuing the previous variation a few times then introducing a subvariation is a useful one. By repeating the previous instruction after a break or rest, you re-establish your students' ability to repeat what they have just learned – did they remember it, or did you have to repeat the instructions over again? This repetition also serves as a bridge or link to what you will teach them next, which is to blend this alternate rounding and straightening movement (with possible orientation or reaching intentions) into a transitional movement from side-lie to supine.

Transitional movements

Transitional movements are one of our seven major categories of function. Balance is about organizing yourself to fall without hitting your head. Orientation is about moving to gather information about your external environment. Transitional movements are about changing positions, moving your center of mass in space. Horizontal transitions are from back to sides to belly, just what we did in the Cherry Turnover. Other lessons are built around transitional movements such as supine to sit, side-lie to sit, prone to sit, left side-sit to right side-sit, to sole sit, to long sit, to lotus, or many dozens of other subvariations of sitting on the floor.

Transitions from floor sitting to hands and knees, prone to hands and knees, hands and knees to three-and-a-half point (hands and knees but one foot forward on the ground), Sit to Stand, three-and-a-half point to stand and prone to stand also have movement lessons that revolve around them. Chair sitting to stand, stand to squat, and even bending over and coming back up again are transitional movements. Most of these movements change the height of the center of mass. This is a very big deal to the developing child.

We might make a transitional movement to better orient our senses (especially sight), to prepare ourselves to locomote, to reach toward and manipulate something for vegetative purposes (get out the easy chair to grab a beer), or to express an idea or emotion. Transitional movements are not usually an end in themselves: they are generally a bridge between different intentional positions or activities. Hence the name, transitional movements. In a motor learning approach, we use transitional movements frequently because:

- It is a good way to access motor pathways learned in childhood that may have been forgotten or long unused.
- It is a discrete movement that has a clearly defined goal (functional context) and that students seem to take pride in accomplishing – they can clearly tell they are doing something.

Box 4.1 Cherry Turnover

Reciprocating global torso flexion and extension movements – spring-loading the antagonists

Introduction of transitional movements – side-lie to supine, supine to side-lie and side-lie to prone

Upper and lower extremities move globally with torso

- Transitional movements, especially movements toward or within a vertical orientation, always necessitate balance reactions and most often include an orientation component. We can file a newly learned or freshly relearned movement into several functional categories at the same time.

Dr Feldenkrais thought enough of the importance to the CNS of transitional movements and enough of their usefulness for teaching that he designed hundreds of lessons around them; you will experience, and I will describe, a sample of them as you progress through this book.

Horizontal transitional movements such as those found in the Cherry Turnover or in Baby Rolls are the main ones that can be performed by the worm. To raise the center of mass up off the floor, we need to differentiate the extremities from the torso, especially the legs. It is for this reason that we could often skip global movement lessons of the worm altogether and go straight to transitional movements that simultaneously train the legs to support and move the pelvis and torso and train the torso to move with 360° competence in balance and orientation contexts (Box 4.2).

In variation G you put the whole thing together by making serial transitions from back to side, from side to belly, from belly to opposite side, from side to back and so on. This is the culmination of a lesson that has already been integrative in nature. This lesson distills all of our previous lessons into one. The lesson as a whole features alternating flexion and extension movements with a side-bending component. It recalls movements from all of our previous lessons, in that we are working the torso muscles against gravity in supine, side-lie and prone positions. The movement at the end, the last variation of the lesson, both reviews the lesson itself and is a microcosm of the whole series of horizontal worm lessons.

Summary/cumulative movements or lessons

These summary lessons and cumulative movements are great for a home exercise program. Teach a lesson in the office and have your students go through the whole thing a few times again at home before you see them next. Then review key parts of the lesson, instruct them on continuing with one or two movements that distill that lesson, then go on to our next lesson from there. That lesson will be practiced, along with a few reminder movements from the previous lesson, until your next session. Here again we are reviewing and moving on, but always having something from each lesson that they will be continuing with. This keeps their learning fresh and their muscles ready to go.

When I first started using movement lessons in my practice, I noticed these summary movements at the end of lessons that previous movements seemed to be leading up to. So I figured

I'd just cut to the chase and teach the finished product to my students. It worked to a certain extent, but people did a lot better once I started teaching them whole lessons, even if they were very simple ones with only three or four variations.

There is something about going through a step-by-step process the first time or two that helps to coordinate and solidify things better in the CNS. Starting with simpler movements and progressing to the more complex, having to choose a preferable pathway and attending to proprioceptive input all make the movements informational. This is what makes an exercise a lesson. Try to avoid the temptation to skip building the foundation and just teach the end result to your students, but do use these integrative movements in a well-rounded home exercise program.

Comparing baselines

We finish the lesson by taking a final look at our static and dynamic baselines. Proprioceptively perceived changes in the length or volume of breath in the two sides, in level of comfort, in ease of movement or in an enhanced ability to sink into the floor are strong arguments for participating in a home program: use them to motivate and inspire your students. In addition to the usual questions about contact with the floor and differences between the two sides while supine, we asked some questions at the end of this lesson pertaining to upright organization and function.

How was your head balanced in standing? How did your shoulders move as you walk? How does it feel to reach one arm overhead? These are questions that were not asked at the beginning of the lesson, but they easily could have been. Having reference points while in upright orientations is in some respects even more important than having static baselines. Vertical is where we spend most of our time. Vertical is where most of our musculoskeletal damage occurs. Ultimately, everything we do in therapeutic or informational exercise has to relate in some way to vertical positions and functions. Why don't we just do all our exercise in vertical and bag the horizontal and transitional orientations altogether?

Working horizontally on the floor or mat table has some definite advantages when working with people who have movement and postural impairments that contribute to musculoskeletal pain. One advantage is that it helps to reduce the volume of neurological chatter from both the sensory and the motor side. When we are upright, our CNS is being flooded with proprioceptive sensations that monitor our balance and regulate muscle tone and antagonist coordination to keep us from falling.

Partner practice – how pressure on the feet increases hip muscle tone

Pressure on the soles of our feet stimulates associative and habituated motor reactions throughout the legs and torso. Try this simple proprioceptive volume experiment. Have a student or colleague lie on the floor on her back. Support one leg with a pillow under the knee and lift the other leg to hold it securely but gently (don't leave any fingerprints) by the sole of the foot and the outside of the proximal tibia. Get your subject to

---

Box 4.2 Transitional movements

Good access to early developmental movement – relearning an old trick

Discrete skill with defined outcome – good measuring stick for progress

Plays well with balance and orientation – juggling an extra ball now

understand that you want her to be relaxed/loose, to give the whole weight of the held leg to you as you move the knee slowly and gently from side to side.

In this position, she will need to recognize effort and let go of the adductors to allow the knee to fall outward into your hand. She will also need to be able to inhibit her hip external rotators and gluteals to allow her knee to fall inward into your hand. Use a little patience, listen for and stop when you feel subtle effort or resistance, and cue verbally. Proceed once your subject has recognized the effort and has given you her full weight again, and you will probably be able eventually to move her knee from side to side without resistance from either adductors or abductors.

If you are able to accomplish this within 5 minutes or so, slowly place her foot on the floor or table so her knee is bent and the sole of her foot is 'standing.' From this position, try tilting her knee in and out again, making sure that your hands are well placed to give her a sense of support. What many of you will notice is that once the sole of the foot hits the ground, either the adductors or the abductors or both will contract to make tilting the knee much harder. For many people, the CNS stimulation provided by the pressure on the sole of the foot elicits a habitual motor response that often mirrors that person's adductor/abductor bias in standing.

If they can't let go of a stereotyped response in the relatively simple context of lying with just the weight of the leg and a trickle of proprioceptive information to deal with, imagine how many other preprogrammed motor responses are present when they are fully weightbearing: sorting out torrents of constantly changing sensory input and having to make constant adjustments throughout their entire body to keep from falling.

Advantages to working on the floor

The problem from a motor learning standpoint is that in working exclusively with someone while they are upright, we are swimming upstream against a very powerful current of preprogrammed motor responses. By putting our students horizontal for some of our teaching, we reduce both the flood of proprioceptive input and the huge volume of outgoing motor instructions that happen while upright. This allows the student to more easily feel herself and to become more fully aware of subtle sensations such as shapes, muscle tone or effort, or side-to-side imbalances.

This position allows our student to reduce muscle effort and allows her to gain better incremental control over muscles and their antagonists. By lying her down, we have cleared the blackboard, we have wiped the slate clean for some fresh writing. This position is a hothouse for our newly germinated and still young and tender budding motor patterns that we are trying to get our students to adopt as substitutes for their damaging, but familiar, movement or postural patterns.

Another advantage of working horizontally, especially initially, is that we can go back in history and work with some earlier, developmentally based movements that are ancestors or precursors to the current dysfunctional movements. If someone is hypermobile in their low back when walking because of a waddling gait and an excessively rotating pelvis, for instance, we can go back to lessons that simulate prone commando

crawls, hands and knees creeping, transition to standing and other transitional movements on the floor that have pelvic force couples as a primary component.

These earlier movements are either progressions or cousins of the locomotor function that can be relearned then blended back into upright locomotion with an awareness of, and an acquisition of, the physical skills of Using the Legs in a fundamentally different way from what they have been doing. If a painter is hurting his neck from looking up all day, we could use some of the lessons we have already performed in this chapter to help him to reconnect his intention to look overhead with a proximal response that emphasizes a proportional extension movement throughout his whole torso (especially his thoracic spine/chest).

Contrast this organic progression of motor learning to a command and control model of gait training, postural instruction or other gross motor retraining that relies on external (and sometimes arbitrary) criteria imposed by the therapist and maintained through constant cognitive vigilance. It would be much better to have our more appropriate or preferable motor responses woven throughout multiple functional categories and ingrained into the subcortical brain through a focused review of some key early learning.

A third reason for working on the floor is simply for the surface it provides. We can use the floor as a passive masseur, rubbing and pressing various parts of ourselves against its untiring (and inexpensive) surface. We can roll our heads on it, rest our legs on it, shift our weight, press our feet, mash our muscles or slide our bones on it. We can learn to give our weight fully to the floor in a number of different positions to enhance both our effort recognition/reduction skills and to earn the trust of the CNS in our bones to support our weight (skeletal weightbearing).

Touch and pressure are key elements of our sensory system and can help to guide us in proprioceptively feeling ourselves more clearly, and in developing a clearer and more complete self-image. Pressing bones against the floor helps you to feel them, to map their size, shape and relationships to other bones; and an awareness of which bones are pressing and which aren't helps you in discerning your overall shape (static baseline). By being creative about how we use gravity and the predictable constraint of the floor, we can design exercises that mobilize restricted joints or passively stretch skin, fascia or muscle (Box 4.3).

The floor is a tool, a teacher, the mother of all movement, and a very unusual place for adults to hang out – and this may be its final advantage. Most adults lie down only to sleep and to dance the horizontal mambo. Most spend zero time on the floor and think it a bit scandalous to do so (I've personally been stalked many times by security guards at theaters when I've

---

Box 4.3 Reasons for exercising on the floor

Reduction of proprioceptive chatter – Weber/Fechner
Go back in history and access earlier developmental movements that current imbalances and inefficiencies are bred from
Touch and pressure main components of the proprioceptive system – maximize surface area

eschewed the seats in favor of the floor.) Most adults have both a smaller movement repertoire and a longer list of neuromusculoskeletal ailments than the average 3-year-old – coincidence, or cause and effect? You be the judge.

Getting people out of furniture, out of their shoes and restrictive clothing and down on the ground for some nitty-gritty rolling around is just what the doctor ordered (though you might think twice about submitting that prescription to the insurance company). For most people, the shear novelty of it forces them to pay attention to what they are doing, and in many cases forces them to relearn how to move on, get up and down from and be comfortable supporting themselves on the ground all over again. This is a good thing!

Applications

For what kind of student might this lesson be useful? Because it is an integrative lesson that provides a summary for the global flexion, side-bending and extension lessons that preceded it, we could use it for the same kind of problems. When I use global or more primitive lessons with my students, I will often try this type of lesson first. If I can skip earlier lessons or blend a number of different directions of movement into one lesson I will do so. Sometimes I will do this entire lesson except for the rolling to the belly part if they are particularly sensitive to extension movements in the low back.

I asked earlier about what everyday movements this might mimic. Infants, especially when they are mad, will alternate between global flexion and global extension patterns. They get a bit hard to hold on to when they do this. How about adults? It may be hard to find real-life movements that adults do that involve this alternating global flexion and extension where the extremities are moving globally, but there are some sports where this happens. Divers and gymnasts may go from a tuck to a layout position, or vice versa.

The butterfly stroke in swimming is an imitation of a dolphin kick, which alternates flexion and extension. Serving and spiking in volleyball involve a windup phase where the torso and legs extend as the arms extend overhead, then an action phase where the arm comes powerfully forward and down to strike the ball as an extension of a powerfully flexing torso. Especially in swimming and volleyball, each global movement provides a spring-loading effect for the antagonists and therefore provides for a stronger and more explosive movement.

In the butterfly stroke, the extension phase prepares the torso flexors for action and the flexion phase prepares the back. This is a classic example of coordinating the antagonists, in this case the torso flexors and extensors. Can you think of any alternating side-bending movements of the torso being used in real life? How about riding a horse? Or paddling a kayak or canoe with waves coming in broadside? How about walking? Although the examples in this chapter deal mainly with the torso antagonists, you will find many more examples of alternating and coordinated antagonists of the extremities in subsequent chapters. Use this lesson at face value to teach bed and floor mobility to neurology and general medical students, or to your patients with Parkinson's disease, MS, heart surgery, total hip or knee replacement, or who have had a stroke.

Variations

The variation on this lesson is really another lesson. Baby Rolls feature the same rolling or transitional movement from back to belly and back again, but this time with the extremities lifted from the floor. This kind of movement always reminds me of otters and how they play in the water. They roll from belly to back, dip down for a dive and porpoise back up again, and generally move in an almost snake-like way when in the water. This can be a pretty strenuous lesson for many people, so move with care and attention yourself while also being selective about whom you use this lesson with. As always, I would recommend that you go through all the movements of a lesson first before teaching it to someone.

The description and number of variations of this lesson will be a bit bare bones. Although there are many ways of approaching the end result of this lesson and there is a lot of detail that can be taught as a lead-up to this, we are doing a condensed version of it that shouldn't take more than 10 or 15 minutes. It is, however, a good integrative lesson that incorporates movement and muscular control in all 360 directions of the worm while in a horizontal orientation. Besides that, it's really fun – enjoy!

Baby Rolls

Variations

A. Lie on your back with your legs long and spread and with your arms on the floor somewhere below shoulder height.

- Scan your contact against the floor. Feel for bumps and hollows through your backside. How is your weight distributed along your back?

- Imagine your torso as a cylinder. Is it a true cylinder, or are you wider than you are deep? Vice versa? Is your cylinder straight or bent? Or twisted?

- Does your breath fill up your cylinder evenly throughout its length from top to bottom? From side to side? From front to back?

B. Lie on your back with your feet off the ground and your knees held up over your belly. Lift your head off the floor to look between your knees and lift your arms off the floor so your elbows are near your knees. Your hands are near but not quite touching your head or face. Knees are spread a bit and your right elbow is near your right knee, while your left elbow is near your left knee. Stay in this position for a moment and then:

- Move both elbows and both knees closer to each other – or touch them if possible. Contract your belly and round your back to do this. Repeat a few times.

- Move right elbow and right knee toward each other a few times, letting yourself bend to the right.

- Then move your left elbow and left knee. Pause in the middle with arms, legs and head still lifted from the floor (Fig. 4.5).

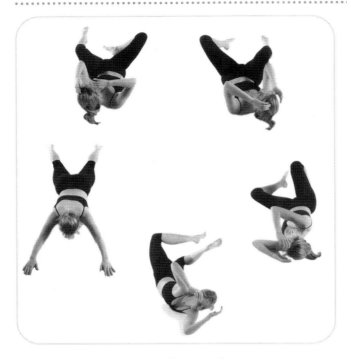

Fig. 4.5 Differing combinations of knees to elbows.

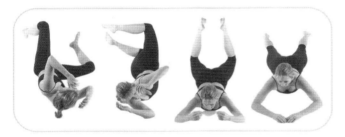

Fig. 4.6 Rolling like a baby.

- Begin a movement of rolling yourself toward your left side. Move your left elbow and left knee away from each other as you do this; both knees and elbows stay bent – don't straighten either knee or elbow.

- The act of moving the 'bottom' or left elbow and knee away from each other while rolling to your left side will cause your torso to straighten or arch (Fig. 4.6).

- Feel where your balance point is. Where do you start to 'fall' on to your side? Or your belly? Return to your back by rounding or curling yourself and bringing left elbow and left knee back toward each other.

- Repeat movement from back to left side several times. Where is your balance point?

- Try the same movement now to the right; the 'bottom' or right elbow and right knee move away

from each other, which again triggers an arching movement of your torso. Your knees and elbows stay off the floor the whole time.

- Repeat this movement several times from back to right side and back again. How controlled is this movement? Do you lose control and fall? How does this side compare to the other?

- Alternate from side to side: back to left side, back through your back and over to your left side, and so on. Look toward the elbow that reaches overhead along the floor. Feel how your cylinder changes its shape, from round to bent to arched.

C. Lie again on your back with arms, legs and head lifted as before.

- Repeat the movement of rolling from side to side a few times. Next time you roll to your left:

- Continue the movement of arching to look along the floor above your head, let yourself 'fall' on to your belly and bring your head toward vertical (Fig. 4.6).

- Remember to keep both elbows and knees away from the floor. You are now on your belly with legs, arms and head all lifted while looking forward toward the wall.

- From here, move left elbow and left knee back toward each other as you roll yourself back through your left side and all the way back to your back again. There is an odd corkscrewing movement of the legs where the left knee moves under and to the right while the right leg moves over and back to the left.

- Your head moves back and to the left as your legs and torso contort to roll you back to your back, with arms, legs and head still held off the floor. Try this movement of rolling from back to belly through your left side several times then:

- Try the same movement of rolling back to belly, but now through your right side. How does this direction compare? Is it generally easier to roll back to belly or belly to back? How are you organizing your breath?

- Rest on your back with head, arms and legs resting fully on the floor and compare your contact against the ground to when you started.

- Do you have any clearer image of the size, shape and dimensions of your cylindrical torso? How evenly is your breath expanding through your cylinder?

D. Lie once again on your back with legs, arms and head all lifted away from the floor as before. If you have enough room on your floor:

- Roll as before across your left side to your belly but now instead of reversing the movement to come back through your left side, continue the roll in the same direction to roll yourself back on to your back through your right side. . .

- Then across your left side to your belly, then back through your right side, and so on. You roll yourself across the floor.

- Reverse direction to roll across the floor the other way. Feel the different aspects of your torso as they contract and work, then lengthen and stretch. Think again of your torso as a cylinder with 360° of movement. Think of yourself as an accordion or a slinky.

- Rest on your back and notice differences from when you started. Stand up and feel the shape and balance of your torso in standing. Feel your breath. Does it fill you like a cylindrical balloon? Walk around and feel the balance or carriage of your head. How tall can you be?

Synopsis – Baby Rolls

This is the culmination of our horizontal worm. It is essentially the same lesson as Cherry Turnover, with the same muscle breakdown and same clinical usage. Its functional context is orientation (as Baby Rolls to belly as an outgrowth of the intention to look overhead), balance (as baby strives to keep from hitting head on the floor) and transitions. We could almost even say that our last variation of rolling across the floor is a primitive form of locomotion.

There are really only three ways a worm or snake can get from A to B. Rolling across belly, back and sides as we did in the last two lessons is one way. Another way is to move like an inchworm, or like an elephant seal on land. They lift their front by extending, then roll back down along their front sides to shift their weight forward while drawing up their back section with a flexing movement to provide the forward movement (Box 4.4).

Do humans move like this? You might see a version of this movement early on, when baby is learning to draw its knees up underneath in preparation for coming up to hands and knees. The dolphin kick or the butterfly stroke in swimming both mimic the alternating flexion/extension inchworm pattern, which is a true locomotion function. A bunny hop or kangaroo hop is also a version of this pattern, and is seen sometimes in children with developmental delay.

Even if your students never have the opportunity to use these rolling or 360° movements in these literal contexts, the skills learned here are precursors to later, more mature movement patterns. This 360° movement of the torso is a basic Lego that you will see many times throughout this book, either as full circles or as partial arcs.

You will see these movements not only in upright orientation and balance, but also in manipulation, matured (leg-centered) transitions and locomotion. We will use these head/tail relationship or worm movements in many different positions to qualitatively stretch and strengthen hip/thigh and shoulder girdle/shoulder musculature, and to help to integrate the torso and the extremities in well-organized whole body movements.

To summarize, this whole section of horizontal head/tail relationship lessons, and these last two integrative lessons in particular, are designed to mobilize, balance and gain motor control over the chest, ribcage and thoracic spine. We do this by deliberately coordinating pelvis and head in balance and orientation functions, and asking for an attention to proportional movement.

This mid-torso mobility is necessary for evenly distributed movement and is very often missing in our students, who will have both flexion/extension and left/right biases that make movements into some directions difficult or even impossible. Lack of mobility and balance here has important ramifications for the health and movement/postural organization of the neck, lower back and arms, and is a major contributor to movement impairments and pain syndromes in these areas.

This whole section is a goldmine for the neurological therapist looking for ways to facilitate trunk control. Work with your stroke patients horizontally at first. Let them gain confidence relearning to move without the fear of falling. Work on moving and rolling to each side to stimulate CNS rerouting around the damaged areas.

We will now leave horizontal orientation and come up to vertical for the next section. The movements in the lessons will still be familiar to you in terms of patterns of movement and of muscular breakdown, described in both the falls from vertical and the horizontal orientation sections. In addition, because we have already introduced many of the concepts or principles involved in working with worm-like movement lessons and have physically experienced something similar to what we do next, we will go through the analysis of each lesson fairly quickly.

Orientation from vertical

Our first lesson in this section is Sitting Circles. Balance and orientation will again be our main themes, this time while upright. Sitting Circles again features the eight main directions and the 360° capability of the worm, but with an important difference relative to our first several lessons. In this lesson, the legs will no longer be able to move globally with the torso (hip extension with back extension and hip flexion with torso flexion). They are now differentiated from the torso, but we will ignore that little detail for now and revisit this lesson later in the chapter on legs.

You may also have noticed that we skipped an important developmental step: how did we get from lying on the floor up to sitting in the first place? How does a worm get from horizontal to vertical? How does a worm stand on his tail? He doesn't: it's impossible. The worm can neither come up to sit nor maintain a sitting position without legs. We will have to wait until our analysis of the legs in Section 3 to examine this question more thoroughly; for now, we can just pretend to stand our worm on its tail and put it through its paces.

Box 4.4 Baby Rolls

Degree of difficulty progression of Cherry Turnover – legs and arms off the floor

Torso as 360° slinky – movements in all directions

Upper and lower extremities move globally with torso

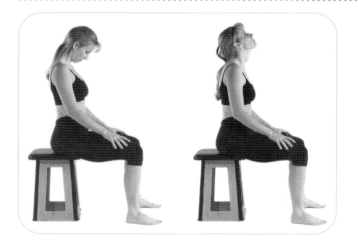

Fig. 4.7 Look up and down – how much of your back participates?

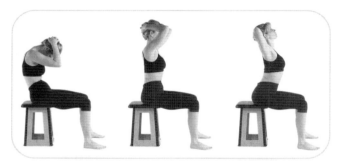

Fig. 4.8 Moving head and arms together is a constraint that requires integrated movement with the back and pelvis.

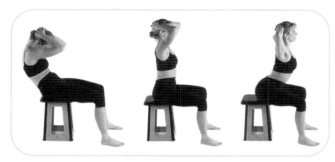

Fig. 4.9 Add in leaning forward and back to looking up and down movements.

Sitting Circles

Variations

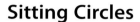

A. Sit in an upright-backed or kitchen-style chair. Sit near the front edge of the seat, so your back is away from the backrest. Sit with your feet flat on the floor and underneath your knees, with feet and knees both between hip and shoulder width apart.

- Notice how your pelvis is balanced on the seat. You may feel two bones on the bottom of your pelvis that are supporting your weight (if you can't feel bones on the seat, sit on your hands and use your hands to help you to feel where those bones are).
- Is your pelvis rolled backward or forward? Is your back rounded or arched?
- Is there more weight to the left or the right sitting bone? Are you longer along one side of your torso and shorter along the other?
- Where are you looking? Up? Down? At the horizon?
- Find the horizon (eyes in the middle of your sockets and looking at a place on the wall in front of you that is at eye height) and from there look slowly and gently down toward your belly button (Fig. 4.7).
- What can you see easily? How proportional is this movement through your back? Does your pelvis move on the seat? Repeat several times, then:
- Look up toward the ceiling (Fig. 4.7). Where on the ceiling can you see easily? How do you organize your pelvis and back with this?
- Alternate looking up and looking down a few times. Which direction is easier? Take care with your neck that you don't strain or try to do it all using just a few vertebrae.

B. Sit on the chair as before; find the horizon. Now interlace your fingers and place them behind your head.

- Point your elbows forward and move both elbows down towards your hips as you look toward your belly button. Let your pelvis roll back on the seat and your whole back round as you do this (Fig. 4.8). Do not pull on your head with your hands.
- Repeat several times, then, as you come back to neutral, continue past neutral to look up to the ceiling (Fig. 4.8). Spread your elbows apart and pinch your shoulder blades together as you roll your pelvis forward on the seat and arch your back.
- Add in leaning back as you round back and look toward your belly button. Move your neck only as long as your back is still moving in cooperation. Add in leaning forward as you roll forward and look toward the ceiling (Fig. 4.9).
- Alternate looking up and down/leaning forward and back. Your elbows point forward when looking down and spread out when looking up. Coordinate head and tail!
- Coordinate your breath. Do you breathe in or out when looking down? Continue this a few times, then start making movements smaller and smaller until you come to stop in a place where your eyes are back on the horizon and your pelvis is balanced forward/back on your seat.

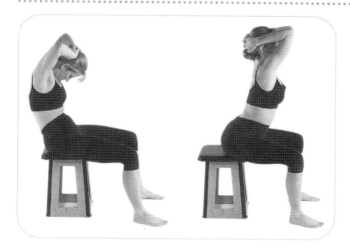

Fig. 4.10 Differentiating the arms from the torso.

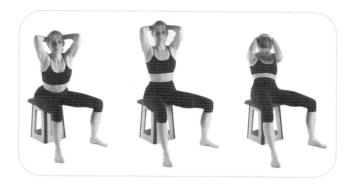

Fig. 4.11 Looking diagonally up and down – pelvis rolls diagonally on your seat.

C. Sit as before on chair. Place interlaced hands behind head.
- Look alternately up and down as before, but this time move elbows forward as you look up and spread them as you look down (Fig. 4.10). Try this version a few times. Which way of organizing your arms is easiest?
- How are you coordinating your breath?

D. Sit again toward the front edge of your seat; interlace your fingers and place hands behind head.
- Turn yourself a little to the right so you are facing your right knee and still looking at the horizon. Elbows are pointed forward over your right knee.
- From here, move elbows downward and look down towards your right hip. Let your pelvis roll back and to the left, and allow the left side of your back to round and lengthen (Fig. 4.11). Lean or 'fall' back when rounding and lean/fall forward when arching.
- Repeat several times, then continue the movement of coming back to neutral to look up and to the right toward the ceiling. Elbows spread apart and shoul-

ders pinch back and down as you roll your pelvis forward and to the right.
- Alternate looking up and down along this diagonal. Your pelvis rolls diagonally on the seat and your arms flap.
- Try this by moving elbows in the opposite direction. Spread arms apart as you look down and to the left, and point elbows forward as you look up and to the right.
- Try timing your breath differently. Inhale with arch and exhale with round, then exhale with arch and inhale with round. Which way works best for you?

E. Sit in the chair with your hands behind your head. Face to left and repeat instructions above to opposite side. Look down toward left hip and roll pelvis back and to the right, then look up and to the left while rolling pelvis forward and to the left. How does this diagonal compare to the other?

F. Sit forward on your seat again. Hands are again interlaced and behind your head with elbows pointed forward.
- Turn a little to the left and do this diagonal again a few times, rolling your pelvis forward and to the left and back and to the right as you look alternately towards left hip and towards the ceiling to the left.
- Next time you look and move elbows toward left hip, swing elbows through middle and over to the right hip, then point elbows up and to the right as you look in that same direction.
- This describes a U-shape. Your pelvis rolls forward and to the left, then back and to the middle, then forward and to the right. Reverse to roll back to the middle and forward and to the left. Your elbows also make a U-shape in space.
- After doing this semicircular movement a few times, complete the circle by moving elbows from up and to the right to up and to the middle, then to up and to the left. Make a circle with your pelvis on the seat, with your elbows in space and with your head in space (Fig. 4.12).
- Change the direction of the circle – go the other way. Gradually make the circular movement smaller and smaller to spiral yourself back to the middle.
- Find that place where your pelvis is balanced on your seat both forward/back and left/right, and where your head is balanced tall on the column of your spine with your eyes on the horizon.
- Go big and spiral smaller and smaller to where your pelvis is rolled neither forward, back, left nor right.
- Feel how your pelvis is balanced on your seat in comparison to when you began. What is the shape of your back? Round? Arched? Straight? Bent to one side or the other? What is your sense of ease in sitting in comparison to the beginning?
- Without your hands on your head, look alternately up and down. How does this movement compare to when you first did it? Can you see farther or more

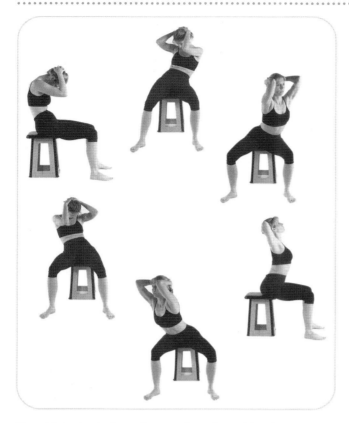

Fig. 4.12 Putting it all together to make circles with head, with chest, with pelvis.

easily? Does your pelvis and whole back move to assist with your intention to look? Is the movement proportioned any more evenly?

Static baselines – Sitting Circles

Here again in variation A are our static and dynamic baselines. The static baseline is now in sitting rather than supine. Contact against the supporting surface is much less, the contact of the ischial tuberosities being our main focus. Get out a model of the pelvis if you have one handy and stand it upright. Roll the pelvis forward and back a little to visualize how, when contact on the tuberosities is more on the posterior aspect, the pelvis is no longer vertical but is falling back. If contact is more on the anterior aspect, the pelvis is falling forward.

Leaving aside for now the question of how we arrest the fall of the pelvis (short answer: the legs), we could say that as the pelvis rolls back, the spine tends to round. What happens if the spine doesn't adjust to the falling-back pelvis? The whole torso remains straight and the center of mass shifts back relative to the pelvis. This is very unbalancing, and is much more effort than to simply round your back in a balance or falling reaction, as described in the falling from vertical section earlier in the book.

The same is true of a forward-falling pelvis. The back tends to arch or extend, both to maintain the center of mass over the base of support and as part of that unspoken intention not to hit one's head. A vertical position of the pelvis is one where the contact on the ischial tuberosities is more or less centered or on the apex of those bones. With a fudge factor of a few degrees in either direction, here is where the spine has its best chance of being neutral and where your bones can best support your weight.

Awareness on the part of the student of where on these bones he is bearing his weight is a critical proprioceptive cue in postural training. Because he is no longer getting feedback from the floor that tells him about the shape of his back, this awareness of ischial tuberosity contact and balance of the pelvis in an anterior/posterior direction is the cue that he now needs to extrapolate to the question of the shape of his back.

We can train our students to recognize this relationship between the falling bias of the pelvis and the habitual shape of the back. It is remarkable how few people have any sense of either the balance of their pelvis or the shape of their back when upright. Frequently, when I ask this question of new students they will either have no idea what I'm talking about or will give answers that are way off – they have a very sketchy self-image of their backsides.

Correct second and ask questions first

I think our first instinct as practitioners is to tell our students what we see, how that is contributing to their problem, and what we're going to do to them to fix it. If we can just hold off for a few minutes and first ask them what they notice, what they perceive, what their reality is, we can pick up some valuable insights into their way of thinking about movement. We might even develop a first impression about the quality of the proprioceptive listening and movement skills of a person. After having asked the question and gotten a response, we can then help him to feel more accurately where he is.

We can sit him on a stool against a wall and use the contact he makes against that wall as a proprioceptive mirror similar to how we have already used the floor. We can roll a foam roller up and down along his back to help him feel where it is round and where it is arched. We can have him roll his pelvis alternately forward and back and direct his attention to the changing contact against his pelvis to help him feel proprioceptively where rolled back is, where rolled forward is, and where a truer middle is.

We use movement to clarify posture. If he has been biased toward falling either back or forward with his pelvis in sitting, his CNS will calibrate his personal neutral to that bias – he feels that he's straight even when he's not. More ominously for us, he will feel out of whack when he really is in neutral.

This is what can make any kind (arthrokinematic, postural, gross motor) of movement behavior so hard to change. When left to its own devices, when put on automatic pilot, the CNS will return to what it knows and what it has been doing. This again is why it is so important to bring self-awareness and proprioceptive acuity training to our exercise prescription.

If our students are just going through the motions of stretching or strengthening individual muscles without achieving the type of organic understanding that can be facilitated by teaching reciprocating movements, by bringing awareness to the relationships between different parts and by using descriptive and inquisitive language, they are far less likely to learn something from the lesson that they can then extrapolate to real life – which is the whole point of most of our exercise in the first place.

Our second reference point in the static scan was left-to-right balance. Feeling weight differences from one ischial tuberosity to the other can be another important clue in helping that person feel more clearly what he tends to do, and to again extrapolate weight shift to side-bending bias through the torso. Did you notice a difference? Are you falling sideways in one direction? If you were sitting on two bathroom scales, would they register the same amount of weight? Unlikely, yet most of our students (and probably most readers) will feel that they are balanced because of the tendency of the CNS to accommodate to the invariance and misinterpret imbalances as neutral.

The practiced eye can observe weight-shifts, even subtle ones. Get behind your students while they sit on a flat, firm surface and visualize the side-to-side balance of the pelvis. You might see one side of the pelvis or one nate flattened to the seat a bit more (nate is a term for your butt cheek; natal cleft is a term for your butt crack). You may see one iliac crest higher than the other. You may see the torso bent in one direction, or be shorter on one side. One handy tip is to palpate the top and bottom of the sternum and sight between your two fingers for its angle relative to vertical.

The bottom of the sternum generally points to the weight-bearing side. This is a general rule of thumb, but has several exceptions. For instance, if weight on the pelvis is to the left we might anticipate the torso being bent to the right as part of our balance response. The angle of the sternum will reveal the bent torso in a much more consistent and accurate way than will visualization of the differences in shoulder height. The shoulders may follow the bend of the torso or may be differentiated, but the sternum has to reflect what the back does.

We might again ask our student to notice which side he bears more weight on and what the shape of his torso is as if looking from the front. He again may either have no idea or be erroneous in his perception. We can ask him to shift weight from side to side, or to lift one hip and then the other, both to assess how accurately he organizes the movement (proportional movement and initiation from legs) and to help him to feel more clearly where he tends to hang out and which direction he moves most easily into.

Everyone has both flexion/extension and left/right imbalances. Part of the game in informational exercise is to help our students be aware of them, how they manifest themselves in a wide variety of daily movements, how those imbalances contribute to their difficulty, and how to soften their invariance with the deliberate introduction of nonhabitual movement patterns throughout many different functional categories. Although this lesson focuses mostly on flexion and extension movements, the introduction of diagonals necessitates a left/right weight shift component that may have a significant effect on side-to-side balance. We will be exploring weight-shift/side-bending relationships in more detail in another lesson in this chapter.

A high horizon facilitates ideal posture

Our next reference point is one not of contact but of orientation – where you are looking? Recall the baby's intention while horizontal to orient to the horizon? To be as tall as possible, to have as high a horizon as possible? The accuracy and height of the horizon is important for two reasons. One is for ease of movement and balance of antagonists. The other is for its implications in postural alignment. We discussed earlier that one of the characteristics of well-organized movement is that we can move more or less equally well in both directions.

Orientation to the horizon involves neither a downward (flexion) bias nor an upward (extension) bias. It is that place from which we can look equally easily either up or down. It is also a place where we can most easily rotate in left/right orientation, as we'll demonstrate in a subsequent lesson. It is the functional context around which we want to organize our heads to balance in neutral over our shoulders, to balance our chests and shoulders on our backs, backs on pelvis and pelvis on seat (or on legs if standing).

The height of the horizon is important in that it serves as a functional context for elongating the spine and for reducing excessive thoracic kyphosis (and excessive lordosis). Many of our students both lack full height and are biased to look down. This inefficiency of movement and this habitual bias are movement impairments that can lead to, or contribute to, an array of neck, jaw and shoulder girdle problems. Clinically, we want our students to associate accurate orientation to a high horizon with good skeletal alignment (Box 4.5).

With a high horizon, I am in my best configuration for supporting my weight skeletally, breathing cylindrically through my torso and being ready to move in any direction equally easily. Here is where my torso flexors and extensors and my left and right side-benders are perfectly balanced in length and tone – all the antagonists are coordinated. From this place, the antagonists actually reciprocate. As you begin to fall forward infinitesimally, your finely tuned CNS picks it up immediately, takes corrective action which probably results in an infinitesimal fall in the other direction, which in turn elicits a prompt response, and so on.

Ideal posture is where falls in all directions are equally possible

This is an ideal situation in which you momentarily achieve equilibrium then fall randomly in any one of 360 directions. If you catch the fall early enough, the muscles don't ever have to

---

Box 4.5 The high horizon

Place where orientation up and down equally accessible

Place where orientation left/right along the horizon moves head best on a vertical axis

Place where bones supporting weight of head and muscle effort minimal – skeletal weightbearing

Developmental imperative – the higher off the ground she can get (prone, prone prop, hands and knees, floor sit and stand), the more the baby can see of her world

work too hard. If you fall randomly, you cycle through a number of different muscle units as their turn comes up, allowing for an adequate rest cycle. In reality, the way most of us organize ourselves is to fall in a biased direction and then arrest the fall there – this leads to muscle imbalances, as you are constantly hanging on one agonist and constantly inhibiting the other.

Some people fall only a little way before they arrest it and hold it there; they are working invariantly but mildly, as some of the weight can still be borne by the bones. Some people allow themselves to fall a long way before arresting it and holding it there; they are working both invariantly and very hard – a deadly combination.

You cannot achieve truly efficient posture if you have any kind of left/right or front/back imbalances, muscular, structural or functional. However, because we all have these imbalances, it is safe to say that none of us will ever achieve this perfect state of balance and that to expect such a degree of perfection from our students is unrealistic. We help them to become aware of their biases or their pattern. We begin with simpler lessons and we don't demand a lot right away: we allow time for learning by approximation.

We increase the complexity and vary context and orientation to gravity. We blend what they've learned about pattern recognition into everyday movements. We help them with pattern- and context-specific home exercise, and with specific instructions on moving or posturing nonhabitually when doing specific daily activities. Motor control is not just a switch you can turn on or off, but a process you cultivate. You systematically cull the weeds and nurture the fruit. There are gradations of right and wrong in motor learning. Teaching is a fine line between expecting too much and demanding too little.

Dynamic baselines

Our next baseline is a dynamic one: look toward your belly button and then toward the ceiling. If we were evaluating someone for neck pain, how would we like to see these movements being performed? When I attended physical therapy school, we were trained to evaluate things in sections. If you are evaluating the cervical spine, let only the neck move because moving elsewhere would be compensatory. However, if you agree with the notion that ideal movement should be integrated and proportional, you have a conundrum.

If, while testing cervical flexion and extension, you disallow movement of the pelvis and whole back, especially the thoracic spine/ribcage, you may be unintentionally reinforcing a pattern of movement that contributes to the problem in the first place. You may be giving tacit approval to the student's poor choices and reinforcing their belief that the problem is in the neck, rather than in the relationship of the neck and head to the pelvis and torso. They will then probably focus their attention and their exercises on their neck in the (often mistaken) belief that the whole problem and the whole solution rest there.

Think of the classic neck stretches we give people: flexion and extension, left and right side-bending, left and right rotation and circles. These exercises are a manifestation of a certain framework for thinking about movement that emphasizes con-

cepts of origin and insertion. One thing moves but the other thing doesn't. Move the head and neck on top of the shoulders. This is how we have created our robots and our Barbie dolls, but fortunately this is not how we ourselves are designed.

Nor is it how we should be teaching movement skills to our students. Although these exercises can help codify the students' poor motor organization, all of them can be made much more effective by making them integrative (coordinating head with tail), linking them to meaningful functional contexts and facilitating student self-awareness.

From a motor control standpoint, we would like to see someone initiate the movement of looking down from their pelvis and to flex evenly through their torso. Alas, this rarely happens. What we will often see is a movement that involves a rounding at the cervicothoracic (CT) junction or a shearing somewhere in the mid-low cervical spine. Most people don't even come close to seeing their belly button until we suggest (or give permission) that they roll their pelvis back and round their back.

Try it yourself right now. Can you see your belly button if you move only your neck? Is it easier or more successful if you coordinate head and tail? It is again this demonstrable ability to do something more easily or more successfully that nudges the habit-driven CNS to change its ways. These habitual shearing stresses leading to low cervical disc degeneration or herniation, or to intersegmental instabilities, are epidemic in the population.

On looking down while erect

I had a student once, Barbara, who had neck pain secondary to a C6 on C7 hypermobility. She had already worked with a good manual therapist who mobilized some upper thoracic hypomobile segments and gave her some postural and strengthening exercises. This helped and she got better, but then plateaued. Something she was doing at work continued to give her grief. One of the things I noticed about her on our first visit was that she sat very erect. Her pelvis was rolled forward and she was extended all the way up through her thoracic spine, only to protrude a bit at C7.

When I asked her to look toward her belly button, she promptly confirmed my suspicion by shearing at C6 and keeping her mid-upper thoracic spine perfectly straight. She struggled to see her belly button, even though she didn't stand a chance, but only succeeded in making her neck hurt. I said, 'let this be a lesson to you, grasshopper,' and proceeded to show her the marvels of integrated movement. I suggested she try rolling her pelvis back and softening her back to let it round. I suggested she try exhaling to facilitate flexion, and suggested moving slowly to better know what she's doing.

I had her compare, contrast and make a qualitative judgment (Goldilocks principle) on which way of looking down was easier and more successful. She was floored. She was flabbergasted. She was dubious: 'Is it legal to allow my back to move?' She had been raised by a mother of the always-sit-up-straight school and had embodied that as an ironclad rule: you are never to bend your back. What she had been doing at work then became immediately apparent to her. She sits rigidly upright at her desk all day and looks down at the papers and reports on her desk.

Since she can't use proportional movement because of her mother's prime directive, and because she still had a functional requirement to look down, C6/C7 became the path of least resistance and became overused. This overuse led eventually to abuse as the delicate muscular and articular elements were asked to repetitively do something that was way more than their job description called for.

Although her manual therapist mobilized her upper thoracic segments to allow more movement in principle, Barbara was not using that available movement in reality because of ingrained postural and movement habits. She needed work on the forest (motor control over whole-body, integrated movement) as well as the trees (manual therapy).

Looking upward is similar. From a motor control perspective we would like to see our student initiate the intention to look upward with a rolling forward movement of her pelvis and an evenly distributed extension movement through the whole torso – global torso extension with the larger muscles initiating and providing most of the power of the movement. Even in our initial evaluation of a person, we can start teaching.

We can put a bee in the bonnet of our student. We will be looking not just at range of movement and how far can she go before it hurts, but at ease of movement, integration, and the relationships of the part with the whole. You can observe quality and proportion of movement just as easily when allowing, or even encouraging, whole-body participation as you can when artificially constraining complementary or integrative movement elsewhere. Try it out and start to look past the range of movement (ROM) of a part to the quality of movement (QOM) of the whole in your evaluations.

You can even start making educated guesses about how someone might move and into which directions they might have trouble from an observation of their posture. Do you think someone will have an easier time looking up if they habitually roll their pelvis back and round their back, or if they habitually roll their pelvis forward and arch their back? Is the person who is always falling back going to be able to orient above herself very well?

Hypermobility/hypomobility pairs

Can you envisage how that movement might be disproportional, with C4/C5 or thereabouts falling on his sword because of the laziness of his squadron mates? We see this repeatedly in our business: someplace that moves too much right next to someplace that doesn't. It is this junction between mobility and rigidity, between a mobile C4/C5 next to an immobile C5/C6 in extension, between a mobile C6/C7 on an immobile C7/T1 into flexion, where train wrecks occur.

We can diagnose the specific tissue being strained and causing the pain using imaging tests, provocation tests and deductive reasoning – but that is only part of our assessment. We also need to ask if this local tissue irritation is a manifestation of some larger picture. Could that C4/C5 degenerating disk possibly be degenerating because of something your student does or doesn't do? How he looks toward the ceiling. How he looks at the road when riding his bike. How he bends over to weed his garden.

In all these situations, if he doesn't or can't extend his thoracic spine, he will most likely be extending somewhere in his mid-low cervical spine and further irritating an already peeved spot. If that is the case, we need to apply the rule of holes: when in a hole and getting deeper, the first thing to do is to stop digging. How can we get him to stop extending primarily at C4/C5? Try to think of the good housekeeping rule when doing your evaluations and in prescribing your exercise.

Is the site of irritation moving too much because of a violation of that rule? What is the relationship of the part with the whole? Where is the hypomobile part that contributes to the hypermobile part? How can I get him to recognize how he damages himself with his behavior? How can I help him to trade in that behavior for the new and improved model we propose? What do I want to teach, and how do I want to teach it?

Applying constraints – flapping

In variation B our first movement variation features a blast from the past. Have you seen this strategy of placing hands on head before? With hands on head and starting with orientation to horizon, look down while reaching elbows toward hips. Then look up while spreading elbows out. Then alternate looking up and down with described directions to move pelvis and change the shape of the back.

In this early variation, we are trying to help our student to associate an intention to look with an integrated, whole-body movement that coordinates head and tail. In this variation, the elbows move forward and the scapulae abduct while the torso flexes. The upper extremities move globally with the torso and the pectorals are synergists with the torso flexors. The elbows then extend back and the scapulae adduct and depress – the upper extremities move globally with the torso and the mid-low trapezii are synergists with the torso extensors.

We are using this flapping movement of the arms as another facilitation device for the movement of the torso. We are also timing the breath as before, with an exhalation to assist flexion and an inhalation to boost extension. We use descriptive language to help him coordinate his pelvis and back with this movement. We are taking advantage of balancing reactions of the torso in response to our instruction to roll his pelvis forward and back and lean himself alternately forward and back. We are facilitating motor control.

We also have an instruction at the end of this variation where we make each reciprocating movement smaller and smaller until you come to neutral – that place where the pelvis is vertical and the eyes are on the horizon. This helps hone proprioceptive acuity, as you have to make finer and finer determinations about where the crossover is between falling forward and falling back. Recall that one of our advantages in using reciprocating movements is that it helps to define a truer middle and a more accurate balance between the antagonists.

Differentiating the arms – achieving core competence

In variation C the story continues, but with a twist. We are now asking the arms to differentiate – move the elbows forward with an extending torso and move the elbows and shoulders back with a flexing torso. Does this movement of flexing the arms forward with an extension movement of the torso have clinical relevance? Absolutely! Coordinating the serratus and the abduction of the shoulder girdle (which contracts synergistically with the torso flexors in global flexion movements) with symmetrical or unilateral extension of the torso is useful for many shoulder, shoulder girdle and upper extremity syndromes.

Does the movement of flexing the torso and extending the upper extremities have clinical relevance? In a way. Sometimes you will see someone who flexes through her back and has developed a habit of pulling her shoulders up and back in a futile attempt to haul the torso upright. What we would like is for the torso to be able to move independently of what the upper extremities are doing – besides, asking our students to do unusual movements helps break up rutted neurological pathways, makes them think about what they are doing and stimulates better proprioceptive self-awareness.

Clinically, although we may start by having the scapulae adduct and depress to facilitate the straightening torso, we don't want our students to be required to continue the pinching back and down of the shoulder girdle to maintain an upright posture. We don't need our students to expend the effort of the arms (to which the mid-low trapezii belong) to achieve or maintain good posture; that is the role of the worm. We can use the arms initially to facilitate movement of the torso, but the arms need eventually to be differentiated from the torso (Box 4.6).

We also don't want the arms to try to substitute for core control, as in the scenario of the student who adducts and elevates the shoulder girdles to create a false sense of being upright. This is what can happen if the prime directive that someone organizes their posture around is to pull the shoulders back. This is a big reason that we added this back-to-back variation of moving the arms both globally with and differentiated from the torso. We need them to be both integrated with and independent from each other.

Diagonal falls and orientation

In variations D and E, we play with diagonal directions. The technique is essentially the same: interlace your fingers behind your head and move arms and head together to facilitate a coordination of head and tail. What is the pattern of movement through the torso when looking up and to the left? Down toward the left hip? These are the diagonal patterns introduced in the section on falling.

- Looking up and left is like falling forward and to the left; right torso extension.

Box 4.6 Sitting Circles

Orientation from vertical – global torso flexion/extension and diagonal movements. Chair sitting

Orientation from vertical identical to forward, backward and diagonal falls

Head moves as extension of torso and pelvis

Change of venue – same 360° slinky movement of the torso in vertical instead of horizontal

---

- Looking down at the left hip is like falling back and to the right; left torso flexion.

- Looking up and to the right is like falling forward and to the right; left torso extension.

- Looking down at the right hip is like falling back and to the left; right torso flexion.

- Same patterns, different intent.

How did your two diagonals compare? Which of the four directions seemed easiest or most familiar? We all have flexion/extension and left/right biases, which means we all have a preferred diagonal direction. We might again play a guessing game with our students: which way do we anticipate they will be able to move easily just from an observation of their posture? What difference does the diagonal movement of the torso make to the organization of the arms? Which way did your right lower trapezius work best? Did you coordinate it with left torso extension or right torso extension?

These are again subvariations of basically the same thing, where we are asking the student to move the arms both globally with and differentiated from the torso, but now outside the cardinal lines. These variations add variety, they add spice, they keep you on your toes, they inform you about your tendencies and they provide a framework for working with your deficiencies.

Comparing baselines

In variation F we have the movement we have been leading up to and that, once adequately learned, makes a handy home exercise. Connect the dots and make a circle. Start with an alternating U-shaped movement of your elbows in space and of your pelvis on the seat. Progress to filling out the top of the U. This is the 360° circle that we saw in Baby Rolls, but in an upright orientation. Which way is it easier to do?

For most people, it will be in an upright position. This is an example of something coming later in the developmental sequence being more readily accessible to the average adult than the more primitive movement. Whereas we might logically say we should teach Baby Rolls before teaching Sitting Circles, this is usually not the case.

This last variation compares our baselines again to the beginning. How was your sitting balance? How was your integration in looking up and down? This last or summary movement features our four cardinal directions: flexion, extension, left side-bending and right side-bending. This movement features our four diagonal directions: left and right torso extension and left and right torso flexion. This movement then fills in the rest of circle by bringing in the other 352 directions. Why do we do this?

Because the neck starts at the pelvis! Because for the neck to move freely and be balanced accurately, the pelvis has to be mobile in all directions and the thoracic spine and ribcage need to be integrated with the neck and be balanced accurately themselves. We are doing this lesson for the same basic reasons we have performed all our previous lessons: we want our students to recognize the advantages of using integrated, well-proportioned movement in balance and orientation functions, and we will use it to teach postural awareness and improvement.

Applications

Who are we going to use this lesson with? We could use it with everyone who needs to learn proportional movement from head to tail and everyone who needs to learn tall orientation. We could use this lesson with everyone that needs to learn trunk control and upright sitting. The people who need these skills may have a degenerated cervical disk or a hypermobile facet joint. They may have neck or shoulder girdle muscular tension or muscle imbalances. They may have headaches, temporomandibular joint (TMJ) syndrome or thoracic outlet syndrome. They may have a lumbar disk or joint dysfunction, lumbar or sacroiliac (SI) instabilities, or any number of thoracic spine or rib joint irritations.

They may have suffered a stroke and tend to slump back in their wheelchair. They may have had open-heart surgery and stopped moving their chest. This is often why you won't get a straight answer from a Feldenkrais practitioner when you ask him what he would do for a particular diagnosis. What he would do would depend less on knowing the exact tissue being strained or the exact tracts of the brain that were affected, and more on knowing what that particular person's postural and movement biases or inefficiencies were that were contributing to that tissue strain or functional imbalance.

That having being said, the observant practitioner might, with experience, be able to correlate certain diagnoses with certain common patterns and eventually be able to guess what he might do for a certain diagnoses; as always, be prepared to be wrong sometimes, and don't get too attached to your initial assessment and plan.

Variations

Variations of this lesson are myriad. There are many different positional variations in which we establish a grid (move forward and back; now move side to side) and then connect the dots to make a circle. Hands and knees, sitting on heels with hands forward on the floor, side-sitting and leaning forward on hands, three-and-a-half point stance, modified plantigrade or three-and-a-half point plantigrade, standing with pelvis on a wall and leaning with hands (or elbows) on knees, or making the circle in that same position but without support from the arms are all belly-down orientations that help integrate the torso with the legs. Toy variations include the use of a long pole as both constraint and reference point (Fig. 4.13). There are also belly-up versions of the circle. I will briefly describe one here and discuss variations of it.

Heads Will Roll

Variations

A. Lie on your back with your legs long and spread and with your arms on the floor somewhere below shoulder height.

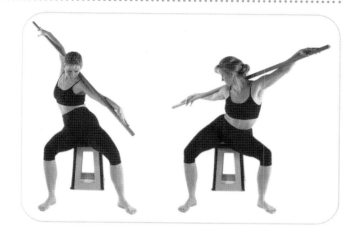

Fig. 4.13 Using toys to facilitate diagonals – move front end of pole down and back, then up and forward.

- Scan your contact against the floor. Feel for bumps and hollows through your backside. How is your weight distributed along your back?

- Imagine your torso as a cylinder. Is it a true cylinder, or are you wider than you are deep? Vice versa? Is your cylinder straight or bent? Or twisted?

- Does your breath fill up your cylinder evenly throughout its length from top to bottom? From side to side? From front to back?

B. Come up to sit on the floor and lean on your hands behind you. Place the soles of your feet together and let your knees hang out to the sides. If this is uncomfortable on your hips or inner thighs, you can cross your legs tailor-fashion, but try with soles together first. Look initially toward the horizon.

- Look down toward your belly button. How do your pelvis and torso participate? How do you organize your breath?

- Try intentionally rolling your pelvis back on the floor and rounding your back. Let your shoulders round forward and slide upward on your back.

- From there, begin to roll your head along your chest to the right, as if bringing your right ear toward your right shoulder (Fig. 4.14).

- Push your belly and chest a bit forward and to the left as you move your left knee towards the floor in cooperation.

- Return to looking down and slumping, then repeat; move in a quarter of an arc. Your pelvis rolls in a quarter-arc on the floor as your head rolls a quarter-arc on your chest. Which of your hands can you press back into the floor to assist with this?

- Roll now in a quarter-arc to the left. Head rolls toward left shoulder as pelvis rolls forward and to the right and right knee reaches toward the floor.

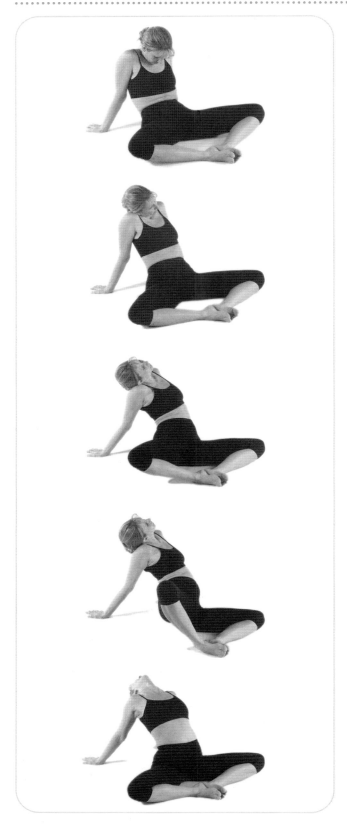

Fig. 4.14 Head rolling sequence to one side – imagine the other half of the circle.

- Alternate from side to side, combining the two quarter-arcs into a half-circle. Pelvis rolls in a half-circle on the floor and head rolls in a half-circle across your chest.

C. Come up to sit again with soles of feet together, leaning again on hands behind.

- Let your head drop toward your chest again and let your whole spine round.
- Now roll your head to the right, then continue in that arc to roll your head backward as if looking toward the ceiling (Fig. 4.14).
- Let your whole back arch, push your belly and chest forward and roll your pelvis forward on the floor. Roll back through right side to slumped/looking-down position. Reverse to make a half-circle to the right.
- Repeat, then pause a moment before doing the same half-circle to the left. How does this side of the circle compare?

D. Come up to sit again with soles of feet together, leaning again on hands behind.

- Combine left and right half-circles into a whole circle. Your head rolls in a circle but not just on top of your shoulders. Your whole back moves around in a circle and your pelvis describes a circle on the floor.
- Reverse the direction of the circle.
- Try circles in each direction while leaning back on your elbows and forearms. How does this differ from leaning on hands?
- Lie on your back again and scan contact, differences from when you started. Can you more clearly feel your torso as a cylinder? How does your breath move in that cylinder?
- Stand up. Walk around. Look around the room. Think of standing inside a 360° sphere. Can you see all around the inside of this imaginary ball?

Synopsis and variations – Heads Will Roll

Here is another lesson that features head-to-tail relationships and which encourages movement of the torso as a 360° slinky. It is very similar to the Sitting Circles lesson except for what happens with the legs and arms. In this lesson, the soles of the feet are together instead of being on the floor – why? You will find in our third section that the legs can control the circular movement of the pelvis, especially if the feet are on the floor, as they are in Sitting Circles.

By placing the soles of the feet together (or sitting tailor-style), we are asking the circular movement of the pelvis on the ground, of the bottom of the sternum in space and of the head in space to be accomplished not by the legs but by the muscles of the torso. It is about as close as you can come to moving like a worm without legs in a vertical orientation (Box 4.7).

Box 4.7 **Heads Will Roll**

Companion lesson to Sitting Circles – sitting on the floor instead of a chair

Upper extremity weightbearing component – upper extremities still moving globally with torso

The arms are also different in this lesson – they are on the ground to create a closed kinetic chain situation. The worm can take advantage of the newly integrated arms to help with the circle, especially the extension half. The arms can press back into the floor, with the lower trapezii being especially useful in assisting and facilitating back extension.

Variations would include changing the position a bit to long sitting, heel-sitting, side-sitting and leaning back on hands or elbows (a particularly diabolical position for anyone with short quadriceps), or sitting in a chair and leaning back on one or both hands. Sitting with one or both knees bent up so the foot or feet are on the floor is a further variation that emphasizes the initiation of the circular motion from the legs – but we're getting a little away from the worm with these.

Lying on your back with the soles of the feet together and rolling your pelvis around in a circle and coordinating your head to roll in a circle but 180° out of phase, is a classic Feldenkrais lesson commonly known as the pelvic clock. There are also subvariations in each of these positions where you make a circle within each quadrant – try them if you feel ambitious. These are all belly-up variations. How many lessons can you construct out of making circles with different positional and orientational variations? I count at least 15!

Are you going to teach them all to each student? No, but having a variety to choose from is useful in case you need to adjust a lesson to accommodate a particular person's limitation or pain. Varying orientation to gravity (belly up vs belly down) is a very important change of venue. Variety is also nice from the perspective of a practitioner – you won't get tired of teaching (and maybe demonstrating) the same thing all the time. Spice up your work life a little bit!

Orientation along the horizon

We have now looked at orientation from vertical: looking up and down, up and to the right and down and to the left, up and to the left and down and to the right and circles.

What are we missing? Orientation left and right along the horizon. This next lesson explores rotational movements as an outgrowth of an intention to look. This again is a variation of a classic Feldenkrais lesson; here we'll call it Side-sit Spirals. This will also be the first lesson in which we deliberately separate the head and neck from the torso and pelvis. Here is where we start to introduce differentiated movements of the worm itself.

Side-sit Spirals

Variations

A. Lie on your back with legs long and arms somewhere on the floor below shoulder height

- Feel your contact against the floor.

- Can you feel any twists through your body? Is your pelvis rolled right or left on the floor? How about your chest and shoulders? How about your head?

- With your eyes closed, move your eyes slowly to the right then back to center. Do this several times then move eyes to left, then alternate. How smoothly do they move? Do they move at an even pace or do they jump from one spot to another?

B. Side-sit right. Sit on the floor with left foot behind and leaning on right hand. Look straight ahead.

- Find the horizon with your eyes open, then close them and move closed eyes to right. How smoothly are they moving here?

- Look over right shoulder and find an 'end-range' reference point. Repeat a few times. Do not strain your neck to see. Move proportionally and protect your neck!

- Put left hand on right shoulder with elbow at shoulder height, pointing forward. From there move left elbow to right and allow pelvis/torso to turn to the right (Fig. 4.15). Left hip moves forward. Keep looking at your elbow. Repeat.

- Come back to looking forward at the horizon and move left elbow forward and back a few times. Your left shoulder blade slides forward and back on your upper back.

- Turn pelvis, torso, elbow to right. Stay there and move elbow forward and back a few times here.

- Move elbow to right and look over right shoulder. What can you see? Deliberately turn your head and move your eyes to the right this time to see behind.

- Move elbow/turn pelvis and torso left and stay there. Then move just the elbow forward and back a few times in that position.

- Alternate moving elbow right and left – turn to look in spirals. Get taller and extend yourself as you twist to the right and get shorter/round yourself as you twist to the left (Fig. 4.15).

C. Repeat steps as in B to left side.

D. Side-sit right. Left leg is behind and you lean on right hand.

- Look over right shoulder; move pelvis, torso, head and eyes. Compare to the beginning.

- Move pelvis, torso to the right but keep head and eyes forward. Try with left hand on right shoulder.

- Do this several times, then move pelvis, torso to the left but keep head and eyes forward (Fig. 4.16).

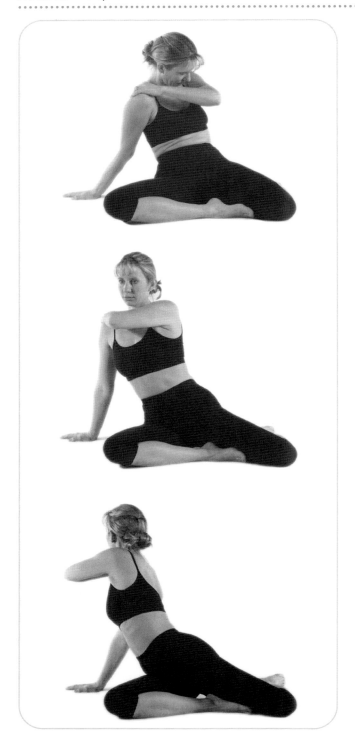

Fig. 4.15 Spiraling shorter and taller – moving head and elbow together.

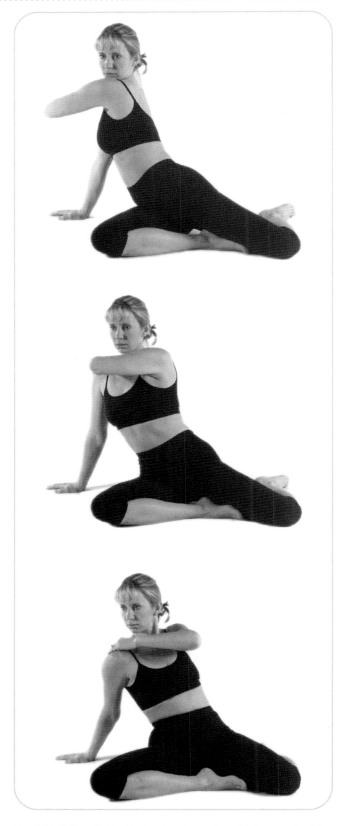

Fig. 4.16 Differentiating the head and neck from the torso and pelvis.

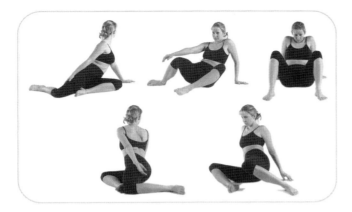

Fig. 4.17 Alternate spiraling to look 360° – or more?

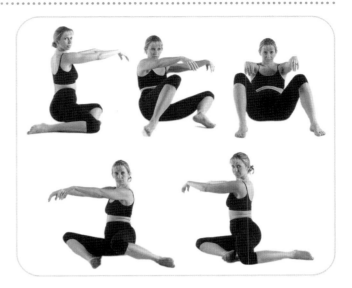

Fig. 4.18 Alternate spirals with more complex variables.

- Do this several times, then alternately turn pelvis and torso right and left while still looking forward.
- Finally, look again alternately over right and left shoulders. Can you see along a 360° horizon? How easy or successful is it to look over your right shoulder now compared to when you started?

E. Same as D, in left side-sit.

F. Same as D and E, except:

- Move eyes with elbow; nose continues to point forward. Move head with torso and elbows, but move eyes opposite. Do this movement in both directions.
- Turn to look over your shoulder once again as you did at the beginning of the lesson. How far or how easily can you see now? Does any more of your body participate in this intention to look than it did at the beginning?
- Now from right side-sitting and looking over your right shoulder, switch everything over to left side-sitting and turn to look over your left shoulder.
- Make the transition from one side to the other by leaning back for a moment on both hands while tilting your knees through the middle (Fig. 4.17).
- Continue by tilting your knees to the other side and lifting the original hand off the floor. Continue this alternating movement of looking over right and left shoulders while making a transition between left and right side-sitting (Fig. 4.17).
- Try continuing this movement but without leaning on your hands (Fig. 4.18). Experiment with turning to look over your shoulder as you spiral taller, and separating your head and neck from your turning torso by continuing to look forward the whole time (Fig. 4.18).
- Find the horizon once again, and close your eyes. Move just your eyes and feel the quality of this movement in comparison to the beginning.

G. Lie on your back again with legs and arms down.

- Scan for contact; compare to the beginning. Feel for whether your head is rolled left or right on the floor.
- Move eyes slowly side to side and compare quality to the beginning.

Static and dynamic baselines – Side-sit Spirals

We start with our familiar supine static baseline again with an emphasis on recognizing rotational bias at the head and pelvis. We also have a dynamic scan while still supine – move closed eyes side to side. Especially when moving slowly, many people will have a difficult time initially with this very important aspect of motor control. With such a close association between the intention to move the eyes and the coordination of the rest of the spinal system, could there be a correlation between the quality of the eye movements and the quality of organization of the rest of the spinal system? Feldenkrais certainly thought so, as he developed many lessons with deliberate movement of the eyes as a major component. Research seems to back this up.[1–9]

The lesson we're analyzing now is one of a number of versions of a classic Feldenkrais lesson that explores coordinating the eyes both globally with and differentiated from the head, torso and pelvis. Adherence to the good housekeeping and proportionality guidelines implies that we want to help our students associate the intention to look left and right with an evenly distributed whole-body movement initiated from the large and all-powerful pelvis.

Other lessons deal with up-and-down orientation and feature up-and-down control of the eyes and their role in coordinating flexion and extension movements and anterior/posterior postural balance of the head and torso. Still others explore circular movements of the eyes within their sockets linked to circular movements of the pelvis and torso (as in

Heads Will Roll). There are even some lessons that ask you to smoothly coordinate the up-and-down movement of your eyes with the side-to-side movement of your head and neck, and vice versa.

Others coordinate and differentiate eyes, tongue and jaw. Some eye lessons deal with distance focus and others coordinate opening and closing of the eyes (sphincter) with opening and closing of the mouth (sphincter), the inhalation and exhalation of breath, or opening and closing of the pelvic floor (Kegel's/sphincters).

Places of disproportionate representation in the CNS

Recall from anatomy and physiology class the concept of the homunculus (the little gnome with huge hands, feet and face and tiny legs and torso that represents proportional representation of these body parts in the sensory and motor cortex) and how disproportionately large some parts of the body are in relation to others. The eyes, mouth/tongue/lips, feet/toes and hand/thumb have a disproportionately large representation in the CNS, whereas the legs, arms, torso and pelvis have relatively smaller representation considering their size. Whereas the muscles of the back or thigh may have one nerve controlling hundreds of muscle fibers in one motor unit, these finer areas might have one nerve controlling a few dozen muscle fibers.

Enhancing control of these key areas of the body helps to enhance control throughout the whole body. It is no surprise that several of our main functional categories revolve around these areas. Movements of the eyes have to do with orientation. Movements of the mouth have to do with eating (vegetation) and talking (communication). Movements of the hands have to do with manipulation of our external environment.

Movements of the feet are concerned with standing (balance) and walking (locomotion). As there are far too many eye lessons to describe here, you'll have to do some of your own research. You might also try incorporating deliberate eye movements into some of our previous lessons.

Be a Better Ball seeks to improve our ability to flex. Start this lessen in supine. As a dynamic baseline, have your student move her eyes down in her sockets to assess quality and control. Have her do some of the lesson with eyes closed and deliberately moving them in their sockets both down (global coordination) and up (differentiated). Reassess smoothness and control at the end of the lesson.

In London Bridges, start and finish with an assessment of the coordination of the eyes moving diagonally up and to the left or up and to the right – again closing eyes for part of the lesson and moving them deliberately both globally and in a differentiated manner. Xs and Os have both up-and-down movements of the eyes, but I doubt you'll be able to spin your eyes 90° in Be a Better Bow. Cherry Turnover and Baby Rolls could have a more prominent role for up-and-down movements of the eyes (Box 4.8).

We will revisit Sitting Circles later in this chapter and play some with eye/head/torso relationships. Heads Will Roll might be a progression of a series of lessons that explores and refines circular movements of the eyes by breaking the circle

---

Box 4.8 Importance of linking exercise to distal intention – places of disproportionate representation in the CNS
Feet – locomotion and balance
Hands – manipulation and orientation (touch)
Lips and tongue – communication (speech and facial expression), vegetation (breathing and eating), and orientation (taste)
Eyes – orientation and balance

down into quarters. Try circling your eyes and head in opposite directions in this one – it's a hoot! Try including the intentional movement of the eyes (and hands, feet and mouth) in your exercise prescriptions: it will make them more effective.

Spiraling from side-sitting

In our first movement variation, come up to right side-sitting on the floor. Your left leg is behind you and your right foot touches your left knee. Lean on your right hand out away from your side. This side-sitting position is an important one from a developmental perspective, as it is from here that as youngsters we spend a lot of time in play, and from which there are a wealth of transitional movements available: side-sit right to side-sit left, side-sit to supine, side-sit to prone, side-sit to hands and knees, side-Sit to Stand, side-sit to three-and-a-half points, side-sit to long sit, etc.

We will be exploring or describing a number of these transitions in Section 3, and will be using transitions from side-sit as functional contexts in which to qualitatively stretch and strengthen the hip, back and lower extremity musculature. Skills used here are also useful in bending, sitting, walking and turning. In this lesson, our focus is still on the movements of the worm, so discussion of lower extremity and upper extremity coordination with the worm will be deferred to the appropriate chapters.

One important detail about this position is the ability to find a place for the hand on the floor where you can allow your weight to be fully supported by the arm. When you are leaning fully on the arm, the torso musculature doesn't have to work as hard just to hold you upright and provides conditions where the torso may be able to move more freely and in a more completely differentiated manner than if those muscles were overly engaged in preventing you from falling. Recall the Weber–Fechner principle and how our ability to discern changes in a sensation is inversely proportional to the intensity of that sensation. Reduce effort in the torso to feel more clearly what you are doing with your torso.

Find the horizon and close your eyes. Move your eyes slowly to the right and back to center several times. How smooth was this movement initially, and how did it change in its quality by the end? Recall the close association of the eyes to the head, the neck and the rest of the torso that we have already explored in horizontal and in sitting. Those orientation movements were primarily of the up-and-down variety, with variations of up and left, down and right, etc.

From horizontal (especially from prone), looking around yourself triggers more of a side-bending movement. For babies and four-legged critters whose torsos are parallel to the ground, looking around a 360° horizon (which is in a horizontal configuration, as opposed to the 360° vertical circle we found in Sitting Circles) takes longer and has a much longer moment arm than looking around with a vertically oriented torso.

Being erect is a unique advantage

This is one of the great advantages of being human. Organizing ourselves from an upright posture allows us to see around much more easily and allows us to change our orientation much faster. Think of bullfighters and how they can keep from being trampled by a provoked bull. They rotate themselves on a vertical axis to get out of the way. The bull, who has to side-bend his whole body to turn, cannot turn fast enough to pin down the little twit.

These movements of the eyes left and right are important ones. We would again like the CNS to associate the intention to turn to look right or left with a whole-body movement that includes an evenly distributed movement all the way through the torso (the good housekeeping rule), with the power, bulk and initiation of the movement provided by the movement of the pelvis (proportionality principal). These questions were part of our second dynamic baseline. Our first dynamic baseline was a question about the smoothness and control of the eye movements.

Smoothness and accurate motor control of the eyes is important for the health of the neck and the postural balance of the head: I have found this to be true both personally and clinically. There is something about smoothing out the eyes that makes the movement of the skeleton better coordinated and better integrated with the eyes. There is something about going through a lesson that deliberately coordinates the skeleton with the movements of the eyes that makes those eye movements smoother. How did this lesson work for you?

How are you going to be able to tell quality of eye movements with your students? You will be able to see it through their eyelids if you are paying attention – look for flutters, jumps or inconsistencies. Many people will have a hard time moving the eyes smoothly, especially with them closed. This will be even more pronounced if head and eyes are moving in opposite directions while the eyes are closed, as you no doubt noticed when doing one of the last variations of the lesson. When teaching this lesson to my students, I ask them to move their eyes as if reading some fine print on the inside of their eyelids (in both directions), to go slowly and focus on control rather than range of motion, and to quiet their jaw, face and eyelids to reduce proprioceptive chatter.

For our second dynamic baseline, find the horizon then turn to look over your right shoulder as if you want to see something behind you. How far can you turn without feeling a strain in your neck? Where do you start this movement? How evenly distributed is this movement? How do most of our cervical students organize this movement? They will move their head and turn their neck, initiating the movement from the top and working on down from there. Head – C1 – C2, 3, 4, maybe C5 or 6 – then somewhere in there they run into their brick wall.

Almost universally, the cervicothoracic junction (C6 or 7 through T3 or 4) will be locked up tighter than Queen Victoria's corset. It is often this interface between segments that move and segments that don't where joint and disk shearing or joint instabilities/hypermobilities occur. It is no wonder that the majority of cervical disks and degenerative articular changes happen between C4 and C7.

When working with these folks, or younger versions of them who organize themselves the same way but haven't been doing it long enough to have those degenerative changes show up on imaging tests yet, we again need to apply the rule of holes. When your student is in a hole and getting deeper, the first thing to do is to stop digging.

Teaching head to tail connections – spiraling

How do we get someone to move more proportionally? To stop moving way too much at one vulnerable spot? How do we get the CT junction to move, to participate in the intention to look? We do this by encouraging initiation or simultaneous activation of the movement from the pelvis. Organize the movement from bottom up, to include the CT junction. Can people move from bottom to top without getting actual intervertebral movement in that area?

Certainly, but to at least set the tone for CT movement we need to get the CNS to associate movement of the head with movement of the tail. We can then progress that to get CT segmental movement by differentiating head and neck from torso (as we begin to do later in this lesson) by bringing the arms and shoulder girdles into the action (as we will do in Volume 2) and by your favorite manual technique. How did we facilitate head to tail coordination in this lesson? 'Put your left hand on your right shoulder and move your elbow to the right.' This movement nearly requires the pelvis to move.

By continuing to look at the elbow and focusing attention and intention on moving (reaching) the elbow, we can begin to help the student's CNS to dissociate an intention to look with top-to-bottom organization. This is another variation of the type of constraint we used in earlier lessons where we put hand and head together to move them as one unit – this time we put arm and thorax together to move them as one. By combining movement of the elbow with the additional intention to look over the shoulder, we are providing the CNS with information about the advantages of integrated movement and the importance of the movement of the pelvis to the movements of the eyes; the neck starts with the pelvis (Box 4.9).

How did we facilitate additional thoracic movement in this step of the lesson? Move your elbow alternately forward and back both in neutral and while turned. This abduction/adduction of the shoulder girdle, especially in a turned position,

---

Box 4.9 Side-sit Spirals

Floor-sitting rotational movements – head moves globally with and differentiated from the torso
Combines spiraling taller and spiraling shorter movements with orientation along the horizon and with orientation fixed forward
Standing and supine variations – hand fixed to shoulder as constraint technique
Use of cumulative movements – combining orientation, balance and transitional movements

nearly requires some movement of the ribs and thoracic spine and helps to achieve a more evenly distributed movement through the torso.

After facilitating rotational movements in one direction, we then have our students turn in the opposite direction, but from the same asymmetrical sitting position. When side-sitting right, is it easier to turn to look over right shoulder or over the left? When in right side-sit, the instructions of the lesson were to intentionally (if you hadn't already figured it out) add in a flexion and extension component to the rotation. Get taller and extend yourself as you turn to look over your right shoulder, and get shorter/round yourself a bit as you look over your left. This spiraling movement is an important one for a couple of reasons.

One reason we would like our students to spiral rather than just rotate in a purely transverse plane is to make sure they are not rotating while flexed. This is a common organization and again puts that interface between segments that move (typically C4 or 5) and segments that don't (typically C6 or 7) at risk for shearing and hypermobile movement. By maintaining a habitually flexed postural pattern, either throughout the entire thoracic spine or just in the CT junction, it makes intersegmental movement in that area much more difficult because the joint play in those segments is already taken up by the movement into flexion.

For most people, the spiraling to get taller movement allows for greater freedom and better distribution of movement. This is because as the thoracic spine or CT junction moves out of chronic flexion toward a more neutral position of the joints it frees up joint play that can now be available for rotation. Get on the floor (or sit in a chair) and try this yourself. Turn to look while staying flexed and notice what you can see. Then spiral taller to look and compare. Most of you will find spiraling more successful in terms of range and less stressful in terms of effort or local tissue strain.

Part of this spiraling movement is a result of weight-shifting to the side you are turning to. Part of the reason we are doing the spiraling movement from a side-sitting position is that the asymmetrical weightbearing is already present. We exaggerate the shift of weight forward and to the right when spiraling taller to look over the right shoulder. This movement may suggest a version of a left torso extension pattern in response to this fall forward and to the right. We also exaggerate the shift of weight back and to the left when spiraling shorter to look over the left shoulder. This movement may suggest a version of a right torso flexion pattern in response to this fall back and to the left.

This reciprocation between left torso extension and right torso flexion is enhanced by the balancing requirements of the torso in response to the weight-shifting of the pelvis. We are using balancing reactions to help link the same torso patterns now to the additional function of orientation (we will use it again later to help link these same torso patterns, these same Legos, to manipulation functions). Our last variation in this lesson has you doing this movement of alternately spiraling down and left and up and right without the support of your hand on the floor.

Many people cannot do this, so don't kill yourself trying it out, but if you can carry it off, feel how the additional demand for balancing in these positions requires additional flexibility

and strength through the torso and legs, compared to what it was like leaning on your hand. Because this is a diagonal reciprocating movement of the torso, it has the same advantages as all reciprocating movements.

1. One, it helps balance the left torso extensor musculature and the right torso flexor musculature, requiring the CNS to orchestrate this cooperative tug-of-war.

2. Two, it helps define more clearly where middle or neutral is. It is a means of improving left/right postural balance.

3. Three, moving reciprocally helps provide contrast and allows our students to repeatedly move into and out of the spiraling taller movement. It helps them to know where they are, how they got there, and how moving in a spiral is advantageous in terms of success (larger range) and ease (less strain in the neck).

Another reason we would like our students to spiral taller to look left or right along the horizon is to facilitate a higher horizon. We use this movement to uncover the murky corners of our brains that once recognized the advantages of looking at the world from as high a vantage point as possible. The extension component of the spiral is crucial in being able to lengthen the spine and to bring the mid-thoracic spine forward and underneath the head to provide the skeletal weightbearing support so desperately needed by our long-suffering cervical students.

Differentiating the head and neck from the torso

In variation D, continue with the same spiraling movement in each direction but with a twist: keep the nose and eyes pointed forward while still turning pelvis, torso and shoulders. This variation features the first intentional differentiation of the head and neck from the pelvis and torso. In all our previous lessons, the head and its orientation apparatus has moved as an extension of the pelvis and the torso. In these early balance and orientation functions, the global relationship between head/neck and torso/pelvis makes perfect sense in light of the good housekeeping rule. Why would we ask someone to move their head and neck opposite to their shoulders and chest? It only makes sense when considering the need of the CNS to execute multiple functions simultaneously.

For instance, I might want to throw a ball. Initially, I might turn sideways to whatever I'm throwing at and look past my left shoulder (if right-handed). As I throw, my pelvis and body twist to the left to provide the power of the legs, pelvis and torso to the movement of my arm. Because I am still looking at what I'm throwing at, my head and eyes stay oriented forward as my torso and pelvis turn underneath (Fig. 4.19). This is a differentiated movement of the head and neck from the pelvis that combines the functions of orientation and manipulation.

Golf is another example of this. Keeping your eye on the ball both as you back-swing and as you swing through (one of an endless series of difficult features in golf that makes this game so maddening yet addicting) again combines orientation and manipulation. Another example involves walking. When walking, we would like to see some turning of the shoulders

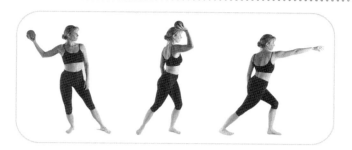

Fig. 4.19 Combining orientation and manipulation differentiates head from torso.

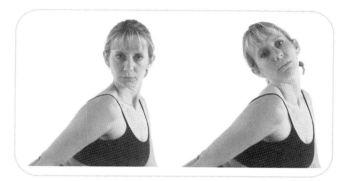

Fig. 4.20 Two versions of organizing the head – vertical or tipped.

and upper back/chest. While still looking forward toward the horizon, the head and neck are again differentiated from the swinging arms and turning shoulders. This differentiation occurs because of the need to juggle multiple functions: orientation and locomotion.

Using this differentiated movement can help us clinically in two ways. One, it is another way to stimulate a high horizon as the torso continues to spiral taller and move into left or right extension. Two, it helps us to mobilize and balance the CT and suboccipital junctions. The ability to keep the head truly vertical and the eyes truly on the horizon is much more difficult than you might at first think. The most common error most people make with this movement is to tilt their head and neck back and to the left when moving the pelvis and torso to the right and keeping the head oriented forward (Fig. 4.20).

This tilting-back or quadrant movement of the head and neck is consistent with the quadrant movement of the torso. The head moves globally as an extension of the left torso extension movement in response to falling forward and to the right. This 'erroneous' movement can actually be a very good way to help someone to reaccess long-forgotten movement capabilities in the CT junction. Clinically, I have especially found using global and differentiated unilateral extension and side-bending movements to be useful in getting someone to feel again how to move the upper thoracic spine and upper ribs.

In this variation, we could use just balance as our sole criterion and actually encourage tilting the head and movement of the neck into left cervical extension. As long as you move

proportionally, this reduces quadrant stresses on the cervical spine and facilitates movement of the thoracic spine and CT junction into left extension.

The rotational component of the movement also encourages independent movement between the often glued-together vertebrae of the CT junction, the mobilization of their facet joints and the emergence of more accurate motor control over the intrinsic and extrinsic cervical and torso musculature. With the head and neck moving in one direction and the torso and shoulders moving in another, we would like the necessary rotational differentiation adjustments to happen over the several segments of the CT junction, rather than just at the hypermobile one. We ensure this by going slowly and by having our students pay close attention to deliberately limiting and protecting the movement of the neck while encouraging movement of the upper back/upper chest.

What happens to the organization of this global movement if we add in the requirement of orienting to a high horizon? The tilting movement of the head back and to the left has to stop to be able to bring the eyes to horizontal. This differentiation of the head from the neck is made at the suboccipital junction, where the head has to tilt back forward and to the right (complex differentiations at occipitoaxial (OA) and atlantoaxial (AA)) in response to the neck tilting back and to the left. Here is one way of facilitating suboccipital mobilization (through requiring the adjustment for horizontal eyes), left/right balance (through alternating or reciprocating movements) and decompression (through the downward nodding or right/left occipital flexion as the head differentiates from the neck).

Try it again several times and see if you can feel and be aware of what I'm describing. Use a mirror to ensure the eyes are level. Mimic the movement with your favorite articulated model of the spine and observe the movements of the head on C1 and C1 on C2. Because I like this movement so much and think it has such positive benefits for my students, you will be seeing it again later in this book linked to other functional contexts.

Spiraling down and to the left while looking forward at the horizon is another differentiated movement that is a version of a very common way that people organize themselves. While the torso flexes, bends to the right and rotates to the left, the head and neck have to extend, bend to the left and rotate to the right. This creates a flexed thoracic and/or CT junction and compresses the suboccipital junction. This is just what we are trying to have many of our students stop doing so much. Why even move them in this direction? Reciprocating movements help the CNS to map where you are on a movement continuum. This spiraling movement can help balance both left/right and anterior/posterior postural balance.

Reciprocating movements help coordinate the diagonal antagonists of neck and torso; they reduce muscle imbalances. Spiraling shorter into flexion stimulates a spring-loading effect of the diagonal extensors and allows a fuller and more complete movement into our (usually) desired direction of spiraling taller. Our students get practice in moving repeatedly into a (usually) desirable direction, and in doing so know more clearly how to get there and why it may be advantageous, compared to how they were doing things. Recall that the art of teaching requires knowing both what to teach and how to teach it. Whereas logic dictates movement only into a desirable direction with total avoidance of a damaging direction, biology has other criteria.

Differentiating the eyes – scrambling the habitual associations

The next variation, F, is a subvariation of the last. Resume moving head and neck with spiraling pelvis and torso but move eyes in the opposite direction. This movement of differentiating the eyes from the head is another one I use for facilitating smooth mobility and postural balance of the neck, especially the upper cervical area. The eyes seem to be most strongly connected to the upper spine, and lessons featuring global and differentiated movements of the eyes and head in various positions and in different directions (up/down, left/right) can be used with people with headaches and other symptoms of upper cervical dysfunction or imbalance.

This is a hard variation for most people. You probably have an appreciation for just how tightly connected the movements of the eyes and the movements of the head and neck are for most people. This instruction to differentiate eyes from head is to further refine motor control over the cervical (especially the upper cervical) spine and to further refine proprioceptive accuracy on the part of your students. Do people ever do this in real life? Notice what you do when using a mirror to shave or to put on make-up.

This eye/head differentiation also occurs when combining another pair of functional categories: communication and orientation. Someone might turn or tilt their head for emphasis (body language) in a conversation while still looking at you, thereby differentiating their head and eyes. I have noticed that children do this more frequently and with more variety than adults. Could the loss of variety of head/eye combinations contribute to neck problems?

This segment of the lesson includes a return to the dynamic baselines of first looking over your shoulder then moving closed eyes left and right. Was it good for you too? What was the experience of the person you taught this to? Will you ask (use inquisitive language)?

This segment also includes a culminating movement, a summation of the whole lesson. It is this sort of movement that we should encourage our students to continue with on a home program. Adding in a transitional movement from side-sitting to opposite side-sit helps bring the pieces together. It incorporates weight-shifting in the direction you are turning and the alternate spiraling taller and shorter. It features reciprocating movements from side to side and allows back-to-back comparisons to be made between the two sides. Once those comparisons are made, your student is in a better position to make motor adjustments needed to lessen any imbalance.

By making the transitional movement a bit quicker, you lessen reliance on upper extremity support and require more balance adjustments to be made by the torso. This necessity for torso mobility and strength so as not to topple over is put to the test in the variation of doing this movement without the hands on the floor at all. This variation requires some serious multitasking; balance, orientation and transitions. It also requires precise and reversible trajectories of movement, or it will become a form of locomotion as well.

You will scoot forward on the floor as you make these transitional movements unless you roll your pelvis back and to the middle as far as you roll it forward and to the side. Differentiating head and eyes from the reciprocally turning torso and pelvis is another cumulative movement that we could prescribe for continuing at home. Differentiating eyes from turning pelvis, torso and head is fun and requires a lot of concentration (trains proprioceptive self-awareness), helps to scramble habitual neural patterns, softens their stranglehold on strained tissues and makes for a great party trick!

Applications

What sort of people might this lesson or its variations be useful for? Any kind of cervical dysfunction where an ability to access a full 360° horizon is compromised, manifesting in or resulting from cervical disk, facet strain or degeneration, muscle imbalance, etc.; any kind of cervical or shoulder girdle postural dysfunction that features a chronically flexed thoracic and/or CT junction, manifesting in cervical disk, facet, muscle imbalance, etc.; any cervical trauma or whiplash where we wish to restore fluidity and spontaneity. Use this with people with headaches to help mobilize, balance and decompress the suboccipital area.

We would use this lesson with various upper extremity dysfunctions for its upper extremity closed kinetic chain and thoracic extension components. We could use this lesson with someone with scoliosis, using the concept of moving equally easily in both directions to recalibrate toward a truer neutral. We could use this with our neurologic population to help restore turning movements or rotational movements of the torso: stroke, MS, Parkinson's disease and other nervous system malfunctions that lead to rigidity or imbalanced movement, or to marked left-to-right imbalances.

In terms of performance enhancement, we might want to think of sports where rotation is a big component, especially when orientation is independent of the turn. Golf is a classic example because of the need to keep your eye on the ball with both the back-swing and the stroke. All racket, batting and throwing sports have this feature. Gymnastics, dance and figure skating are other examples.

Variations

Variations of this lesson can be performed while sitting, standing or on hands and knees. If sitting on a mat table or bench, your student can still lean on a hand to the side that they spiral taller towards. When in a chair, you can either dispense with leaning on a hand altogether or can place a hand on the seat behind you. All the same variations can still apply in terms of moving pelvis, torso, head and eyes in various combinations of global and differentiated patterns.

The weight-shifting component is still applicable, as we often want our students to do this when turning. Try turning a few times to look over your right shoulder while turning pelvis and shifting weight to the right. Then try it while still turning your pelvis to the right but shifting your weight back

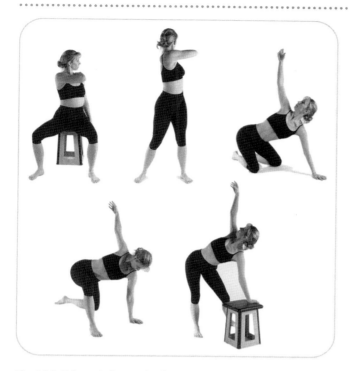

Fig. 4.21 Other spiraling and differentiation opportunities.

to the left instead. You will probably find that shifting weight to the right facilitates our desired extension bias by spiraling to get taller, whereas shifting weight to the left suggests more of a flexion bias. Compare and contrast turning with weight shifts toward the side you are turning to, away from the side you are turning to, and with no weight shift at all – the classic Goldilocksian triple choice (Fig. 4.21).

In standing, the basic idea is the same. Without a hand to lean on, we could either continue to place one hand on the opposite shoulder or we could spread the arms out to the sides like an airplane and move them as if there were a stick all the way through them (or put a pole across your shoulders). This constraint serves the same purpose as the hand on the shoulder as it links head and eyes with torso and pelvis. Try out the weight-shifting options here; you will probably again find that shifting weight in the same direction as the turn is more successful.

You can facilitate this weight shift by adding a variation about lifting the back heel (left heel if turning right) and pivoting on the ball of the left foot. The spiraling movements and the intention to see around with a high horizon helps to improve standing posture in the same way that it did in sitting. The differentiations of head from torso and eyes from head also serve to mobilize and balance the CT and suboccipital (SO) junctions, as described in sitting (Fig. 4.21).

On hands and knees, we could ask our student to reach her right hand toward the ceiling, looking at it the whole time. Encourage a shift of weight to the right, a turning of the pelvis to the right around the hips, and another version of a left torso extension pattern through the torso. Initially, looking at the hand as it reaches makes for a global pattern of move-

ment where the head and neck are turning with the pelvis and torso.

Later, we can differentiate the head by continuing the same movement but looking instead at the hand on the ground. Add in variations about differentiating eyes and head or doing the same thing from a three-and-a-half point stance and you have another version of the same basic lesson. This could also be performed in a modified plantigrade position, or a three-and-a-half point variation of this (Fig. 4.21).

This lesson and its variations explores global spiraling patterns linked to horizontal orientation and to differentiated patterns linked to combinations of orientation and manipulation, orientation and locomotion and orientation and transitional movements. What seems to give people the most trouble clinically is the combination of orientation and balance. It is this combination that we will address in this next section.

Combining balance and orientation

This section features both global and differentiated sidebending and flexion/extension movements. The context for differentiation will be the sometimes deadly combination of balance and orientation to the horizon. I say deadly because it is this combination that gives people so much grief relating to neck and shoulder girdle pain. Nobody has perfect posture in either an anterior/posterior or a left/right direction: we all tend to fall in a habitual direction.

These habitual pelvis and torso imbalances combine with adjustments made in the CT and SO junctions to keep the head vertical and the eyes horizontal. The results are invariant compressions, gaping and shearing of articular structures, and invariant antagonist relationships where one of the pair is chronically weak and long and the other is short and hypertonic. The first lesson is entitled Eskimo Rolls and explores side-bending relationships. The second lesson is really just a continuation of the Sitting Circles lesson, this time with additional variations that differentiate head and torso.

Eskimo Rolls

Variations

A. Sit on a kitchen-style chair and be aware of the balance of your pelvis on the seat left and right.

   • Is one shoulder higher than the other?

   • How is your head balanced on top of your spine?

   • Is your head tipped left or right?

   • Bend your head to the right as if to read imaginary vertical writing (Fig. 4.22). How much of your spine participates in this movement?

   • Do the same thing to the left. How does this side compare? Alternate this movement.

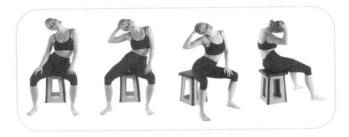

Fig. 4.22 Test movement – move head and hand together – stay side bent to round/arch.

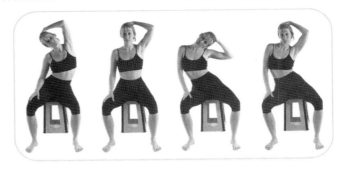

Fig. 4.23 Going both ways, then differentiating head from torso.

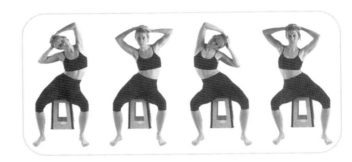

Fig. 4.24 Putting it all together to make an undulation.

- Which way does your head bend most easily? Do you sense movement of your pelvis on the seat? Do your ribs move?

B. Sit with your right hand on top of your head, right elbow pointing out to the right.

- Let your torso bend as you reach your right elbow toward your right hip. Lift your right hip to meet your right elbow – let your weight shift on to your left hip (Fig. 4.22). Repeat several times, then –

- Bend and stay there; round and arch slightly in this bent position (Fig. 4.22). Where are you centered? Where you are neither arched nor rounded in your bend?

- Bend and exhale; wheeze. Repeat this several times.

C. Sit with left hand on head, left elbow pointed to the left. Repeat instructions from B; do the same as above but to the opposite side.

D. Sit with your left hand on top of your head.

- Reach your left elbow to the ceiling. Let your head and torso bend to the right and lift your right hip (Fig. 4.23). The whole left side of your torso gets longer as you shift your weight to your left hip.

- Return to the movement of reaching your left elbow toward your left hip as above, still letting weight shift to the right and your torso bend to the left.

- Alternate between reaching your elbow up and down, bending left and right and shifting weight from side to side (Fig. 4.23).

- Pause for a moment, then reach your left elbow to the ceiling again while bending to the right and with weight toward your left hip. Now lead the movement back to center with your head (Fig. 4.23).

- Bring your head back to vertical, then follow with your pelvis and torso. Repeat moving head and torso together to bend to the right, but separate your head from your torso by bringing it back first.

E. Same thing as D to the opposite side: right hand on top of your head and bending alternately from side to side. Differentiate head and neck from torso by returning head to vertical first.

F. Sit with both hands on top of head.

- Alternately bend right and left, allowing coordinated movement of pelvis, torso, head and arms. Repeat this alternating movement several times.

- Then continue to bend and shift weight from side to side, but keep your head vertical and your eyes on the horizon. Your head and neck end up bending opposite to your torso. This is another differentiated movement.

- Can you turn this movement into an undulation? Imagine yourself as a snake and wave your head, neck and torso from side to side (Fig. 4.24).

G. Resume your seat; this time let your arms hang down by your sides.

- Look up and down; let your back round and arch and your pelvis roll forward and back on the seat.

- Bend right and left as if reading vertical writing; allow pelvis and torso to assist. How does this movement compare to how it was at the beginning?

- Connect the dots; make a circle. Your pelvis makes a circle on the seat. Your head makes a circle in space.

- Simply sit and observe pelvis contact on seat. How are you balanced from side to side? How are you balanced front to back? Where on the circle are you?

- Stand up and walk around. How is your head balanced on top of your spine? Do you allow your ribs to bend from side to side as you walk?

Static and dynamic baselines – Eskimo Roll

The baselines in this lesson concern left and right differences. The static baseline questions were about differences in distribution of weight on the ischial tuberosities, height of the shoulders and left/right balance of the head. The dynamic baseline questions were about ease, balance and integration while bending your head from side to side as if reading vertical writing.

What we would like this dynamic baseline to look like should be obvious by now. We would like to see an evenly distributed global side-bending movement where head and tail are coordinated in what is essentially a balance reaction. As you bend your head to the right, we would expect your right hip to lift and the whole torso, CT junction and neck to bend to the right. You should shift your weight to your left ischial tuberosity.

The first part of the lesson was devoted to communicating this idea of integrated and evenly distributed movement, initiated from the pelvis, relating primarily to the function of balance. Placing your hands on your head and deliberately moving your elbow and hip towards and away from each other is yet another variation of that frequently used constraint: attach head and hand and move them as a unit.

The second part of the lesson deals with separating the movement of the head and neck from the pelvis and torso, exploring differentiated movements in side-bending directions. Why would we do this? What is the functional and clinical relevance of this movement? To begin to answer these questions, let's look back at our static baseline for a moment.

If the weight of your pelvis is shifted more to the left, we could say functionally that you are in an arrested state of falling to your left. We would expect that the torso would then bend to the right as part of a balance reaction; this is most often the case in sitting. We might then expect the left shoulder to be higher than the right and the head tipped to the right, with the left eye higher or closer to the ceiling than the right. Whereas this would be true of a well-organized system if balance were the sole criterion, this is not really how people do things.

Although the height of the shoulders is usually predictable from an awareness of differences in weight distribution left to right on the pelvis, the head rarely is held in this side-bent position. The strongly conditioned desire to keep the head vertical and the eyes horizontal results in differentiated movement that counters bending the torso in response to the falling pelvis. Balance and orientation to the horizon combine to make this a differentiated posture.

CT and SO differentiations

As a schematic, we can think purely in terms of side-bending movements, though we know that side-bending and rotation are linked. As a schematic then, if the pelvis were rolled to the left we would expect the torso to be bent to the right. The right shoulder girdle would be lower, as it follows the bending of the torso to the right. The differentiation required to keep the head vertical can happen in one of two basic ways. First, the neck can continue to bend to the right as an extension of the right side-bending torso and the differentiation happens in the suboccipital area.

This results in gapping strains of the right OA and AA complex and compression strains on the left. What this might look like to the observant practitioner is a translation of the head in space to the right. With your student sitting, standing or supine, visualize the vertical midline of the face and note where it is in relation to the sternal notch. In this scenario, the midline will be to the left of the sternal notch. Think of an 'Egyptian dance' and the translatory movement of the head from side to side in space.

On visual observation of this relationship in supine, the practitioner with the fine touch might pick up the aforementioned head and gently suggest this same translatory movement from side to side. You will probably find that movement in the nonhabitual direction is restricted at some or many levels. The experienced practitioner can assess mobility, bias and relationships if she goes slowly and listens for subtleties as she works her way down the neck.

The second common pattern we see is that the initial differentiation happens somewhere around the CT junction as the neck side-bends opposite the torso. This often manifests itself in an offset of the facial midline to the left – the same kind of translatory or 'Egyptian head' movement as above, but in the opposite direction. This sometimes happens at the C6/C7 level (my own personal Waterloo), or it can happen a few segments up (most common) or down (more rarely).

As the neck bends to the left, we get yet another differentiation at the SO junction as the head has to bend back to the right again to compensate for the leftward-bending neck, which was compensating for the rightward-bending torso, which was compensating for the leftward-falling pelvis and which is a reflection of hip and pelvic girdle muscle imbalances. Could imbalances of the iliopsoas groups contribute to headaches? Can the organization of the forest as a whole increase the likelihood of damage to individual trees? Let me tell you a story.

A tragic story

I have had a historically strong pattern where I habitually bear weight to the left, bend my torso to the right and bend back to the left again at C6. This has contributed to a vulnerable spot at the left C6 facet joint as it was constantly being compressed into a close-packed position. When I turned to look over my left shoulder, I quickly ran C6 into C7, as C7 would stick with the torso and refuse to participate in orientation. This would hurt. For the same basic reason, it also hurt when I side-bent my head and neck to the left.

I was 'surfing' my sea-kayak on some small breaking waves near the outer Washington state coast some years back and had the misfortune (or inadequate motor skills – you be the judge) of dumping. As I felt myself falling to the right, I needed to brace with my paddle and bend back to the left to get my center of mass back over my boat. The brace was woefully inadequate and in my attempt to bring my head back over my boat, I bent in the only place I really knew how.

I quickly and forcefully side-bent left at C6/7 and could feel the error of my ways in my neck even before hitting the frigid water. Ouch! If only I had known then what I know now.

Box 4.10 The history preceding the accident

Historic biases predispose to certain injury
Forces travel path of least resistance – injuries funnel to already hypermobile places

I should have followed the good housekeeping rule and bent evenly throughout my whole torso instead of bending at that one spot. The trouble, of course, is that left torso side-bending is my nonhabitual and more difficult direction. Maybe next time I'll bias myself to dumping to the left so I can bend my torso in my habitual/easier direction.

In the heat of battle, of course, it's not likely you'll have the time to think it through and make less damaging choices. All the more reason to teach people integrated from an organic and functional standpoint rather than from a strictly cognitive and logical one. Make these movement patterns ingrained so they are available at all times (Box 4.10).

The other issue this story illustrates is the connection between injuries and habitual biases. My historic bias predisposed me to injuring myself at the particular spot, especially as a result of left rotation, left quadrant or side-bending stresses. The stress in the kayak story is falling to the right. What do you think the outcome would be if I were hit broadside from the left while in my car? How about if I'm lying on my right side and lifting my head to peer groggily at the intruding alarm clock? Or if I'm sitting on the floor looking at and talking to someone to my left, and my son comes up in a stealth charge behind me and nails me in the back? Or if I fall asleep on my belly with my head turned to the left?

Habitual biases make us more likely to injure certain places. Forces causing injury tend to go for the path of least resistance. They tend to stress the weakest link in the chain, and they go right for the hypermobile segment. When seeing someone with a neck injury, don't assume that their history starts on the day of their accident. Look for patterns or biases, and make guesses as to whether they precede or come from an accident. In reality, trying to sort out historical patterns from compensations and protective mechanisms as a result of the injury is tough. All the more reason to prescribe exercise that moves our students progressively and organically toward more ideal movement and postural organization.

Applying constraints and subvariations

Variations B and C feature a familiar strategy: place your right hand on your head and move your right elbow and right hip toward each other. This facilitates torso side-bending. The instruction to lift the right hip to meet the right elbow is designed to facilitate our desired weight shift to the left and to reawaken (sometimes) ancient balance reactions.

The exploration of flexion and extension movements while in a side-bent position is to help the CNS find a truer or more accurate side-bend without inaccurately incorporating that person's habitual flexion or extension bias. This is another example of reciprocating movements designed to find a neutral. The instruction to wheeze, to force your air out, is a way to facilitate a fuller lateral intercostal contraction. By bringing in

another function (vegetation), we are helping the CNS to diversify – to put the same motor information in several different folders.

The instruction in variations D and E was to place your left hand on top of your head and reach your left elbow toward the ceiling. You were encouraged to allow full torso side-bending to the right and weight-shifting to the left. The emphasis has changed from shortening the sides, as it was in the first variation (bring elbow and hip toward each other), to lengthening the side (with reaching upward being the context). The next variation in this section combines the two movements into one alternating one.

Here again we have our reciprocating movements and cooperative antagonists. We are connecting weight-shifting with side-bending and movement of the head in one direction with the movement of the pelvis in the other: the classic balance reaction. This is a global pattern of movement and you will find that many lessons are structured this way. We often introduce global patterns first in a lesson to re-establish the more primitive response and to simplify pattern recognition. We then progress to differentiated and more complex patterns later.

Falling sideways and orienting to the horizon

The last variation is this section is where this progression begins. Here, we are asking our students to remain bent to one side and then to bring the head back to vertical without moving the rest of the pelvis/torso yet. This is the variation that most closely resembles the incongruent combination of balance and orientation described earlier. By incongruent, I mean that in a well-organized system the pelvis and torso would be balanced left/right to support the intention to orient forward to a high horizon, whereas in real life we are all falling in some direction and staying there while the neck and head have to make the adjustments necessary to keep the eyes horizontal. The CNS is letting the pelvis and torso fall into their accustomed spots and has left the neck and head to fend for themselves.

Let's say we have a student with left-sided neck pain who presents with an elevated left shoulder girdle, short left upper trapezius and levator, and pain on left cervical quadrant testing. In our simplified schematic, we might anticipate that she is bearing weight predominantly on the left side of her pelvis and is bending her torso to the right. This would account for at least part of the elevation of the left shoulder girdle and the probable depression of the right shoulder girdle. Her neck will be bent in some fashion to the left, with many possibilities of CT and SO compensation.

We could prescribe exercises to stretch the left upper trapezius and levator and strengthen the right. We could prescribe stretches for the right lower trapezius and latissimus dorsi, and strengthening exercise for the left. We could strengthen the left lateral intercostals, lateral abdominals and quadratus lumborum and stretch the right. Stretch the left scalenes and strengthen the right. The list is already pretty daunting, and we haven't even discussed the legs yet. Do we really want our students to do 16 different home exercises to address these various imbalances?

Alternatively, we could do more complex but more meaningful movements designed to simultaneously train

Box 4.11 Eskimo Roll

Chair-sitting side-bending movements – head moves globally with and differentiated from the torso

Combines left/right falls with intention to orient to the horizon to create a differentiation of the head from the torso

Standing, supine and floor-sitting variations

Use of cumulative movements

proprioceptive self-awareness and pattern recognition, to balance antagonist pairs of muscles and oppositional postural relationships, and to mobilize stuck places to reduce the necessity for movement at a hypermobile segment. We could give them a lesson that features first global then differentiated patterns of side-bending movements couched in functional contexts of balance and orientation – the very same functional combination that probably contributed to their symptoms in the first place.

What particular differentiation combination do you think we might want to get them to recognize and minimize? (Shift weight left, bend torso right, bend head left.) Which combination would be particularly therapeutic? (The exact opposite.) In what daily contexts can they use this movement? (Manipulation or locomotion combined with orientation to a high horizon). If we can bring this nonhabitual differentiated pattern of movement into gait and reaching, we have a mechanism both to stop digging holes and to turn a walk in the park or left-handed bowling into a therapeutically effective exercise for the neck (Box 4.11).

This last variation, F, contains a couple of cumulative movements that distill the lesson and are suitable for continuing with in a home program. The first cumulative movement has you placing both hands on top of your head and bending alternately from side to side. This reviews and condenses the global side-bending aspect of the lesson. The second cumulative movement has you continuing to bend and shift weight from side to side but this time keeping your head vertical.

The net effect is to do alternating differentiated movements that result in a translatory movement of the head from side to side in space (Egyptian head). These are fine home exercises and the movement into the nonhabitual differentiated direction (left Egyptian head for me) is one that I do dozens of times during the day to keep things variant and to keep the hounds of cervical hell at bay.

Undulations of the snake

The third cumulative movement was the undulation. An undulation has both global and differentiated movements in it, but emphasizes a sequential movement of alternate side-bending that invites the CNS to smooth over the rough edges. It puts together a seamless movement where before there were steps. An undulation has a certain grace and rhythm to it that is difficult to explain. Try it yourself and with your students, but don't be too disappointed if complete success is not immediately attained.

We return once again in variation G to our dynamic baseline with instructions to bend the head from side to side as if reading vertical writing. We would like our students to spontaneously adapt what they learned in the lesson to this test movement, but this does not always happen. Sometimes you will have to specifically give them permission to allow their whole body to participate, as they may again interpret the instruction to mean move only your head. I call this the 'Simon says' phenomenon. Once they have been prompted, most folks will be able to recognize the differences between an initial compartmentalized attempt at bending and the final integrated product; they then have a choice to make concerning which is easier, which is more successful and which they like better.

The next variation in this segment reviews something we have already performed in a previous lesson. Looking alternately up and down along with a rolling forward and back of the pelvis and a rounding and arching movement of the torso is reminiscent of Sitting Circles. The cumulative movement of making circles is then revisited as you connect the dots of right and left side-bending with flexion and extension. Is the side-bending component of the circle any clearer or more evenly distributed than it was when you did this during Sitting Circles?

Comparing baselines and applying the lesson

We then come back to our static baseline and compare it to the beginning. How is your weight balanced left/right on your seat? How close to level are your shoulders? Is your head tipped? These are some of the proprioceptive cues our students need to be aware of for them to change damaging postural behavior. We then brought an awareness of possible differences to standing and asked about standing balance and side-bending movements of the ribs when walking. Did your head glide or translate from side to side at all when you walked?

Clinically, we would use this lesson as a continuation of, and for the same purposes as, Be a Better Bow. In addition to enhancing the slinky properties of the thoracic spine and ribcage and helping to mobilize the upper back and upper chest, we could use it for any unilateral cervical or lumbar pain where the compression or gapping strains in either area are contributing factors. Versions of the cervical scenarios described above are pretty common, and this is one of the lessons I might use with them.

Unilateral lumbar compression secondary to habitually asymmetrical weight distribution on the pelvis is also pretty common, and again this lesson is useful with these sorts of folks. It stretches the upper trapezii, scalenes and levator (especially with the differentiation of head and shoulders), stretches the latissimi and the lateral intercostals, and helps the left and right abdominals and quadratus lumborum balance the pelvis more accurately.

The possibilities really are endless when you consider the possible number of musculoskeletal pain syndromes that are related to left/right imbalance in sitting or standing posture. As a general rule of thumb, if you have predominantly unilateral headaches, TMJ syndrome, neck pain, shoulder girdle pain, glenohumeral pain or lumbar or SI pain, it is a pretty safe bet that their habitual left/right imbalance is contributing to it.

Sometimes the relationship is obvious, sometimes you can puzzle it out, and sometimes you will have no idea why a particular way of organizing oneself leads to one-sided pain. To a certain extent, you don't have to know. If you are going to take a motor control approach to exercise, you are going to be doing alternating global and differentiated movement patterns anyway and, hopefully, everything just comes out in the wash. If on your initial assessment you picked up on some individual muscle imbalances, try starting out with some integrative lessons to begin with and see if by accessing accurate movement of bones you can facilitate a waking up of slacker muscles and a toning down of the over-eager ones.

If then you find no change in the individuals, be specific with therapeutic exercise and then fold back again into the bigger picture. You really have nothing to lose by delaying individual work and seeing if the shortcut works! This is an approach that starts with the overview and progresses to the particulars. Another approach would be to start with the particulars and work to the general. Use this lesson as described in previous head/tail lessons for your performance, neurologic and general medical population as well.

Variations

Variations of this lesson can be performed in side-sitting, standing and on hands and knees, and can be facilitated by toys and with movements while supine. Side-sitting variations are nearly identical to chair-sitting, except that side-to-side weight-shifting here will not be equally accessible to either side. The side-to-side movement of the pelvis on the floor in this position requires the back knee (left knee if right side-sitting) to slide alternately towards and away from your pelvis as you bend alternately from side to side. You can still do global and differentiated movements and can change the venue by leaning to the side on your elbow and forearm instead of your hand.

You could complete this lesson by sliding your weightbearing hand out away from you and coming back up again by dropping your head and lengthening the top side (left side of torso if coming to sit from lying on your right side). This variation is not for the delicate. Be careful and go slowly until you figure it out (Fig. 4.25). Culminating movements (global and differentiated distillations) can be performed from tailor-sit or from long-sit.

Standing variations also include the hand on the head constraint and instructions to lift a heel rather than lifting a hip. Don't forget the weight-shift or the undulation. From hands and knees, you can shift weight to one knee while bending head and neck in the opposite direction. Progress by differentiating head and neck. This is great CT mobility stuff!

Toy variations include the use of a rolled-up towel or smallish foam roller in sitting. Start with a rolled-up towel under the left sitting bone and your right hand on top of your head. Bring right elbow and right hip toward each other and shift weight up and on to your left sitting bone. Figure out how to move your pelvis uphill! Coming back down again encourages side-bending left as the right ischial tuberosity drops lower to the seat than the left. Do this in mirror image to the other side, then place the rolled towel centrally to allow falls equally easily in either direction.

This toy exaggerates the need to balance and can give people a better sense of the relationships between pelvis and head and

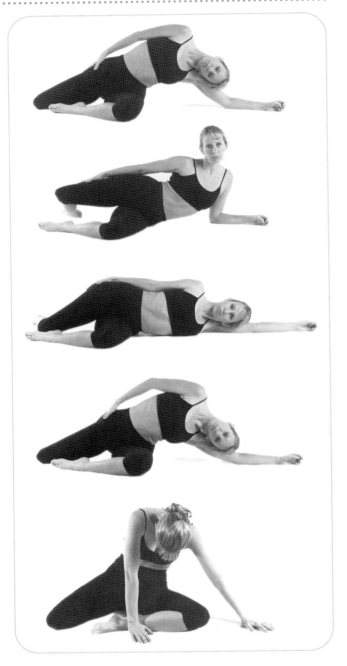

Fig. 4.25 Other positions – variations – segue into transitional movement.

of differences in their habitual and nonhabitual sides. A word of caution here: there is a lot of pressure on and around the pelvic floor. There may be physical sensitivity or emotional associations with this. Another favorite toy is a long pole. Place the pole across your upper back and hold on with both hands. Make side-bending movements rather than the diagonal movements you made with the pole in Figure 4.13.

We can facilitate these side-bending relationships in supine as well. Lie on your back with your knees bent and feet apart.

Place your interlaced fingers behind your head with your elbows on or near the floor. Slide elbows, head and hands (the whole Lego) first right several times, then left, then alternately. Does your pelvis roll from side to side on the floor? Is there a weight-shifting component to this intention to side-bend? Now lift your pelvis and lower back off the floor in a bridging position, and from there slide elbows together to the right several times, then to the left. Finish up by alternating sliding your elbows right and left.

You will probably notice a tendency of the pelvis to translate in space in the opposite direction of where the head and hand Lego is moving. Do this a few times to recognize the pattern, then continue to move your pelvis from side to side but keep head/hand/elbows Lego where it is. This differentiated movement can be a great CT and intrascapular spine mobilizer, and again suggests an Egyptian translatory movement of the head. This once again combines weight-shifting with side-bending, and explores first global then differentiated movements of the head/neck and torso/pelvis.

For our last lesson of this section on the worm, we will be revisiting Sitting Circles. In this thrilling conclusion to our first episode, we will pick up the story where we left off by adding in differentiated movements that simulate balance and orientation relationships in an anterior/posterior direction.

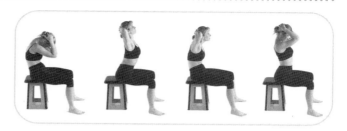

Fig. 4.26 Moving head and torso together, then differentiating.

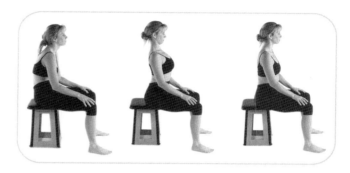

Fig. 4.27 Pecking – orientation to a high horizon.

Sitting Circles II – differentiating the head

Variations

A. Sit in a kitchen-style chair and feel the forward/backward balance of your pelvis on the seat. Feel the shape of your back and the balance of your head on your spine.

- Find the horizon with your eyes open.

- Look up and down. What is your easy range of movement? What else moves beside your eyes?

B. Interlace your fingers and place them softly behind your head. Make sure that you don't pull on your head with your arms. Be careful of your neck.

- Move your elbows towards your belly and look down towards your belly button. Let your pelvis roll back and your whole back round as you do this (Fig. 4.26).

- Spread your elbows out and look up toward the ceiling. Let your pelvis roll forward and your whole back arch (Fig. 4.26). Be careful with your neck by moving it as an extension of how fully your mid to upper back can bend back.

- Alternate between rolling your pelvis forward and back. Time this rolling movement with the in-and-out movement of your breath and with looking alternately up and down, and continue this while you add in –

- Leaning/falling back as you look down and leaning/falling forward as you look up.

C. Drop your arms down now.

- Look alternately up and down again as at the beginning. Is it any easier now, or does more of your back and pelvis contribute to the movement than did at the start? Continue to roll your pelvis and alternately round and arch back, but now –

- Move head and eyes in opposite direction from torso. Look up when rolling/rounding back and look down when rolling/arching forward (Fig. 4.26). This differentiates head and eyes from pelvis and torso.

- Continue this rolling movement but allow your head to move with your torso. Move only your eyes in the opposite direction, to differentiate eyes from your head and spine.

- Now keep your eyes and nose on the horizon as you continue to alternately round and arch your back. Your face moves forward and back in a pecking movement (Fig. 4.27).

D. Interlace fingers behind head as before.

- Turn your head, torso and elbows to orient toward your left knee and look alternately up and down in a diagonal. Let your pelvis roll forward and to the left as you look up and back and to the right as you look down. Add in leaning/falling forward and left and back and to the right.

- Drop your arms as you continue in this diagonal, but differentiate head and neck. Look down when rolling forward and left and look up when rolling back and to the right.

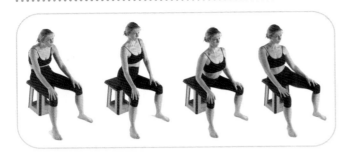

Fig. 4.28 Sitting Circles with head differentiated – eyes stay horizontal and on the horizon.

- Resume moving head with torso, but move just eyes now in the opposite direction (extra credit).

- Do the same movement but now oriented toward your right knee. Do the same variations of falling/leaning and the same variations of dropping your arms and differentiating your head from your torso and your eyes from your head.

- Put your hands on your head again and try connecting the dots to make a circle! Your pelvis makes a circle in space and your elbows do the same.

- Drop your arms once again and make a circle with your pelvis and torso but keep your head vertical and your eyes on the horizon (Fig. 4.28). Circle in both clockwise and counterclockwise directions.

E. Sit with arms hanging down.
- Look up and down. Compare to the beginning.
- Feel postural balance on your seat front to back. Compare to beginning.
- Stand up and observe the balance of head on your spine and the balance of your pelvis on your legs. Look up and down from here. How is this movement organized now?

Static and dynamic baselines – Sitting Circles II

There is not much to add here to the analysis of the original Sitting Circles lesson, as it is nearly identical except for the differentiation of the head and neck from the pelvis and torso and the differentiation of the eyes from the head. This again combines balance (falling forward or back) with orientation (eyes horizontal and on the horizon).

The differentiated movement of falling/rounding back then extending at the cervical spine and suboccipital space is a common one and one that contributes to a host of head, neck, shoulder, shoulder girdle and low back pain syndromes. Does that mean we should avoid moving at all in this direction? Not if we take motor learning into account and want to train our students to recognize where they tend to hang out and how to move out of it. The differentiated movement of falling/arching forward then flexing at the cervical spine and suboccipital area is one that we frequently try to get our students to

do. It decompresses the SO junction and reduces forward shearing at the mid-low cervical segments.

It approximates a high horizon and facilitates a better skeletal weightbearing support for the head and shoulder girdles, lessening the need for muscular effort. It provides better support for a reaching arm and reduces any inferior orientation tendency of the glenoid fossa and attendant impingement stresses of the subacromial tissues. It provides better potential for movement of the ribcage and belly with breathing. It reduces posterior ligament or annular stresses in the low back and SI joints.

Multidimensional differentiations of the head

The global diagonal patterns are the same as in the first installment of the lesson, but the differentiated movements are a bit more complex, combining flexion/extension with left/right movements. This results in diagonal nodding movements that alternately compress and decompress the suboccipital space unilaterally. If you have a student with one-sided headaches, figure out which diagonal upper cervical nod (up/down and left/right combo) is habitual and emphasize the mirror image as a home program.

For instance, if her pelvis falls back and to the left and her whole torso bends forward and to the right, we might anticipate the neck bending back and to the left (to keep the eyes horizontal) and might have left lower cervical facet closed-pack stresses (or right low cervical gapping stresses) or left suboccipital compression with left sided headaches.

We might want to teach her to recognize this pattern and have her move in her nonhabitual direction of having her pelvis fall forward and to the right. This would encourage a left torso extension pattern and would perhaps achieve our desired movement of the head and neck into right flexion, resulting in better balance of the CT junction and in left suboccipital decompression.

In reality, the compensations and balance adjustments through the SO and CT junction are both three-dimensional and very complex. There will probably be imbalances of the pelvis and torso in all three planes; someone with a flexion, right side-bend and right rotation bias is required to make a cervical adjustment of extension, left side-bend and left rotation. To make this even more complex, there is often a differentiation between the pelvis/lower back and the mid-upper back/chest. We will look at this further in Section 3.

For now, just appreciate the three-dimensional complexity and interweaving functional contexts of posture and try not to despair. Even if you can't tell exactly what someone is doing, they will benefit from proprioceptive learning experiences that ask for reciprocating global and differentiated patterns of movement in a number of different relationships to gravity and linked with a variety of functional contexts. You will have to trust that their CNS will be able to glean useful information from those experiences.

Variations

Variations of this lesson can again be performed in side-sitting and on hands and knees. Standing is a bit more difficult because

Box 4.12 Sitting Circles II – differentiating the head

Continuation of Sitting Circles – orientation up/down and diagonals in chair-sitting

Differentiation of head/neck from pelvis/torso – combining falling forward/back and diagonals with orientation to the horizon

Another 360° movement in vertical – complex head/neck adjustments

Supine facilitation of thoracic and cervical differentiation – of thoracic and lumbar differentiation

of the additional requirements to access both anterior and posterior tilt of the pelvis on top of the legs – something few people can do equally easily in both directions. Both the side-sitting and hands and knees variations are pretty straightforward and are much like the sitting version, except that you can't facilitate the movement by placing hands and head together. Both of these variations can be linked to transitional movements – hands and knees to sitting back on heels, and side-sitting to hands and knees. Continue with global and differentiated circle combinations here (Box 4.12).

Supine is a good position to start with when first exploring these differentiated movements. Lie on your back and feel the spaces under neck and lower back. Bend your knees up and start to rock your pelvis alternately up and down on the floor. This moves your pelvis alternately into posterior and anterior tilt and alternately flexes and arches your lower back. The low back alternately presses into and lifts away from the floor. If you allow it to do so, your head will also roll alternately up and down on the floor in the same direction as the pelvis.

For example, when rolling the pelvis upward into posterior tilt, the head will roll upward in an upward nodding direction (if you let it). There is then a reciprocal relationship between the space under the lower back and the space under the neck. As the space under the lower back flattens, the space under the neck increases. When rolling the pelvis downward into anterior tilt, the opposite occurs. The space in the low back increases while the space under your neck flattens as your head rolls into downward nodding; here again is a reciprocal relationship between the spaces (Fig. 4.29). These are both differentiated patterns of movement very similar to what was happening in sitting – back flexion with cervical extension and back extension with cervical flexion.

This alternate rocking movement of the pelvis is an excellent way of facilitating freedom of movement of the head and effort recognition skills in the neck. To allow the head to respond to the movement of the pelvis, there has to be some transmission of force from the pelvis through the torso. If that force were able to penetrate the sometimes rigid ribcage/chest, how would the head behave if the neck were passive?

The head would roll rather than slide on the floor, and we would get a nodding movement of the head and a pumping effect of the SO junction. If the head is sliding, or not moving at all, there is unwanted effort going on somewhere. Your mission, if you decide to accept it, is to search out and destroy that effort. Try timing the up-and-down movement of the eyes with the up-and-down rolling of the head. Try differentiating your eyes from the still freely rolling head (easier said than performed).

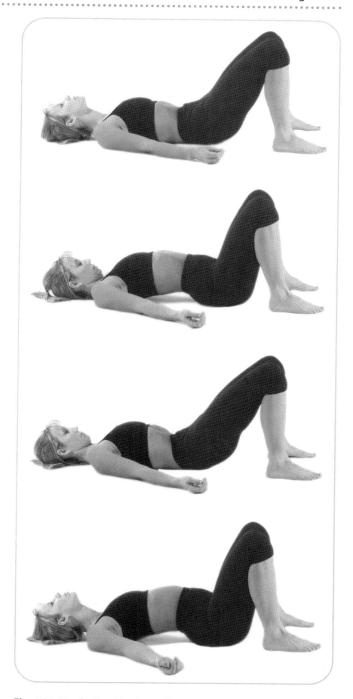

Fig. 4.29 Head rolls with, then differentiates from, the pelvis.

Try moving your eyes from side to side in their sockets as you continue to allow free movement of your head rolling up and down on the floor. You might actually end up moving your head in a zigzag. These are great ways of 'lubricating' the upper cervical spine and helping to create an impression of your head moving like a gyroscope or as if sitting on top of ball bearings.

Now change the movement a bit by reversing the reciprocal relationships of the spaces. Instead of allowing the head to roll downward and the neck to flatten as the pelvis rolls downward, move your eyes upward in their sockets. For most of you, this will slide your head back to arch your neck. This simultaneously lifts both the space under the neck and the space under your lower back. Going in the other direction, move your eyes downward in their sockets while rolling your pelvis upward. For most of you, this will slide your head downward and tuck your chin to flatten your neck. This simultaneously flattens both the space under your neck and the space under your lower back (Fig. 4.29). This second movement is an extremely important one.

To simultaneously flatten both spaces, you have to flex both your neck and lower back while your thoracic spine is required to flatten, in this case by extending. This movement differentiates the thoracic spine and ribcage from the lower back and pelvis. This movement also asks for a differentiated movement of thoracic extension and cervical flexion. It is a movement much like the one we want when orienting to a high horizon, and this supine variation is another good way to facilitate it. Both CT and SO mobility and differentiation are required.

This movement also facilitates motor control of what are getting to be recognized as important cervical intersegmental stabilization muscles: the longus colli and the rectus capitis. People who have performed studies in this area are now indicating the importance of these muscles in treating neck pain, and have advocated training motor control over these muscles by doing small and slow nodding movements that emphasize contracting the longus colli and rectus capitis independently of the superficial anterior cervical musculature.[10–12]

The teaching method for this has involved the use of a pressure-sensitive cuff under the neck while supine and progressively pressing and holding the back of the neck on the cuff at prescribed pressures. This facilitates individual muscle control, but how do we then get those muscles to work appropriately in various functional contexts and as a part of larger synergistic relationships?

We can train them initially in the same supine position but with the infusion of some pattern specificity. By requiring the thoracic spine to extend and the cervical spine to flex at the same time, we require the anterior intrinsic muscles of the neck to work simultaneously along with the thoracic and ribcage extensors. This coordinates the cervical flexors and thoracic extensors in a (usually) nonhabitual differentiated pattern that accrues the benefits of a high horizon:

- Enhanced skeletal weightbearing;
- Reduction of muscular effort in postural support; and
- Reduction of shearing and compression stresses in the neck.

This variation is a place where you can simultaneously train for both individual muscle control and integrative and relational movement patterns. This very important movement can be further facilitated with some toys. Place a rolled-up towel crosswise across your back at about the level of the apex of your thoracic kyphosis and interlace your fingers behind your head. Use your hands to lower your head back toward the floor.

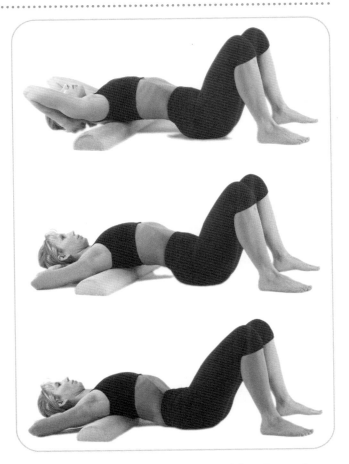

Fig. 4.30 Using toys to encourage differentiated thoracic extension.

Keep your face parallel to the ceiling as much as possible, rather than letting your chin come away from your chest. If you simultaneously flatten your lower back to the floor, this requires an even more exaggerated differentiated extension of the thoracic spine – just what the doctor ordered (Fig. 4.30)! Use your imagination and think about how you might do a diagonal version of this.

Bring the movement back up to sitting on a stool or bench with your back to a wall. Use the wall initially to assess the relationships between the spaces, then make a movement similar to what you did on the floor where there was the reciprocal relationship between the spaces – one space lifts as the other space flattens. Progress to flattening both spaces simultaneously and facilitate that by placing a rolled towel or small rubber ball on the wall at the apex of the thoracic kyphosis. Do the same reverse pecking movement here as you move the back of your head toward the wall while still orienting to the horizon, then roll your pelvis back on the seat to flex your lower back. Demand that the thoracic spine extend independently of the cervical and lumbar areas (where most extension occurs for most people, to their eventual chagrin).

References

1. Ivanenko Y, Grasso R, Lacquaniti F. Effect of gaze on postural responses to neck proprioceptive and vestibular stimulation in humans. Journal of Physiology 1999;519:301–14.

2. Heuer H, Owens DA. Vertical gaze direction and the resting posture of the eyes. Perception 1989;18:363–77.

3. Hill SG, Kroemer KHE. Preferred declination of the line of sight. Human Factors 1986;28:127–34.

4. Owens DA, Leibowitz HW. Perceptual and motor consequences of tonic vergence. In: Schor CM, Ciuffreda KJ, eds. Vergence eye movements: basic and clinical aspects. Boston, MA: Butterworth Scientific; 1980: 25–74.

5. Berthoz A. Reference frames for the perception and control of movement. In: Paillard J, ed. Brain and space. New York: Oxford University Press; 1991: 81–91.

6. Gurfinkel VS, Shik ML, Kotz YM. The control of the human posture. Moscow: Nauka; 1965.

7. Wolsley CJ, Sakellari V, Bronstein AM. Reorientation of visually evoked postural responses by different eye-in-orbit and head-on-trunk angular positions. Experimental Brain Research 1996;111: 283–8.

8. Popov KE, Smetanin BN, Furfinkel VS, Kudinvova MP, Shlykov VY. Spatial perception and vestibulomotor responses in man. Neurophysiology 1986;18:779–87.

9. Lund S, Broberg C. Effects of different head positions on postural sway in man induced by a reproducible vestibular error signal. Acta Physiologica Scandinavica 1983;117:307–9.

10. Jull GA. Cervical headache: a review. In: Boyling J, Palastanga N, eds. Modern manual therapy of the vertebral column. Edinburgh: Churchill Livingstone; 1996: 333–47.

11. Jull GA. Headaches of cervical origin. In: Grant R. Physical therapy of the cervical and thoracic spine, 2nd edn. New York: Churchill Livingstone; 1994: 261–85.

12. Boyd-Clark LC, Briggs CA, Galea MP. Muscle spindle, morphology, and density in longus colli and multifidus muscles of the cervical spine. Spine 2002;27:694–701.

The tyrannosaurus rex

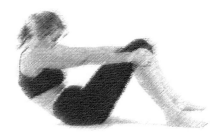

"Where's the Rex?"

JULIANNE MOORE IN *JURASSIC PARK 2 –*

THE LOST WORLD

CHAPTER FIVE

The worm acquires legs

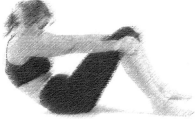

Chapter outline

Postural types

1. The *full round* features posterior pelvic tilt, lumbar flexion, thoracic flexion and cervical extension. The whole worm is falling backwards and the head is differentiating to maintain orientation to the horizon. No high horizon or skeletal weightbearing. Violation of proportionality; cervical extensors working too hard. Predict difficulty in looking upward (and spiraling to look left and right).

2. The *full arch* features anterior pelvic tilt, lumbar lordosis and flattening, or even lordosis of the thoracic spine and cervical flexion. Pelvis and torso fall too far forward, extending torso globally in response and flexing neck to keep orientation to the horizon. Predict difficulty looking down.

3. The *half arch* posture type is characterized by a differentiated pattern of anterior pelvic tilt, lumbar lordosis, thoracic kyphosis and cervical lordosis. Very common – to the point of being thought of as normal/ideal rather than normal/average. Clinical conundrum: how to extend the thoracic spine to help with cervical support and movement without extending the lumbar spine.

4. Another differentiated posture is the *half round*. This somewhat rarer pattern features posterior pelvic tilt, lumbar kyphosis, thoracic extension and cervical flexion. Clinical conundrum: how to extend the lumbar spine while differentiating the thoracic spine into flexion.

5. A *columnar* postural pattern would feature a vertical pelvis. It is falling neither forward nor back. The lumbar spine is neutral; it is neither flexing nor extending. The thoracic spine is neutral; it is neither flexing nor extending. The cervical spine is neutral; ditto. The head is vertical with eyes on a high horizon.

Legs as prime movers of the pelvis and torso

1. The legs as central to orientation and balance (both AP and left/right).

2. Necessity in gaining a deeper understanding of how the organization, or disorganization, of the legs resonates through the whole body and in developing tools with which to influence any imbalances or inefficiencies.

3. Lesson 1: *Sitting Circles III – Using the Legs.* Balance as functional context.

   - Lesson identical to Sitting Circles but language and attention emphasis on legs.

   - Fall back controlled by lengthening hip flexors – return to neutral powered by shortening hip flexors. Fall back is a differentiated pattern of hip extension and torso flexion; bilateral gluteal pattern. Return to neutral is a differentiated pattern of hip flexion and torso extension; bilateral iliopsoas pattern.

   - Fall forward controlled by lengthening hip extensors; return to neutral powered by shortening hip extensors. Fall forward is a differentiated pattern of hip flexion and torso extension; bilateral iliopsoas pattern.

Return to neutral is a differentiated pattern of hip extension and torso flexion; bilateral gluteal pattern.

- Fall back and to the right (left gluteal pattern) and back to neutral controlled by left hip flexors. Mirror to other side. Belly-up orientation emphasizes lengthening and strengthening of the hip flexors.

- Fall forward and to the left (left iliopsoas pattern) and back to neutral controlled by left hip extensors. Mirror to other side. Belly-down orientation emphasizes lengthening and strengthening the hip extensors.

- Hip flexors pull pelvis towards leg or legs; hip extensors push pelvis away from leg or legs. Hip extensors constrain anterior pelvic tilt; hip flexors constrain posterior pelvic tilt.

- Falling of vertical pelvis controlled by lengthening contractions – pelvis always rolling down slope. Movement of horizontal pelvis controlled by shortening contractions; always pushing uphill.

4. Lesson 2: *Pelvic Tilts*. Balance as functional context – keep from hitting the back of your head.

- Hip extensors push pelvis into posterior tilt (with lumbar flexion) and pull the pelvis into anterior tilt (with lumbar extension) when supine.

- Belly-up explorations of the use of the legs to control movements of the pelvis and back. Emphasis on stretching and strengthening the hip flexors in differentiated patterns.

- Why use legs to control anterior pelvic tilt? Inhibition of diaphragm, leading to scalene breathing. Using chest instead of the floor as an anchor from which to move the pelvis pulls the chest down and forward, leading to upper back and shoulder girdle imbalances. Abdominal contraction can be part of the somatic manifestation of an anxiety pattern. Muscle size and mechanical advantage goes to the legs.

5. Lesson 3: *Side-sit Bending*. Balance as functional context; keep from rearranging your face. Additional intention to reach (manipulation).

- Belly-down exploration of the use of the legs to control movements of the pelvis and back. Emphasis on stretching and strengthening the hip extensors.

- Side-sit position dovetails with diagonal movements. Good place to start teaching forward bending mechanics.

- Two basic errors in bending: either the pelvis doesn't rotate far enough forward on the legs or it falls too far forward. The former requires too much lumbar flexion, whereas the latter requires too much lumbar extension and too much work for the lumbar extensors.

- Side-sitting position important developmentally: a place to play and many transitions possible from here. Link handedness to asymmetrical pelvis, torso, leg musculature in this position.

- Using a 'hamstring constraint' to strengthen the thoracic extensors/differentiating from the lumbar extensors.

- Using reciprocating movements to find spinal neutral, then bending and coming back to vertical while keeping that neutral spine.

- Rotational component to bending for the purpose of reaching with one hand. Rotation of pelvis should occur around the legs rather than rotation of lumbar vertebrae around the pelvis.

Pelvic force couples

1. Cooperative use of opposite side hip flexors and extensors to create a weight shift or turning movement of the pelvis.

2. Lesson 4: *Wishbone*. Supine exploration of 'scissoring' movements of the legs.

- Pelvic force couples central to turning the pelvis (golf, tennis) and to locomotion (walk, run, bike, swim, crawl).

- 'Doll body' gait – very little pelvis or torso movement.

- 'Waddle' gait – rotational movements around lower back as pelvis turns in the direction of the push off leg.

- 'Swish' gait – lateral shear of the pelvis underneath the torso creates shearing at the lower back.

- 'Force couple' gait – rotational movement around hips as pelvis turns in direction of stepping leg.

- Many of the pelvic asymmetries we see clinically are related to pelvic force couple imbalances.

- In a pelvic force couple gait, the pelvis turns in the direction of the forward/stepping leg – developmental progression of this phenomenon.

3. Lesson 5: *Side-lie Transitions*. Exploration of pelvic force couple movements in context of transition from lying to sitting.

- Orientation to gravity places more emphasis on hip abductor/short and stubby use.

- Benefits of simultaneous abductor use in standing: enhances vertical support of pelvis (reduces lumbar lordosis), enhances pelvic stability in the presence of lateral, rotational or centrifugal forces and enhances vertical organization of legs (reduces knee valgus and foot pronation).

- Lots of opportunity for spring-loading of force couple muscles. Did whole sequence to one side first to exaggerate left/right contrasts.

4. Lesson 6: *Cat/Camel*. Exploration of pelvic force couple movements in context of transition from hands and knees to side-sitting.

- Belly-down version of the same circle we did previously in sitting circles. Plantigrade variation of same movements.

- Degree of difficulty progression from Lesson 5. Poor man's splits as transitional position to/from sitting and hands and knees. Link to Side-sit Bending.

5. Lesson 7: *Side-sit Transitions*.

- Exploration of pelvic force couple movements in context of transitions from side-sit to side-sit.

- Belly-up orientation emphasizes lengthening and strengthening the hip flexors. Links back to Pelvic Tilts – rolling to back then up again diagonally.

6. Lesson 8: *Sit to Stand*. Final transitional exploration – continuation of sitting circles.

   - Facilitation of improved standing and sitting, as well as bending/lifting.

   - Approach is modular. Look for similarities, connections, relationships, common denominators.

   - Variations off the main path, ways of building one lesson on top of another and new ways of constructing a learning environment.

Postural types

The purpose of this chapter is to explore the role the legs play in organizing the whole skeleton to move. We will be demonstrating the use of the legs in balance, orientation, manipulation and transitions. We will be demonstrating the cooperative use of opposite side hip flexors and extensors in gait movements. We will be discussing the central role the legs have to play in movements of both the trunk and the legs, describing use of 'cornerstone' muscles.

Before we go on to talk about the legs, let's take one last look at the worm, viewing a vertical worm from the side. We looked at movements of the worm in the last chapter and described global patterns of movement of the torso: global torso flexion, extension, side-bending, right and left extension, and right and left flexion. But do people always organize themselves globally with their posture? No, there are some differentiated patterns here as well. We could describe five basic postural types when looking at anterior/posterior balance.

The full round

In sitting, the *full round* features posterior pelvic tilt, lumbar flexion, thoracic flexion and cervical extension. The whole worm is falling backward (global torso flexion) and the head is differentiating (cervical extension) to maintain orientation to the horizon (Figs 5.1 and 5.2) Clinically, we know that some possible consequences of this habitual organization might include lumbar or sacroiliac (SI) ligament overstretching, lumbar disc degeneration or herniation, or radicular irritation because of flexion stresses acting on the vertebral structures.[1-5]

Cervical shearing stresses (the lower cervicals shear forward on the upper thoracic segments as the spine makes a sharp turn from thoracic flexion to cervical extension), prevalent in this type of postural organization, may lead to mid-low cervical disc degeneration or derangement, to cervical facet hypermobility with attendant capsular and ligamentous overstretching, or again to radicular irritation. Thoracic outlet syndrome, shoulder girdle myofascial syndromes, shoulder joint impingements/tendinitis/bursitis and even elbow tendinitis and the various forearm/wrist/hand repetitive stress syndromes may have this less than efficient postural pattern as a possible causative or contributing factor.[6-9]

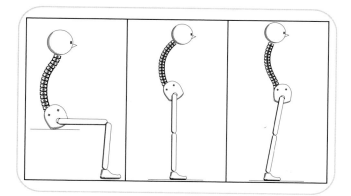

Fig. 5.1 The full round in sitting and standing – ski jumper variation – the pelvis falls backward on the legs.

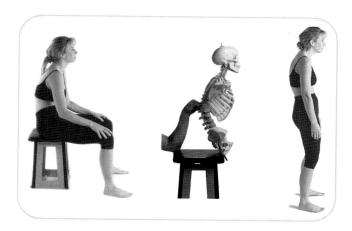

Fig. 5.2 The full round – flesh and bone.

Suboccipital compression may lead to headaches and upper cervical pain, and the chronic lengthening of the infra- and suprahyoid and the deep anterior neck muscles and the changing relationship of head, mandible and gravity can contribute to temporomandibular joint pain syndromes.[10-15] What can we say about this type of organization if we look at it from a motor control perspective?

We can say that she is not supporting her weight skeletally. She is relying on the ligaments of her SI joints, lumbar and thoracic regions to prevent her from completely folding in half and then relying on her poor neck to make a sharp turn into extension to orient to the horizon; this is a violation of the good housekeeping rule, as the only part of her spine contributing to horizon orientation is the neck.

She is also requiring the smaller and more delicate muscles of her neck to do all the work of supporting the weight of the head; this is a violation of the proportionality principle, as the larger and stronger torso extensor musculature is off on holiday while the cervical extensors and tiny little posterior suboccipital muscles are left at home to toil in the fields. How do you think the longus colli and rectus capitis are faring in this environment? Do you think you can regain longus colli and rectus capitis control without addressing the relationships between head, thorax and pelvis?

We can also say that she isn't orienting to a high horizon. Although this is another way of saying that she isn't supporting her weight skeletally, it also implies probable errors in how she organizes her head and neck for movement. For instance, can you hazard a guess about how this person might organize herself to look up? Probably she will organize herself to move from the top down and do most of her extension at the already chronically extending cervical spine.

It is unlikely that she will have recognized the advantages of rolling the pelvis into anterior tilt and arching the whole spine in a global torso extension pattern. This particular way of performing this particular movement exacerbates and amplifies her habitual postural stresses. In looking over her shoulder to see behind her, it is unlikely that she will have recognized the advantages of turning her pelvis and spiraling taller through her torso.

She will probably organize herself again from the top down and will crash her vertebrae into her immovable object somewhere around the cervicothoracic junction. Movement stresses can often be predicted from an observation of postural biases. Start playing the game yourself but, as always, be prepared to be wrong some of the time and be willing to change the course of treatment if your original estimations prove to be inaccurate.

We could extrapolate what might happen at the lumbar spine while bending. How do you think this person might organize herself to bend over? She will probably keep flexing at her back instead of flattening her back to neutral; this again might stress posterior lumbar and SI ligaments through overstretching, and puts the lumbar discs at risk for shearing stresses that may contribute to degeneration or herniation. What is she likely to do with her neck when she bends?

Because she will probably be looking at something as she reaches for it, she will effectively have to extend her cervical spine even more to maintain orientation forward to the floor while bending. Another version of this is present in riding a bike. If she bends over to put her hands on the handle bar (manipulation) but still has to look upward to see the road (orientation), she is again hyperextending her neck. These are further examples of how postural strains and movement strains are related.

How might this person organize herself in standing? There are two basic ways. One is nearly identical to the sitting organization. The pelvis falls backward on the legs and the whole spine rounds (Fig. 5.1). We see this type of organization more among the elderly, though that is not to say that most of the elderly people we see have this organization. Their weight is carried way back on their heels and their gait is shuffling.

The other way this person might stand is to throw her hips forward to 'hang' on her anterior hip ligaments, then allow her chest to fall backward into a long thoracic kyphosis (Fig. 5.1). This often results in a short and compressed lumbosacral area, as it has to make a sharp turn into extension. These folks may have pain on both flexion and extension, as they may be habitually overflexing in sitting and bending and overarching in standing.

How are the various antagonist pairs balanced in this postural type? The suboccipitals and cervical extensors will be hyperactive and shortened, while the longus colli and rectus capitis will be long and hypoactive. The thoracic and lumbar

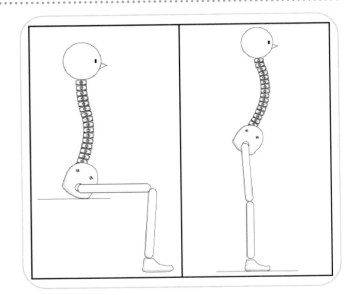

Fig. 5.3 The full arch in sitting and in standing – the pelvis falls forward on the legs.

extensors and posterior intercostals will be long and weak and the anterior intercostals, internal/external obliques and rectus abdominis will be tight and contracting. Recall in Chapter 2 the schematics of antagonist imbalances and how the habitually weaker of the pair allows the bone it controls to move too far. This is essentially what is happening in all the above scenarios. What can we say about the legs and any probable muscle imbalances there may be in this postural type? We will address this question after our first experiential lesson of the chapter.

The full arch

Our next basic postural type in sitting is the *full arch*. This organization features anterior pelvic tilt, lumbar lordosis, and flattening or even lordosis of the thoracic spine and cervical flexion (Figs 5.3 and 5.4). The student is allowing her pelvis and torso to fall too far forward, is extending globally in response to the fall, and is flexing her neck to keep her orientation to the horizon.

What might be the clinical manifestations of this type of organization?[16,17] In the low back, we might expect some facet joint and articular structure irritation as the facets are in their close packed position. This means that the joint surfaces compress together and the facet joint capsules are at maximum tension. SI joint shearing may be occurring and the lumbar and thoracic extensor musculatures are working very hard to keep the torso from toppling over. This further compresses the spine while in extension and contributes to back pain in its own right through myofascial syndromes. The posterior annulus of the disc is under invariant compression and is vulnerable to forward shearing stresses. This could lead to annular breakdown and disc dysfunction.

These folks will often have a very short kyphosis at a stiff CT junction as the spine changes its shape from a lordotic

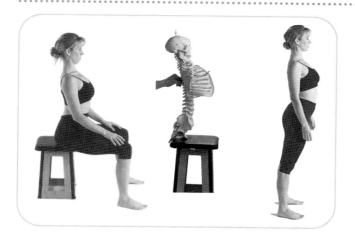

Fig. 5.4 The full arch – flesh and bone.

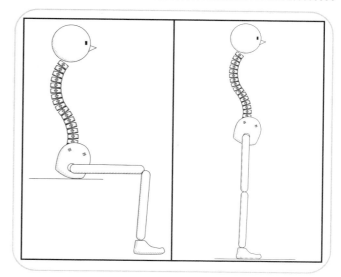

Fig. 5.5 The half arch in sitting and standing.

thorax to a neck that flexes to orient forward or downward. We may again have cervical hypermobilities above or even below the CT junction secondary to disproportional movement and poorly stacked vertebrae creating asymmetrical weightbearing stresses. What can we say about this type of organization from a motor control perspective?

We can say that she is not supporting her weight skeletally. She is allowing herself to fall too far forward and is holding herself in that falling position with considerable muscular effort of the back extensors and posterior intercostals. We can also say that she is not orienting herself to a high horizon, even though this is higher than for the people who engage in the full round.

She may again, as in our first scenario, organize herself from the top down in orientation. In particular, looking down might be a big stressor for her neck as she flexes it further to look down while keeping the rest of her torso rigidly upright. This may result in anterior shearing forces on the facet joints and discs at the mid-low cervical segments.

Looking over her shoulder may involve some torso extension, but often there is that clump of undifferentiated bones at the CT junction that may contribute to hypermobilities above or even below that wad. In bending over, she may allow her pelvis to fall too far forward and rely too heavily on the lumbar extensors, not appreciating the advantages of bending with a nearly neutral spine. These people may especially experience discomfort in their low back on return to sitting or standing after having bent over.

Have you noticed how both rounded and full arch students may have back pain on sitting and bending? Whereas the stressing activity is the same for both, the underlying organization that contributes to their pain is not. When training your students in sitting posture and proper bending, you will need to keep in mind what their particular error is and will have to emphasize different patterns and directions of movement for each of the types. One size does not fit all!

How would this person probably organize herself to stand? Most often, it will be nearly identical to sitting, but exaggerated. She will allow her pelvis to fall forward into anterior tilt on her legs and she will extend globally throughout her torso. Subvariations include either anteriorly tilting her pelvis on top

of vertical legs or anteriorly tilting her pelvis and hyperextending her knees while shifting her weight forward on her toes (ski-jumper pose). Why might this basic full arch pattern be accentuated in standing? Blame the legs.

How are the torso antagonists balanced? The lumbar and thoracic extensors and posterior intercostals will be short, strong and tight, and the abdominals and anterior intercostals will be long and weak. The cervical spine may be markedly flattened, with anterior cervical muscle shortening.

The half arch

Whereas our first two postural types featured global torso patterns with differentiation of the head and neck, our next type features differentiation of different parts of the torso. This differentiated or *half arch* posture type is characterized by anterior pelvic tilt, lumbar lordosis, thoracic kyphosis and cervical lordosis (Figs 5.5 and 5.6). This type is like an accordion because of the appearance of pleating throughout the spine. If we take a straight spine and push down on top of the head, the first pleat is the cervical spine as it moves into extension.

The second pleat is the thoracic spine as it folds in the opposite direction to create the thoracic kyphosis. The third pleat is the lumbar spine as it again folds back on itself to create the lumbar lordosis. The pelvis is falling forward and dragging the lumbar spine along, but the chest is differentiating to fall backward and flex. The head and neck then find themselves falling forward and needing to extend to bring the eyes back forward to the horizon. The whole effect is one of compression – like an accordion or a bellows.

This pattern is a bit of a chameleon. It comes in different flavors. One version features a long kyphosis and a short and compressed lumbar lordosis. Another version features a long and deep lordosis and a short and round kyphosis. Where does a half arch with a long kyphosis start and a full round with an

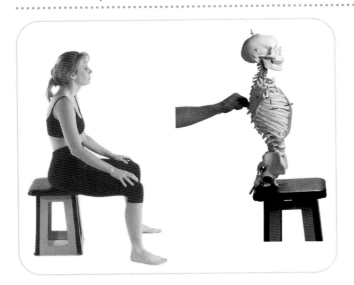

Fig. 5.6 The half arch – flesh and bone.

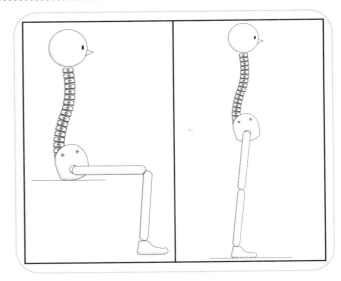

Fig. 5.7 The elusive half round.

anterior pelvis and lumbar extension in standing end? You be the judge.

Clinically, the lumbar spine and SI joint manifestation of this postural (and movement) type will be similar to those of the full arch. They will be subject to extension strains. The neck, shoulder girdles and upper extremities will be subject to movement and postural strains similar to those described in the discussion of the rounders. The worst of both worlds!

Is this person bearing weight skeletally? Nope. Is she orienting to a high horizon? No. How would she organize herself to stand? Basically the same as in sitting, but again probably even more accentuated. Why would the relationship of the legs to the pelvis make a difference? The hip flexors become a factor.

Antagonist imbalances may be as follows. There will probably be posterior cervical and suboccipital muscle tightness and shortening, and longus colli and rectus capitis weakness and disuse. The thoracic extensors and posterior intercostals will be weak and the anterior intercostals and upper belly will probably be shortened and contracting. The lumbar extensors and quadratus lumborum will be working hard and the lower belly might be low toned.

This is a very common postural pattern and can be a particularly challenging one in which to facilitate change. For the health of the neck, shoulder girdles and arms, we need to move into extension. For the health of the lower back, we need to move into flexion. If we do global flexion movements for the lower back, we may end up just emphasizing thoracic flexion as the CNS defaults the movement to the path of least resistance. If we do global extension movements in hopes of getting thoracic extension, we may end up just emphasizing lumbar (and cervical) extension as the CNS defaults the movement to the path of least resistance.

What we really need to do with these folks is to have a way to constrain lumbar extension while encouraging thoracic extension and to constrain thoracic flexion while encouraging lumbar flexion. We need to find ways of training them to move into a nonhabitual differentiated torso pattern. We need pat-

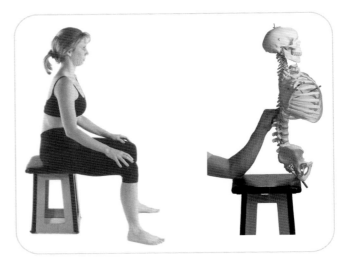

Fig. 5.8 The elusive half round again.

tern specificity in our exercise. How do we do this? There are many ways and I will describe several, but they all require an understanding of the role the legs play in movement and balance of the pelvis and torso.

The half round

The fourth basic postural pattern is another differentiated pattern – the *half round*. This somewhat rarer pattern features posterior pelvic tilt, lumbar kyphosis, thoracic extension and cervical flexion (Figs 5.7 and 5.8). The pleats just fall in the opposite direction to its more commonly seen cousin. The pelvis is falling backward, and the thorax is trying hard not to be dragged along with it into flexion. Clinically, we see move-

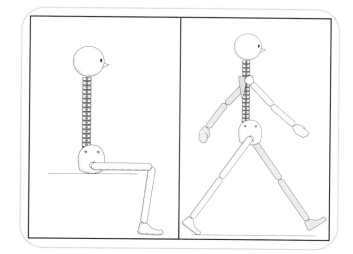

Fig. 5.9 A columnar posture in sitting and walking/standing.

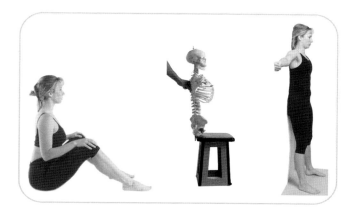

Fig. 5.10 A columnar posture – flesh and bone.

Box 5.1 Postural types
Full round – posterior pelvic tilt, global torso flexion and cervical extension as head differentiates
Full arch – anterior pelvic tilt, global torso extension and cervical flexion as head differentiates
Half arch – anterior pelvic tilt and lumbar extension, thoracic flexion and cervical extension as head differentiates. Variations of long and short kyphosis
Half round – posterior pelvic tilt and lumbar flexion, thoracic extension and cervical flexion as head differentiates
Columnar – pelvis balanced forward/back, neutral lumbar and thoracic spine, long and vertical neck

straight spine is ideal? Although I wouldn't exactly say that a completely straight spine and horizontal pelvis is best, reaching toward that goal would greatly benefit many people.

I think we have artificially determined that a certain degree of lumbar lordosis and a certain degree of thoracic kyphosis are normal or even ideal.[18–21] This assessment is based on the best available hard science and is rooted in biomechanics, mathematics and statistics. But nobody has thought to ask swimmers, divers, gymnasts, skaters, martial artists and other people from nonwestern cultures with straighter spines than we consider ideal what that organization *feels* like (Box 5.1).

I've got to tell you: it feels really good, especially in comparison to a half arch. Anyone I've ever talked with or worked with who has the physical skills to transition back and forth between a scientifically set ideal and a more columnar posture invariably chooses to minimize the curves. Granted, you'll not find many people with that movement skill, but try to keep your mind open to the possibility of personal change in that direction as you proceed through the book and decide for yourself whether to curve or, as the tai chi practitioner says, to 'be the curved line seeking straightness.'[22]

The shock absorption rationale

You've probably heard the argument: a curved line absorbs shock better than a straight line. Take a straight stick and jab it vertically into the ground and feel the shock vibrate up the stick and into your arm. Take a curved stick and jab it vertically into the ground and feel the give through the stick, not through your hand. If that was really the way we absorb vertical shock in real life, I might agree that curved is better. But this isn't the case.

Whether it be a meteor or the occasional errant box that falls on your head, you don't have to worry overmuch about absorbing shock coming down from above. The earth is for all practical purposes immobile unless you live in southern California, so you don't have to worry much about shock coming from below. That leaves jumping, stepping down, running and walking as the main vertical shock stressors, and you should not be absorbing shock vertically through your spine in these contexts!

Have you ever stepped down into a hole or off a curb without expecting it? When your CNS has not prepared the ankles, knees and hips to bend to absorb the shock? This is

ment and postural flexion stresses on the low back and a lot of upper back, cervical and posterior shoulder girdle muscular tension, and possible myofascial pain as a result.

The upper body is doing all the work of staying upright to orient to a high horizon while the pelvis pulls the rug out from underneath the rest of the spine to rob it of the possibility of bearing weight skeletally. These patterns are subtle – look for a rolled-back pelvis in sitting but an erect torso. These folks need to learn how to better organize the relationship of their pelvis to gravity.

The columnar

The fifth type is a neutral or *columnar* posture. A neutral postural pattern would feature a vertical pelvis. It is falling neither forward nor back. The lumbar spine is neutral: it is neither flexing nor extending. The thoracic spine is neutral: it is neither flexing nor extending. The cervical spine is neutral – ditto. The head is vertical with eyes on a (high) horizon. Weight is born skeletally (Figs 5.9 and 5.10). Does this mean that a completely

what it is like to absorb shock through accentuated lumbar lordosis and thoracic kyphosis. It is a real teeth rattler! The same thing applies to jumping. You don't jump up then come back down vertically with knees and hips straightened into extension. You'll give yourself a concussion. The shock is absorbed again here with ankles, knees and hips and by the bending forward of your torso *out* of a vertical position.

When walking and running, bouncing on your spine like a pogo stick is not in your best interests. Shock is taken again by ankle and knee flexion, by hip horizontal adduction, flexion and internal rotation, and by side-bending movements through the spine and ribcage. Just say no to vertical shock absorption through your spine.

Although the legs are best able to handle vertical shocks (and asymmetrical vertical shock absorbers also include torso side-bending movements) there are also horizontal shocks to contend with. What if we have to absorb shocks coming at us from in back or in front, from the left or the right? What if we got hit in a car while sitting at a stoplight?

Think of the analogy of your car's antenna and how it would respond to the blow. If hit from the front, the antennae would bend forward initially then whip back and forth in a dampening oscillation. The antenna is stiffest and most stable lowest down; this is analogous to the connection of the spine to the pelvis. It is thinnest and weakest higher up; this is analogous to the neck. The medium stiffness and strength is in the middle; this is analogous to the chest and ribcage.

With impact, the bending of the antenna would be distributed proportionally along its whole length. No one section of the antenna is asked to absorb more than its fair share. Once it has returned to vertical, it is ready to absorb shock again from another direction. Because of the columnar nature of the antenna, it can absorb shock coming from any direction equally well. Although the same would be true for the passenger in the car who has selected the columnar posture option, this would sadly not be the case for any of our other options.

- Whereas a full arch posture might do relatively well if being hit from the back because of its ability to extend evenly throughout the torso, getting hit from the front would tend to exacerbate flexion stresses in the lower neck.

- Although a full round posture might do well getting hit from the front because of an ability to flex evenly throughout the torso, getting hit from behind would tend to exacerbate extension stresses in the low to mid neck.

- The half arch posture is most susceptible to getting nailed from behind. The flexing and stiff thoracic spine absorbs no shock and the extending neck and lower back get creamed.

- Given the preponderance of half archers in our culture, it's not surprising that we see so many more mid to lower neck and so many more mid to lower back strains in people who get rear-ended than in people who do the rear-ending.

The increased interdiscal pressure rationale

Studies show an increase in interdiscal pressure going from extension toward flexion.[23,24] Look at a model of a spine and observe for yourself how, as you anteriorly tilt the pelvis and increase lordosis in the lower back, more weight will be borne

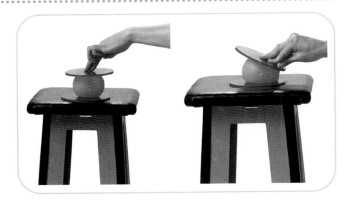

Fig. 5.11 Incompressible disc creating space between vertebral bodies – moving from a balanced place spreads the work around whereas invariant positions create invariant stresses.

posteriorly through the facet joints and less will go anteriorly through the discs and vertebral bodies. Let's just say it's a given that interdiscal pressure is greater in a columnar posture than in a half arch posture.

What if it was designed that way? Aren't the vertebral bodies better designed for vertical compression than the facet joints are? Isn't the nucleus of the disc an incompressible fluid that transmits forces from vertebral body to vertebral body?

Imagine a ball between two boards (Fig. 5.11). With the boards arranged anywhere out of vertical, compression on the nucleus (and therefore on the annulus) is asymmetrical. This results in invariant and unremitting stresses to the same section of the annulus, accelerating degenerative changes over time. This is true whether the habitual postural organization is lumbar flexion or extension.

With the boards arranged near vertical, compression forces on the nucleus and annulus are more evenly distributed out into the annular walls. Moving from a balanced place allows movement stresses to be spread out in several directions and allows the tissues a rest cycle they won't get with either habitual flexion or extension postures. Could it be that interdiscal pressure itself is not the culprit, but that invariant compression stresses and habitual directional shearing stresses are to blame for disc breakdown?

Additionally, even though flexion increases interdiscal pressure, many more people relate an increase in low back pain to extension (73.2%) than to flexion (43.4%) according to Jacobsen.[25] More people felt a consistent preference for flexed postures in Dolan's study,[26] which he suspected was because of the reduction of compressive forces on the posterior annulus. Horst and Brinckmann[27] confirmed this supposition. There is even evidence to suggest that the incidence of lumbar disc disease is very low in people who habitually sit or squat in positions that flex the lumbar spine.[28] This was a comparison of more primitive populations with North Americans and North Europeans. Guess who had healthier backs?

We'll cover this more in the lumbar stability chapter, but there are also many more categories of potential extension stress than of flexion stress. They are as common as the dandelions in my yard and are endemic in the real world, partly because we habitually focus most of our intention to orient and manipulate in front of us.

In reality, there is no way of resolving this question of ideal anterior/posterior postural alignment. We might as well argue about what the best breakfast cereal is: both decisions are arrived at subjectively. Differing genetic makeup and body types affect alignment. What your functional intention is, and what the arrangement of affordances in your environment is, influences alignment. In theory, alignment constantly changes to meet a varied environment, and tissue load is evenly distributed throughout the whole spine. In this scenario there are no good movements or bad movements, only successful or unsuccessful ones.

Sadly this is not a typical scenario, and for most of us there are such things as bad movements. Bad movements, damaging movements, movements that create tissue strain and eventual breakdown are ones of our own making. We make them bad by doing them so often. The answer to the question 'What is ideal posture?' most often turns out to be: 'Whatever you aren't *habitually* doing.' For most people, that will mean a reduction of anterior pelvic tilt and lumbar lordosis.

Benefits of a posture approaching columnar

What happens to a habitual half-archer when she rolls her sitting pelvis into posterior tilt and reduces or eliminates her lumbar lordosis? She will end up looking down and rounding her shoulders further forward. She will feel like she is slumping. When you cue her to return to her half arch, observe as she does the whole movement with anterior pelvic tilt and lumbar extension. There will be little or no change in the shape of the thoracic spine because she moved in an unevenly distributed manner, using only the lower back.

Half-archers often have a limited ability to mobilize their chest and thoracic spine into extension. Because of its length and the added complexities and constraints that the attachment of the ribs on to the thoracic spine provides, it is a part of the spine that is easy to just forget. Why figure out how to use this more complex part of my spine when I can much more easily move at my lower back and neck? Many people will choose this strategy. The caveat is that in electing to forfeit movement in one area in favor of concentrating the movement somewhere else, you have put yourself on the path of self-destruction.

What could be the advantage of a rounded mid back? Besides the fact that it is average,[29] which is not the same as saying it is ideal, it would be great for looking downward and for falling backward, but not for much else.

- A columnar organization would be much more efficient in skeletally supporting the weight of the head and neck. A round mid back necessitates a sharp transition at the lower cervical spine with anterior shearing stresses at the lower vertebrae and extension stresses on the facets and intervertebral foramen a bit higher up.

- A columnar organization gives you the advantage of seeing your world from a higher horizon. A round mid back robs you of height and compresses your internal organs.

- A thoracic spine that is habitually neutral when straight will have a much greater ability to move into extension than a thoracic spine that is habitually neutral when rounded.

Lack of thoracic mobility into extension necessitates overextension of the lumbar and cervical spines, both posturally and in movement.

- A head balanced on a columnar structure can rotate to orient left and right along the horizon with better participation from the thoracic spine. Rotation and side-bending through the thoracic spine occurs much more easily from a columnar organization than from thoracic joints engaged in a prior commitment to flex.

- A columnar organization balances the head over a vertical support, like the guy with the poles and the dishes at the circus. A half arch pushes the head forward and necessitates a compressive backward bending at the suboccipital junction and a constant firing of the suboccipital muscles to prevent the head from falling forward.

- A columnar organization invites breath to move evenly throughout the torso and to mobilize the chest, belly and back. Breath moves, expands and contracts the trunk like a cylindrical balloon. A half archer constrains her breath, often chronically holding the anterior intercostal and upper abdominal obliques and rectus abdominis tight to maintain her thoracic flexion. The diaphragm is constrained by chronically holding the upper belly, and breath defaults to upper chest and the scalenes.

- A columnar organization supports the shoulder girdles naturally in a more adducted or posterior position compared to shoulder girdles saddled to a round back. This facilitates better shoulder girdle muscle balance. Glenohumeral movement is improved through the contribution of superior thoracic extension abilities in reaching up, out or forward.

One nice thing about having a columnar organization as an ideal is that it is almost completely unattainable. Few among us can get their pelvis to vertical in standing or organize the vertebrae of their lumbar and thoracic spine in a straight line. Fewer still can avoid that little block of chronically flexed vertebrae in the upper few thoracic vertebrae that still provides for a bump in an otherwise straight road they may make of their spines.

I say this to assuage your fears that I am somehow whipsawing my patients to contort into unnatural poses in their struggle to attain postural nirvana. Not at all! I only edge them in a direction I think would help them to best achieve their goals of comfort, function or efficiency. How far we travel in that direction is up to them. For many of us, that will mean in a direction of reducing AP spinal curves. Decide for yourself as you progress through this book whether to recalibrate your definition of spinal neutral to one that is longer and straighter.

Assessing AP postural balance and correlating to movement bias

When assessing your students, try observing them while in sitting or on hands and knees. Have them look alternately up and down and direct them to coordinate their head and pelvis as in sitting circles I. The full-rounders will probably be able to round well throughout the whole torso but have difficulty moving fully into extension. The full-archers will probably be able to arch well but have difficulty moving fully into flexion.

The half-archers will probably round most in their thoracic spine while staying flat or even remaining a bit extended in their lumbar spine. They will probably arch most in their lumbar spine while staying rounded in the thorax. These folks very often can't even get their thoracic spine to neutral, let alone move into true extension.

Our half-round folks will show a decent ability to round all the way through but difficulty in anteriorly tilting their pelvis and moving especially the lower lumbar segments into extension. Hands and knees is a particularly good position to make this assessment if knees and wrists can tolerate it. The columnar will show an ability to be more equally mobile throughout each part of the spine, with a balanced proportion of AP movement at each section. These are even more rare than the half-archers.

It is easier to visualize the proportion of movement and you can easily use a short foam roller to rock along their spine to help them to feel proprioceptively what you notice visually. Use the edge of the roller to provide the tactile and proprioceptive information that will help your students assess their AP postural bias. Try mimicking all five postural types yourself, though some may escape you. What is your type?

Legs move the pelvis in balance and orientation

What do you get if you put legs on a worm? A Tyrannosaurus Rex with a big torso, large legs, huge jaws and itty-bitty little arms. Let's move on now to a discussion of the legs and how they control movements of the torso. We will return now to the sitting circles series and repeat each variation of the first lesson, but with slightly different language that directs your attention more to the role of the legs. It is the legs, and more specifically the muscles that cross the hip joints to connect the femur to the pelvis and lower spine, that are the prime movers of the pelvis and torso.

The legs act to balance the pelvis and spine in sitting and standing posture both front to back and left to right, and by extension are responsible for AP and left-to-right imbalances of the pelvis.[30,31] They act to control the position of the pelvis and the shape of the lower spine in bending, and are responsible when bending activities create tissue strain.[32] They act to stabilize the pelvis on the legs and contribute directly and indirectly to lumbar and SI stabilization.[33–35]

They act to turn the pelvis in space to initiate rotational movements, and are largely responsible for controlling rotational stresses at the lower back. The legs act to shift the weight of the pelvis left and right in sitting and standing. When organizing the head and arms to move as an extension of the torso and pelvis in orientation and manipulation functions, it is ideally the legs that initiate and control these movements.

Martial arts and eastern movement disciplines emphasize the importance, nay, the central role of the pelvis and lower abdomen in movement, and it is the legs that provide that power. Martial artists call this 'Moving from your one point.'[36] The one point, *tan tien* in Chinese and *hara* in Japanese, is the center of mass of your body. It is located 2 or 3 inches below your navel and centrally located front to back and left to right. This center of mass does not move itself: it is moved by the muscles that cross the hip joints.

Legs are the remote control devices for the pelvis and lower spine and need to be addressed in more detail and with more specificity when we deal clinically with neurological trunk control, lower back pain, neck and shoulder girdle pain and so on. Hip muscles are the remote control devices for the feet and how they interact with the floor, controlling the position of the knees in space and the shape and orientation of the feet on the floor.

Properly trained, those key muscles that cross the hip joint can reduce valgus and recurvatum stresses on the knees, provide some needed power to assist the quadriceps in walking, jumping and climbing stairs, and reduce knee rotation and foot pronation stresses. The curious practitioner may wish to gain a deeper understanding of how the organization or disorganization of the legs resonates through the whole body, and may want to develop tools with which to influence any imbalances or inefficiencies. Now put on your student cap and revisit the sitting circles lesson proprioceptively, listening this time for what the legs are doing. Illustrations are as in previous sitting circle variations.

Sitting Circles III – Using the Legs

Variations

A. Sit in an upright-backed or kitchen-style chair. Sit near the front edge of the seat so your back is away from the backrest. Sit with your feet flat on the floor and directly underneath your knees, with feet and knees both somewhere between hip and shoulder width apart.

- Notice how your pelvis is balanced on the seat. You may feel two bones on the bottom of your pelvis that are supporting your weight.
- If you can't feel bones on the seat, sit on your hands and use your hands to help you to feel where those bones are.
- Is your pelvis rolled backward or forward? Is your back rounded or arched?
- Is there more weight to the left or the right 'sitting bone?' Are you longer along one side of your torso and shorter along the other?
- Where are you looking? Up? Down? At the horizon?
- How are your feet contacting the floor? Are your toes pointed inward or outward? Is more of your weight to the inside or the outside edge of your feet? Are there any differences between the two sides?

B. Sit on chair as before, find the horizon. Now interlace your fingers and place them behind your head.

- Point your elbows forward and move them both down towards your hips as you look toward your

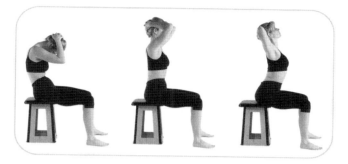

Fig. 5.12 Does the weight on your feet change as you fall back – or when you fall forward?

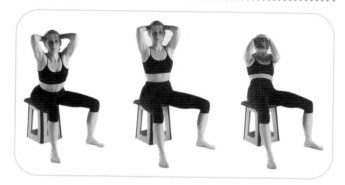

Fig. 5.14 Rolling and falling along a diagonal – feel the pressing and lightening of your right foot.

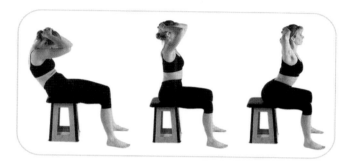

Fig. 5.13 Does adding in leaning forward and back make the pressing and lightening of your feet more obvious?

belly button (Fig. 5.12). Let your pelvis roll back on the seat and your whole back round as you do this.

- Do not pull on your head with your hands. Does the weight of your feet against the floor change at all as you do this?

- Repeat several times, then as you come back to neutral, continue past neutral to look up to the ceiling (Fig. 5.12). Spread your elbows apart and pinch your shoulder blades together as you roll your pelvis forward on the seat and arch your back.

- Move your neck only as long as your back is still moving in cooperation. Does the weight of your feet against the floor change at all as you do this?

- Add in leaning way back as you round your back and look toward your belly button, and leaning way forward as you arch forward and look toward the ceiling (Fig. 5.13). You will now find that as you roll back/lean back, your feet will lighten away from the floor.

- As you arch forward and lean forward, your weight will get heavier through your feet. Alternate back and forth several times and pay attention to the pressing and lightening of your feet against the floor.

- Alternate looking up and down/leaning forward and back – elbows point forward when looking down and

spread out when looking up. Coordinate head and tail!

- Continue this a few times, then start making movements smaller and smaller until you come to stop in a place where your pelvis is balanced forward/back on your seat and where your feet are somewhere evenly between pressing heavily and lightening.

C. Sit again toward the front edge of your seat; interlace your fingers and place your hands behind your head.

- Turn yourself a little to the right so you are facing your right knee and still looking at the horizon. Elbows are pointed forward over your right knee. From here –

- Reach your elbows downward and look downward toward your right hip (Fig. 5.14). Let your pelvis roll back and to the left and allow the left side of your back to round and lengthen. Lean or fall back when rounding and lean/fall forward when arching.

- Continue the movement of coming back to neutral to look up and to the right towards the ceiling. Elbows spread apart and shoulders pinch back and down as you roll your pelvis forward and to the right.

- Alternate looking up and down along this diagonal; your pelvis rolls diagonally on the seat and your arms flap. Notice change of weight on right foot.

- Pay attention to how you alternately bring weight on to your right foot as you arch and lean forward, then lighten your right foot away from the floor as you roll back and lean back and to the left. Repeat several times.

D. Sit in a chair with your hands behind your head. Face to the left and repeat instructions above to opposite side.

- Look down and reach your elbows towards your left hip and roll your pelvis back and to the right, then look up and to the left while rolling your pelvis forward and to the left.

- How does this diagonal compare to the other? How does your weight change on your left foot as you do this reciprocating movement?

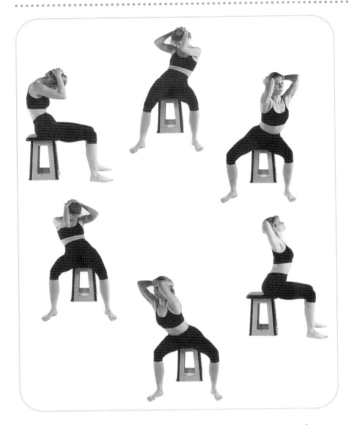

Fig. 5.15 Make U-shapes then circles – how are you using your legs to move your pelvis?

E. Sit forward on your seat again. Hands are again interlaced and behind your head with elbows pointed forward.

- Turn a bit to the left and do this diagonal again a few times, rolling pelvis forward and to the left and back and to the right as you look alternately toward left hip and toward the ceiling to the left. Lean way forward and back as you do this. Next time you look and reach your elbows toward your left hip –

- Swing elbows through middle and over to the right hip, then point them up and to the right as you look in that same direction (Fig. 5.15).

- This describes a U-shape; your pelvis rolls forward and to the left, then back and to the middle, then forward and to the right. Reverse to roll back to the middle and forward and to the left.

- Your elbows also make a U-shape in space. Exaggerate the leans back and forward and feel the use of your legs as they alternately catch you from falling all the way forward and then catch you from falling all the way back.

- After doing this semicircular movement a few times, complete the circle by moving elbows from up and to the right to up and to the middle, then to up and to the left.

- Make a circle with your pelvis on the seat, with your elbows in space and with your head in space.

- Change directions of the circle; go the other way. Gradually make the circular movement smaller and smaller to spiral yourself back to the middle.

- Find that place where your pelvis is balanced on your seat both forward/back and left/right, and where your head is balanced tall on the column of your spine with your eyes on the horizon.

- Go big and spiral smaller and smaller to where your pelvis is rolled neither forward, back, left nor right.

- Feel how your pelvis is balanced on your seat in comparison to when you began. What is the shape of your back? Round? Arched? Straight? Bent to one side or the other? What is your sense of ease in sitting in comparison to the beginning?

- Without your hands on your head, look alternately up and down. How does this movement compare to when you first did it? Can you see farther or more easily?

- Does your pelvis and whole back move to assist with your intention to look? Is the movement proportioned any more evenly? Do you have any clearer sense of how your legs participate in these movements?

Static and dynamic baselines – Sitting Circles III

The static baseline or proprioceptive scan is the same as for the original sitting circles but with less emphasis on position of eyes and more inquiries about the organization and weight distribution of the feet on the floor. In essence, the whole lesson is the same but with fewer directions to pay attention to breath and eyes, fewer variations involving the differentiation of the arms, and more instructions to notice weight and orientation of the feet on the floor. Few people think of sitting as something that should involve the legs, but indeed they should.

We already know what happens to the worm when falling backward. Moving your elbows down toward your belly button while rolling your pelvis backward, especially when adding in the leaning backward, simulates a backward fall. We know that the torso rounds, the torso extensors are inhibited/stretched and the torso flexors are excited/strengthened. What are the legs doing?

As the pelvis and torso fall backward, the hip joints are moving in the direction of extension. Does this mean that the hip extensors are actively shortening? No, in this relationship to gravity, the fall back is being arrested by the lengthening contraction of the hip flexors (Fig. 5.16). The psoas major, iliacus and rectus femoris have to pay out the line to catch the pelvis from falling back and then have to powerfully shorten to haul it back up to vertical.

Falling back then coming back to neutral features alternating lengthening and shortening contractions of the bilateral hip flexors. Feel how, as you roll and lean back, your feet get lighter on the floor. That is a result of the hip flexors contracting and

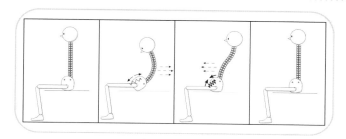

Fig. 5.16 The hip flexors control the fall of the worm backward and pull the pelvis and torso back upright again.

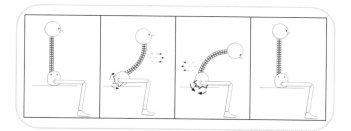

Fig. 5.17 The hip extensors control the fall of the worm forward and push the pelvis and torso back upright again.

using the weight of the legs as a counterbalance to the backward-falling torso. This is why a worm is so rarely seen standing on his tail – without legs, sitting is impossible.

As the pelvis and torso fall forward, we know that the torso extends, the torso flexors are inhibited/stretched and the torso extensors are excited/strengthened. We can also observe that the hip joints are flexing. This is controlled by a lengthening contraction of the hip extensors. The gluteus maximus, hamstrings and hip short and stubbies (piriformis, internal and external obturators, inferior and superior gemelli and quadratus femoris) have to pay out the line to catch the pelvis from falling forward, and then have to powerfully shorten to push it back up to vertical (Fig. 5.17).

Falling forward then coming back to neutral features alternating lengthening and shortening contractions of the bilateral hip extensors. Feel how, as you roll and lean forward, your feet get heavier on the floor. Again, sitting is impossible without legs. By extension, imbalanced sitting posture results from imbalanced hip musculature.

Let's go through one complete cycle of alternate falls. Starting from being leaned backward, you are in a position of hip extension and back flexion. This is a differentiation of the legs and back. Recall that in the chapter on movements of the worm, we mostly did lessons in which the extremities and torso were moving globally into either flexion (Be a Better Ball) or extension (Xs and Os). We described those lessons as primitive: they happen earlier on in the developmental sequence. Once having come upright, though, those global patterns of movement are less useful. Matured, upright function requires competence and balance of differentiated movements.

Box 5.2 Bilateral iliopsoas pattern

Basic differentiated relationship of lumbar extension and hip flexion

Hip flexors do lengthening contractions to control/prevent falls backward

Hip flexors do shortening contractions to pull pelvis/lower spine back upright from falling-back position

Hip flexors pull the pelvis toward the legs – creating anterior tilt and constraining the movement of the pelvis into posterior tilt

Bilateral iliopsoas and gluteal patterns

To come back upright from a falling-back position we will need a differentiated movement of hip flexion and back extension. The bilateral hip flexors do a shortening contraction that pulls the pelvis toward the legs. We will call this basic movement relationship a *bilateral iliopsoas pattern*. We are naming the pattern after the muscle that does a shortening contraction to flex the hips and extend the back. As you pass over the top of the ischial tuberosities, the relationship to gravity changes and you begin to fall forward. The basic differentiated pattern is still the same (hip flexion and back extension), so we will continue to call it a bilateral iliopsoas pattern even though it is now a lengthening contraction of the hip extensorss (Box 5.2).

To come back upright from a falling-forward position, we have some choices. Although the hips have to extend, the torso could continue to stay arched, could move to neutral and stay there, or could move into global flexion. For our current purposes, we will direct the movement in such a way as to encourage a combination of hip extension and back flexion. The bilateral hip extensors do a shortening contraction that pushes the pelvis away from the legs.

We will call this basic movement relationship a *bilateral gluteal pattern*. We are again naming the pattern after the muscle that does a shortening contraction to extend the hips and flex the back. As you pass over the top of the ischial tuberosities, the relationship to gravity changes and you begin to fall backward. The basic differentiated pattern is still the same (hip extension and back flexion), so we will continue to call it a bilateral gluteal pattern even though it is now a lengthening contraction of the hip flexors.

When falling backward (i.e. when belly up), we are emphasizing the lengthening and strengthening of the hip flexors. When falling forward (when belly down), we are emphasizing the lengthening and strengthening of the hip extensors. In this lesson, we are doing alternating lengthening and shortening contractions of oppositional muscle groups. We are coordinating the antagonists. We would like the iliopsoas and gluteal groups to be balanced and, in being balanced, to hold the pelvis in a vertical or neutral position in sitting.

We would like the iliopsoas to do much of the work of keeping the pelvis from falling backward and keeping the back from falling into flexion. This can take much of the load off the back extensors. We would like the gluteals to do much of the work of keeping the pelvis from falling forward and keeping the back from falling into extension. This also relieves strain on the back extensors. Coordinated pelvic girdle antagonists are crucial to effortless sitting posture and uncoordinated pelvic girdle antagonists are responsible for postural imbalances.

Bilateral gluteal or iliopsoas bias determines pelvic tilt

The gluteals, hamstrings and short and stubbies are responsible for posterior pelvic tilt. If they are too short, what happens to posture and movement? In sitting, short hip extensors result in posterior pelvic tilt and lumbar flexion. Short hip extensors and short torso flexors tend to go together. We have already discussed some of the clinical manifestations of these full- and half-round postural types. In bending over from sitting or standing, the hip extensors will disallow full hip hinge or anterior pelvic tilt and necessitate too much flexion at the lower back; clinical manifestations are the same as listed previously.

What happens in posture and movement if the hip extensors are too weak? In standing and sitting, the hip extensors may not be working appropriately to push the anteriorly tilting pelvis back to neutral. Weak hip extensors and weak torso flexors tend to go together. We have discussed possible clinical manifestations of full arch and half arch postural types. In bending, the hip extensors may allow the pelvis to fall too far forward on the legs and necessitate too much back extensor work, with resultant compression forces acting on close-packed facets.

The psoas, iliacus and rectus femoris are responsible for anterior pelvic tilt. If they are too short, what happens to posture and movement? In sitting, but especially in standing, the iliopsoas may prevent the pelvis from being pushed back to vertical. Short hip flexors and short back extensors tend to go together. We get full arch or half arch patterns. What happens if the iliopsoas is too weak? We get full- or half-round patterns. Weak iliopsoas and weak back extensors tend to go together.

Through reciprocal inhibition, we can surmise that with short hamstrings, gluteals or short and stubbies we might also have weak iliopsoas and back extensors. With short iliopsoas, we can surmise weak hip extensors and abdominals. With weak iliopsoas, we get tight hamstrings. With weak gluteals, we get tight iliopsoas. These relationships are not set in stone and sometimes you get someone where everything is tight or everything is weak, but in general you will see one of these two basic types in your office. Having a gluteal bias may result in full-round or half-round patterns because of hip extensor tightness and hip flexor weakness. Having an iliopsoas bias may result in either the full arch or the ever-popular but dreaded half arch pattern.

Which of these two reciprocating movements (falling back or falling forward) would be best for the iliopsoas-dominant folks in our practice? They need both! The iliopsoas-dominant (hyperlordotic) student needs to learn to allow the pelvis to fall backward. This lengthens the back extensors and hip flexors and strengthens the abdominals (killing three birds with one stone). The iliopsoas-dominant person needs to learn to push her pelvis back toward vertical from a belly-down orientation. This strengthens the hip extensors and the abdominals while lengthening the back extensors and turning off the iliopsoas.

Which of these two reciprocating movements (falling back or falling forward) would be best for the gluteal-dominant folks in our practice? They also need both! The gluteal-dominant (posterior tilted pelvis and kyphotic spine) student needs to learn to allow the pelvis to fall more completely forward in a belly-down orientation. This lengthens the hip extensors and

Box 5.3 Bilateral gluteal pattern
Basic differentiated relationship of lumbar flexion and hip extension
Hip extensors do lengthening contractions to control/prevent falls forward
Hip extensors do shortening contractions to push pelvis back upright from falling-forward position
Hip extensors push pelvis away from legs – creating posterior tilt and constraining the movement of the pelvis into anterior tilt

abdominals while strengthening the back extensors. The gluteal-dominant person needs to learn to pull her pelvis back toward vertical from a belly-up orientation. This strengthens the hip flexors and back extensors and lengthens the abdominals and hip extensors (Box 5.3).

By reciprocating movements, we are coordinating the antagonists and allowing a more neutral posture to emerge organically. By doing reciprocating movements, we are stretching what needs to be stretched and strengthening what needs to be strengthened. Clinically, we would usually teach the lesson as a reciprocating movement for informational purposes, then have each student emphasize the appropriate nonhabitual direction of movement in a home program while de-emphasizing the mid-to-end range of movement into the habitual direction.

An understanding of the way the legs work in both belly-up and belly-down positions and an understanding of the clinical consequences of gluteal and iliopsoas dominance are critical to understanding the rest of this section and to understanding the section on the arms and shoulder girdles. Make sure this information is clear in your mind before you read on!

Unilateral gluteal and iliopsoas patterns

Our next variations, C and D, are diagonal patterns. The movement of falling forward and to the right, as you no doubt recall, is a left torso extension pattern. What moderates this fall (Fig. 5.18)? The right hip extensors do a lengthening contraction to arrest the fall of the pelvis and torso forward and to the right – the right leg acts as a kickstand. These same muscles do a shortening contraction to push the pelvis back and to the left towards vertical (Box 5.4).

This movement of pushing the pelvis and torso away from the right leg, where the right hip is extending and the torso is moving toward right flexion, we will call a *right gluteal pattern*. As the pelvis goes over the top of the ischial tuberosities and begins to fall back and to the left, we will still call the pattern of right hip extension and right torso flexion a right gluteal pattern even though the movement is now controlled by a lengthening contraction of the right hip flexors (Fig. 5.19).

From this position of having fallen back and to the left, the right iliopsoas group has to do a shortening contraction to pull the pelvis and torso back upright (see Fig. 5.9). The right hip is flexing and the torso is moving toward left extension. We will call this a *right iliopsoas pattern*. As the pelvis goes over the top of the ischial tuberosities and begins to fall forward and to the right again, we will still call the pattern of right hip flexion and

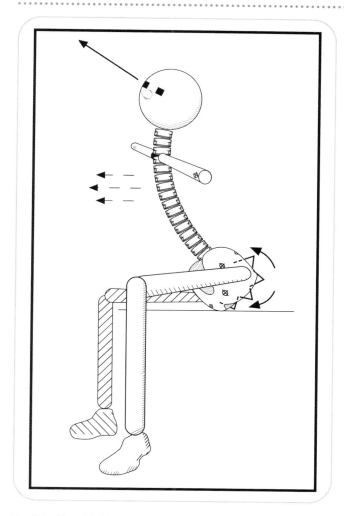

Fig. 5.18 One-sided hip extensors control a diagonal fall forward with a lengthening contraction, then push the pelvis back upright again with a shortening contraction.

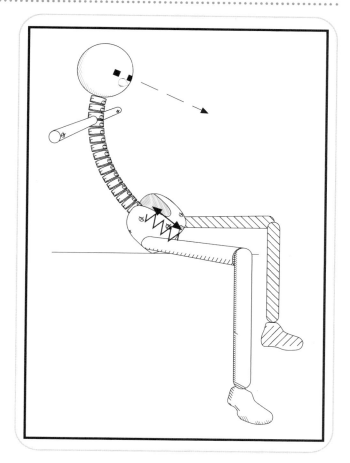

Fig. 5.19 One-sided hip flexors control a diagonal fall backward with a lengthening contraction, then pull the pelvis back upright again with a shortening contraction.

Box 5.4 Right gluteal pattern

Basic differentiated relationship of right lumbar flexion and right hip extension/abduction/external rotation

Right hip extensors do lengthening contraction to control/prevent falls forward and to the right

Right hip extensors do shortening contractions to push back upright from falling forward and to the right

---

Box 5.5 Right iliopsoas pattern

Basic differentiated relationship of left lumbar extension and right hip flexion/adduction/internal rotation

Right hip flexors do lengthening contractions to control/prevent falls back and to the left

Right hip flexors do shortening contractions to pull back upright from falls back and to the left

---

left torso extension a left iliopsoas pattern, even though the movement is now controlled by a lengthening contraction of the right hip extensors.

The belly-down half of this reciprocating movement emphasizes the length and strength of the right hamstrings, gluteals and short and stubbies. The belly-up half emphasizes the length and strength of the right iliopsoas, iliacus and rectus femoris. Observe again for yourself how your right foot lightens from

the floor when falling back to the left and how your right foot presses into the floor when falling forward to the right. This movement helps to balance and coordinate the right hip flexors and extensors (Box 5.5).

Let's look at the opposite diagonal: falling forward and to the left and then back and to the right. The movement of falling forward and to the left is a right torso extension pattern. The left hip extensors now do a lengthening contraction to arrest the fall of the pelvis and torso forward and to the left. Here is our kickstand again. These same muscles do a shortening contraction to push the pelvis back and to the right toward vertical.

> **Box 5.6   Left gluteal pattern**
>
> Basic differentiated relationship of left lumbar flexion and left hip extension/abduction/external rotation
>
> Left hip extensors do lengthening contractions to control/prevent falls forward and to the left
>
> Left hip extensors do shortening contractions to push back upright from falling forward and to the left

> **Box 5.7   Left iliopsoas pattern**
>
> Basic differentiated relationship of right lumbar extension and left hip flexion/adduction/internal rotation
>
> Left hip flexors do lengthening contractions to control/prevent falls back and to the right
>
> Left hip flexors do shortening contractions to pull back upright from a falling back and to the right

This movement of pushing the pelvis and torso away from the left right leg, where the left hip is extending and the torso is moving toward left flexion, we will call a *left gluteal pattern*. As the pelvis goes over the top of the ischial tuberosities and begins to fall back and to the right, we will still call the pattern of left hip extension and left torso flexion a left gluteal pattern even though the movement is now controlled by a lengthening contraction of the left hip flexors (Box 5.6).

From this position of having fallen back and to the right, the left iliopsoas group has to do a shortening contraction to pull the pelvis and torso back upright. The left hip is flexing and the torso is moving toward right extension. We will call this a *left iliopsoas pattern*. As the pelvis goes over the top of the ischial tuberosities and begins to fall forward and to the left again, we will still call this a left iliopsoas pattern even though the movement is now controlled by a lengthening contraction of the left hip extensors.

The belly-down half of this reciprocating movement emphasizes the length and strength of the left hamstrings, gluteals and short and stubbies. The belly-up half emphasizes the length and strength of the left iliopsoas, iliacus and rectus femoris. Observe again for yourself how your left foot lightens from the floor when falling back to the right, and how your left foot presses into the floor when falling forward to the left. This movement helps to balance and coordinate the left hip flexors and extensors (Box 5.7).

Unilateral bias determines pelvic weight shift and rotation

Whereas the bilateral use of the iliopsoas resulted in pulling the pelvis straight forward, the asymmetrical use of one iliopsoas group results in a movement of pulling the pelvis forward and toward the side of the working iliopsoas. This goes along with the diagonal torso patterns we introduced earlier. Whereas the bilateral use of the gluteals resulted in pushing the pelvis straight back, the asymmetrical use of one gluteal group results in a movement of pushing the pelvis back and away from the side of the working gluteals. The iliopsoas group pulls, the gluteals push. These four cornerstone muscles are responsible for positioning, moving and stabilizing the pelvis in space through the constantly adjusting coordination of these pushing and pulling actions.

Whereas a bilateral iliopsoas pattern tends to be linked to global torso extension pattern (full arch) or to the differentiated pattern of lumbar extension and thoracic flexion (half arch), the asymmetrical use on one iliopsoas group is associated with asymmetrical torso extension. For instance, if the left iliopsoas is dominant, we would anticipate some variation of right torso extension.

The left iliopsoas may be pulling the weight of the pelvis to the left; this mimics falling forward and to the left and stimulates the worm to extend back and to the right to avoid hitting his head. In the full-arch types there might be a global right extension. In the half-arch types there may be right lumbar extension and right thoracic flexion. If the right iliopsoas is dominant, we would anticipate some variation of left torso extension.

Whereas the bilateral gluteal pattern tends to be linked to global torso flexion (full round) or to the differentiated pattern of lumbar flexion and thoracic extension (the reclusive and rarely seen in the wild half-round), the asymmetrical use of one gluteal group is associated with asymmetrical torso flexion.

With a right gluteal dominance, we'll probably get right torso flexion. The right gluteals are pushing the weight of the pelvis back and to the left, which mimics a fall back and to the left, which stimulates the worm to round forward and to the right. With a left gluteal dominance, we might see either the global or the differentiated versions of left torso flexion.

If someone has some short iliopsoas muscles, we might anticipate short and hard-working lumbar extensors and quadratus lumborum. They could be considered to be synergists in many functions. That would make the left iliopsoas and right quadratus/lumbar extensors synergists. Ditto for the right iliopsoas and left quadratus/extensors. Observe, palpate and test for these relationships in your students. What happens above the lumbothoracic junction is dependent on what the thoracic extensors and posterior intercostals do. The most common pattern is for the chest to fall back into flexion.

If someone has short hamstrings, we might anticipate short and chronically contracting rectus abdominis and abdominal obliques and, most often, short anterior intercostals. They are usually synergistic. That would make the right gluteals/hamstrings/short and stubbies synergists with the right abdominals and usually the right anterior intercostals.

The pelvic clock

Thinking schematically, imagine the pelvis as a ball sitting on the face of a clock with a convex surface (Fig. 5.20). The top of the convex clock would be directly in the center, equidistant from 12, 3, 6 and 9. The front of the pelvis (pubic side) faces 6 o'clock and the back of the pelvis (sacral side) faces 12 o'clock. That would make 3 o'clock to the left and 9 o'clock to the right. Because the surface of the clock is convex, this means that any movement from center will be downhill. The ball will fall in one of 360 possible directions. This is a schematic representation of a vertical pelvis in sitting.

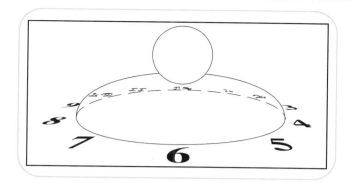

Fig. 5.20 Ball on a convex clock – it can fall equally easily in all directions.

If the ball starts rolling straight forward, we could say it is falling toward 6 o'clock. For the pelvis, we could call this direction of movement an anterior tilt. We could also call it a bilateral iliopsoas pattern. If the ball rolls back, we could say it is falling toward 12 o'clock. This would be posterior pelvic tilt or a bilateral gluteal pattern. If the ball falls back and to the left, this is 1.30 or a right gluteal pattern. Back and to the right is 10.30 or a left gluteal. Forward and to the left is 4.30 or a left iliopsoas. Forward and to the right is 7.30 or right iliopsoas.

What is responsible for moving the pelvis straight side to side? Who does 3 and 9 o'clock? We will address this after a few more lessons emphasizing front to back and the two diagonal patterns; we will continue to work with just six of the eight primary directions of movement for now.

With falls going forward, there is a lengthening contraction of the gluteals to stop the fall and a shortening contraction of those same gluteals to push the pelvis back to center. These belly-down falls (especially 4.30 to 6–7.30) lengthen and strengthen the gluteals but are still variations of iliopsoas patterns (left, right and bilateral). With falls going backward (especially 10.30 to 12–1.30), there is a lengthening contraction of the iliopsoas to stop the fall and a shortening contraction of those same iliopsoas to pull the pelvis back to center.

Note that whereas a true ball can fall as easily to the right and left as it can forward and back, the same cannot be said about the pelvis. With the two ischial tuberosities to balance on, front to back stability is much more problematic (at the same time that front to back mobility is easier) than left-to-right balance. It's just like trying to balance on an unmoving bicycle, except that in that situation front/back stability is good and right/left stability is problematic.

Posture isn't static

It is important to remember that there is no stable platform upon which the pelvis can balance statically in vertical. Your pelvis is always falling. In a well organized system, there is a constant wobble between falling almost imperceptibly forward, catching the fall with the gluteals, pushing the pelvis back to vertical, catching the resultant fall backward with the iliopsoas, pulling the pelvis back to vertical and so on. This small recip-rocating movement keeps the pelvis from falling too far off center and from constantly activating some muscle groups while constantly inhibiting others.

This ideal contrasts with the average. Most of us fall either forward or backward, catch the fall too far off center to be able to easily bring it back, and hold it there with long habituated muscular effort. The hours and months and years of this repetitive behavior helps to create and maintain structural and muscular imbalances and puts certain overstretched, overcompressed or overworked tissues at risk.

Note how there is a rotational component to all of the diagonal movements as well as right/left weight shifting. The pelvis turns to the left in a left iliopsoas pattern and turns to the right with a left gluteal pattern. You will find clinically that people will not have just nice clean front/back imbalances but will also have left/right asymmetries. Observe first in sitting, standing and supine for front/back imbalances. Imagine there are eyes on the front of the pelvis of the person you are assessing.

Are they looking up or down? Are they iliopsoas or gluteal dominant, and to what degree? Observe in sitting, standing and supine whether one side of the pelvis is further forward of the other one. Are the eyes of the pelvis looking right or left? Which side of the pelvis is further forward? Palpate the antero-superior iliac spine (ASIS) bilaterally in standing, sitting and supine and visualize depth differences. In standing and sitting, you can also palpate and visualize the relative depth of the posterosuperior iliac spine (PSIS). It is sometimes easier to see the rotational component of a diagonal bias more easily than differences in weight distribution.

The person who turns her pelvis to the left may be left iliopsoas dominant. The person who turns her pelvis to the left may be right gluteal dominant. Part of the game clinically is to observe for biases and start predicting muscle imbalances. Are they going to have tighter hamstrings on the left or the right? Tighter left or right iliopsoas? Piriformis? Quadratus lumborum? Anterior intercostals?

When looking at these rotational imbalances, you may often find a consistency of relationships throughout the various positions, though sometimes you'll be surprised or confused. If you just think of normal developmentally based imbalances, these described biases are what we would expect to see consistently. Because movement and posture are also influenced by past injuries, occupation, emotional history, communication style and other factors that we can only barely glimpse, there will always be odd subvariations and weird permutations of the basic patterns and relationships described.

Cutting the Gordian knot

You could spend time trying to track down the exact whys and wherefores of odd variations, or you could (perhaps more effectively) spend your time training your students towards better integrated and more efficient movement patterns, incorporating global and differentiated patterns, using reciprocating cardinal and diagonal planes, linking those patterns to a variety of functional contexts and performing in a variety of relationships to gravity. Train them in head-to-tail relationships and in controlling the movements of the worm from the legs, and trust the CNS to make sense out of it. Cut the Gordian knot, rather than trying to untangle it!

When working with pelvic imbalances, look for cornerstone imbalances in addition to your assessment of bony landmarks. Look for high or low iliac crests, ASISs or PSISs. Diagnose upslips, downslips and outflares. Suspect innominate rotations and sacral torsions. But be aware that the legs are not affecting the pelvis the same way from side to side. How much of what appears to be a displacement of the sacrum relative to the two innominates is because of an imbalance of the pelvis as a whole relative to the legs? At the least, the direction in which muscular imbalances of the legs torque the pelvis is probably contributing to and consistent with the direction of SI dysfunction.

Pelvis balancing on legs rather than on a seat

What is the difference between standing and sitting? The pelvis is now balanced on top of two legs instead of on a flat surface. The relationships between pelvis, torso and head generally stay essentially the same, but the relationship between the legs and the pelvis has now changed dramatically. Instead of being bent at about a 90° angle, the hips are now extending. Although it is relatively easy for most people to allow their pelvis to fall backward in sitting, for most people once standing it is much harder. Why is this?

In standing, a vertical balance of the pelvis requires near or at end-range hip joint extension. If the iliopsoas is too short or the hip extensors and abductors are not completing their shortening contraction, the pelvis will be held in a constant state of falling forward. As discussed earlier, this may result in lumbar joint compression or disc shearing stresses and necessitates constant compressive contractions of the back extensors. For many people, moving their pelvis over the top of their hip joints and allowing their pelvis to fall even a little bit backward is simply not possible in this position.

For these folks standing may be painful, and they may seek respite by sitting, squatting, leaning against a wall, bending their knees (one can tilt one's pelvis posteriorly in standing by bending the knees, but the relationship between pelvis and thigh bone remains the same), side-lying in a fetal position or lying supine with hips bent (supine with legs long will often be very uncomfortable).

These folks need to learn to more fully extend their hip joints in standing to take extension stresses off their lower back. They need to lengthen the iliopsoas and strengthen the gluteals, and be able to recognize how to use that newfound length and strength for that particular function. Whereas a comfortable majority bias their pelvis toward falling forward in standing, there are some people with very strong gluteal bias who actually do spill their pelvis back. Look for these folks in your office, the mall and the grocery store. They will generally be characterized by a very long and pronounced thoracic kyphosis.

As in sitting, there will also be left-to-right imbalances in standing. Observe here for depth differences at ASIS and PSIS to visualize rotational asymmetries. The basic bias may even be evident in walking. Is your student walking with her pelvis turned always in one direction, or is her pelvis only turning in one direction from center and not the other?

Is it clear to you how imbalances of the four cornerstone muscle groups that cross the hip joint can contribute to lower back pain? Gluteal bias leads to flexion stresses. Iliopsoas bias leads to extension stresses. Left iliopsoas bias leads to right extension – probably compression – stresses on the right lower back. Right gluteal bias leads to overstretch stresses, especially on the left lower back. Though somewhat less common, left iliopsoas bias can lead to left low back gapping or overstretching stresses, and a right gluteal bias can lead to right low back compressive stresses.

Distal compensations leading to injury

Could imbalances of these four cornerstone muscle groups have an effect on the organization and health of the head and neck? I once had a man come to me complaining of left neck pain and shooting pains down his left arm. He would experience his arm pain when looking up, looking over his left shoulder or reaching overhead. He rode a desk in his executive position and had such difficulty sitting and working at his computer that he would have to lower his head and look at his computer screen out of the top of his eyes.

During our initial interview I took the opportunity to observe, without him specifically knowing that he was under observation, the way he sat (balance) and engaged in conversation (orientation and communication). I noticed that he allowed his pelvis to roll back and to the left (right gluteal pattern) and that he was flexed and bent to the right through his torso (right torso flexion). Because he had to orient forward and to the horizon to engage with me (or to see his computer screen), he had to bend his head and neck back and to the left to compensate for the right torso flexion/right gluteal bias. This resulted in narrowing the left low cervical intervertebral foramen and compression on the C6 nerve root.

He held his neck effectively in a position of left side-bending, rotation and extension. As we carefully assessed mobility and organization, I asked him to look up, down, left and right, and to bend his head from side to side. Not surprisingly, he had limited motion and mild to moderate reproduction of pain on left side-bending, left rotation and especially extension (these all act to narrow the left low cervical intervertebral foramen). What really gave him a jolt, though, was when he moved into a combination of left rotation, left side-bending and extension. This is the classic quadrant test. We could also call it left cervical extension and can predict its presence when we see a right torso flexion/right gluteal bias.

How did we treat this individual? We helped him to become aware of where his pelvis was on his seat, the consequences of the organization of his pelvis on the shape of his torso, and how his head and neck were required to compensate for these habitual imbalances by moving into the exact direction that causes him so much pain and anguish. We helped him learn to use his legs to move his pelvis and how to coordinate his head and tail globally in balance and orientation functions.

We helped him to identify his nonhabitual direction of movement (left torso extension/right iliopsoas pattern, with differentiation of head and neck into right flexion), gave him pattern-specific and functionally relevant home exercise, and guided him in finding ways to incorporate this movement into daily activities. As part of his training in proprioceptive self-awareness and pattern recognition, he stretched the muscles that needed to be stretched: right hamstring/gluteals/

short and stubbies, right abdominal obliques and anterior intercostals, right pectoralis major and minor, left upper trapezius and levator scapulae, left cervical paraspinals and suboccipitals.

As part of his learning process, he strengthened muscles that needed to be stronger: right iliacus/iliopsoas/rectus femoris, left quadratus lumborum, left lumbar and especially thoracic spinal extensors, left posterior intercostals, right sternocleido-mastoids (SCM) and scalenes and right rectus capitis/longus colli. Depending on how you count, we could have sent him home with 15–20 different exercises and hoped that his CNS would make some sense of it. Or we could teach him global and differentiated patterns of movement, in cardinal and diagonal planes, with different relationships to gravity and with differing functional intentions. Think through what might happen at the neck in various scenarios involving other diagonal pelvic biases.

This lesson introduces the use of the legs in controlling the movements of the pelvis and, by extension, the movements of the torso, in balance and orientation. The movements of the worm are identical to those described in Section 2, but the emphasis shifts to an inquiry into the role of the legs. The next two lessons will continue to focus on themes of controlling balance and orientation through the bilateral or unilateral use of the four cornerstones.

First we will look in more depth at a lesson featuring a belly-up orientation. We will then work with more detail in a belly-down position. After these three introductory lessons, we will look at the simultaneous and cooperative use of the two legs working to move the pelvis in transitional movements and locomotion. Learn well the patterns and relationships described here, as much of the rest of this section is designed to help the practitioner to influence the balance of, and to facilitate the efficiency in using, these four cornerstones in a variety of functions.

Revisiting circles

In variation E we blend our front to back cardinal plane and our two diagonal patterns into first a U-shape movement then a full circle. The circular movement of the worm is the same as in the original Sitting Circles. The four cornerstones blend together in varying amounts to fill in the rest of the circle.

When in a straight falling-back or 12 o'clock position, both iliopsoas are working equally. As you move toward a falling-back and to the left or a 1.30 position, the right iliopsoas pays out a little line and the left iliopsoas starts to reel in his line. The left iliopsoas continues to take more of the load and the right iliopsoas eases off as the pelvis moves toward 3 o'clock. As the pelvis moves over the top of the left ischial tuberosity, the gluteals catch the now forward-falling pelvis (Box 5.8).

The left gluteal is lengthened and contracting while the right gluteal is shorter and contracting. The left gluteals now begin to shorten and the right gluteals lengthen to allow the pelvis to fall towards 6 o'clock. From 6 o'clock the left gluteals push harder to move the pelvis back and to the right toward 9 o'clock, where the pelvis begins to fall back and to the right and the left iliopsoas takes over again. The left iliopsoas then

---

Box 5.8 Sitting Circles III – Using the Legs

Using the Legs to move the pelvis in falling and orientation from vertical

Legs differentiating from pelvis and torso

Cardinal plane and diagonal torso movements – segue into circles again

From vertical, falls in all directions downhill – lengthening contractions to control fall and shortening contractions to return upright

---

shortens as the right iliopsoas lengthens to allow the pelvis to again fall back to 12 o'clock.

Moving in both directions of the circle allows the four cornerstones to work cooperatively in a variety of combinations. We will look at this circle again with the pelvis lying supine and will dissect its muscular coordination in this horizontal orientation to gravity. We will also look at directions we glossed over in this lesson – towards 3 and 9 o'clock.

Variations and applications

Positional variations for this lesson include straight, diagonal and circular variations with one ischial tuberosity off the edge of the seat. This variation requires the leg on the same side of the unsupported ischial tuberosity to push into the ground to keep from falling off the chair to that side, and is a good way to illustrate the advantages of being active with one's legs while sitting. The variations described in the original sitting circles using rolled towels can also be of benefit when focusing on lower extremity control of the pelvis in sitting. They act to magnify the falls.

Balancing and developing competence in using the four cornerstone muscles is important for treating lumbar dysfunction. Full-round and half-round folk benefit from back and hip flexor strengthening and hip extensor and abdominal lengthening. Full-arch and half-arch folk benefit from hip flexor and lumbar extensor lengthening and hip extensor and abdominal strengthening. One-sided back pain and pelvic imbalances benefit from balancing of the right and left cornerstones.

Balancing and developing competence in using the four cornerstone muscles are important for treating cervical or shoulder girdle dysfunction or pain syndromes. This lesson features head-to-tail elements useful for balancing and integrating the neck and shoulder girdles with the thorax and pelvis. Asymmetrical neck and shoulder girdle symptoms often correlate to left/right pelvic imbalances.

Use this lesson for treating lower extremity dysfunction or pain syndromes. Training the competence and balance of the cornerstone muscles assists in balancing the position of the knees in space and of the feet on the floor. Use in patients with total knee or total hip replacements to mobilize and reconnect the affected part and to provide early weightbearing. Use similarly for knee or ankle sprains, ligament tears or lower extremity fractures and postoperative rehabilitation.

Use this lesson for treating neurologic problems such as stroke or MS. Use this lesson to enhance trunk control, to balance hip antagonists on the unaffected side, then to reaccess and rebalance hip flexors and extensors on the affected side using the appropriate diagonal pathway. Work with upright-sitting balance and controlling the upright position of the pelvis from the iliopsoas and gluteals. Work with early weightbearing linked to contexts of reaching orientation or beginning a transitional movement from sitting to standing.

Use for general medical rehabilitation and geriatrics. Get your students active in sitting: challenge their balance, get their blood flowing, get their minds involved in self-care, self-exploration and problem solving. Mobilize the spine, ribcage, neck and hip joints, and facilitate deeper breathing and movement of the breath into different areas of their torsos.

Legs controlling the pelvis and back in belly-up orientation

Let's look now at supine and belly-up versions of this lesson. Pelvic Tilts are reminiscent of, but in important ways fundamentally different from, the classic exercise of the same name that is part of the William's Flexion series.

Pelvic Tilts

Variations

A. Lie on your back with your legs long and straight and with your hands somewhere on the ground below shoulder height.

   - Scan for contact against floor, especially your pelvis and lower back.
   - Is there a space between your lower back and the floor? If so, how high is it? How long is it? Is it higher on one side or the other?
   - How fully do your legs contact the ground? Are there spaces under the back of your knee? Is one leg more fully supported by the ground than the other?
   - Is there more weight to one side of your pelvis or the other? Is your pelvis rolled left or right?
   - In what direction do your toes point? Are your feet parallel to each other, with the toes pointed toward the ceiling? Are your legs rolled outward so the toes point outward? Are your legs rolled inward? Is there a difference in degree of roll out or in between one leg and the other?

B. Lie on your back with both knees bent and with the soles of both feet standing on the floor somewhere between hip and shoulder width apart.

   - Roll your pelvis gently and slowly upward on the floor away from your feet. Allow it to roll rather than lift. Your tailbone lifts toward the ceiling but the weight of your pelvis stays supported by the ground. Your lower back will flatten and press toward the floor (Fig. 5.21).

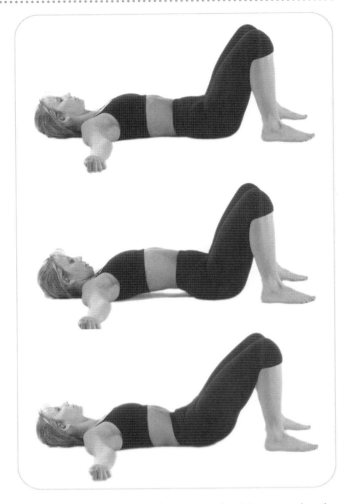

Fig. 5.21 Alternating rolling pelvis downward and then upward on the floor.

   - Where do you notice effort as you do this movement? Belly? Pelvis and legs? Do your feet press into the floor as you do this?
   - Repeat several times, then change the direction to roll your pelvis slowly and gently down towards your feet. Your tailbone presses into the ground and your lower back lifts away. Be careful while moving in this direction if you have any sensitivity in your back (Fig. 5.21).
   - Where do you notice the effort as you do this movement? Back? Front of your hips? Do your feet lighten away from the floor as you do this? Repeat movement in this direction several times.
   - Then, alternate rolling your pelvis up and down on the floor. Your tailbone alternately lifts and presses and your lower back alternately flattens and arches.
   - Notice the ease/difficulty of each direction. Which direction seems most familiar? Which is the most comfortable? Do you organize this movement mostly with effort in your torso or in your legs?

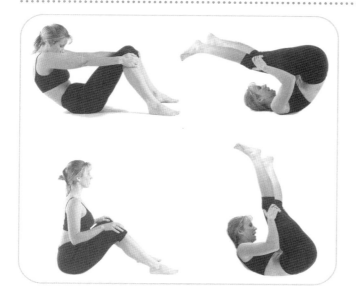

Fig. 5.22 Same rolling of the pelvis forward and back – segue into rolling to back.

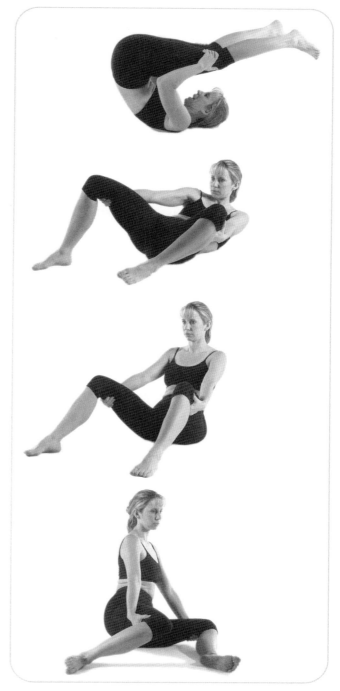

Fig. 5.23 From back, rolling back up along a diagonal.

C.   Sit on the floor with the soles of your feet on the floor somewhere around shoulder width apart. Hold on to the backs of your thighs near your knees (reaching from the outside).

   • Resume this same basic movement of rolling your pelvis toward and away from your feet.

   • As you roll your pelvis forward, allow your whole spine to arch or straighten and push your belly and chest forward between your knees; look up a bit towards the ceiling.

   • As you roll your pelvis backward, allow your whole spine to round, your elbows to straighten and your head to drop toward your chest; look towards your belly button.

   • Feel the sinking, widening and lengthening of your whole back as you roll backward. Let your elbows straighten and your lower back reach toward the floor. Straighten your back and bend your elbows to roll back forward; get taller!

   • Continue rocking forward and back and add in falling on to your back then swinging back up to tall sitting again (Fig. 5.22). Round your back to fall backward to roll your spine along the floor then arch again to come forward.

   • Roll up along your back as you fall back. Swing your feet above your head so your pelvis lifts off the floor. Roll back down along your spine and back up to sitting tall again.

   • Push your belly and chest forward between your knees and push the top of your head taller toward the ceiling. How slowly can you do this movement? How much momentum is needed?

D.   Sit on the floor with your hands holding your thighs behind your knees again.

   • Rock/fall back, then swing back up to sit as before; just a brief review of our previous variation.

   • Now change the basic movement a little to rock/fall back and to the left and swing yourself back up and to the right.

   • Repeat then reverse to 'fall' back to right and swing up to get tall to the left (Fig. 5.23). Use momentum as needed. How does one diagonal compare to the other?

- Make a circle with your pelvis on the floor, still holding on to the back of your thighs near your knees (Fig. 5.24).
- Change the direction of the circle.

E. Sit on the floor with knees bent, soles of feet on floor at shoulder width. Your hands are on the front of your thighs near your knees. This time you can't help with your hands!

- Continue with the same basic movement of rolling your pelvis forward and getting taller/straighter then rolling/falling back while rounding.
- Feel for any effort or signs of fatigue in your legs. Continue the same rocking movement but start to add in –
- Extending your legs straight out in front as you sink back and down while allowing your hands to slide upward on your thighs (Fig. 5.25).
- When rocking forward to come back up to sit, bend your knees back up and slide your heels on the floor toward your pelvis.
- Rest for a moment in sitting, and then try a diagonal version of this. Roll your pelvis back and to the right and take your right hand off your thigh to lean back on your right elbow and forearm (Fig. 5.25).
- Then, roll back up and to the left as if reaching for something forward and to the left with your right hand.
- Do this a few times keeping your knees bent, then do it several times by straightening your left leg as you 'fall' back and to the right, then bending your left leg up again as you come back forward and to the left.
- Try the same thing to the other side. Roll your pelvis back and to the left to lean on your left elbow and forearm, then roll back forward and to the right as if reaching with your left hand across and up to your right.
- Try this while keeping both knees bent. Then by straightening your right leg to fall back and bending it up again to come back forward.
- Now lean back on your left elbow, place your right elbow back on the floor, lift your left elbow and come upright. Go around in a circle leaning first on one elbow, then both, then the other, then upright again. Do the circles in both directions.

F. Lie on your back as before with your legs bent up and with your feet somewhere between shoulder and hip width apart.

- Roll your pelvis alternately toward and away from your feet. Alternately lift and press your tailbone.
- How does this movement compare to when you first tried it? Is it any easier? Smoother? Is there more or easier movement through your torso? Do you have any clearer idea of where your effort is in doing this movement?
- Rock your pelvis rapidly now; set up an oscillation.

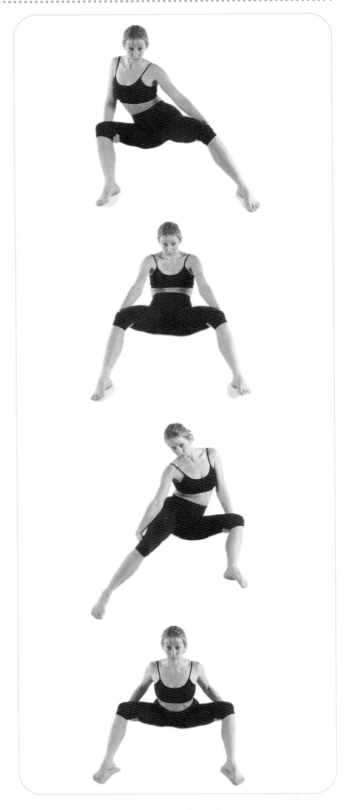

Fig. 5.24 Combining diagonals to make circles.

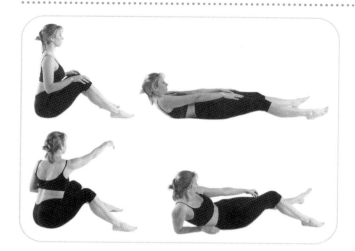

Fig. 5.25 Straight and diagonal variations of straightening legs while falling back.

G. Lie flat on your back once again and be aware of your contact against the ground.

- Are any of your spaces flatter?
- How is the balance of your pelvis and legs from side to side?
- Where are your toes pointed?
- Stand up. How is your pelvis balanced on top of your legs? Is your pelvis vertical? Spilling forward? Spilling back? Turned to the left? To the right? Walk around and feel your hips. How completely do they straighten?

Static baselines – Pelvic Tilts

This initial static baseline scan features questions about contact against the ground of the legs, pelvis and lower back. What does this observation of contact tell us about muscle tone or imbalances?

If the pelvis is rolled downward on the floor toward the feet and the lower back is arched away from the floor, we could say that the pelvis is anteriorly tilting. It could be that the lumbar extensors are contracted and shortening. It is also very possible that the hip joints have not fully extended to allow the pelvis to lie completely horizontal. What might be responsible for this?

Do you recall how the iliopsoas group is responsible for moving the pelvis into anterior tilt and for preventing it from moving into posterior tilt? The iliopsoas is the most common reason for continuing lumbar lordosis while supine. With a short iliopsoas creating an anterior pelvic tilt and lumbar lordosis, the space under the lower back will flatten markedly when you bend the knees up. This puts the iliopsoas on slack and allows the lumbar vertebrae to fall or flatten to the floor.

When your student puts her legs back down long again, her short iliopsoas will drag her pelvis and lower back along with

it into anterior tilt and lordosis. This may be a clue that helps us determine if she is iliopsoas dominant. With some people, the iliopsoas is so short that not only is the lower back lifted away from the floor, but the hip joints are so flexed that the back of the knees and even much of the back of the thighs will be off the ground.

If, when she bends her knees up, her lower back doesn't flatten markedly, the fault may lie elsewhere. Usually there will be a rigidly rounded thoracic spine that is very resistant to flattening into extension. Because the bottom of the kyphosis is the apex of the lordosis, a rigidly kyphotic thoracic curve will necessitate a continued lordotic lumbar spine even when the legs are bent.

If the pelvis is rolled upward on the floor away from the feet and the lower back is close to or pressing into the ground, we could say that the pelvis is approaching a posterior tilt. The hip joints have extended enough and the thorax has flattened sufficiently to allow the pelvis to lie horizontally with the lumbar spine close to neutral. Can we surmise a gluteal bias? Probably. Another clue that may be suggestive of a gluteal bias is if there is excessive external rotation of the legs. The toes pointing markedly outward may indicate this.

What is an excessive amount of hip external rotation while supine? In this position, gravity will act to roll the lower extremities into external rotation. This is normal and desirable for this position. If the legs don't roll outward, the person to whom those legs belong is actively engaging in muscular effort to internally rotate her hip joints. She is probably contracting her adductors and tensor fascia latae. This is a very common pattern and most often tends to go along with an iliopsoas bias, anterior pelvic tilt and a lordosing lumbar spine.

The adductors and iliopsoas groups both act to pull the pelvis toward the legs, so you will often see internally rotating hips with iliopsoas-dominant folks. These folks also tend to rest with their legs relatively close together because of the often-synergistic relationship of the iliopsoas to the adductors. Try getting on the floor for a moment and gently internally and externally rotate your hips while lying with your legs long. Feel for the effort in your adductors and tensor fasciae latae (TFL) when rotating inward. Do you find your lower back lifting off the floor a bit?

Feel for effort in your gluteals or short and stubbies when moving your hips into external rotation. Is there a subtle movement of your lower back toward the ground? What, then, is an excessive amount of hip external rotation in this position? It is hard to say, but certainly if her little toes touch the ground, you can bet that her gluteals and short and stubby hip external rotators (piriformis, internal and external obturators, inferior and superior gemelli and the quadratus femoris) will be short and contracting. Manual assessment of hip movement will usually show limitations on hip internal rotation and horizontal adduction.

There may also be a tendency to rest the legs farther apart on the ground with a gluteal/hip external rotation bias as the hip abductors tend to be synergists with the gluteals. They will both push the pelvis away from the legs (though sometimes the posterior adductors will team up with the gluteals and the anal sphincter to keep a clamp on the lower end of the digestive tube). Differences between the two sides in terms of one side being more externally rotated than the other can also give us clues about pelvic muscular imbalances, as does a difference in weight distribution from side to side.

The leg that is rolling farthest outward probably has more active gluteals than the other side. The leg that rolls farthest inward probably has a more active iliopsoas than the other side. This is not always the case, though. Often, the pelvis will be pulled or rolled to the side with the more active iliopsoas and adductor and pushed away from the side with the more active gluteals and abductors. For instance, if the pelvis is biased to roll downward on the floor and you observe the right ASIS as being closer to the ceiling and the left ASIS as being closer to the floor, you might surmise a left iliopsoas bias.

Think again of the clock and how imbalanced cornerstones might position the horizontal pelvis. If the pelvis is rolled straight downward, we call this a bilateral iliopsoas pattern. If the pelvis is rolled down and to the left (towards 4.30), we call this a left iliopsoas pattern. If the pelvis is rolled down and to the right (towards 7.30) it could be a manifestation of a dominant right iliopsoas. If rolled up and to the left (1.30) it may be a dominant right gluteal, with a left gluteal pattern doing a mirror image.

Often, the pelvis will be turned or rolled on the ground to the left, the left leg will be relatively more internally rotated and the right leg will be relatively more externally rotated. In this situation, the internal rotation of the left hip and the external rotation of the right hip are in reality more pronounced than they appear. Sometimes this will be reversed. When observing your students supine, look both at the position of the pelvis relative to an imaginary clock and at the relationship of the pelvis to the internal/external rotation and flexion/extension differences in the legs.

Observation of your student lying supine with legs long can be a handy way to assess relationships and biases that may translate to standing. Standing and lying supine with legs long are nearly identical patterns, but with different relationships to gravity. One of the advantages of making observations while supine is that the floor makes a handy backdrop. The space between lower back and floor (amount of lordosis) can be pretty easily assessed, and visualizing the pelvis and how it is rolled up/down and left/right on the floor is easier here than in standing.

Try reconciling what you see in standing with what you see in supine. Although it is often consistent, you will be confused enough to keep you appropriately humble. Looking at whole-body patterns and making sense of their sometimes conflicting cues is an acquired skill. As movement teachers, we are already trained in eyeballing the pelvis for imbalances at the iliac crests, ASIS, PSIS, ischial tuberosities or even the sacral sulcus. We look at foot pronation, knee recurvatum, squinting patella, scapular abduction and so on; we already see the trees. Further insight and information can be gained by looking for relationships; try taking a wider view of the forest.

Dynamic baselines – Pelvic Tilts

The first movement of this lesson in variation B is one of rolling the pelvis on the floor in such a way as to lift the tailbone. This is the classic Pelvic Tilt. More accurately, it is a posterior pelvic tilt. It is also a differentiated pattern of movement that features lumbar flexion and hip joint extension. It is also a direction

of movement and a relationship between thigh, pelvis and low back that we called a bilateral gluteal pattern using the description of the last lesson. Why? Why not call it a bilateral abdominal pattern?

This movement presents us with a choice. We could pull the pubic bone upward with the rectus abdominis and the abdominal obliques. We could also push the pelvis upward on the floor using the hip extensors: the gluteus maximus, hamstrings and the deep hip arthrokinematic muscles (short and stubbies). Which method of controlling excessive anterior tilt do we want to teach? Although abdominal tone can certainly contribute, it is not an adequate substitute for the legs.

With iliopsoas shortness being a prime culprit in anterior pelvic tilt and its resultant extension stresses on the lower back and SI joints, it only makes sense to treat this postural type by addressing control and movement of the hip joints. If the iliopsoas are too tight, we need to teach movements that help the student to balance them with their antagonists.

Coordinating the antagonists in this case means simultaneously inhibiting the iliopsoas and activating the gluteals. If we take a fresh look at this golden oldie, it may make more sense to emphasize pushing with the feet rather than pulling with the belly. By using the gluteal group to push the feet, we are simultaneously creating an excitation of the hip extensors and inhibition of the hip flexors.

Although the strengthening part of this movement is not exactly the sweat-popping, vein-bulging make-it-burn popular image of strengthening exercises, in motor control terms it is just what the doctor ordered. This movement, when initiated from the legs, combines our desired activation of the hip extensors with an equally desirable inhibition of the lumbar extensors (you will need to observe carefully here – the back extensors are not automatically inhibited).

One-leg standing experiment

What you will commonly see when supine and pressing one foot into the floor is a lifting of the pelvis and back as one unit – the back and hip extensors are undifferentiated. You will probably need to manually cue your iliopsoas-biased students to lift their tailbone and roll their pelvis into posterior tilt because of their tendency to substitute pushing their feet into the floor with their back extensors rather than their hip extensors and hip flexors. It is also simulating a functional context we are trying to influence while standing: we need to teach our hyperlordotic students to press their feet into the ground.

Try the following experiment. Stand up and shift most of your weight over to your left leg (maybe even put your right foot up on a stool). Keeping your left knee straight, make yourself taller and shorter. Let the right side of your pelvis drop toward the ground as you make yourself shorter and raise the right side of your pelvis back up to get taller (Fig. 5.26) This is a movement of pivoting your pelvis around your left hip joint.

Notice the tendency of your pelvis to spill forward into anterior tilt as you drop your right hip to get shorter. Notice also the tendency of your pelvis to move in the direction of posterior tilt as you get taller. This movement is performed by alternately pushing your left foot into the floor then letting go of that effort. This is a shortening and lengthening contraction

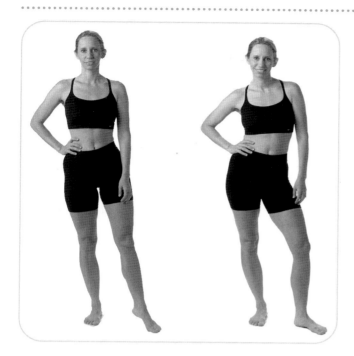

Fig. 5.26 Pushing taller – and sinking lower in one-legged stance.

of the left hip abductors and extensors. Do this movement slowly and repeatedly to feel clearly how you are alternately pushing yourself away from the floor and letting go of the push to let yourself sink on to your hip.

Observe people standing when they are not aware they are being observed. Notice how some people shift their weight to one side or the other and then hang on that hip. The greater trochanter sticks out to the side and the pelvis spills into anterior tilt. This is just what you did in your experiment. What these folks are not doing is actively pushing their foot into the ground. Although this is probably more obvious when doing this movement while supporting most of your weight on one leg, the same thing happens when you look at your students who lordose even when bearing weight more or less equally on both feet. They are allowing their pelvis to fall too far forward on their legs and are necessitating a movement of the worm into extension. They are not grounding their feet on the floor. Training your students to push the feet into the floor and to use the legs to move the pelvis and low back provides them with a meaningful functional context for improving their posture. Sucking in the belly has no such corresponding contextual framework.

A common mistake

When you push your feet into the floor in supine with knees bent, the floor is not going to move (appreciably). What will move is the pelvis, as it is much lighter than the earth. When pushing the feet into the floor while supine, the pelvis can either lift from the floor or roll on the floor. Which do we want to happen? If the pelvis lifts from the floor when pressing the

feet, we can surmise a simultaneous contraction of the gluteals and the lumbar extensors. The hip and lumbar extensors are synergists and the hips and low back are extending.

This is a global pattern of movement, with the hips and low back being undifferentiated. If our intention in exercise is to change the postural motor behavior of anterior pelvic tilt and lumbar lordosis, we will need to guide our students toward rolling their pelvis on the floor rather than lifting it. Rolling the pelvis is a differentiated pattern of lumbar flexion and hip extension. This is just what we would like to see our hyperlordosing students learn how to do. Although we may also do an exercise of lifting the pelvis off the floor, this bridging also needs to be performed with pattern specificity and some eye toward functional context.

Disadvantages of using belly to control pelvis

What might be some of the disadvantages of relying only on the abdominals to tilt the pelvis posteriorly? One is that chronic abdominal contraction inhibits the diaphragm. Breathing is compromised when the belly is not free to move or expand on an inhalation. We can think of the rectus abdominis and obliques, and even to a somewhat lesser extent the transversus abdominis, as being antagonists to the diaphragm. Whereas the diaphragm expands or rounds the belly as it domes downward into the abdominal cavity on inspiration, the abdominals flatten and harden the belly.

Try hardening your belly and breathing into it simultaneously: good luck! Chronic abdominal effort makes the diaphragm weaker through reciprocal inhibition. Disallowing expansion of the belly on inhalation necessitates movement elsewhere. Other possibilities include breathing with the intercostals or breathing with the scalenes. Intercostal breathing features lateral expansion of the ribcage through a 'buckethandle' phenomenon and can often be a desirable movement for people to learn, though it certainly takes more effort than belly breathing.

Scalene breathing features an expansion of the thoracic cavity upward: the scalenes and related muscles pull the top of the ribcage upward to increase the vertical dimensions of the chest. Although scalene breathing can be useful as a method of last resort during very strenuous physical activity, it is not desirable as a primary method. Many people who are always contracting their abdominal muscles, either as a way to posteriorly tilt their pelvis or for artificial aesthetic purposes, are defaulting their breath to their scalenes.

When performed constantly, this type of upper chest breathing has some negative consequences. Because the scalenes attach on to the cervical vertebrae, they compress the cervical spine and pull the head and neck down and forward every time they contract. This can manifest itself in cervical segmental dysfunction or shearing, thoracic outlet syndrome, temporomandibular joint (TMJ) syndrome or headaches as the suboccipital area extends and compresses.

Another disadvantage in relying solely on the abdominals to support the pelvis and lower back is because of the direct pull of the abdominals on the lower ribs and the associative connections of the abdominals with the anterior intercostals. The rectus abdominis and the obliques connect to the sternum and lower ribs and, when exerting force to pull the pubic bone upward into posterior tilt, also act to pull the sternum and lower ribs downward.

This contributes to thoracic kyphosis and the often-resultant shoulder girdle abduction (protraction), forward head posture and internal rotation bias of the upper extremities. These postural imbalances may contribute to cervical facet or disc dysfunction, headaches, TMJ syndrome, glenohumeral tendinitis/bursitis/impingements and even elbow/forearm/wrist/hand repetitive stress syndromes and tendon irritations.

In terms of movement, chronic abdominal contraction can lead to an inability to extend the thoracic spine, making looking and reaching overhead much more difficult and putting additional strain on the neck and shoulders. An inability to extend in the thoracic spine also makes rotational movement very difficult: recall the spiraling taller movements you did in the second section and how the extension component of turning assisted with and reduced strain on the cervical spine.

We can think of the anterior intercostals as continuations of the abdominals in terms of their contribution to thoracic kyphosis and its sequelae. The intercostals are really just abdominal muscles that happen to have some bones embedded in them; they even have the same layering and fiber orientation as the belly. This association of simultaneously contracting abdominals and intercostals will then disallow both diaphragmatic and bucket-handle breathing and further limit options to scalene breathing.

Although the kyphotic effects of abdominal and anterior intercostal contractions can be offset by simultaneous contractions of the thoracic extensors, this also has consequences. This simultaneous use of torso flexors and extensors is a co-contraction. It is compressive, it still disallows choice in breathing, and it has a rigidifying effect on the chest/ribcage/thoracic spine. This contributes to shoulder girdle tension syndromes and neck problems as the neck and upper extremities are left to do the work of orientation and manipulation on their own, without the assistance of an integrated torso.

Another disadvantage of training our students to always use their bellies to control the position of their pelvis is that abdominal contraction can be part of the somatic manifestation of an anxiety pattern. Although we will discuss this in a bit more depth in Section 5, you should be aware of some common physical characteristics of stress. When someone is fearful/anxious/stressed, they tend to react physically by flexing and pulling inward.

They may adduct and internally rotate their hips, flex their chests, adduct and internally rotate their arms, elevate and abduct their shoulder girdles and pull their head down and forward.[37] Think of a falling reaction: we will pull in and round ourselves to minimize injury. This is a protection mechanism. We see the arm go into a flexion/protection pattern after injury or in the presence of pain. The lower extremities exhibit an inhibition of extension and push-off and bias toward withdrawal after injury or in the presence of pain (Box 5.9).

This is a stereotypical reaction to physical strain that for many people has made the associative leap to a reaction to emotional strain. The abdominal muscles are part of this flexion/protection mechanism. Are we contributing to the perpetuation of anxiety on the part of our students when we ask them to always tighten their bellies? Are we getting unintentional spillover into other muscles (adductors, hip flexors, pelvic floor, scalenes, pectoralis major and minor) that are part of the flexion/protection pattern? Are we reinforcing shallow upper chest breathing? Might it not make more sense to teach someone how to ground herself to the floor with her legs to control her pelvis?

Box 5.9 Disadvantages of using the abdominals to control the pelvis

Inhibition of diaphragm – funnels movement to scalene breathing
Pulls chest and shoulder girdles down and forward – using the chest as an anchor instead of the ground
Link to anxiety patterns
Smaller muscles and mechanical disadvantages relative to hip musculature

---

Move the pelvis with the legs

The position of the pelvis in space in terms of anterior or posterior tilt is best controlled from the legs, which are in turn anchored to the floor. The chest and ribcage have no such anchor. Movements in general, but especially of the pelvis, are best organized from the ground up rather than from the top down. An image we as physical therapists sometimes use is that of a sky-hook. We teach our students to visualize a hook pulling them up from the top of their head, elongating and straightening their spine. I'm going to let you in on a little secret: there is no sky-hook!

You cannot pull yourself up with air and clouds, you can only push yourself away from the floor. Many people I have observed when they are trying to get taller will attempt this by pulling up their pelvic floor and belly, raising their shoulder girdles with upper trapezial effort and lifting their chest with scalenes and SCMs. Attempting to organize the pelvis exclusively from the belly is a version of the same idea: they are pulling the pelvis up with their belly and trying to use their chest as an anchor, rather than pushing their pelvis toward vertical with their legs and using the ground as an anchor. This is not good body mechanics!

A final reason for de-emphasizing our near-obsession with the abdominals and teaching control of the pelvis from the legs instead is simply one of size and mechanical advantage. The gluteus maximus, medius, minimus, hamstrings and short and stubbies make up a far greater mass than the abdominals; they are potentially much more powerful. Postural support muscles should be capable of contracting submaximally over extended periods of time.

Stronger and more massive muscles have a much better chance of doing this without fatigue. With the hip extensors and short and stubbies both crossing and being much closer to the axis of rotation (a line across the hip joints) for pelvic anterior and posterior tilt, they are in a much more advantageous position than the belly. They have a *mechanical advantage*.

Although I am advocating a nearly heretical concept of de-emphasizing the abdominals when working with people with lower back pain, try to hold off sending me before the Inquisition quite yet. I do teach transverse abdominis control for lumbar intersegmental stabilization and will address how to better facilitate that control later in this section. I also encourage abdominal contraction during certain functional activities, especially falling back, controlling side-bending movements in response to right/left balancing, lifting and accelerating, decelerating or disallowing trunk rotation.

I teach use of the abdominal muscles as a way to control the relationship between pelvis, lower spine and chest. Abdominals are necessary in controlling rotational stresses at the lower back. Where I diverge is in teaching control of movement and position of the pelvis: I believe it is best directed through the legs, and will spend most of the rest of this section trying to convince you of that. Think of layers:

- The legs control the position and movement of the pelvis and are the first line of defense for the lower back.

- The belly and back muscles control the relationship of the chest to the pelvis and are the second line of defense.

- The intrinsic muscles (transverse abdominis and multifidi) control the movement of individual vertebrae relative to each other and are the third line of defense.

Historically, we as physical therapists have focused on the extrinsic abdominal muscles. Recent studies have highlighted the importance of the intersegmental stabilizers, and we have begun to focus our attention more on motor control of these intrinsic muscles rather than on the frank strengthening of extrinsic trunk musculature.[38] What we are still missing is an understanding of and a way of influencing the role of the legs in the movement and control of the pelvis and lower back. We need better and more effective ways of facilitating motor control over both local and synergistic extrinsic muscles.

Without motor control over the gluteal muscles and without an understanding of how to control excessive anterior tilt of the pelvis on the legs from the legs, the relatively tiny transversus abdominis and multifidi, making relatively tiny contractions, have little hope of controlling intersegmental stability in the presence of grosser postural and movement stressors.

The first instruction of this lesson was to roll your pelvis in such a way that your tailbone lifted away from the floor. This is one of our dynamic baselines. Did we use descriptive language? Yes: 'Allow your pelvis to roll rather than lift – your tailbone lifts toward the ceiling but the weight of your pelvis stays supported by the ground. Your lower back will flatten and press toward the floor.' Did we use inquisitive language? Yes, 'Where do you notice effort as you do this movement? Belly? Pelvis and legs? Do your feet press into the floor as you do this?'

We are asking our students to be aware of how they do this movement. What was your choice? Did you control the movement of your pelvis from belly or legs? Can you do either one independently of the other? I have worked with many people who were initially totally incapable of dissociating their belly from this movement – others have not been able to use their belly at all.

Part of the game in motor control is to be able to do the same movement a number of different ways. Try training yourself and your students to do this movement nonhabitually. This is how we both recognize choices and develop the proprioceptive criteria to select that which works best for us. This is how we go from being a trained circus bear to a fully developed and self-regulating Goldilocks (Box 5.10).

Box 5.10 Pelvic Tilts

Belly-up movements emphasize lengthening and strengthening of the hip flexors and abdominals

Supine rolling the pelvis into anterior and posterior tilt – facilitated by controlling falls backward

Train rounding students to sit up straight and control balance falling backward

---

Choices in pressing the feet

Even in how you press your feet into the floor, there are choices. You could press in such a way as to emphasize straightening the knees and contracting the quadriceps. This results in an almost sliding of the feet on the ground away from your pelvis; if the surface were slippery, your feet would slide forward. Even with a high-friction surface you can feel your foot bones slide forward relative to the skin.

This way of pressing your feet is less desirable both from the standpoint of the health of the knees (examined later in section on lower extremities) and from the standpoint of synergistic push-off (hamstrings working with gluteals to straighten the hip). The other choice is to press your feet straight back into the floor so there is no sliding effect. You could do the movement this way even if lying on a sheet of ice. The hamstrings and gluteals are further emphasized. This is a crucially important distinction that we will continue to work on facilitating throughout the rest of this chapter.

Psit up straight with the psoas

The next movement that we used as a dynamic baseline was that of rolling your pelvis downward on the floor and pressing your tailbone. We again used descriptive and inquisitive language. Of particular interest is whether you did this movement with effort originating in your back extensors or from your legs. Did your feet lighten relative to the floor? Did you use your hip flexors to roll your pelvis into anterior tilt? Why would I want to strengthen my iliopsoas – aren't they supposed to be the bad guys?

Let's review one of our four major postural types, the full round. These people sit with their pelvis rolled/falling backward, their whole torso rounding into flexion and their neck and head differentiating into extension to keep orienting to the horizon. Review for yourself the possible clinical manifestations of this postural type. What is this person neglecting to do?

Perhaps most obviously, she is neglecting to straighten her back. We might prescribe exercises to strengthen her back muscles but, while this is certainly one of the things that need to be performed, it will not address a major component of this postural type. Perhaps less obviously, what this person is neglecting to do is to pull her pelvis upright – she is not anteriorly tilting her pelvis to neutral. She is not flexing her hips. She is not familiar with accessing a bilateral iliopsoas pattern.

Why not just use the back muscles to anteriorly tilt the pelvis? It can be performed in prone, supine and side-lie – but can the back muscles anteriorly tilt the pelvis in sitting? No. A worm cannot stand/sit on its tail, nor can it bring itself back upright again from a falling-back position. Our student needs her legs to act as a counterbalance to the falling of her pelvis backward. She needs her hip flexors to pull her pelvis upright.

What many people who slump do when they try to sit upright is to overuse their back extensors. They have a poor understanding of how to use their hip flexors and use them minimally to come upright. They then attempt to maintain that position with back extensor effort and will often give up after a time because it is too hard (even if they know cognitively that letting themselves slump contributes to their pain and that their physical therapist will be on their case when they do). We as physical therapists might think that they give up because their extensors are too weak and might prescribe exercises to strengthen the back.

Although logical, this thinking is not entirely accurate. Using the back extensors predominantly to sit upright is very inefficient and very tiring. Because the angle of the back extensors relative to the spine is nearly parallel, much of the effort of the back extensors actually goes into compression. Contrast the angle of pull of the back extensors with the angle of pull of the iliopsoas. The iliopsoas runs forward and down from the anterior vertebral bodies and the iliac fossa of the pelvis, and as such has a much more efficient angle. Recall vector forces from physics class and imagine that whereas the most efficient angle of pull would be straight forward, there is nothing directly in front of the lumbar spine or pelvis to act as an anchor.

Instead, the hip flexors compromise to angle forward and down to attach on to the relatively heavier legs, which can and do act as an anchor from which the iliopsoas can bring the top of the pelvis and the lumbar spine forward. The hip flexors are also much larger and (potentially) stronger and, as in the case of the hip extensors, both cross and are much closer to the axis of rotation of the pelvis for anterior/posterior tilt. They have a great mechanical advantage over the back extensors.

With this person and with people with the half-round postural type we need to have a mechanism for progressively strengthening the iliopsoas. Although we could do this in chair sitting, starting in supine has some advantages. While sitting, the pelvis is vertical and can easily fall in any direction; this necessitates a constant effort to prevent the fall and may make effort recognition more difficult. While supine, the horizontal pelvis is more stable and requires effort to make it move. Effort recognition is easier when one is able to contrast the effort of movement from the cessation of effort on a return to neutral.

While sitting, the CNS is already preprogrammed toward a certain bias or homeostasis. The need to balance in upright and the pressure of the ischial tuberosities against the chair stimulates a habitual motor response and creates a strong undertow that moves us to a position of familiarity. When supine, gravity is more neutral in terms of its pull on the pelvis and in terms of relieving the torso musculature of the need to maintain balance. This strategy of starting with a clean slate and minimizing both the complexity and the effort of a movement is common and is one of the main reasons that so many Feldenkrais lessons are performed lying on the floor.

In our full round and half round postural types, the iliopsoas group will probably be long and weak. What musculature might we anticipate as being too short? The next time you are working with someone who tends to slump, or who you

notice sits relatively erect but whose pelvis seems to be falling a bit back (half round), have them roll their pelvis into anterior tilt while sitting on a chair and make note of the range and apparent ease. Then have them sit on the floor with legs crossed. This will probably exaggerate the posterior tilt and make movements into anterior tilt more difficult. Then have them sit with their legs long. This will almost certainly exaggerate the posterior tilt and make movements into anterior tilt nearly impossible. Why? The hamstrings are probably going to be short. This relationship will be obvious in long sitting, but the short hamstrings, gluteals and short and stubbies that we might anticipate as being short in the presence of weak hip flexors also contribute to habitual posterior tilt in sitting and standing. We could say that someone who slumps has weak iliopsoas.

We could anticipate tight hamstrings and gluteals. We could say this person has a habitual gluteal bias. We might want to simultaneously strengthen the iliopsoas, stretch the hamstrings and gluteals and train them to come more fully upright in sitting while also addressing torso muscle imbalances by strengthening the back extensors and stretching the abdominals and anterior intercostals. Half of this lesson is designed to do just that – but which half?

Reciprocating the cornerstones

The final variation of our initial inquiry was to put the two directions together and roll your pelvis alternately up and down on the floor. This is a question of how to reciprocate and coordinate antagonists. Though balancing and coordinating the front and back of the torso is part of this, the main focus of this movement is on reciprocating between use of the gluteals and use of the iliopsoas. Think again of the pelvis as lying on the face of a clock, but this time with the face of the clock being concave (Fig. 5.27).

When in sitting, we used the image of a convex clock surface where movement in any direction was downhill. Movement away from the center was through the lengthening contractions of bilateral or unilateral gluteal or iliopsoas, and the return to neutral was through a shortening contraction of the same muscles.

When supine, movement in any direction is now uphill. Movement away from the center is through a shortening con-

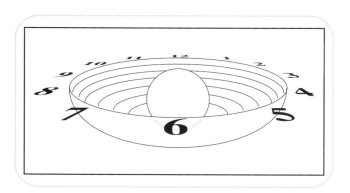

Fig. 5.27 Ball on a concave clock – rolls uphill in all directions.

Box 5.11 The pelvic clock – cardinal planes

Six o'clock equals anterior pelvic tilt equals bilateral iliopsoas pattern – goes with (global or differentiated) torso extension

Twelve o'clock equals posterior pelvic tilt equals bilateral gluteal pattern – goes with (global or differentiated) torso flexion

Three o'clock equals pelvic weight shift left equals left pelvic force couple – goes with (global or differentiated) torso right side-bending

Nine o'clock equals pelvic weight shift right equals right pelvic force couple – goes with (global or differentiated) torso left side-bending

Box 5.12 The pelvic clock – diagonals

One-thirty equals posterior pelvic tilt and left pelvic weight shift equals right gluteal pattern – goes with (global or differentiated) right torso flexion

Four-thirty equals anterior pelvic tilt and left pelvic weight shift equals left iliopsoas pattern – goes with (global or differentiated) right torso extension

Seven-thirty equals anterior pelvic tilt and right pelvic weight shift equals right iliopsoas pattern – goes with (global or differentiated) left torso extension

Ten-thirty equals posterior pelvic tilt and right pelvic weight shift equals left gluteal pattern – goes with (global or differentiated) left torso flexion

traction of gluteals or iliopsoas, and movement back to center is through a lengthening contraction of the same muscles. Movement towards 12 o'clock, or rolling the pelvis upward on the floor into posterior tilt, is performed with the gluteals. Movement towards 6 o'clock, or rolling the pelvis downward on the floor into anterior tilt, is performed with the iliopsoas (Box 5.11).

Recall the advantages of reciprocating movements: they help to establish a truer center or neutral posture, they help to coordinate the antagonists, and they help the student with pattern recognition (relationships between pelvis and spine, recognition of habitual and nonhabitual directions, recognition of direction of comfort and discomfort). How were your antagonists coordinated at the end of the lesson in comparison to the beginning? Most people will find it much smoother. Did you have any clearer idea of how you could use your legs to do this movement by the end of the lesson?

Were you able to confirm or did you freshly discover what your personal direction of bias is? I can't emphasize enough the pivotal nature of the gluteal and iliopsoas groups, how important it is to be competent moving in both directions, and how important it is that they be well balanced and coordinated. These four cornerstone muscles play a central role in the position and movement of the pelvis and torso and, by extension, of the arms and head, as well as in the movement and efficiency of the lower extremities.

Whether working with someone with a sprained ankle, patellar tracking problems, hip joint replacement, low back pain, stroke, neck pain or glenohumeral impingement, there is a link to cornerstone musculature imbalance or inefficiency. Begin to look for the threads of those imbalances and inefficiencies as they weave themselves through to distal skeletal components.

If the bilateral contraction of both iliopsoas pulls the pelvis straight downward on the floor towards 6 o'clock, what do you think would happen if just the left iliopsoas fired? The left iliopsoas pulls the pelvis down and to the left, towards 4.30. The right iliopsoas pulls the pelvis down and to the right, toward 7.30. If the bilateral contraction of both gluteals pushes the pelvis straight upward on the floor towards 12 o'clock, what do think would happen if just the right gluteus was firing?

The right gluteus pushes the pelvis up and to the left, towards 1.30. The left gluteus pushes the pelvis up and to the right, towards 10.30. Although we will be exploring this experientially in another lesson in this chapter, be aware of how

here, as was the case earlier in sitting, the unilateral iliopsoas pulls the pelvis towards while the unilateral gluteal pushes it away from itself. Look for right/left imbalances in supine, sitting and standing, both with you and with students. Develop an eye for recognizing where the pelvis is on the imaginary clock (Box 5.12).

Now that we have established static and dynamic baselines, we progress into the meat of the lesson. We are trying to establish better motor control over the iliopsoas and gluteal groups. Is this particular lesson useful more for the hyperlordotic student or for the rounding student? Is it better for the person with gluteal bias or the student with an iliopsoas bias? These are trick questions: the real answer is that this lesson is useful with both types!

Falling back

In the movements described in variation C, you sit on the floor with your feet about shoulder width apart and hold on to the back of your thighs near your knees. Resume this same basic movement of rolling your pelvis toward and away from your feet. As you roll your pelvis forward, allow your whole spine to arch or straighten and push your belly and chest forward between your knees; look up a bit towards the ceiling. As you roll your pelvis backward, allow your whole spine to round, your elbows to straighten and your head to drop toward your chest; look towards your belly button.

We are now linking this rolling movement of the pelvis with two functional contexts. Looking up and down links anterior and posterior tilt, along with torso flexion and extension, to orientation. Rolling back and coming back upright again links pelvis and torso coordination and reciprocation with controlled falling or balance.

Falling partially back is a lengthening contraction of the iliopsoas and a shortening contraction of the abdominals and anterior intercostals. Coming back upright again is a shortening contraction of the iliopsoas and the back extensors. Falling back inhibits the back extensors. Coming forward inhibits the belly and anterior chest along with the gluteals, hamstrings and short and stubbies. Holding on to the back of the thighs with the hands allows an initial assist from the arms. This provides initial pattern recognition and an extra layer of support and safety until later in the lesson, when you have learned enough in earlier variations to recognize how to use the iliopsoas accurately.

Assessing lumbar flexion

Falling all the way back and rolling along your spine to swing your feet overhead then using some momentum to swing yourself back upright again is a change of venue and a handy reference point for your ability to round evenly through your back. The changes of venue are to complete the movement into a full fall and to introduce a faster speed and the use of momentum. The faster speed helps to enlarge and complete the movement coming forward and getting taller; momentum helps the back to extend and the hips to flex.

Rolling back along your spine is a handy reference point for assessing lumbar flexion. Although most people round well along their thoracic spine, there are many who cannot round their lower back. These folks will have a flat spot that they roll over. There will either be a bump, or they will move slowly through the flat spot so they don't bang their lumbothoracic area coming back or the base of their sacrum coming back up. Did you have a flat spot?

This movement can actually be a nice assessment tool for your nonacute low back pain students. It is both clearer and is in a more meaningful functional context than trying to assess lumbar flexion by having your student bend forward from a sitting or standing position. Whereas bending forward can be performed appropriately in a number of ways, including flexing, extending or staying neutral at the low back, falling backward should stimulate lumbar flexion if the low back is at all capable of rounding. When bending forward, the CNS may interpret the movement as a version of falling forward. This may stimulate a movement of the worm into extension as part of an intention to keep from hitting one's head.

This tendency will be exaggerated if you disallow movement of the pelvis backward in space. Whereas the idea of blocking pelvic movement might be to try to localize the flexion movement to the lower back and see how the spine bends on a stable pelvis, the effect for the student is disconcerting. She will feel as if she is falling forward, as she is violating one of the main principles of balance she learned growing up: when moving something in one direction, something else has to move in the opposite direction.

When bending forward, you are shifting your center of mass forward as the weight of your head, arms, shoulders and chest moves forward. The pelvis needs to – should ideally – would most appropriately – move backward. By disallowing this movement of the pelvis backward when we are assessing lumbar mobility, we are doing an organically foolish thing.

Try standing against a wall with your heels close to and your pelvis touching the wall. Bend over from here and feel how unsafe this feels. Feel how your toes have to grip. Step away from the wall and bend over while allowing your pelvis to move backward. Feel how much safer and less tense you are when you can move in such a way that your center of mass is still over your base of support. When assessing lumbar flexion, try it in chair sitting or floor sitting.

Have your student roll back or even do a controlled fall back and observe the shape of the back and the proportion of rounding throughout the spine. You could also have her on hands and knees and ask her to round her back to look at her belly button. There are many alternatives to assessing lumbar flexion with standing or sitting bends; please use the alternatives.

Using the same exercise for opposites

How is this movement useful for the rounding student? For her, coming forward and getting taller is a nonhabitual differentiated pattern of lumbar extension and hip flexion. She is strengthening her iliopsoas and back extensors while simultaneously stretching her abdominals, anterior intercostals, hamstrings, gluteals and short and stubbies. She is learning how to, is recognizing the pattern of, and is gaining competence in an ability to haul herself upright from her habitually fallen-back position.

How is this movement useful for the full arch or hyperlordotic student? For her, falling back and rounding herself in anticipation of landing on her back is a nonhabitual differentiated pattern of lumbar flexion and hip extension. She is stretching her iliopsoas and back extensors and strengthening her abdominal muscles. She is learning how to, is recognizing the pattern of, and is gaining competence in an ability to allow her pelvis to fall backward from her habitually falling-forward position.

For her, allowing her pelvis to fall back in sitting is much easier than allowing her pelvis to fall back and allowing her lower back to lengthen and decompress while standing. Why? Because in standing her iliopsoas are near end-range. It is the full arch, and especially the half arch, postural types that will exhibit the most marked flat spot on rolling back.

Why not just have our half-rounders hold an upright position and our full-archers hold a falling-back position? Why not just train them in their nonhabitual direction? The beauty of reciprocating movements is in their ability to help our students recognize patterns and relationships, to recognize habitual and nonhabitual directions, and to gain competence in moving from the familiar to the unfamiliar. It is not just the position we are training, but also the skill of being able to move into that unfamiliar position. We train better posture by training better movement.

After a rest on your back and an assessment of contact and balance against the floor, variation D brings you back upright again and briefly reviews the last variation of rolling/falling back and bringing yourself back forward again. This provides a bridge to, and a reminder of, the last variation and segues into the next. This time, instead of falling straight back, you are falling back and to the left or right. Falling back and to the right is a lengthening contraction of the left iliopsoas and a movement of the trunk into left torso flexion.

Coming back forward and to the left is a shortening contraction of the left iliopsoas and a movement of the trunk toward right torso extension. Falling back and to the left and coming forward and to the right is a mirror image moderated by the right iliopsoas. This should be familiar from the sitting circles analysis earlier in this chapter.

What movement might be especially useful for a student with an iliopsoas bias, left more than right? A left iliopsoas-dominant person would habitually be forward and to the left, towards 4.30. This person could especially benefit from falling back and to the right, towards 10.30. This would lengthen the left iliopsoas, the right quadratus lumborum and the right back extensors while simultaneously strengthening the left abdominals. This would be her direction of first aid.

What movement might be especially useful for a student with a right gluteal dominance? This person would be habitually back and to the left, towards 1.30. She could especially benefit from movements coming forward and to the right, towards 7.30. This would lengthen the right gluteals, hamstrings, short and stubbies and the right abdominals and anterior intercostals while simultaneously strengthening the right iliopsoas and the left back extensors.

Connecting the six dots into a circle further refines and coordinates the legs, pelvis and torso into all 360 directions. The circle is a blending of bilateral, unilateral and asymmetrical use of the two iliopsoas in both lengthening and shortening contractions. This whole lesson is performed in a belly-up orientation and emphasizes lengthening and strengthening the hip flexors. Think back to the sitting circles lesson.

That lesson alternated between belly-up and belly-down orientations, whereas this lesson is a refinement of and a more challenging progression of the belly-up parts of sitting circles. The next lesson will explore in greater detail the belly down parts of sitting circles and will emphasize lengthening and strengthening the gluteals, hamstrings and short and stubbies. The three lessons taken together make for a balanced exploration of the role of the legs in orientation and balance.

Belly burners

Variation F is essentially the same as the last variation but with additional complexities. By placing the hands on the front of the thighs rather than holding behind the thighs near the knees, we are disallowing assistance from the arms. You can no longer pull yourself upright or lower yourself back by helping with your arms; this requires the hip flexors to work harder. By straightening the legs when rolling back and bending them up again when coming forward, we are exaggerating and making more deliberate the lengthening and shortening of the hip flexors.

Describing the movement of rolling back by asking the student to reach for the ground with her lower back and the back of her knees simultaneously is a way of encouraging the differentiated movement of hip extension and lumbar flexion. The floor then becomes a target for both thighs and back. This full lengthening contraction of the iliopsoas (moving both origin and insertion away from each other) in a functional context of controlling one's fall backward is an excellent way of creating hip flexor length. Did you notice a further flattening of the space in your lower back after doing this variation (if you had a space to begin with)?

Describing the movement of rolling forward by asking the student to slide her feet toward her pelvis and moving belly and thighs toward each other makes for another target that further encourages the differentiated movement of hip flexion and back extension. This full shortening contraction of the iliopsoas (moving both origin and insertion toward each other) in a functional context of hauling oneself upright from a falling-back position is an excellent way of stimulating hip flexor strength.

This is a movement that mimics what we want our rounding students to do. Do you think the CNS might more readily recognize how the hip flexors contribute to upright sitting as a result of doing this movement? Or would our students be better served by strengthening the hip flexors with straight leg raises or by resisting hip flexion in standing with theraband or rubber tubing?

What is problematic about this more traditional approach? It lacks pattern specificity. The hip flexors can be strengthened, but not in a way that anteriorly tilts the pelvis or extends the spine. It also lacks functional context. What motor behavior is probably to change as a result of a straight leg raise? Is there any emphasis on proprioceptive self-awareness; what are you asking your student to pay attention to? What are your static and dynamic baselines?

Is there a demonstrable change in habitual posture or movement as a result of the exercise? Are you using descriptive or inquisitive language? Although we will be exploring a motor control version of a straight leg raise and a motor control version of standing hip flexion later in this chapter, it will be for different purposes than training the hip flexors to move the pelvis into anterior tilt in sitting.

We also did a diagonal version of this variation. Rolling back and to the right to lean on your right elbow simulates a controlled fall back and to the right. Here again we have a lengthening contraction of the left iliopsoas and a movement of the torso into left flexion. Adding in sliding the left foot away from your pelvis further lengthens the left iliopsoas and provides a longer lever arm and an effectively heavier anchor from which the iliopsoas can pay out to lower the pelvis back and to the right, and from which the iliopsoas can winch the pelvis back up and to the left. Is it obvious by now what controls the movement of rolling back to lean on your left elbow?

What is the torso pattern? Coming upright with the additional intention to reach across and forward stimulates a completion of the diagonal by encouraging full unilateral iliopsoas shortening and a movement of the pelvis forward in a diagonal. Going around in a circle by leaning on one elbow, then across to the other, reinforces our earlier circle but with a higher degree of difficulty.

How could we progress this? We could do both the rolling straight back and the rolling back in diagonals with the legs long and straight in front the whole time. This requires additional hamstring length while coming upright and additional iliopsoas length when rolled back. We can progress this movement even further by rolling back to lean not on the elbow, but all the way back to place a shoulder on the floor.

We could even do a circular variation of this by leaning back on one shoulder, rolling across the upper back to the other shoulder, then back up in yet another progression of the circles we performed earlier. Get on the floor and check this out. How's the belly doing? How are your hip flexors doing? These last variations and described progressions are cumulative movements that I encourage my students to practice, refine and continue as home exercises.

Comparing baselines

In variation F we repeat a variation that brings us full circle, back to where we started. Roll your pelvis upward on the floor, downward on the floor and alternating between the two. We used some inquisitive language to focus attention on differences in dynamic baselines from when we started: 'How does this movement compare to when you first tried it? Is it any easier? Smoother? Is there more or easier movement through your torso? Do you have any clearer idea of where your effort is in doing this movement?' The questions have to do with quality of movement, integration of movements of your pelvis with movements of your torso, and initiation of movement from your legs.

How did you do? How might this movement have gotten easier or smoother? Could it be that your CNS has cleaned things up a bit? Is it more accurately inhibiting muscles that don't need to be used and that might have been getting in the way of the movement when you first started? Could it be that you are initiating the movement from more powerful and centrally located muscles? Could it be that you are in compliance with the proportionality principle? Could it be that your CNS has re-established better coordination of torso and pelvis? Could it be that you are in better compliance with the good housekeeping rule?

The final movement variation is really just a simple change of venue: do the movement faster and set up an oscillation. An oscillation is like pushing a kid on a swing. There is a slight pause on change of direction, but movement doesn't really stop. Timing is the key to making an oscillation. Push too soon and you inhibit movement. Push too late and you'll lose power. If you push at just the right time, not much effort is required to keep the swing going. The same is true when oscillating the pelvis on the floor.

The timing of the pushing from the gluteals and the pulling from the legs is crucial – otherwise a fast movement will feel awkward. This oscillatory movement is very difficult to do with alternating contractions of belly and back. Try it yourself on the floor and feel the difference in quality between doing this from the legs or from the torso. This variation is yet another way of funneling our students in such a way that they learn the advantages of moving the pelvis from the legs.

The last instruction of this lesson is to return to our static baseline and compare contact against the ground and balance from side to side to when you started. Many people will feel flatter to the floor. Why would that be? The hip flexors might have gotten longer and allowed the pelvis and lower back to rest more fully on the ground. The anterior intercostals and upper abdominals may have relaxed and allowed the thoracic spine and the back of the ribcage to flatten to the floor.

The CNS may have recalibrated muscle tone throughout the whole body, and muscles that may have been contracting unintentionally may now be matching more accurately your intention. They are resting, and are allowing the bones they control to sink on to the ground.

Many people will feel less of a difference in weight distribution or perception of length from side to side. Why would that be? The diagonal and circular variations in this lesson are designed both to further coordinate the lengthening and shortening contractions of the iliopsoas and to enhance balance of both iliopsoas and of both sides of the torso. Doing full lengthening and shortening contractions of both iliopsoas enhances the coordination and balance of both and results in a reduction of asymmetrical pulls on the pelvis and lower back. The asymmetrical iliopsoas bias that all of us have may be reduced.

Doing movements into both left and right torso flexion helps the CNS discover differences between the two sides and make adjustments to lessen those differences. The result is a recalibrated neutral that comes as an outgrowth of an ability to do movements competently in both directions. Movements into right and left torso extension have the same rationale. Circular movements are the icing on the cake and are great home exercises once learned and refined.

The rest of the story

I started a story about my son earlier where I described how he learned through bitter experience the advantage of rounding himself and dropping his head forward when falling backward. I left off in that story with him getting competent in his ability to fall back without hitting his head, and hinted that the next step of the progression was to arrest the fall and bring himself back upright again without actually rolling all the way back to the floor. What he learned to do is exactly what you were just practicing in this lesson.

One day when I walked into the room, he looked up and started to fall back as usual but was able to stop his fall about halfway back. From there, he started to wobble a bit with his pelvis on the floor forward and back. He struggled a bit but was able to slowly bring himself back upright again. He was very proud and got a very smug look on his face. He deliberately started to fall back again, brought himself back upright again and repeated this sequence until he was too tired to do it any more. Over the course of the next few months, he would do this rocking movement at every opportunity.

He would do it sitting on the floor, sitting in his high chair, in the car seat and when sitting on a lap. He rocked forward and back and got progressively more coordinated, more integrated and stronger. He would do it slowly while he played and would do it fast and furious when he got excited. Sometimes he would get so wild with it that he would topple over, but that never seemed to dampen his enthusiasm. What is interesting is that his older sister never did this, and I can see differences in their organization to this day.

Whereas my son is much more erect in sitting, my daughter tends to allow her pelvis to roll back and relies on her mid to upper back to bring her upright – she is gravitating toward a half-round pattern. Whereas my son flexes and abducts at his hips and sticks his pelvis out behind when he bends over, my daughter tends to stay rounded in her lower back and disallows full hip flexion and tends toward hip adduction as she bends. The moral of the story is that the habitual organization we see in our students when they come to see us for some ache or pain is very probably very old, very ingrained, and woven throughout their entire tapestry of movement and posture.

These ingrained patterns are resistant to intellectual arguments and to exercises that localize individual muscles for stretching and strengthening. Changing whole-body motor behaviors requires teaching whole-body patterns of movement. Although it may seem logical and is certainly easier to think of conceptually and remember cortically, our traditional framework of using unidirectional, nonintegrated and cardinal plane movements in an attempt to change complex motor behaviors is, I believe, misguided. We need to update and modernize our method of exercise. We need to bring our exercise into the information age.

Applications

This is a degree of difficulty progression from sitting circles III. All falling-back benefits accrue to this lesson: lengthening and strengthening of the hip flexors, lengthening the lumbar extensors and strengthening the abdominals. Use as in sitting circles III for orthopedic, neurologic or medical rehabilitation. The same diagonal and circular patterns of movement are explored here as in sitting circles III, and all left-to-right balancing benefits from that lesson accrue to this one.

In addition, this is a nice way to work with differentiated thoracic extension. When pulling back upright again from a falling-back position, the instruction is to push your belly and chest forward between your knees and to push the top of your head taller. When you do this movement with both knees bent and the soles of your feet on the floor, you are constraining anterior pelvic tilt with the hamstrings and gluteals.

By using this *hamstring constraint* to disallow movement of the lumbar spine into extension, we are funneling the extension movement needed to push taller into the thoracic spine. This is a nice place to work with safely strengthening the thoracic extensors in folks who half arch. The fact that you are working also on lengthening those predictably short hip flexors is an added bonus. Two exercises for the price of one!

Falling variations

What are some variations on this lesson? I am going to break them down into two categories. Most of the lesson was about falling back, and I'll describe more variations of this iliopsoas emphasis. A small but important part of the lesson was about rolling the pelvis into posterior tilt using the gluteals. Although we will be doing much more on this theme in subsequent lessons, I will describe many variations of this pushing movement now. All of these variations will be of the belly-up variety.

There are hundreds of subvariations of rolling or falling back and coming back to sit in the Feldenkrais Method. As a class of lessons, I call these them psoas psit-ups. The shear volume of these movements precludes me from including all of them, but I'll describe a representative sample. Some of the variations are the controlled fall-back movements you already did in this lesson, but with different hand placements.

A great variation of this lesson involves holding on to the front of your knees with your hands. Start in sitting, knees bent, left hand on the front of your left knee and right hand on the front of your right knee. Start rolling back but keep the soles of your feet on the ground. Let your elbows straighten, your shoulder blades pull forward and your whole back and neck round. How far back can you go? Continue from here to slow roll on to back, then reverse to come back up again. Don't use momentum. Slowly push your feet toward the floor. This will push your hands into your knees and pull you back upright again.

Go back and forth a few times between rolling to your back and coming back up again very slowly; control this movement

with your legs. After a rest, come back to the same position except hold your right knee with both interlaced hands. Resume the rolling-back movement and continue to use your right leg to control your roll back. Add in sliding your left foot away from you, using your left leg as an additional counterweight to the fall back. Come back upright by pushing your right foot toward the floor and bending your left leg back up. Do to the other side, then rest and do the other side. Come back to holding both knees again and compare. Vary hand placement and be creative.

When falling straight back, you could place your hands around the back of your thighs or on the front of your thighs as you did earlier. You could also place your hands around the front of your knees, or hold on to the outside edge of your feet with both elbows to the inside of your thighs. Hands could also be on the floor by your sides, crossed over your chest, or interlaced and placed behind your head.

When falling back diagonally to the right, try holding on with your left hand around the front of your right knee. This emphasizes a turning movement of the pelvis to the right. The mirror image is true to the left side. Try the diagonal roll back on to your elbow or shoulder while holding on to a foot with your opposite hand. Try rolling up a towel or placing a roller lengthwise under your pelvis while sitting upright and rolling back.

The roller provides a reference point for rolling straight back, and provides immediate feedback. If you are using your muscles in an imbalanced way, you will fall off the roller either left or right. Use a roller horizontally across your pelvis in supine and roll your pelvis alternately anteriorly and posteriorly. Using the roller (or rolled-up towel) allows for a falling movement of the pelvis anteriorly and posteriorly (ball on a hill). Cue to lighten the feet to train awareness of the use of the iliopsoas in anterior tilt and lumbar extension and to train differentiation of the hip flexors from the abdominal flexors. This is very difficult for many people.

Some of the variations involve starting on your back, holding on to knees or feet and using a pushing movement of the legs to help you to come back to sit. Lie on your back and lift your feet off the floor. Hold on to the front of your knees with your hands and move both feet back down toward the ground. This movement pushes your knees into your hands. The gluteals fire and the hands now act as the ground. This presses your lower back into the floor.

It is possible to roll yourself along your spine and get your feet on the ground without contracting your belly at all — though this will be beyond most of you to start with. From there, you'll need to use your hip flexors to come all the way upright. You could move one foot at a time toward the ground with your head lifted. This again pushes the knee into the hand, fires the gluteals, rounds the back and flexes/side-bends your torso. You could hold on to your opposite knee with that foot lifted and drive your knee into your hand to help drag you up toward side-sitting in a diagonal, rolling across your other elbow as you do this.

There are further subvariations on hand placement. Holding behind the thigh, holding the knee or thigh from the outside, and placing the other hand behind your head. All of these variations are also great ways of mobilizing the upper chest and upper back as the shoulder girdles are dragged down, forward and into flexion/rotation or flexion/side-bending by the powerful legs.

Pushing variations

Let's switch our emphasis now to exploring variations and refinements of using the gluteals to push with the feet. In this lesson, you were lying supine with legs bent up and pushing the feet into the floor to push the pelvis into posterior tilt. Try this movement with your feet as far away from your pelvis as possible and still have the soles of your feet flat. This requires the hip extensors to work in a range closer to full hip extension and requires the hamstrings to work much harder at the same time as facilitating pushing the feet with the hamstrings instead of with the quadriceps.

By the way, with all these movements of pushing the feet into the floor when supine, watch out for hamstring cramps: they are pretty common with people who don't normally use those muscles. For people who have a difficult time conceptualizing the rolling movement of their pelvis, try rolling up a towel or placing a small roller crosswise under the middle of their sacrum. This makes movement into both anterior and posterior tilt downhill and provides a fulcrum and a reference point.

For people who have a half arch postural type, we could use a modification of this movement to help differentiate lumbar and thoracic areas. The conundrum with these folks is that global torso extension movements tend to default to the lumbar spine and global torso flexion movement defaults to the thoracic spine. What we would especially like to see is a simultaneous ability to flex the lumbar spine and extend the thoracic spine.

Use a small roller or roll up a towel and place it crosswise under the apex of your thoracic convexity. A small, soft, air-filled plastic or rubber ball is another toy that works well for this. Interlace your fingers and place them behind your head. With your knees bent and with your feet on the floor, roll your pelvis into posterior tilt and lift your head with the assistance of your hands.

Lift both ends of your spine and round your whole back so the apex presses into the roller. Now roll your pelvis downward into anterior tilt and lower your head gently towards the ground. Press both ends of your spine and arch your back so the apex presses less heavily into the roller.

Alternate this movement a few times then pause for a moment with your pelvis rolled into anterior tilt and your head and hands resting on the ground. From there, keep your head and hands where they are and gently and slowly press your feet into the floor to roll your pelvis into posterior tilt. The pelvis has to stay on the floor and roll rather than lift. The movement of the pelvis into posterior tilt has to be performed from the legs, so make sure you know how to do this before progressing to the roller.

If you use your belly, you will also be contracting your anterior intercostals and pulling your chest downward into kyphosis. For most people, a small movement is sufficient to create an intense sensation in the mid back or even the front of the chest. The idea is to constrain thoracic flexion with the roller, reduce effort in the abdominals and anterior intercostals

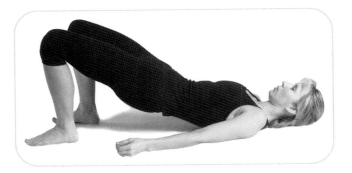

Fig. 5.28 Bridging, but with details – move sequentially.

to allow the chest to move into extension, and to flatten the lower back with the legs. This movement and asymmetrical variations of it are big hits with my students.

Bridging is another continuation of this pushing movement while supine. When bridging, though, make sure you don't lift pelvis and low back at the same time. This is hip and back extension happening together. Try rolling up your spine one vertebra at a time and lowering back down one vertebra at a time. Lifting the tailbone, pelvis, low lumbars, mid lumbars and upper lumbars sequentially emphasizes our desired differentiation of hip extension and lumbar flexion and makes the gluteals work both much harder and in a position closer to full end-range of hip joint extension than if you allow the back to arch right away (Fig. 5.28).

You can extend this movement to roll along your spine all the way up to the upper shoulder girdles and cervico-thoracic (CT) junction (we'll be doing more bridging in the chapter on upper extremities and will discuss effects on the CT junction there). At what point in the lifting do you run out of room in your hip joints and have to extend your back? The higher up you can go without kicking in your back, the better. This demands fuller hip joint extension and fuller gluteal contraction. At some point, though, you'll have to arch if you roll all the way up. When coming back down, you may notice a place where it is difficult to round through one vertebra at a time. This is usually at the lumbothoracic junction.

Many people will have difficulty differentiating the lower thoracic and lumbar vertebra and will roll along this area like a flat chunk. To make this movement smoothly, you will have to learn to allow the thoracic spine to extend while flexing the lumbar spine. This is another way of facilitating this differentiation. Imagine the thoracic spine as it lowers to the floor. To place one vertebra down at a time it has to extend from its (possibly) chronically flexed position.

When you get to the lumbothoracic junction, the ability to lower one vertebra at a time switches to become dependent on an ability to flex the lumbar spine. Try doing a few full bridges to assess accuracy and ease. Then use the roller or small ball as described above to facilitate that oh-so-desirable thoracic and lumbar differentiation. Then come back to the bridge again. Did the use of the toy help in your ability to do an accurate bridge?

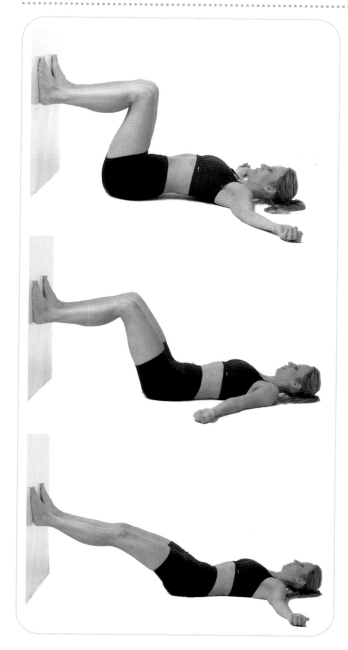

Fig. 5.29 Lie supine with feet on wall – a degree of difficulty regression.

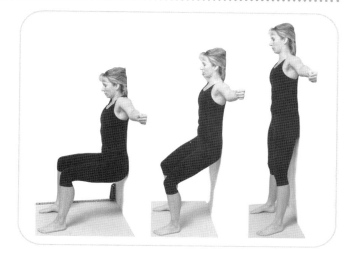

Fig. 5.30 Teach the same basic movement against the wall – roll into anterior tilt, then push into posterior tilt. Progress by moving feet closer to the wall.

Wall variations

Try lying supine and placing your feet up on a wall with hips and knees bent at 90° (Fig. 5.29). This position more closely approximates the relationship of the feet to the floor when upright in sitting or standing. Press your feet into the wall and release. Did your pelvis roll upward on the floor? Repeat several times to familiarize yourself with the movement in this position, then scoot yourself away from the wall so your hips and knees are straighter. Do this pushing movement several times here, then scoot farther away.

Moving progressively farther away from the wall moves you gradually towards fuller hip extension and gets you closer and closer to a position that approximates standing. We described this progression briefly and illustrated it in Chapter 2. You will have to be clear about pushing the feet into the wall with the hip extensors rather than the quadriceps. This is a common error, and you will find yourself sliding unintentionally away from the wall rather than rolling your pelvis on the floor.

Feel for (or visualize when working with your students) the sliding effect of the feet upward on the wall. To facilitate an awareness of this difference, try doing a few bridges from these positions. Bridging from here without sliding away from the wall requires you to use your hamstrings and gluteals. Try pushing the wall with an additional intention of almost sliding your feet up the wall – this emphasizes the quadriceps. Try pushing the wall with an additional intention to almost slide your feet down the wall – this emphasizes your hamstrings. Feel for differences in these two strategies in terms of familiarity, and in terms of accurately rolling your pelvis rather than sliding your pelvis on the ground.

Change orientation to gravity altogether and stand with your back and pelvis against a wall and your feet on the floor out in front of you. Roll your pelvis up and down on the wall without bending or straightening your knees. This constraint emphasizes using the hip extensors rather than the knee extensors in this pushing into the ground movement. Progress by moving your feet closer to the wall and add diagonal subvariations (Fig. 5.30).

Legs controlling the pelvis and back in belly-down orientation

Now that we have explored movements in a belly-up orientation, let's turn our attention to movements performed in a belly-down orientation. Put on your proprioceptive hats again and find a place on the floor.

Side-sit Bending

Variations

A. How do you bend? How do you go about reaching toward the ground from a standing position? Stand for a moment before lying down and simply reach toward the ground with both hands – anything is fair game except for squatting.

- How far apart do you put your feet?
- Are they side by side or is one in front of the other?
- What is the shape of your back as you bend? Is it round, arched or straight?

B. Lie on your back with your legs long and comfortably spread and with your arms somewhere on the floor below shoulder height.

- Feel the contact you make against the floor. How much of yourself is on the floor? Observe whether there is a space between your lower back and the floor.
- How is your weight distributed across your pelvis? Is your pelvis rolled left or right on the floor?
- Notice how your legs are resting on the floor. Are they narrow or wide? Are the toes pointed away from or towards each other? Is there a difference in the two sides?

C. Come up to sit on the floor – place your right foot and leg behind you on the floor and place your left foot on the floor near your right knee. This is a left side-sitting position (Fig. 5.31). Your weight is mostly on your left hip. Lean with both hands on the floor just a little in front of your left knee, one hand to either side of that knee.

- Keeping both elbows straight and leaving the left hand where it is on the floor, slide your right hand backward on the floor towards your right thigh.
- How do you do this movement and still keep your right elbow straight? Does your back move? Or your pelvis?
- Try rolling your pelvis backward a bit and rounding your back. Try reaching your right sitting bone toward the floor behind you. Try looking toward your right hip.
- Reverse the movement to slide your right hand forward on the floor. Slide and reach your right hand out on the floor in front of your left knee. Look at your hand as it slides. How do you organize your back and pelvis to assist with this?
- Try rolling your pelvis forward and straightening your back a bit; lift your right sitting bone away from the floor behind you. Try looking forward toward the wall in front of you. Repeat this several times.
- Now alternate sliding your right hand forward and back on the floor (Fig. 5.31). Alternately roll your pelvis diagonally on the floor, forward and to the left and back and to the right. Your back alternately straightens and rounds.

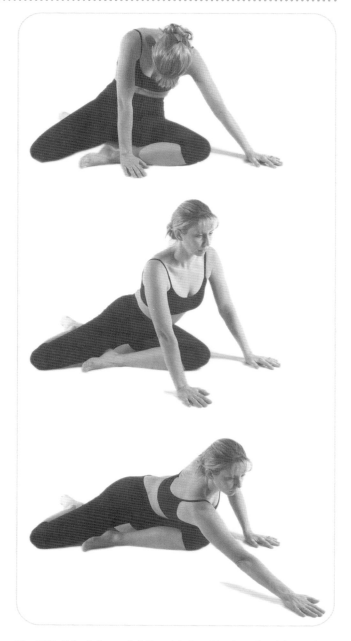

Fig. 5.31 Side-sitting and sliding right hand backward and forward.

- Keep looking at your right hand as it slides and make sure to keep your elbows straight. Rest on your back and compare contact to when you started. Compare also your two sides.

D. Come up to sit in the mirror image of B. Side-sit right with your left foot behind you and your weight mostly on your right hip. Repeat the same instructions as in B to the opposite side. Then rest on your back and compare left and right sides again.

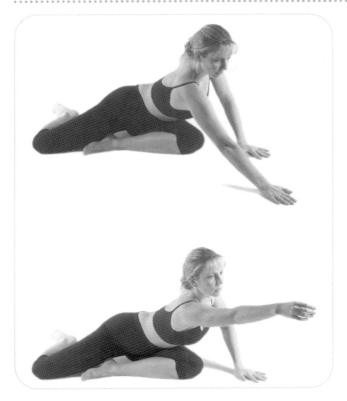

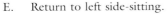

Fig. 5.32 Make things more challenging by lifting your hand off the floor.

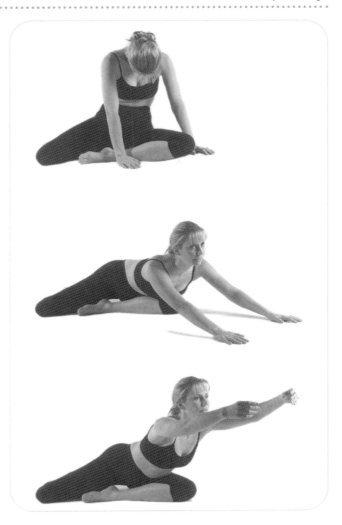

Fig. 5.33 Sliding both hands together – lift them both for extra credit.

E.   Return to left side-sitting.

*   Resume the movement of sliding your right hand forward and back on the floor, coordinating it with the rolling of the pelvis and the movements of the back.

*   Now enlarge the movement of sliding forward by lifting your right hand off the floor and reaching it forward and toward the ceiling (Fig. 5.32). Stay with your left hand on the floor, and don't let your chest twist to the right.

*   Your mid-upper back has to arch back to do this. Continue to look at your hand so you don't over-strain your neck.

F.   Return to right side-sitting. Repeat instructions as in D. Lift the left hand now to the ceiling in front. How do the two sides compare?

G.   Return to left side-sitting.

*   Slide both hands alternately forward and back on the floor. Keep both elbows straight and allow your pelvis to roll forward and back on the floor.

*   Because you can't support your weight so much on your sliding hands, you'll have to use the left knee and thigh on the ground to support you. Push with

the left leg against the floor to slide your hands back and use the same leg to control your fall forward when sliding hands forward.

*   Would you care to lift both hands from the floor once you have reached them forward? Be careful not to strain your back and use your legs for support (Fig. 5.33).

*   Place your hands to either side of your knee again and roll your pelvis forward and back without sliding your hands. Let your back fully round and arch as you roll your pelvis backward and forward, and use this movement to find neutral, that place where your back is neither rounded nor arched.

*   Find that place and stay there. From there, slowly lift both hands away from the floor and, keeping your back in neutral, push yourself up to sitting upright (Fig. 5.34). Reverse the movement to slowly put your hands on the floor.

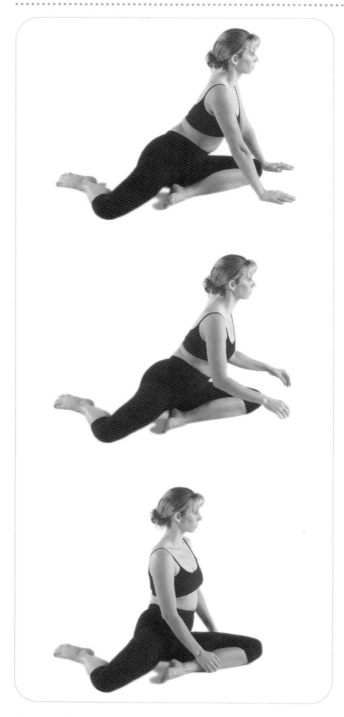

Fig. 5.34 Keeping a neutral spine while bending and while pushing back upright again.

- Alternate bending over and coming back upright several times. Make sure your back is neither arched nor rounded, as if there were a stick between head and pelvis.

H. Return to left side-sitting. Repeat instructions as in F. How do your two sides compare?

I. Return to left side-sitting but this time with your left leg long out in front of you. Your left knee is nearly straight, but not quite. Let your left leg roll outward on the floor so your toes point out to the left. Lean back on your left hand behind.

- Place your right hand on the inside of your left thigh and begin to slide your right hand down along the inside of your thigh and lower leg toward your foot. Roll your pelvis forward and to the left as before and straighten or arch your back.

- Slide your hand back up again by again rolling your pelvis backward on the floor and rounding your back. Alternate sliding your right hand up and down the inside of your left leg (Fig. 5.35).

- Don't force this movement. Allow your pelvis to roll on the floor as before. Allow your left knee to bend a little and roll even farther outward on the floor.

- Would you like to try this movement with your left hip lifted away from the floor? If you try this, make sure that your left knee and lower leg stay on the floor. You will have to let your left knee bend a little.

- Return once again to our original side-sitting position with the left knee bent again and your left foot touching your right knee.

- Slide just the right hand forward and back on the floor a few times to compare ease, quality and organization of movement now to when you started.

J. Return to right side-sitting and repeat instructions as in I to the opposite side. Compare sides.

K. Return to lying on your back. Scan and compare contact against floor to the beginning and compare balance of pelvis left and right.

L. Stand up. Walk around. How do your legs, hips and back feel? Reach towards the ground; how are you bending now? Do your hips bend any more easily?

M. Can your back be more neutral? Do you have any clearer sense of how your legs control this movement?

Static and dynamic baselines – Side-sit Bending

We started this lesson a bit differently from the others. We began with a dynamic scan related to bending from a standing position. How should one bend? How do we go about teaching someone how to bend? Bending is one of the main stressors of the lower back. Conventional wisdom admonishes us to squat down, keep our back straight and use our legs. Although squatting to lift something of substantial weight or awkward bulk is an excellent idea, bending to lift something heavy is only a small part of why we bend.

Even squatting to pick something heavy off the floor requires bending. Your back cannot remain vertical if you need to get your hands to the floor. Try this yourself. Squat down and try to keep your back straight and vertical while you try to bring your hands to the floor. Although the back itself can stay straight or neutral, you will have to angle your torso forward to get your hands to the floor: you have to bend.

Bending as a transitional movement

At what other times do we bend in the course of our daily lives? We bend to pick up the shampoo bottle off the floor of the shower. We bend to pick up a magazine off the coffee table, or to get the cereal box out of the bottom cupboard in our kitchen. We bend to load and unload the dishwasher, or to get the apple out of the crisper in our refrigerator. We bend to put on our pants, our socks and our shoes. We bend to scratch an itch on our knee or foot. We bend over to kiss our children.

We bend to get a drink of water from a water fountain. We bend over to get a closer look at something. We bend when we get in and out of our cars, or when we get up and down from a chair. We bend over when we sit in a chair to reach into the bottom drawer of our desk, or to reach the pen and pencil holder at the far edge of our desk. We bend over the bathroom counter to get a closer look in the mirror when shaving, primping our hair or putting on makeup. We bend in reaction to losing our balance backward (witness the jackknife that babies do when they lose their balance and fall on their bottoms).

We bend over when we're slurping soup or biting into a sloppy piece of barbecued chicken (or tofu). We bend forward when we have to take a big step up while hiking, or while taking two stairs at a time. We lean forward in our chairs when we want to emphasize a point in conversation with someone, and we bend over to wag an admonishing finger at our kids. We bend hundreds of times a day.

We bend to balance ourselves in a gravity field, to orient ourselves to get a closer look at something below our head and to grasp and manipulate objects. We bend to make transitional movements, to locomote, to punctuate our communication, and to bring our mouth somewhere for vegetative purposes. If all seven of our functional categories can involve bending, into which of those seven categories do we place bending?

I would call bending a transitional movement. We are transitioning from one posture to another for the purpose of balance, orientation, manipulation, locomotion, communication and vegetation. We are bending and coming back upright again to raise and lower our center of mass. Most people have no idea how much they bend in the course of their daily life – and many people have no idea how to bend in a well-organized way.

Although showing our students posters on proper lifting and demonstrating good body mechanics is helpful, it is seldom enough. We run into the problem of situation-specific learning. They can mimic good technique when picking up a box on the floor but don't carry the principles over to putting on their socks or getting up from a chair. They may also lack the physical skills required to bend without undue tissue strain.

Tools for well-organized bending

What are the physical skills (strength, flexibility, coordination, proprioceptive self-awareness) necessary for efficient bending? Bending with a neutral spine would usually be a good idea, but what if someone has been bending their whole life with a back either too arched or too round? To them, they are bending with a neutral back. How do we get them to recalibrate neutral? Having hamstrings and hip extensors that can elongate adequately to allow a full hip hinge would be nice.

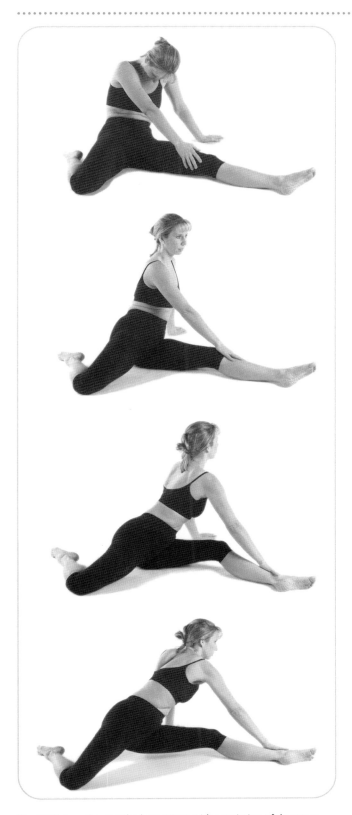

Fig. 5.35 Lengthening the hamstrings with a variation of the same pattern of movement – do it with lifted hips for extra credit.

How can we incorporate principles of pattern specificity and functional context to make our stretching exercises carry over into the bending our students do on a daily basis, and which they do for a variety of different reasons? Having legs that are strong enough to support the weight and control the angle of the pelvis in space is critical. Which specific muscles need to be stronger, and how can we get our students to recognize the advantages of using those muscles to protect their lower back when bending?

We start this lesson with a dynamic scan. How do you bend? How do you go about reaching toward the ground from a standing position? How far apart do you put your feet? Are they side by side, or is one in front of the other? What is the shape of your back as you bend? Is it rounded, arched or straight? Did the way you organized yourself to bend change at all by the end of this lesson?

Using real-life movements and postures as reference points both before and after a lesson is a great way of helping our students make the conceptual leap from doing exercise to doing movements from which they can learn better how to do mundane tasks. Start a lesson by having your students sit in a chair, stand, walk, reach forward or overhead, bend, step up on a stool, look over their shoulder or toward the ceiling, get up and down from a chair, shift weight from foot to foot in standing or from cheek to cheek in sitting, or any number of other upright and real-life functions.

Ask them questions about what they notice, how they are doing things, if there are differences between right and left side, and so on. I would highly recommend using this concept with your students regardless of the technique you use. Whether doing manual therapy and joint mobilization, myofascial release or deep soft tissue releasing, muscle energy, proprioceptive neuromuscular facilitation (PNF), craniosacral therapy, strain–counterstrain, progressive resistance exercise (PRE), or any of the myriad tools available in our bag of tricks, there should be a change in movement: range of movement, quality of movement, organization of movement, degree of comfort of the movement, where the movement is initiated or how the movement is proportioned.

What you want your students to feel is a qualitative difference in how they are moving before and after your intervention. It is this awareness that something feels better that provides the trigger to the CNS to make a change and to adopt a different and less stressful way of moving.

Getting clues from supine observation

In variation B we return to our familiar static baseline while lying supine. Although the awareness of contact points and spaces has been a recurring theme, an awareness of weight distribution across the pelvis may hold particular interest. Lie on your back for a moment with your legs long. Slowly pinch/contract your right cheek/gluteals. Does your pelvis roll on the floor to the left? Could a pelvis that is rolled on the floor to the left be a result of a difference in tone of the two gluteals?

Now try lifting your left heel, leg and thigh off the floor just a smidge. Does your pelvis shift its weight to the left? Could a pelvis that is rolled on the floor to the left be a result of a difference in tone of the two iliopsoas? You may have noticed during the course of this lesson how much the back of the hips was worked. Did the muscle tone around the two hips change as a result of these explorations? Was your pelvis lying on the floor any differently at the end of the lesson from the way it was at the beginning?

We also inquired about the distance between the legs and the orientation of the toes. The side-sitting position requires external rotation of the front/weightbearing hip and internal rotation of the back hip. If you or your students start with habitual hypertonus in the adductors/TFL, the toes will be pointing more toward the ceiling or even inward a bit. If the toes are angled more outward at the end, it probably happened as a result of a reduction of adductor/TFL tone which allowed the hip joints to roll into external rotation.

If you started with habitual hypertonus in the piriformis, gluteals and other hip external rotators, the toes would have pointed more outward toward the walls. If the toes were a bit more inward at the end, it probably happened as a result of a reduction of tone in these muscles.

There are nearly always differences between the two sides both in terms of the degree of rollout of each leg and in terms of the roll of the pelvis one way or the other on the floor. Figuring out and making sense of what you are seeing is a gradually learned skill that will never be mastered. There are just too many ways in which people organize themselves and too many factors involved to make this an exact science.

Just start making observations, make your best guess in terms of anticipating muscle imbalances, and confirm or disprove those guesses when watching your students move during the lesson. In the end, what we are trying to do is to get our students to move better and to have better proprioceptive awareness. When you get confused, just train them in efficient movement patterns and demonstrably more comfortable ways of moving.

Side-sitting creates a diagonally falling worm

We start the action phase of the lesson in variation C. We start in a left side-sitting position. This is where the right leg is bent behind, the left leg is bent in front and the left foot touches the right knee or distal thigh. You lean forward on your hands a little in front of your left knee, with one hand on either side of that knee. This is a belly-down orientation, as your torso is leaned forward to allow you to place your hands on the floor.

Think back to the balancing movements of the worm. What would be the pattern of the torso? Because the worm is falling forward and to the left, we could anticipate some variation of right torso extension. Ideally, the left anterior torso is longer and the right posterior torso is shorter. Some folks who have strong global torso flexion tendencies and a gluteal bias may still be rounded here.

Those people who tend toward a half arch type posture might be extended in the lower back and still rounded through the thorax. What we would like to see, however, is an evenly distributed right torso extension. Most of your weight is on the left side of your pelvis and your left hip is flexed and externally rotated. Your right hip is extended and internally rotated.

Side-sitting is a classic developmental posture. Kids spend a lot of time in this position, and it is one from which a number of transitional movements are possible. Movements from side-sit to supine, side-sit to prone, side-sit to hands and knees and side-Sit to Stand are great contexts around which we can build lessons. We will be doing several later in this chapter. It is a position that many adults no longer choose or are able to get into easily, which is a shame.

As mentioned in the first chapter, we should encourage people to spend more time on the floor as a way of introducing greater complexity and variety to what, for most people, are greatly constrained movement lives. It requires a degree of flexibility in the hips and torso that many people have lost as a result of too much sitting in chairs, too many modern conveniences and too much movement invariance. It can therefore be a tool for regaining that lost mobility. Get your students on the floor!

Your first movement from this position is to slide your right hand backward on the floor toward your right thigh while keeping both elbows straight. The 'curse of the doll body' version of this movement is to elevate and adduct the right shoulder girdle: moving the hand (manipulation) without recognizing the advantages of moving that hand in an integrated way as an extension of the movement of the pelvis and torso.

Much of what we do in motor control exercise is to help our students link the intention to move distally (eyes, hands, feet, mouth) with a proximal initiation. How would we like to see our students do this movement? We are looking for a diagonal version of a differentiated movement, left hip extension with left torso flexion.

Are instructions to roll your pelvis backward a bit and round your back, reach your right sitting bone toward the floor behind you and look toward your right hip examples of descriptive language used to direct your students toward moving their pelvis and rounding their back? The intention to look toward their right anterior hip adds another functional context, another trigger. The intention to reach the right sitting bone to the floor behind requires an intention to move the pelvis.

Again, we are helping their CNS to link an intention to move distally with proximal integration or, better yet, a proximal initiation. We would like them to move their biggest bones and to contract their strongest muscles first. Which is the biggest bone? The pelvis. Which are the strongest muscles capable of rolling the pelvis backward and rounding the back? Those muscles that extend/abduct externally the left hip: the gluteals, hamstrings and short and stubbies.

Pushing against the floor to control bending

Get on the floor and try this movement again. What if, as you slide your hand back by rolling your pelvis back, you intentionally push your left knee and thigh into the floor? You would push your pelvis back and to the right, away from the left leg. Feel the effort of pushing – where is it? Maybe we should ask what is happening at the hip joints? The left hip is extending, abducting and externally rotating. The left extensors, abductors and external rotators are pushing the pelvis backward.

This is a closed kinetic chain exercise that I use not only for spinal problems, but for biomechanical knee and foot dysfunction and early rehabilitation for lower extremity injuries. With both lower extremity biomechanical faults and injuries, it is

often the ability to engage the powerful push-off muscles in an efficient way that needs to be retrained. If your left knee and thigh are lifting from the floor as you roll back and to the right, you are not pushing with your left leg.

What is happening at the right hip? It is flexing, adducting and internally rotating. The right iliopsoas, tensor fascia latae and adductors could be used to pull the pelvis back and to the right. Try this movement again and notice if you can perceive effort in the medial and anterior hip and thigh. Although pushing back with the left leg and pulling back with the right hip are possibilities, they are not necessary yet.

One could push with the hands and contract the belly and leave the legs completely passive, though the range of movement will probably be incomplete. Which of these choices would we prefer our students to learn? The pushing-back function of the left leg is what we want to emphasize, but what we would be truly delighted with is a cooperative motion of the two legs – one pushes and one pulls to make a *pelvic force couple*. More on this later too!

How do you get back forward to our starting point again? For many, it will just be a matter of letting go of the effort of pushing the pelvis back. Gravity can roll you back forward again, so is decelerated by a lengthening contraction of the same muscles that got them there. For some, it will require some effort to get back to our starting position. How could the legs initiate this movement? The left hip is flexing and adducting when rolling forward; the left iliopsoas and adductors could pull the pelvis forward.

The right hip is extending and externally rotating; the right gluteals could be pushing the pelvis forward. Try getting into this position of rolling yourself back from left side-sitting. Pinch/contract your right cheek/gluteals and see if that drives the right side of your pelvis forward. If you pinch your right cheek and the right side of your pelvis doesn't move forward, you are doing something else to prevent that from happening.

Make sure you aren't resisting the movement of the pelvis by tensing your left gluteals or your abdominal muscles. Part of the game in motor learning is to do a movement and feel where the effort is. The flip side of that experiment is to do an effort somewhere and ask what the consequence of that effort is in terms of movement of bones, and to gain competence in inhibiting the antagonists. Let the games begin!

Our next movement is to slide your right hand forward. To help you to recognize how to coordinate the intention to slide your hand with a proximal movement, we again used some descriptive language: 'try rolling your pelvis forward and straightening your back a bit – lifting your right sitting bone away from the floor behind you and looking forward toward the wall in front of you.'

This again directs your intention to moving your pelvis and extending your back. We again added another functional context (orientation) to the original intent (manipulation) and to the unspoken, but always present, intention not to strike your head against the floor (balance). We are helping our students' CNS to link an intention to move distally with proximal integration or, better yet, a proximal initiation. We would like them to move their biggest bones and to contract their strongest muscles first.

What is the biggest bone? The pelvis. What are the strongest muscles capable of rolling the pelvis forward and arching the back? Although normally we would think of the iliopsoas, in this belly-down position we might instead expect to see a lengthening contraction of the gluteals, hamstrings and short and stubbies, along with a shortening contraction of the right torso extensors. This relationship becomes much more obvious once you start sliding both hands.

What movement are we looking for here, ideally? We would like to see a differentiated pattern of movement again: hip flexion with back extension. What are we stretching? In the torso, we are stretching the left anterior abdominals and intercostals. At the left hip, we are asking the hip rotators to lengthen, not because we are internally rotating that left hip but because of the horizontal adduction and flexion component of this movement.

The left piriformis, inferior and superior gemelli, internal and external obturators and the quadratus femoris are all arthrokinematic muscles. They control the slide and glide of the head of the femur inside the acetabulum. They also have a contribution to make in hip extension or in posterior pelvic tilt. By extension, they will limit hip flexion when their muscle spindles (tripwires) are set by the CNS at too short a length. The gluteals and hamstrings also limit hip flexion and are also stretched by this differentiated movement. This inability to allow a full hip hinge movement is detrimental to efficient bending.

Bending errors – pelvis falls too much or not enough forward

There are basically two errors that people make when bending. They either don't allow their pelvis to rotate far enough forward on their legs or they allow it to fall too far forward. If they don't allow their pelvis to fall far enough forward and if the gluteal group doesn't allow a full hip hinge, the lower back will be required to take up the slack. This results in too much flexion at the SI joints or lumbar spine, and ligamentous overstretching or disc shearing can occur.

If they let their pelvis fall too far forward on their legs and if they can't adequately catch their pelvis with their legs, the worm goes into a forward falling response, the lower back extends too much and the lumbar extensors are required to work too hard while the joints are close packed. Bending is one of those activities that can be a major stressor for both iliopsoas-dominant and gluteal-dominant people.

When training someone how to bend, then, we have to recognize what error that particular person is making and emphasize different strategies for each of the types. With both types we want to encourage a more or less neutral spine while bending, though we may want to bias an iliopsoas-dominant person in the direction of back flexion and the gluteal-dominant person in the direction of back extension. We will revisit this idea in discussion of later variations of this lesson and in subsequent lessons (Box 5.13).

Alternating back and forth between sliding the hand forward and backward introduces our information-rich reciprocating movement. How do the two directions compare? Which direction is easiest? By alternating back and forth with an emphasis on the use of the legs, we are alternating back and

Box 5.13 Bending

Transitional movement – done hundreds of times a day

Leaning, bending forward and lifting – different spectrums along a continuum

Errors in bending – letting the pelvis fall too far forward or not letting it fall forward enough

forth between a lengthening and a shortening contraction of the – especially – left gluteal group.

Just as in the last lesson, where we were using a lengthening contraction of the hip flexors while rounding/falling backward to stretch the hip flexors, we are doing the same thing in a belly-down orientation and are using a lengthening contraction of the hip extensors to stretch the hamstrings, gluteals and short and stubbies. Lengthening contractions are one of the best ways to get neurological lengthening of muscles: resetting the muscle spindle to a longer length.

After having explored this alternating movement of sliding the right hand forward and back while in left side-sitting, we then went through the same exploratory process to the other side in variation D. Was there a difference between the two sides? Why did we start in left side-sitting? Although everyone will have differences in flexibility, strength and familiarity between the two sides, not everyone will necessarily notice the differences.

Handedness gives clues about anticipated hip muscle imbalances

Some differences will be subtle and will not be noticed by casual observation. Some will be huge but will still not be noticed by the proprioceptively challenged. Recall our factors contributing to imbalances: development, injury, occupation, emotional history and cultural influences. Development is the 800 pound gorilla of imbalance factors. Handedness in particular will influence muscle imbalances all through the body.

In a left side-sitting position, which hand tends to be the weightbearing side and which hand is free to move? Most right-handed people will gravitate more toward a left side-sitting position because it leaves the right hand freer. This is why we started in left side-sit. Think of a right-handed person swinging a tennis racket in a forehand stroke. She will ideally turn her pelvis and torso to the left and shift her weight forward on to the left foot.

The left hip flexes, adducts and internally rotates while the right hip extends, abducts and externally rotates. Why do so many people have difficulty coordinating and getting power from their backhand? Because both the direction of movement and the use of the hip musculature that is responsible for turning the pelvis in that direction are unfamiliar. The movement of the pelvis in the backhand direction is essentially the movement a left-handed person would do when hitting a forehand: throwing, reaching, pushing, etc.

It is now the left hip that has to extend, abduct and externally rotate. It is now the right hip that has to adduct, flex and internally rotate. Might we expect right-handed people to be a bit stronger or more competent with their right gluteals, hamstrings and short and stubbies? Might we also expect them to be more familiar with the use of their left hip flexors and adductors? Could we then anticipate right-handed people being tighter/shorter/more restricted in their right hip extensors and external rotators and in their left hip flexors and adductors?

Although this is very often the case, it is not universally true. If the only factors in imbalance creation were early development, this is the pattern we would nearly always see. Because injury, emotion and culture also play a role, we can expect to see a certain percentage of right-handed people where these developmentally predictable imbalances are modified or even reversed. What we could say is that if we don't see this pattern of imbalances, we can assume another factor has influenced or superseded the predictable one and that we would want to work to uncover and reduce imbalances.

If someone is left-handed, however, all bets seem to be off. Although many right-handed people are very right-handed (they do almost everything with the right hand and are nearly incompetent at throwing, brushing their teeth or mousing with their left hand), many left-handed people are a bit ambivalent about their handedness. They may write and eat left-handed but swing a golf club or a hammer with their right. Or they may mix and match fine and gross motor skills by putting on mascara with the right hand and pushing open a door with their left.

Their pattern of pelvic asymmetries and pelvic/lower extremity muscle imbalances also seems to be much less predictable than with right-handed people. Perhaps this comes from being a left-handed person in a right-handed world: you need better adaptation skills. Again, don't get too hung up with trying to figure out exactly why you see the imbalances you do. Work towards proprioceptive awareness of the consequences of their particular imbalances on their presenting complaint and on improving quality and balance of movement.

Is having a level pelvic base reasonable – or prudent?

With these asymmetrical whole-body patterns of movement and their concurrent muscular imbalances being tied up so intimately with handedness, is it reasonable to expect geometrical perfection in our students' posture? Should we really expect the pelvic base to be level? How much energy are we going to put into making the ASIS, PSIS, iliac crests, greater trochanters, inferior scapular angles and acromions level? How much asymmetry of bony landmarks would be considered normal?

I don't think we can quantify this, but we sure can't call a level pelvis normal! Does this mean we should never work on reducing asymmetries and imbalances? Not at all! It is actually much of what I do. I just don't go into it with the idea that there is still something wrong if, after a few lessons, their pelvic base (or other bony landmark) is not level.

Left/right imbalances we should expect, though we try to get our students to recognize them and reduce them through deliberately nonhabitual exercise, nonhabitual positioning and deliberate use of their nondominant hand in gross motor activities (bending, pushing and non-precision reaching/manipulation).

Anterior/posterior imbalances we should also expect, but will work harder to balance. There is no biologically driven reason for them to be present. As a general rule of thumb, when working with people with lower back pain we first want to determine whether they tend toward back flexion (gluteal bias) or extension (iliopsoas bias) and if their pain is reproduced or accentuated by moving farther into their habitual direction; this is very often the case.

Focus initial teaching strategies on these anteroposterior (AP) imbalances, especially if their symptoms are central or bilaterally equal. If they have more unilateral symptoms, observe for clues to left/right habitual imbalances both statically in sitting, standing and supine and while doing functional movements involving some left/right movement component.

These functional movements might include weight-shifting in sitting and standing, one hand reaching forward or overhead, walking, stepping on to a low stool, rolling to one side from supine, or turning to look over one shoulder. Then combine the emphasis on the nonhabitual and/or more comfortable AP direction with the nonhabitual and/or more comfortable left/right direction to emphasize one of the four diagonal directions.

For instance, with someone with an iliopsoas bias and a typical right-handed pattern, we would probably stress the importance of movement back and to the right. Think of our left side-sitting position again. This is a movement of the pelvis forward and to the left, is consistent with being right-handed, and would guide us toward movements to the right. With an iliopsoas bias, this guides us to movements backward – connect the dots and we have movements back and to the right.

Extrapolate to muscle imbalances and we might want to emphasize strength of the left hip extensors/abductors/external rotators and to some extent the right iliopsoas and the lengthening of the left iliopsoas/hip flexors. We would want to strengthen the left anterior abdominals and anterior intercostals, and stretch the right posterior intercostals, right back extensors and right quadratus lumborum.

For all practical purposes, we strengthen the nonhabitual differentiated pattern and stretch the habitual differentiated pattern using principles of proprioceptive self-awareness (enhanced by reciprocating movements) and functional context (enhanced by developmentally based activities). This is precisely what we are doing in this lesson!

In variation E you first review the previous variation of sliding your right hand forward and back to refamiliarize yourself with the integrated pattern. After doing this a few times, you now segue into sliding your right hand forward on the floor as far as you comfortably can, then lifting that hand away from the floor and toward the ceiling. Why is this variation included? The intentional link to a specific functional context is the same – reaching/manipulation.

Constraining anterior pelvic tilt to train thoracic extensors

The movement in variation E is a progression of the last in terms of difficulty. It takes more effort to lift the arm than to slide it. One very important benefit we can gain from this type of movement is that it helps to differentiate thoracic extension from lumbar extension. Think back again to the common half arch postural type: anterior pelvic tilt, lumbar lordosis, thoracic kyphosis, cervical lordosis and forward head posture.

If our half-arched student has low back pain related to extension, we could say that she is violating the good house-keeping rule by being unable to extend in the thoracic spine. This inability to extend the mid and upper back necessitates too much arching in the lower back and too much arching in the neck, where we commonly see another differentiated relationship of cervical extension and thoracic flexion.

Our clinical conundrum is this: if we try to strengthen the thoracic extensors through traditional (global) means, we run the risk that our student will just default to extending where she already knows how to (the low back or neck) and will use the muscles she already knows how to use (the lumbar or cervical extensors). What we would like to do is constrain her ability to move into extension in her low back and neck while encouraging a differentiated extension movement in her thoracic spine. That is what this and related movements can help us do.

By leaning way forward and rolling the pelvis anteriorly to near end-range, we are fully flexing the left hip joint. We are using the left hamstring, gluteals and short and stubbies to constrain movement of the pelvis into more anterior tilt and therefore limit movement of the lumbar spine into extension. By lifting the right hand in this position, we are safely limiting the habitual and potentially damaging extension movement of the lumbar spine and are requiring the thoracic spine to move into extension and the thoracic extensors to wake up and get into the game.

Instruct your students to place their belly or lower sternum on or near their left thigh and to keep it there as they lift their hands. Ask them to continue to look at that hand to bring in the additional functional context of orientation. Encourage them to move proportionally with their neck, moving their head only as long as their mid and upper back are still moving, but not to strain their cervical spine with too much extension.

Have them place that reaching hand on the back of their head and reach with the elbow to constrain cervical extension. We are constraining their ability to move either end of their spine to get the movement to happen in the middle – that place that for so many people is out of sight, out of mind and out of the loop of nearly any movement they do, especially movements that require extension.

Language needs to be specific – there are lots of ways to interpret

I am asking that you don't allow your chest to turn relative to the floor. Why not? It is a fine movement and one we could use with people, but by disallowing a rotational movement we are requiring more accurate extension. Try both variations yourself and feel which is easier. Which is more successful? Clearly, turning the chest to the right allows you to more successfully reach higher to the ceiling. Hopefully, it is just as clear to you proprioceptively how turning here reduces the requirement for thoracic extension.

We now have two basic ways to differentiating thoracic and lumbar extension. We could use belly-up positions and constraining toys: let gravity assist you in extending the thoracic spine over a ball or roller, then use the legs to push the pelvis into posterior tilt. This stretches the thoracic spine into extension and lengthens the abdominals and anterior intercostals.

We can now also use belly-down positions and a constraining hip. Flex one or both hip joints fully and use the hamstrings/gluteals/hip rotators to limit lumbar extension while you lift head or arm against gravity in manipulation, orientation or transitional functions to require thoracic extension. This strengthens the thoracic extensors.

Variations on using a hamstring constraint

In what other positions could we do this type of movement (Fig. 5.36)? Sit back on your heels and lean with your elbows on the floor in front of your knees. Look forward, reach forward, or place hand and head together and move them as one. Move to three-and-a-half point stance or half kneeling and bend fully over the forward thigh. From here do the same thing. Sit in a chair and lean either straight over both or diagonally over one thigh.

Stand and bend over to place hands on tabletop – chair seat – low stool – the floor – or, for the contortionists out there, place your elbows on the floor. Kneel, sit back on your heels, sit in a chair, or stand and place both hands on the wall while bent over – push your belly and chest toward the floor and look forward toward the wall. Subvariations include placing one hand on the wall or on the chair, stool or floor.

Subvariations involve asymmetrical torso and pelvis movements that side-bend or rotate you in one direction first – then perform movements similar to those described above. The possibilities, although not quite endless, are considerable. Try some out yourself with colleagues and with students. Be creative by keeping in mind the behavior you are attempting to influence, the specific pattern you are trying to create, and the principle of constraining lumbar extension with the flexed hips and strengthening the thoracic extensors.

Our next variation is a mirror image of variation E. Side-sitting is an asymmetrical pelvic and torso position. Could you feel a difference in how the left and right posterior intercostals and thoracic extensors worked when you went to variation F? Could you predict the weaker side from an awareness of your own habitual pattern? Can you predict which side your student will be stronger on, and will you start her off on her stronger side? Is the weaker side for thoracic extension linked to her shorter opposite hamstring?

Lift the hands to require the legs to push

Coming to variations G and H, our next movements raise the ante a bit. You are now asked to slide both hands forward and back at the same time. You have eliminated the possibility of bearing a significant amount of weight through your left hand – there go the training wheels! Can you feel proprioceptively and can you envisage intellectually how much more your left leg has to work to support your weight?

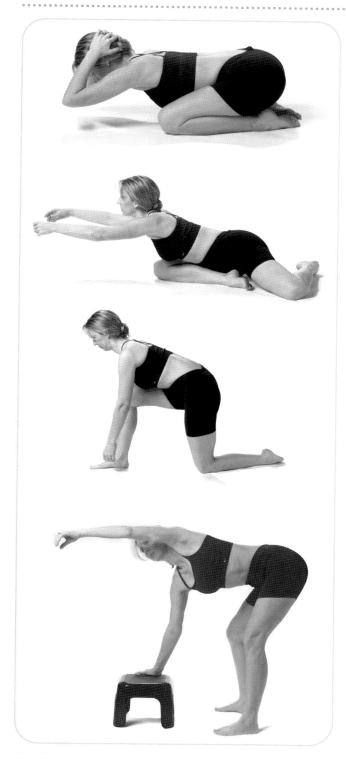

Fig. 5.36 Constraining anterior pelvic tilt with the hip extensors in various positions.

How many hundreds of these do you think you could do before your left hip extensors/rotators get tired? I rarely give my students back or lower extremity exercises to do at home that require either weights or resistive tubing. I tell them that they can strengthen most muscles in their body using gravity, body weight, a floor, a wall, something to pull against (such as stall bars, doorways, railings or ropes) and a little creativity.

You might have noticed yourself, or probably will notice when you do this movement with some of your students, that the right tensor fascia latae also is working hard. It might in fact go into a cramp. This is partly a result of needing to use the right leg as a counterbalance to keep you from toppling over to your left. It may also be driven by the internal rotation component of the right hip when sliding the hands backward. The TFL may be contributing by pulling the right side of the pelvis back and to the right when coming back, or paying out line to control the fall of the pelvis forward and to the left. As you refine your ability to do this movement, the cramping sensation should subside. If not, try placing a couple of folded towels under the left hip and thigh to reduce this strain.

There is an extra credit problem here as well. 'Would you like to lift both hands toward the ceiling from this position?' Many will opt out – that's OK. Having an extensive selection of motor control exercises and an understanding of how to provide a progressive learning experience means that you will have movements in your arsenal that some people simply will be unable to do. For those higher-level students and for athletes, however, you should be able to progress them beyond even what you can do.

The reverse is also true. You should have an understanding of how to modify any of these movements so that those of your students with more limited physical abilities can also participate in a motor learning program. You may have to modify the position, might have to use props, might have to regulate pace and intensity, or might have to limit a lesson to two or three simple variations. You will need to have a clear enough understanding of function to accommodate them.

We asked some questions about bending at the beginning of the analysis of this lesson. We asked about the physical skills (strength, flexibility, coordination, proprioceptive self-awareness) necessary for efficient bending. I hinted that having hamstrings and hip extensors that can elongate adequately to allow a full hip hinge would be nice. How have we stretched the hamstrings in this lesson?

By sliding the hand or hands forward and back, we have been doing reciprocating movements that emphasize lengthening and strengthening of the hamstrings and other hip extensors. This muscle length has been particularly enhanced by sliding the hand/hands forward and by directing a differentiated movement of hip flexion and back extension. This physical skill would be particularly useful for someone who makes the error of flexing too much at the lower back/SI joints when bending.

I hinted that having legs that are strong enough to support the weight and control the angle of the pelvis in space is critical. I asked about which specific muscles needed to be stronger. The advantage of this particular skill might not be as readily apparent as the need for long hamstrings. What many people do when they bend over, or when they lean over to do dishes or cook, or when they transition from sitting to standing, is to incompletely extend their hips and over-rely on their lower back for support. In bending and leaning over, they allow their pelvis to fall too far forward. In coming back to upright, they will lead the movement and make most of the effort of the movement from their back.

Walk in your students' shoes

Get back on the floor and try the following. From left side-sitting, slide both hands forward to about 75% of maximum. From there, bring yourself back upright by first rolling your pelvis backward and rounding your back and then straightening your back to come fully upright only at the end. Do that a few times to get a sense of ease and comfort in your lower back. Now the next time you slide your hands forward, keep your pelvis where it is and bring yourself upright by arching your back. Do this movement a few times to get a sense of ease and comfort in your lower back. Using this concept of trying on your students' habitual movement and postural patterns is one that accelerates your learning and deepens your insight into the workings of the human body. Just don't overcook it and strain yourself!

Can you feel and appreciate how, for someone with a habitual iliopsoas bias and a tendency toward extension stresses, this strategy for bending and coming back upright might be a problem? So, which specific muscles need to be stronger? The hip extensors! Are people going to learn to use them better from doing prone leg lifts or standing theraband? I'm dubious. Doesn't it make more sense to strengthen them in a pattern that looks something like the motor behavior we are trying to change, and to teach it by incorporating a functional intention that bears some resemblance to their reason for bending in the first place?

Bending with a neutral spine

Bending with a neutral spine would be a good idea, but what if someone has been bending with a back either too arched or too round their whole life? To them, it feels as if they are bending with a neutral back. How do we get them to recalibrate neutral? Reciprocating movements. The next part of this variation asks you to alternately slide your hands a little bit forward and back to recognize when your back is arched and when it is round, and to find a place that splits the difference.

It is this ability to find, through movement, where neutral is that enables our students to reproduce a neutral spine during the hundreds of times a day that they bend. From that proprioceptively found rather than habitually programmed neutral position, you then pushed yourself to upright sitting without changing the shape of your back. This is a movement of extending the hip joint, moving the pelvis around the thigh while keeping the spine immobile.

Repeating this movement several times will give you an appreciation for the ability to and the advantage of using your leg both to decelerate your fall forward and to push yourself back up to sitting. This appreciation will be further enhanced by doing the movement very slowly and by pausing at several points along the way to reassess whether you have maintained a neutral spine. Do you have a tendency to err

> **Box 5.14 Side-sit Bending**
>
> Belly-down orientation emphasizes lengthening and strengthening of hamstrings, gluteals and short and stubbies
> Sitting and rolling the pelvis into anterior and posterior tilt – facilitated by controlling falls forward
> Train students to control forward bending stresses – and half arch and full arch students to sit up straight

toward rounding your back too much and not allow your pelvis to spill far enough forward, or do you tend to err toward relying too much on your back extensors and allowing your pelvis to spill too far forward?

Or are you, like Mary Poppins, practically perfect in every way? We will generally teach bending with a neutral spine, but will allow some wriggle room in a nonhabitual direction. For iliopsoas-dominant folks we might suggest they bias themselves a bit toward flexing their back, and for gluteal-dominant folks that they err on the side of extending. There may even be advantages to bending, coming up from bending, lifting from a bent position and pulling something toward you with a flexed back, using myofascial structures to stabilize the back as long as your student isn't habitually biased (gluteal dominant) to do so (Box 5.14).

Change of venue challenges the hamstrings

These final movements in variations I and J challenge the hamstrings a bit more. By doing the same basic movement but with the knee more extended, we are simulating a pattern of movement that more closely approximates a bend from a standing position. The initial variations of this lesson were to establish coordination, pattern recognition, and strength and length of the gluteals and short and stubbies. By straightening the knee, the hamstring is further emphasized.

Note the instructions to allow the thigh to roll into external rotation and to allow the knee to bend as you reach down your leg. Do this because of the tendency of many people to tense their whole thigh when they are trying to stretch their hamstrings. What we don't want is for people to be contracting the muscle they are trying to lengthen: we don't want them driving with the brakes on! We would like them to recognize how to reduce their effort and to discover how to inhibit/relax muscles they are trying to stretch.

We would like them to reset their muscle spindles to a longer length. The roll outward of the thigh is consistent with the rotation of the pelvis in the direction of the straightened leg. If the thigh doesn't rotate outward as the pelvis turns, they are doing something (contracting their adductors or TFL) to prevent it from doing so.

The instruction to allow the knee to bend is what shocks many of my students – 'Is that leee-gul'? It is much more functionally relevant for the hamstring to be long enough to allow free hip flexion with the knee bent at less than 90° than it is to have a fully straightened knee when bending. For most sport and daily activities, it is the proximal hamstring that needs improvement. It is only after achieving complete hip flexion with a slightly bent knee that we should progress the lesson by fully extending the knee.

Contrast this method of hamstring lengthening to traditional means. The traditional versions of sitting on the floor with one leg straight and the other bent and in front, of standing with a foot up on something while bending over to touch the toes or to put head on knee, have some problems. One: without specifically directing our students to do this with an anterior tilt of the pelvis and a straightening of the back, we run the risk of allowing people to flex in the back while flexing also at the hip.

This global relationship, although it may be useful for some functions, doesn't match the differentiated relationship between hips and back that we are most often striving for and that makes up the bulk of matured function. Two: the position of the bent leg on the floor doesn't allow the pelvis to turn fully in the direction of the hamstring we are trying to stretch. Why would we want the pelvis to turn? Why do we want to introduce a horizontal adduction component to this movement?

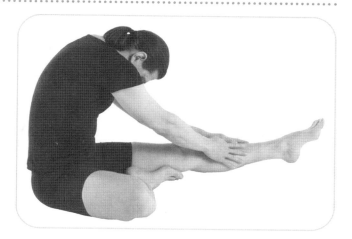

Fig. 5.37 Sitting with bent leg in front constrains rotational and anterior tilt movement of the pelvis – not a good position to lengthen the hamstrings.

Asymmetrical bending requires hip flexion/horizontal adduction hybrid

Although traditional body mechanics instruction has focused on bilaterally symmetrical bending, much of real-life bending involves reaching downward with one hand. When reaching with the right hand toward the ground, for instance, there will be a rotational component as the shoulders and chest turn to the left. Where do we want that rotational movement to occur? Not around the lower back! Perhaps we could train our students to recognize the advantages of turning their pelvis to the left instead; they could learn to rotate their pelvis around their hips rather than twist their lower back around their pelvis.

Just as they did when learning to keep their back neutral in an AP direction when bending, they could also learn to recognize the proprioceptive difference between twisting around their hips with a rotation-neutral spine and twisting at their lower back. We could start them on a learning process of how to recognize neutral spine and how to turn their pelvis to the left when bending by starting in this side-sitting position. Notice the similarities, the pattern specificity, of doing this movement of reaching the right hand toward the left foot while in side-sitting to a movement of reaching toward the floor with the right hand from a standing position.

Contrast this pattern-specific way of coaxing hamstring length while side-sitting to a more traditional posture for stretching the hamstrings – floor-sitting with the bent leg in front (Fig. 5.37). This position constrains movement of the pelvis in rotational and anterior tilt directions. Disallowing movement of the pelvis on the thigh is not a good idea. The side-sitting, or 'hurler's' position, was once used but discontinued because of concerns about the knee of the leg that is bent back.

Whereas it is true that the back knee can be at some risk of being torqued into too much external rotation, there are modifications you can make or precautions you can take that greatly reduce that strain. The first thing to do is to watch out for the orientation of the back foot. If it is dorsiflexed, it is probably pointed outward, creating an external rotation movement at

the knee. Try having your student plantarflex her ankle and turn her heel toward the ceiling as much as possible. This greatly reduces knee rotation. If that is not possible, try propping the inner heel with a small ball or rolled towel. This reduces knee rotation as well.

You could also raise her pelvis with foam blocks or folded towels. If push comes to shove, just don't have her move as far backward. Stay in the forward part of the movement. This reduces demand on the internal rotation mobility of the back hip and reduces strain on the knee. Performed carefully and with attention to detail, this movement from a hurler's position can actually be very beneficial for that back knee. Improving hip and ankle mobility reduces rotational and lateral stresses at the knee.

Let's look at another example: throwing. When a right-handed pitcher throws, he steps forward with the left foot and then powerfully rotates his pelvis to the left. He bends or leans forward as he does this. The whole pattern of movement is again nearly identical to this movement of side-sitting left with the left leg straightened and sliding the right hand toward the foot. Pitching, like bending, requires the hamstrings to be adequately long.

If the hamstrings are not long enough, the ability of the pelvis and legs to contribute their power to the pitch is compromised. This may result in overuse and strain of the shoulder or elbow. This is yet another example of insufficient movement distal to the site of pathology contributing to the onset of that pathology. These are some important reasons to position your student in some variation of this side-sit position when working toward getting more hamstring length. Blocking the rotational movement of the pelvis by placing one foot in front of your pelvis is denying a critically important trajectory in real life movement.

Extra credit assignment

We finished this variation with another extra credit assignment. Would you like to lift your left hip away from the floor and do this same movement? By lifting your left hip, you have to use your left hip extensors, external rotators and abductors to maintain the lift. You are now doing lengthening contractions of those muscles as you slide your right hand toward your left foot. This is just another nuance in gaining motor control over the hip musculature.

It is also another way of making the exercise approximate the activity. This lengthening contraction of the hamstrings and other hip extensors while engaged in vigorous activity is what happens in bending as well. The back leg (right leg if the left leg is straightened) also has to work hard to maintain the lift. If you try this movement again and feel carefully, you will notice how the alternate sliding of the hand up and down the leg and the alternate turning of the pelvis left and right requires a cooperative tug-of-war between the right and left hip extensors.

Neither group of muscles ever really relaxes: they just cooperatively shorten and lengthen by tensioning against each other. It's almost as if the two legs are playing catch with the pelvis! You will need to keep your nearly straightened knee and lateral calf and lateral knee on the floor to avoid varus or rotational stresses at your knee.

After getting increasingly complex and increasingly strenuous during the course of this lesson, we come back once again to our original dynamic baseline. Side-sit and slide one hand forward and back. How does this movement compare to the beginning? Is it smoother and better controlled? Is it easier to lengthen your gluteals, hamstrings and short and stubbies as you slide forward? Is it clearer to you how to use those same muscles to push your thigh and knee into the floor to slide your hand backward? Does this movement seem somehow simpler now? How does that happen?

Story of the farmer and the rabbi

I have heard a few different variations of this story, but I'll tell you the one I heard in my Feldenkrais training program from my trainer, Anat Baniel. There was once a farmer who had a wife, five children and a very small house. After the birth of their fifth child, the farmer went to his local rabbi and complained to him that his house was too small to hold two adults and five children, and he did not have enough money to build a new house. It seemed like an insoluble dilemma. The rabbi thought for a moment then asked the farmer, 'Do you have any chickens?' Perplexed, the farmer answered, 'Of course I have chickens, I am a farmer.' The rabbi then told the farmer to bring the chickens inside the house and to come back to talk with him again the following week.

The farmer was puzzled but did as his rabbi said. The following week the farmer came back in an even more harried state. Not only was the tiny house crowded with two adults and five children, but now 20 chickens, their nests and their deposits were gracing the floors, cupboards and rafters of his tiny abode. Sure that the rabbi had made a mistake, the farmer sought him out again for further advice. The rabbi, instead of admitting his mistake, asked the farmer if he had any goats.

The farmer, a little leery by now, answered yes and cringed at the rabbi's response: bring the goats into the house and

come see me again next week. The resigned farmer did as he was told. By the next week, the frazzled farmer came back to the rabbi who, seeing that the farmer wasn't quite at the end of his rope yet, told him to bring his milk cow into the house. Exasperated but unwilling to openly defy his rabbi, the farmer did as he was told. By now, the house was packed from wall to wall and ceiling to floor with people and critters, and the smell – you can just imagine.

After that week, the worst of his life, he dragged his sorry pelvis back to the rabbi to beg for mercy. The rabbi, seeing the state of the farmer, then told him to go home and put the chickens back in the pens, the goats back in the pasture and the cow back in the barn. The farmer hurried to comply and by the following week was ecstatic. He returned to the rabbi to report how happy he was now that he had so much extra room in his house, and thanked the rabbi profusely.

We have applied the moral of this story both to this lesson and to previous and subsequent lessons: simply, move toward more complex and demanding movements, then come back to the simpler movement again. It will nearly always seem easier than it was at the beginning, even if the more demanding movements were not performed entirely accurately. This is where the rule of allowing approximations comes in. With this approach, perfection is not necessary to make improvements!

Comparing baselines and applications

In this final section, we return to earlier baselines. How was your contact against the floor? How was your weight distributed across your pelvis? How were your legs oriented in external or internal rotation? What was the shape of your back? Once on your feet, how did you organize yourself to bend? How far apart were your feet? What was the shape of your back when bending? When coming back up? How did your hips move as you walked around?

With bending being such an important and potentially damaging function, we will be addressing it again in later lessons, where we will explore ways of facilitating proper bending from chair-sitting and standing. In general, what we would like to see with well-organized bending is a wide base of support, either front to back or side to side, and an ability to create the bulk of the range and power of the movement from the hips.

What type of people might we use this lesson with? Use this with people who complain of low back or SI pain on bending, leaning over (sink, workbench, etc.) or getting up from sitting to standing. Determine whether that person is gluteal or iliopsoas dominant, and do this lesson with both types, but with different emphasis in language and intent, as described above. Use this lesson with people who come to you with posture-related neck and shoulder girdle pain, especially if they have a half arch postural type. You will want ways to facilitate thoracic extension without letting them default to lumbar extension in the way they always do.

Use this lesson with people who have various shoulder and upper extremity tendinitis. Again, we want to facilitate thoracic extension and control over the thoracic extensors and posterior intercostals, in a bilaterally symmetrical but especially in a diagonal or unilateral manner. Use this lesson with various lower extremity injuries or biomechanical faults – ankle sprains, plantar fasciitis, shin splints, patellar tracking dysfunction, hamstring or adductor strains or post acute tears, various knee ligamentous and meniscal strains or post surgical repairs.

Many of our neurologic students would again benefit from this lesson by enhancing trunk control, use of the legs in supporting/controlling forward falls, to reconnect the intention to reach and orient with the pelvis and torso, and as part of a progressive reapplication of lower extremity weightbearing functions. More advanced owners of total hip replacements could use these movements to reaccess the short and stubby arthrokinematic muscles, and can learn to recognize and control movement into end-range horizontal adduction. I wouldn't suggest doing some of these variations with someone with a fresh or problematic total hip replacement.

What sort of athletic or artistic performance could be enhanced with this lesson? We could use this to facilitate the coordination of pelvis, legs and arms in throwing sports such as baseball, football, discus, javelin, shot put or bowling. We could again coordinate pelvis and legs with the upper extremities in racket sports such as tennis, racquetball or squash. The forehand movement, especially when reaching for a lower ball, is very much like bending and throwing. Speed skating, roller-skating and roller-blading are performed in a bent-over position and require long hamstrings and strong hip extensors and abductors. Dancing, gymnastics, figure skating and various martial arts all have motor control over hip musculature in a belly-down orientation as a major component.

Variations

Kneel for a moment then sit back on both heels. Place your hands on the floor in front of your knees. This position requires full knee flexion and full ankle plantarflexion. Some people will be incapable of staying in this position for long, but for those who can it is a dandy place to progress the original lesson.

Start by alternately rounding and arching your back. Can you get a sense of pushing your knees into the ground to round and letting go of the push to arch? Is it possible for you to have enough motor control to do this rounding movement without contracting your belly? How far apart should your knees be? Be Goldilocks. Try it with knees together. It will constrain your ability to anteriorly tilt your pelvis and arch your back. Try it with knees very wide apart. It will constrain your wriggle room from left to right. Try it somewhere around or just barely wider than shoulder width. Is this a nice compromise?

Now as you round, begin to slide both hands toward your knees. Reverse to slide your hands away from your knees as you arch. Alternate several times back and forth to proprioceptively find neutral. From there, lift your hands barely away from the floor. Can you feel your legs push into the ground to support the leaned weight, or do you do this all with your back?

Progress by continuing the movement of lifting your hands and pushing yourself to upright sitting on your heels without changing the shape of your back. Repeat this movement of bending and coming upright several times – bending around your hips and keeping your back neutral. Rest for a bit then come back to the same position. Place both hands on the floor a little in front of your left knee and slide both hands forward and to the left, then back and to the right, by sliding your hands up the front of your left thigh toward your belly.

This is a diagonal version of the same basic movement. Do the same thing to the other side. Now blend the two sides together to make a circle. Slide both hands up the front of your left thigh to your belly, across and down the front of your right thigh to the floor, then along the floor forward and to the right. From there, slide both hands across to the floor directly out in front of you, over to the left, back to your left thigh and so on. Do circles in both directions. You could also work with finding and maintaining a neutral spine in the diagonal variations.

Add in variations of lifting hand or hands when sliding forward to facilitate differentiated thoracic extension. Place one, then both hands on the wall in front of you with both elbows straight and do the AP, diagonal and circular movements with your pelvis and torso. This is a nice latissimus, pectoralis and anterior intercostals stretch. Try working with this position slowly and with attention to detail. Be creative and have fun!

Another version of this same basic lesson can be performed standing. Stand up and lean against a wall so your pelvis is resting on the wall and your hands are supporting the weight of your upper body on your thighs near your knees. Alternately round and arch your back in this position, maybe even link this movement to an intention to look alternately down towards your belly button and forward to the wall in front of you. Can you round without tightening your abdominals?

Add in sliding your hands up the front of your thighs as you round and sliding your hands down the front of your shins as you arch. Find a neutral back with the help of these reciprocating movements, and stay there as you lift your hands away from your thighs a few times. Then, keep your back the same shape as you push yourself upright so your whole back is against the wall. Bend and straighten yourself several times, rotating around your hip joints and keeping your back neutral.

Rest for a bit then resume the same starting position, but this time with both hands on the front of your left thigh. This should turn your pelvis a bit to the left and your right hip should come away from the wall. Slide both hands up the front of your left thigh to your belly while rounding back and to the right in a diagonal movement. Slide both hands back down your left thigh and lower leg as you straighten your back.

Repeat a few times then do the same thing to the other side. Combine the two movements into a circle as in the previous variation of this same basic lesson. You could also work with finding and maintaining a neutral spine in the diagonal variations. Add in variations of lifting one or both hands when slid downward to facilitate differentiated thoracic extension. You can do/teach this same lesson without leaning on the wall behind, though it does provide nice proprioceptive feedback initially. When you do this, you could now place one, then both hands on the wall in front of you with both elbows straight and do the AP, diagonal and circular movements with your pelvis and torso.

This completes our initial section on the role of the legs in balance and orientation. This next section introduces what, for lack of any previous description of this phenomenon that I could find, I call pelvic force couples.

Pelvic force couples

Recall from physics class what a force couple is. It is the action of two separate forces, with opposing directions of pull, acting cooperatively to move a common object. One example would be two people working together to turn a piano to face in the opposite direction. One person stands at the front side of the piano and pushes on the right side while the other person stands at the back of the piano and pushes on the left side. Their forces are in exactly the opposite directions, but the action on the piano is complementary.

Another example would be in turning a canoe. The bow/front paddler does a draw stroke to pull the front of the canoe to the left while the stern/back paddler does a pry stroke to push the back of the canoe to the right. The forces are in opposite directions, but the result is movement of a common object in a desired direction.

There are several examples of force couples in the human body. The serratus anterior and lower trapezius work together to rotate the scapulae upward. The left sternocleidomastoid and the right splenius capitis work together to turn the head to the right. The hip extensors and abdominal muscles work together to move the pelvis into posterior tilt. The hip flexors and back extensors work together to move the pelvis into anterior tilt.

What I mean by a pelvic force couple, however, is the cooperative use of opposite-side iliopsoas and gluteals to rotate the pelvis and to shift weight laterally (Figs. 5.38 and 5.39). The simultaneous activation of the diagonally related cornerstone

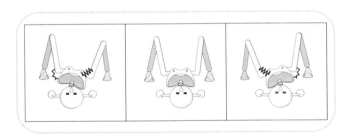

Fig. 5.38 The pelvic force couple – coordinationg the opposite psoas and gluteal groups to shift weight and to turn the pelvis.

muscles provides the power and support for most of the functions that we perform every day. Let's get back down on the floor and see what we can do once we get both paddles in the water at the same time!

Wishbone

Variations

A. Stand for a moment with your legs a comfortable distance apart and with your arms hanging down at your sides.

- How is your weight distributed between your two feet? If you were standing on a pair of bathroom scales, which one would register more weight?
- Notice how your pelvis is balanced on top of your legs. If your pelvis were a bowl filled with liquid, would that liquid be spilling forward or backward? Is your pelvis turned more to the left or right? Is one side of your pelvis higher or lower?

B. Place a low stool in front of you while still standing.

- Slowly lift your left foot to place it on the stool in front of you. Reverse the movement to put your foot back down on the floor. Repeat this several times. Notice:
- How smoothly your weight shifts to the right foot. Do you get taller or shorter?
- Does your pelvis turn left or right as you do this? Do your shoulders turn left or right?
- Where does your left knee end up relative to your hip? Is it to the inside or the outside?
- Where does your left foot end up relative to your knee? Inside or outside? Where does your left foot end up relative to the stool? Are your toes pointed inward, outward or straight forward (Fig. 5.40)?
- Now switch to doing this stepping movement to the other side. Slowly lift your right foot and place it up on the stool. Do this side several times and ask the same questions as above. How does this side compare to the other?

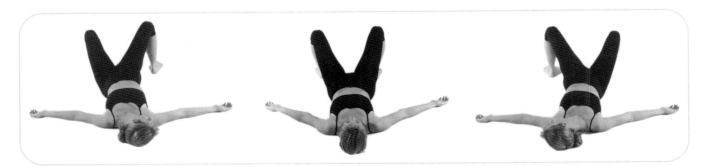

Fig. 5.39 Pelvic force couple – cooperative use of opposite side gluteals and iliopsoas.

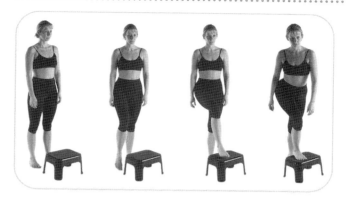

Fig. 5.40 Stepping up on a stool – what do you notice about how you do this?

C. Lie on your back on the floor with your legs out long and straight and with your hands somewhere on the ground below shoulder height.

- Notice your overall sense of contact or support against the floor. Where are you pressing against the floor most heavily, and where are you lifting your bones away from the floor?

- Notice how your weight is distributed across your pelvis. Is there more weight to the right or the left hip?

- Notice where your toes point. Does one leg roll further outward than the other?

D. While still lying on your back, bend up your right knee and place the sole of your right foot flat on the floor. Place your arms on the floor out away from your sides as close to shoulder height as you can. Your left leg is still straight and resting on the floor, angled outward away from your midline.

- Begin to make a small movement of tilting your right knee alternately inward and outward. Feel how the weight shifts on the sole of your right foot alternately towards the inside and outside edges.

- Go back and forth a few times to help you determine where center is – that place where your weight is evenly distributed between your inside and outside edges, and where your knee is balanced in as close to an effortless way as possible over your right foot.

- From there, gently press your right foot into the floor, then slowly release that effort. What is the consequence of this pressing of your foot? What lifts? How does your pelvis move? Does your right foot stay centered (Fig. 5.41)?

- As you press your right foot, allow your right hip to lift away from the floor and your whole pelvis to roll on the floor to your left. Keep your weight evenly distributed across your right foot and keep your right knee pointed still toward the ceiling.

- More specifically, use this pushing movement of your right foot into the floor to roll your pelvis up and to

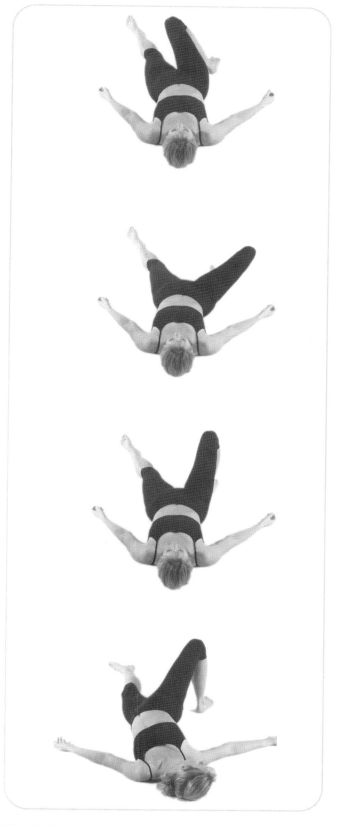

Fig. 5.41 Find center, then press your foot to lift your hip.

173

the left. The left side of your lower back will press into the floor.

- What happens higher up through your back? Do your shoulders or head move? Try pressing your right foot into the floor to roll your pelvis to the left; simultaneously roll your head on the floor to the right as if you wanted to see your right hand.

- Coordinate the movement of your head and pelvis in this movement of rolling in opposite directions.

- Imagine you are wringing out a washcloth. Both ends twist in opposite directions and the movement happens evenly throughout the whole length of your torso.

- Find a way to get your ribcage, chest and mid-upper back to move! Do this movement many times. Coordinate head and tail so they roll in opposite directions, then come back to center at the same time. Pause for a moment.

- Begin a small movement to lighten your right foot from the floor. You don't actually lift your foot, but the intent and the initial effort of lifting will have an effect on your pelvis and back.

- Allow your pelvis to roll down and to the right and your lower back to lift away from the floor a bit (Fig. 5.42). Do this several times.

- Alternate back and forth between pressing and lightening your right foot. How do you coordinate your chest, shoulders and head with this?

E. Bend your right leg up again as before: the left leg is still long and your arms are out at about shoulder height.

- Resume this same movement of pressing your right foot into the floor and rolling your pelvis up and to the left. Coordinate this with your upper body by rolling your head to the right and looking toward your right hand.

- As you continue this movement, begin to add in a movement of bending your left knee and sliding it outward and upward on the floor (Fig. 5.43). Your left hip and knee bend as you drag the heel of your left foot toward your left hip.

- Your left knee will probably lift away from the floor at some point, but keep the left knee hanging out toward the floor as much as possible.

- You are now combining a pressing of your right foot into the floor with a bending of your left hip and a sliding of your left leg up and out. Continue to coordinate the movement of your head and chest with this.

- Do this movement several times then, when you have brought your left foot near your left hip, tilt your left knee up to point toward the ceiling and lower your right hip back to the floor (Fig. 5.43).

- You will pivot across the sole of your left foot and end up in a position where both hips and both feet are on the ground and where both knees are pointing toward the ceiling.

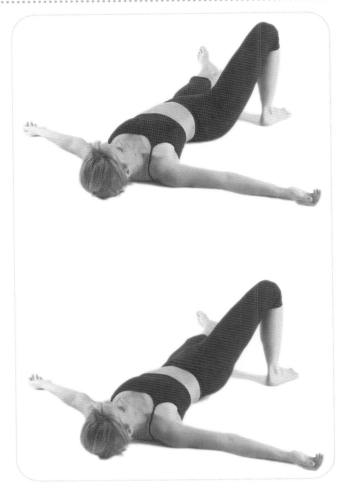

Fig. 5.42 Find center, then lift your foot to press your hip.

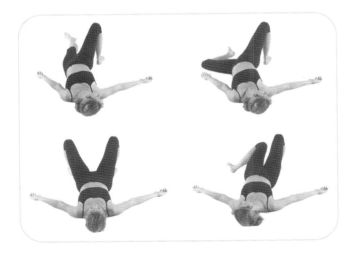

Fig. 5.43 Drawing the knee up – to standing – to tilt inward.

- Reverse this movement to tilt your left knee back outward, pressing your right foot to roll your pelvis to the left, and slide the outside edge of your left leg and foot back down on the floor to straighten your left leg again.

- Repeat this movement of dragging up your left leg, bringing the left foot to standing, then tilting it back outward and straightening it back down again several times.

- Now add in tilting your left knee inward to the right, still keeping your right foot centered on the floor, then tilting the left knee back to center, over to the left and down long again as before (Fig. 5.43).

- The movement is the same but with the addition of tilting the left knee also to the right. Blend these movements together into a seamless whole and coordinate legs, pelvis, chest and head. Try it a few times quickly.

F. Lie on your back and bend up your left leg. Your right leg is straight and arms are out to your sides. Repeat instructions D and E now to the opposite side.

- How does this side compare? Is the pressing left leg stronger or weaker than the right? Is your ability to keep your left foot centered more or less accurate?

- Does your head roll and your chest contort more or less easily to this side?

G. Lie on your back again with your arms away from your sides, but this time with both legs bent up, both feet centered on the floor and both knees pointed toward the ceiling.

- Keeping your right knee upright and your right foot centered on the floor, tilt your left knee toward the floor to your left. Feel free to press your right foot into the floor and roll your pelvis to the left. Reverse to return your left foot to standing and your right hip back to the floor.

- Do the same movement to the other side. Tilt your right knee to the right while keeping your left foot centered. Press with the left foot to roll your pelvis to the right. Do this movement to this side several times.

- Then alternate from side to side (Fig. 5.44). Compare the two sides. Continue to coordinate rolling your head in the opposite direction to your pelvis.

- Pause for a moment with both legs bent.

- Roll your pelvis alternately from side to side but keep both feet centered and both knees pointed to the ceiling (Fig. 5.44). Continue to push a foot into the floor to roll your pelvis. Continue to roll your head and contort your chest and ribcage.

- As you continue this movement alternately from side to side, start to add in lifting one foot a little bit off the floor. When rolling your pelvis to the left, lift your left foot. When rolling right, lift your right foot. Alternate back and forth in this marching movement several times (Fig. 5.44).

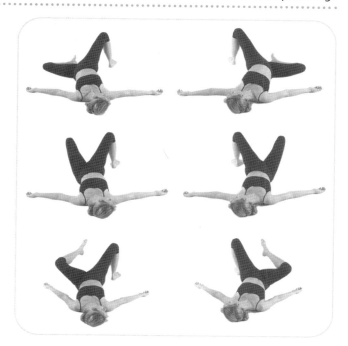

Fig. 5.44 Variations of the same pelvic force couple movements.

H. Lie on your back with your legs long and scan for differences in contact and balance from side to side in comparison to when you began.

- How is your pelvis balanced on the floor side to side? How are your legs arranged?

I. Stand up.

- How is your weight distributed between your two feet? If you were standing on a pair of bathroom scales, which one would register more weight?

- Notice how your pelvis is balanced on top of your legs. If your pelvis were a bowl filled with liquid, would that liquid be spilling forward or backward? Is your pelvis turned more to the left or right? Is one side of your pelvis higher or lower?

- Slowly lift your left foot to place it on the stool in front of you. Reverse the movement to put it back down on the floor.

- Repeat this several times and notice how smoothly your weight shifts to the right foot. Do you get taller or shorter?

- Does your pelvis turn left or right as you do this? Do your shoulders turn left or right?

- Where does your left knee end up relative to your hip? Is it to the inside or the outside?

- Where does your left foot end up relative to your knee? Inside or outside? Where does your left foot end up relative to the stool? Are your toes pointed inward, outward or straight forward?

- Now switch to doing this stepping movement to the other side. Slowly lift your right foot and place it up on the stool. Do this side several times and ask the same questions as above – how does this side compare to the other?

- Walk around a little bit and notice how your pelvis moves. Does it turn at all as you walk?

Deferring the baselines discussion – Wishbone

Because of the complexity of these initial static and dynamic baselines in standing, we are going to defer discussion of them until the end of the lesson. These concepts will be easier to grasp after having some intellectual exposure to the experiential learning you just did. Let's start in the middle, progress to the end, and return to the beginning to finish this off.

The starting position for variation D is supine with the left leg straight and the right leg bent up. Arms are out away from the sides at about shoulder height. The first movements were to press the right foot into the floor and to feel how your pelvis rolls and how your back twists while keeping the right foot centered.

To find center for the foot, we did some reciprocating movements (what a surprise!). Alternately tilting the right knee inward and outward creates sensations of pressure changes on the sole of the right foot and helps you to feel proprioceptively where center is, rather than assuming center to be where you habitually place it. That place where the weight on the foot is evenly distributed between inner and outer edge closely approximates that place where the knee is balanced over the foot and the right hip abductors and adductors are more or less balanced.

Pressing the foot and differentiating hip and lumbar extensors

Once an approximate balance of the right leg is found, you now press your right foot into the floor. Recall the difference between pressing with the quads and pressing with the hamstrings. You have no doubt already figured out that this requires the right hip extensors to work to push the pelvis up and to the left towards 1.30 – this is a right gluteal pattern. Why do we want to keep the foot centered and the knee upright?

This approximates a more accurate skeletal weightbearing arrangement for the lower extremity than if you allow, as many people will do spontaneously, the knee to drift inward. We will revisit this movement in greater detail when we discuss the knee and foot later in this chapter. What this requirement to keep the foot centered does around the hip is to require the hip abductors and external rotators to work along with the extensors – we want this to happen in gait and stepping movements.

Remember the premium we placed on differentiating hip extensors from lumbar extensors in the pelvic tilt lesson and the subsequent bridging variations? This unilateral variation tends to be a place where it is much more difficult for most people to differentiate. We will use this movement diagnostically. We want to determine whether my student is able to fully extend her hip joint. How long does she allow her iliopsoas to become, and how fully can she use her gluteals when unilaterally pushing a foot into the floor?

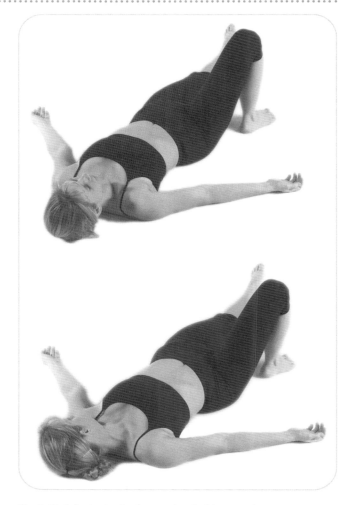

Fig. 5.45 Substituting back extension for hip extension.

We want to determine whether she tends to substitute back extension for hip extension, and can frequently correlate that substitution to unilateral lower back pain (Fig. 5.45). We want to find out whether she is biased toward using her adductors when her intention is to press her foot. Does her knee drift medially and does her weight shift toward the medial edge? We want to determine whether the leg that stays long can be differentiated from the leg that is pushing.

Does she simultaneously contract either the opposite gluteal (both sides of the pelvis will lift forward toward the ceiling) or the opposite adductors (the opposite leg won't roll outward into external rotation – the toes of that foot stay pointed in the same direction as they started)? We want to see if she can move sequentially and in an integrated way from pelvis to head. How does she coordinate head and tail?

Did you find yourself making any of these errors? Can you pick up some of these errors by observing your students do this movement? Once you start watching your students doing complex, noncardinal plane and functionally relevant movements with some understanding of what those errors mean, your observation skills will sharpen and your teaching skills will expand exponentially. Test locally but observe globally.

We also want to connect the movement of the pelvis into a right gluteal direction with a movement of the torso and head – we still want to integrate head and tail. By asking you to roll your head to the right while rolling your pelvis to the left, we are looking for a movement that bends and twists the torso to the right. This would be consistent with a balance reaction. Recall one of the basic rules of balance: as something moves in one direction, something else moves the other way.

This is a basic head-to-tail relationship. Bending the torso to the right would also be consistent with the shift of weight of the pelvis to the left. Be Goldilocks again for a moment and try this movement of rolling your pelvis to the left but rolling your head to the left and bending to the left in coordination. Which way of organizing your head and tail seems most congruent?

Which way of doing this movement goes together like strawberries and cream? Which way goes together like milk and grapefruit juice? Performed accurately, this movement of rolling the pelvis to the left and head to the right will result in a movement of the bottom of the sternum to the left. Move your head in the opposite direction to your pelvis! The bottom of the sternum will point toward the weightbearing hip.

Lifting the foot and differentiating hip and lumbar flexors

The next movement in this variation asks you to lighten your right foot from the floor just a tad. You no doubt recognize this as a right iliopsoas pattern. The iliopsoas group pulls the pelvis down and to the right towards 7.30. The requirement to keep the right foot centered is designed to maintain the skeletal weightbearing integrity of the lower extremity and to require the right adductors to fire with the iliopsoas to assist in pulling the pelvis toward the leg. The left side of the lower back lifts from the floor; the torso could bend to the left and the head could roll to the left in a nearly mirror image of what happens with a right gluteal movement.

Alternating back and forth between pressing and lightening your foot is a reciprocating effort between the right gluteal/abductor/external rotators and the right iliopsoas/adductors. Although this is not really a new movement, it isn't exactly easy either. There is a lot to juggle and a lot of muscles you could be unnecesssarily contracting that are getting in your way. You'll probably have to take some time to figure this one out.

Pay particular attention to an ability to lighten the foot/contract the iliopsoas while inhibiting the belly. Pay particular attention to your ability to press your right foot and to contract your gluteals while inhibiting your back extensors. Pay particular attention to your ability to differentiate!

Pressing one foot and lifting the other – scissoring the legs

So far, this has been a review of unilateral cornerstone use. In variation E, we start making combination movements of the two legs by having an intention to lift one foot while pressing the other. When in real life do we do this? Any time we take a step: walking, running, climbing stairs, stepping up on a stool or anytime we lift one foot away from the ground while standing. This applies to stepping movements in martial arts, dance, tennis, javelin or speed skating. This even applies to swimming and cycling. We are now starting to get into the critically important function of locomotion.

What is the best way to walk? To run? What are some common errors in gait/locomotion that people make? How do those errors manifest themselves in overuse injuries? How do people make walking a repetitive stress injury? How do those errors manifest themselves in performance inefficiencies? How do they provide a drag on speed or endurance? How can we design an exercise program that progressively teaches someone to walk/run/climb/step better? What are some fundamental principles common to the large number of locomotion versions that we do?

Locomotion is central to our ability to get around, to be independent. It is a skill nearly everyone (with an intact CNS and neuromusculoskeletal system) can do, so we tend to take it for granted. And if we don't possess the ability to locomote, we are severely compromised in our independence. Walking is a big deal to people with hip or knee replacements, lower extremity injuries or surgery, stroke, balance problems or amputations.

Gait types – grossly simplified

However, not everyone possesses the same level of skill. There are many different versions of walking: go to a mall or an airport and just watch people for a while as they walk. There is an incredible variety of gait and body types. Are the feet parallel as they walk? Duck-footed? Pigeon-toed? Are the knees bowed? Knocked? Are the stride lengths the same? How does the pelvis move? Does it rotate in space? If so, does it rotate symmetrically to each side? Or is it rotated to one side and stuck there?

Does the pelvis side-bend – do one or both sides drop with each step? Does the torso side-bend? Does it rotate? Do the arms swing? If so, do they swing from the elbows? Shoulders? Shoulder girdles? Or as an extension of the movement of the mid-upper back? How is the head balanced? Do the eyes stay horizontal? Are they on the horizon? Is there any rotational or side-bending movement at the cervicothoracic (CT)s or SO junctions?

Gait is incredibly complex and no one does it 'right.' We all have imperfections and imbalances that are woven into this function as surely as they are woven into balance, orientation and transitional functions. With no owner's manual for growing up, we all stumble upon a way of doing things that works, call it good, and continue the same basic patterns throughout the rest of our lives. Retraining gait patterns is difficult and perfection is impossible. But people can and do change, sometimes quite quickly.

Even if they improve the quality of their gait just a little bit or even just some of the time, it is definitely worth the effort to teach them some basic proprioceptive awareness and pattern recognition skills around this function. And for people who have lost the ability to walk, starting them on the floor where they can safely explore stepping movements without fear of falling can be just the ticket.

Locomotion – training the pelvic force couples

Let's start to look at some basics on how locomotion might be organized, and answer some of the questions about gait that we just asked as we go along. Some of the answers will be provided in the analyses of this lesson. Some answers we will get to subsequently in this chapter. Some of the questions, especially on the role of the upper extremities and the movements of the head, we will defer to the next section.

This first combination movement features a continuation of the movement of pressing the right foot into the ground and rolling the pelvis on the floor to the left with a movement of bending the left knee outward and dragging the outside edge of the left foot up on the floor toward the left hip. We know pressing the right foot is the responsibility of the right gluteal group.

You have no doubt already figured out that dragging the left heel toward the left hip is the responsibility of the left iliopsoas group. It is this combination of one-sided gluteals with opposite-sided iliopsoas that we will call a *pelvic force couple*. Where on the imaginary clock will this combination move the pelvis? If the right gluteal pushes the pelvis to 1.30 and the left iliopsoas pulls it to 4.30, 3 o'clock would split the difference – if the iliopsoas and gluteals were perfectly balanced.

With an iliopsoas-dominant person, the pelvis might gravitate downward a bit on the clock, to 3.45 or 4.12, say. With a gluteal-dominant person, the pelvis might gravitate upward a bit, to 2.32 or 1.58. Regardless of the bias, we would expect the pelvis to turn to the left in some manner when the left iliopsoas and right gluteal groups are working together.

Put another way, we would like to see the pelvis turn to the left when stepping with the left foot. Let's take a look at gait from a developmental standpoint for a moment to see if this general tendency of the pelvis to turn in the direction of the stepping leg is present in precursor movements to walking.

In a commando crawl, when drawing up the left knee in a stepping movement the left hip flexes, the right hip extends and the pelvis turns to the left (Fig. 5.46). The left side of the pelvis moves back toward the ceiling and the right side moves

forward toward the floor. From here, the left hip extends to help propel you forward, the right hip flexes up and out as the right knee is drawn up on the floor, and the pelvis turns to the right. Therefore the commando crawl, as an early form of locomotion, exhibits this general tendency of the pelvis to turn in the direction of the stepping leg.

In creeping or hands-and-knees crawling, the same tendency is present. When lifting the left knee from the floor to take a step forward with that knee, the left hip flexes, the right hip extends to help propel you forward and the pelvis turns to the left (Fig. 5.46). The left side of the pelvis moves backward toward the ceiling and the right side drops and moves forward toward the floor. From here, the left hip now extends to take the next step forward, the right hip flexes and the pelvis turns to the right. Therefore creeping, as an intermediate form of locomotion, exhibits this general tendency of the pelvis to turn in the direction of the stepping leg.

In the transitional movement from hands and knees to standing, the same tendency is present. When placing the left foot on the ground near the left hand, the left hip flexes, the right hip extends and the pelvis turns to the left (Fig. 5.46). Are you starting to see where this might lead? In locomotion, we want the pelvis to be turning in the direction of the stepping foot (Fig. 5.46). This would be consistent with the evolution of gait during the developmental sequence, would reduce many of the repetitive stress injuries we see related to gait, and would be biomechanically more efficient and allow for more powerful stepping movements and for faster and more energy-efficient locomotion.

Because we have just reviewed the evolution of gait and have seen this general tendency of the pelvis to turn in the direction of the stepping leg, let's take a look at how this might contribute to the reduction of overuse injuries. We will defer the effects on the knees, ankles and feet until later in the section. For now, let's talk about the effects around the lower back.

Every part is an island – the doll body walk

Although there are tons of individual quirks and subvariations in walking, there are four common types. The first is the 'curse-of-the-doll-body walk.' The doll body, you may recall, has a solid plastic torso/pelvis with arms, legs and neck that move from their articulations relative to an immobile torso, rather than being integrated with a moving torso. This type of walk tends to look stiff, with a relatively short stride length. There is little to no movement of the pelvis either laterally or in dropping or rotational directions (Fig. 5.47).

The arms, if they swing, will probably do so from the elbows or shoulders. The shoulder girdles and ribcage are relatively immobile, and the head doesn't move much in rotational or translatory directions. The consequences of this gait type on the lower back is to lock in AP and left/right imbalances, and to provide additional scaffolding for invariant joint, connective tissue and muscular strain.

In other words, it doesn't matter much whether they are walking, standing, sitting or dancing the mambo. Tissue strain on the lower back is the same because no variable movements are present. This type also tends to have a bit of a jarring walk. Because there is no give or shock absorption in the hip joints

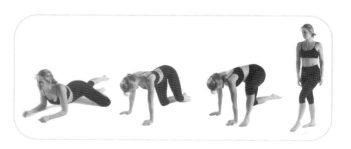

Fig. 5.46 Pelvic force couples in action – each step borrows from the previous one.

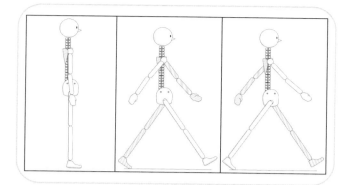

Fig. 5.47 Controlling rotational and lateral stresses through compartmentalization – the doll body walk.

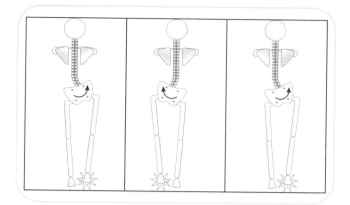

Fig. 5.49 Lateral shear gait stresses – the swish walk.

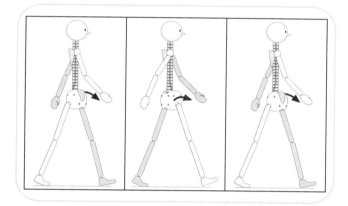

Fig. 5.48 Rotational gait stresses – the waddle walk.

or throughout the ribcage on heel-strike, compression might be another irritant at the lower back.

Rotational shearing – the waddle walk

Another common gait type is the one where people rotate a lot around their lower back. This waddling form of locomotion has as its outstanding characteristic the rotation of the pelvis in the direction of the push-off leg (Fig. 5.48). For instance, when stepping forward with the left foot, they will rotate their pelvis to the right. Think for a moment of the contralateral nature of walking: as the right leg pushes off, the left arm swings backward. As the left leg swings forward to step, the right arm swings backward.

Stand up for a moment and try walking homolaterally: swing left leg and arm forward at the same time as you move your right leg and right arm backward. While it makes for a convincing Frankenstein walk, it won't get you around very fast or very efficiently. Given that to have an integrated contralateral gait you need to twist somewhere, we might want to be aware of where we and our students rotate.

In a waddling gait, the legs are swinging from the torso and there will probably be a lot of rotation happening around the lower back. To make matters worse, we will also often see an immobile chest and thoracic spine ribcage that goes along with this. Without some movement contribution from farther up, it puts even more demand for movement at the lower back.

In more extreme cases, what you might see is a completely immobile head, shoulder girdles, arms and back, with a pelvis that is twisting around the mid-lower lumbar segments. To stabilize these folks, you will have to provide them with another alternative to movement at the lower back. The multifidi and transverse abdominis are incapable of stabilizing intersegmentally in this kind of environment.

Lateral shearing – the swish walk

Another version of a waddling gait and with very similar consequences is lateral shearing (Fig. 5.49). On heel-strike, there is too much of a drop of the opposite hip through an under-utilization of the abductors on the weightbearing side. The pelvis shears laterally, again very often underneath a torso that contributes not a whit of side-bending. This is also not a good idea!

We will very often see unstable SI and lumbar ligaments/ joint capsule and shearing, degenerating or blown discs with this sort of gait as well. These folks need to be stabilized too, not just with intersegmental torso strength but with an understanding of how to stabilize and to properly mobilize their pelvis on top of their legs. These folks, as well as the waddlers, could benefit from learning a force couple gait.

The pelvic force couple walk

A force couple gait features a rotation of the pelvis in the direction of the stepping leg (Fig. 5.50). Think again of our contralateral gait. In an integrated system, as the left arm swings back the shoulders and chest will turn a little to the left. As the right arm swings forward, the chest and shoulders will turn a little to the left. We will be working with the upper extremity contribution to gait in the next volume, but for now keep in

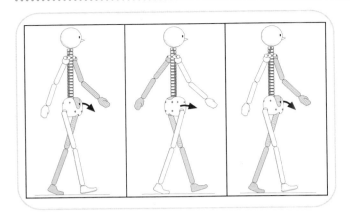

Fig. 5.50 Controlling rotational and lateral stresses through integrated movement – the force couple walk.

mind that we would like the shoulders and chest to turn in cooperation with the swinging arms.

If the chest turns to the left when the left arm swings back, what is happening at the legs and pelvis? When the left arm swings back, the left leg is stepping forward and the right leg is pushing off. In a force couple gait, the pelvis is turning in the direction of the stepping leg: the pelvis is turning to the left. In this type of gait, we have the pelvis and shoulders/chest turning in the same direction. This reduces rotational and lateral shear strains at the lower back as the turning of the pelvis now happens around the hip joints rather than around the lower back.

I think it is not coincidental that whereas most degenerative low back conditions result from too much movement, most degenerative hip conditions derive from not enough movement. Too much movement overstretches ligaments and joint capsule, strains and shears the annulus fibrosus, and mashes articular cartilage as the physiological limits of the joint are violated. Too little movement creates compression invariance on articular cartilage. Because cartilage requires intermittent compression and decompression to spread and work into the tissue the synovial fluid that is responsible for oxygen and nutrient delivery to the chondroblasts, invariant compression is damaging.

Those places that are always compressed can't get enough synovial fluid. Those places that are seldom compressed don't get synovial fluid delivered to them through the spatula effect of one bone moving on another. So much of what we see clinically is this combination of too little movement at the hip joints and too much at the lower back. Although the trend towards lumbar stabilization has been a positive development in the treatment of lower back pain, we also need to take a larger view.

In the presence of imbalanced, immobile or inefficient hip joints, it will be much more difficult to stabilize the low back using worm strategies. The Tyrannosaurus is much more competent. Training belly and back to support the lumbar spine while moving in the right direction is not even close to the whole story. Training our students to have

fully functioning and (more or less) balanced pelvic force couples can make the work of those intersegmental stabilizers much easier.

Advantages of a force couple gait

Does a pelvic force couple gait have any biomechanical advantages? Yes. Much of the power of a truly propulsive gait comes from the largest muscles in the body: the gluteals and hamstrings. You may have noticed that when contracting these bad boys to press your right foot into the floor, the right side of your pelvis moved forward. Lie supine for a moment with your legs long. Contract your right gluteals; pinch your right cheek. Does your pelvis roll to the left?

Come up to sit on the floor with your legs long – lean on your hands behind you. Pinch your right cheek. Does your pelvis turn to the left? Come up to kneel and pinch your right cheek. Does your pelvis turn to the left? Come up to stand on both feet and pinch your right cheek. Do you allow your pelvis to turn to the left? Alternate a few times between left and right cheeks while standing (or any of these positions). Get a rhythm going and turn your pelvis alternately from side to side. Can you discern a difference from side to side?

Try placing your left foot forward on the floor when standing and pinch your right cheek. Does your pelvis turn to the left? Here's the point. When contracting the hip extensors powerfully, the foot pushes off backward against the floor and that side of the pelvis moves forward. Powerful gluteal use results in a turn of the pelvis away from that leg as part of its external rotation component.

External rotation of the femur relative to the pelvis occurs with gluteal contractions with the foot free; in an open kinetic chain environment, the femur is the insertion and the pelvis is the origin. However, when the foot is on the ground, the origin and insertion reverse and it is the pelvis that moves by turning away from the side of gluteal contraction.

Full contraction of the gluteals and a turn of the pelvis away from that side also result in lengthening the iliopsoas on that side. One benefit is that we can repeatedly stretch a tight iliopsoas with more gluteal emphasis when walking. Another benefit is that the lengthened iliopsoas becomes spring-loaded. A fully extended hip and a fully contracting gluteal complex set up the next part of the reciprocating movement: a powerful iliopsoas-driven step forward.

As the right iliopsoas swings the right leg forward, it acts in concert with the left gluteal group to turn the pelvis now to the right. The right hip flexes and does a hybrid version of hip horizontal adduction/internal rotation to provide a soft landing for the right foot. As the right heel strikes the floor, the right hip is in a position to absorb shock through a lengthening contraction of the right abductors/extensors/external rotators. This in turn spring-loads the right gluteal group again and facilitates the next part of the reciprocating movement: a powerful and gluteal-driven push-off. What an incredibly elegant design!

Full gluteal use facilitates full iliopsoas use and vice versa. I sometimes use a particular image with my students. Pretend your feet are like hands and you are reaching out to actively grab the floor, and that you are then pushing the floor behind you with that foot as you simultaneously reach out to grab the

Box 5.15 The pelvic force couple

The cooperative use of opposite sides – left gluteals with right iliopsoas and vice versa

Two oppositional forces having a common effect on an object – left gluteals push and right iliopsoas pulls to turn pelvis to the right

Central to locomotion – walk, run, bike, climb and swim

Central to manipulation – push, pull, throw, punch or swing bat/club/racket

floor with the other foot, which pushes the ground behind you and so on.

This makes walking more intentional, more dynamic, more active, more aggressive and somehow less civilized. This makes for a longer stride and a faster step. This reciprocating scissoring movement of a well coordinated pelvic force couple gait is central to both reducing overuse strains at the lower back and lower extremities and to improving the grace and efficiency of performance activities involving reciprocating steps, such as running, cycling, swimming, skating and cross-country skiing.

Keep in mind that although this has been a description of four common gait types, there are many subvariations. The most common of these involve left-to-right imbalances. These people may walk by turning their pelvis in only one direction; this could be a half-waddle or a manifestation of a dominant force couple. They may walk with their pelvis constantly turned in one direction. Sometimes the pattern you see will make no sense at all. No matter! Train them toward balanced force couple movements in stepping, bending, reaching, transitions and gait, and cross your fingers (Box 5.15).

Changing motor behavior in another human being will always be an inexact science. Don't get too attached and don't feel too responsible for a certain outcome. Our job is to teach, to provide a framework for learning. Although the skill of the teacher certainly matters, the willingness and ability to learn on the part of the student is paramount. You will save yourself a lot of grief and hand wringing if you accept this fact.

Force couples rule!

After our little digression into gait, let's return now to an analysis of this lesson. Keep in the back of your mind how this lesson and much of the rest of this chapter is devoted to facilitating pelvic force couples. Keep in mind also that the pelvic force couples are not only central to walking/running/stairs, but are also linked to many transitional movements, reaching movements, and even balance and orientation.

Look back to the Side-sit Spirals lesson on orientation left and right along a horizon, and you will recognize the central role of the pelvic force couple. Look back on the sitting circles lesson and you'll recognize how combining opposite iliopsoas and gluteals gets your pelvis to move around the clock from 1.30 to 4.30 and from 7.30 to 10.30. Pelvic force couples are central to left–right weight shifting and side-to-side balance reactions.

Look forward to Side-sit Transitions and recognize the central role of the pelvic force couples in some transitional movements. Look forward to reach to roll and the archer to

see how pelvic force couples are linked to reaching/manipulation. Force couples are rampant in both sports and everyday activity. Force couple imbalances contribute to or even lead to structural and muscle imbalances through lower extremities, torso, shoulder girdles, neck and arms.

Ignore the relationships of pelvic AP and force couple imbalances to lower back movement impairments at your own peril. Ignore the relationships of pelvic force couple inefficiencies to lower extremity biomechanical faults to the detriment of your students. Ignore the contribution of pelvic and force couple imbalances on the shoulder girdle and neck and be prepared to suffer the consequences.

Ignore the pelvic force couples incompetence with total hip, total knee, lower extremity prosthesis or quad cane owners and prepare to ask their forgiveness. Pelvic cornerstone and force couple balance is central to the healthy and efficient organization of the entire musculoskeletal system! Don't ignore it!

Slide the foot to simulate the step

We left off our review of this lesson with a combination of pressing the right foot into the ground and sliding the left leg up on the floor. Why slide the left leg up in this exaggerated external rotation of the left hip? One reason is that the iliopsoas will not only flex the hip but externally rotate it as well.

We are emphasizing the flexion/external rotation of the left hip to facilitate activation of the left iliopsoas. Another reason is that this way of flexing the hip harkens back to an earlier developmental movement: it mimics the movement of the leg in a commando crawl. Another reason to do this is to get a wide separation of the two legs – the adductors on both sides, especially the left, have to lengthen.

Why the emphasis on sliding the left heel toward the left hip? A very common error that many people make when doing this movement is to slide the left heel toward the right hip. This emphasizes more the bending of the left knee. The left hamstring is used rather than the left iliopsoas; the focus for the CNS is more to bend the knee than to bend the hip.

Get back on the floor and feel the difference yourself: that way, when you see one of your students make what appears to be a minor error in this movement, you will more readily be able to recognize it and direct them toward more focused hip movement. As you reverse the movement to slide the left leg back down long, you are extending your left hip, flexing your right hip and turning your pelvis relative to where it was to the right. This is a version of the force couple movement too!

The next movement in this variation is to slide the left leg up again on the floor and then to tilt the left knee to point toward the ceiling. This brings the left foot to standing on the floor. To lift the left knee, the left adductors have to fire. How come the left adductors don't pull the pelvis to the left? How is it that you are able to roll your pelvis back to the right again to get your right hip back on the floor? Although there are possibilities that involve the use of the abdominal obliques, a more elegant solution and one that we are trying to facilitate is contraction of the right adductors. This pulls the pelvis to the right and drives the right side of the pelvis back toward the floor. This might become clearer in our next movement.

Pulling the opposite leg toward the standing leg with the adductors

Tilting now the left knee to the right while still keeping the right foot centered and the right knee pointed to the ceiling requires the use of the right adductors in pulling the pelvis across to the right. Rolling the pelvis to the right on the ground is required to fully tilt the left knee inward to the right. This is best performed by the right iliopsoas. Returning the left knee to standing could involve the left hip abductors and external rotators, but would preferably involve pressing again with the right hip extensors/abductors/external rotators to roll the pelvis back to the left.

The left knee tilts back to the left by simply going along for the ride. Tilting the left knee outward stretches both adductors. Tilting the left knee back up to standing strengthens both adductors. This is another reciprocating movement that helps to lengthen, strengthen and balance antagonists. Tilting the left knee to the right lengthens the hip external rotators on both sides and strengthens the right adductors and iliopsoas. Tilting the left knee back to standing from this position strengthens both (preferably mostly the right) abductors and external rotators. This is yet another possible reciprocating movement. This adductor/abductor coordination is both linked to our iliopsoas/gluteal-based pelvic force couples and makes up an auxiliary pelvic force couple itself.

Putting the whole thing together into a seamless whole, especially when mindfully integrating your head/neck/upper torso with movements of the legs/pelvis/lower torso, requires some concentration. We have added in some chickens and some goats. Try this faster to see if the coordination of the movement can become more spontaneous, more automatic, less trying to do five separate things at once and more doing one thing with many interrelated parts.

In variation F we have a repeat of the instructions of the last two sections, but to the opposite side. How was your ability to accurately and fully press your left foot into the floor in comparison to the right? Could we expect a right-handed person to be stronger and more accurate in pressing the right foot? Yes, unless some other factor besides normal development changes things, such as injuries past or present. Could we expect a right-handed person to bend/twist through her torso more easily to the right while pressing that right foot? Probably, again with a few disclaimers. How are your own comparisons and awareness of personal idiosyncrasies going?

Reciprocating force couples – tilting and marching

In variation G we start out with a review of the single knee tilts to both sides and then progress to alternating movements. This sets the scene for the alternating force couple movements that we are leading up to. After alternately tilting one knee then the other to the outside and coordinating it with the pushing of the opposite leg, we segue into a movement that is nearly identical but with an important twist.

While still rolling your pelvis from side to side and alternately pressing one foot into the floor, you now keep both knees upright instead of tilting one knee to the outside. This requires the adductors on the side the pelvis is rolling toward to fire to keep that knee from falling outward and is a variation on a pelvic force couple: one leg is pushing the pelvis away while the other is pulling the pelvis toward. This allows both feet to remain centered.

Think of our stepping movement at the beginning and the end of the lesson. If we did a literal translation of our first force couple version, where we pushed with one leg and dragged the foot and leg out wide on the floor, we would end up with the toes of the stepping foot pointed markedly out to the side. This is not what we want. The responsibility for keeping the legs from going into external rotation when stepping lies with the adductors, which we are conveniently training in this variation.

The culmination of this lesson, the *coup de grace*, is the marching movement at the end. We do another segue, this time from rolling the pelvis from side to side while keeping both feet centered to lifting the foot that the pelvis is rolling toward. This marching movement is a pelvic force couple that simulates what we would like to have happen in stepping and walking. By lifting a foot, we are getting the iliopsoas to fire.

By keeping the knee pointed to the ceiling, we are getting the adductors to fire with the iliopsoas. This is what needs to happen in walking and stairs if you are going to keep the feet oriented forward instead of pointing outward (abducting) with each step (this would happen if it were just the iliopsoas that worked). By doing this as an alternating or reciprocating movement, we are not only coordinating antagonists through both hips and torso, but also are coordinating oppositional pelvic and torso movement patterns. This silly movement looks something like real life! You will also see other versions of this silly movement throughout the rest of this section.

Comparing baselines

Let's now take a look at our beginning and ending static and dynamic baselines after getting a glimpse into the workings of pelvic force couples. Starting in supine, could the roll of the pelvis toward one side or the other be a reflection of pelvic force couple imbalances? Could the angle of the legs and feet tell us something about adductor tone?

We then move to standing and ask some questions about static and dynamic baselines. Where is your weight? Proprioceptively, one can feel differences in weight from side to side. As a practitioner, you can visualize a plumb line from the middle of the pubic bone hanging down toward the ground. If the plumb is closer to the left foot, there is more weight to the left. The opposite is true to the other side.

You can also gently palpate the greater trochanters or iliac crests and just barely suggest a weight-shift left and right. This needs to be a whispered suggestion rather than a shouted demand. What you are feeling for is what direction moves most easily initially. You'll have to practice this with several people to get an idea what to feel for. Sometimes it's obvious to both you and your student, and sometimes not. Try it anyway and gather what information you can.

You may notice that when weight shifts markedly, there is a lowering or dropping of the opposite side of the pelvis. As you shift weight to the right, the left side of the pelvis tends to drop. This happens as well with subtle differences

---

Box 5.16 Wishbone

Supine facilitation of pelvic force couples

Variations sliding and lifting the leg – simulates taking a step

Variations tilting knees in and out – stimulates pressing and lightening opposite foot

---

in weight distribution. This may call into question the reliance on X-rays to assess bony landmarks and true leg length discrepancies.

Are bony landmarks really what they seem?

Some of the assessment tools used in physical therapy, osteopathy and chiropractic come from the assumption that both legs are supporting the pelvis evenly and that the four cornerstone muscles are balanced. From here, we assess levels of ASIS, PSIS, ischial tuberosities and so on. Although this is neither a primer nor a critique on this type of assessment, if imbalanced bony landmarks are what you base your assessment of up-and-down slips, in-and-out flares and other SI structural imbalances on, they could be leading you astray.

Differences in gluteal, hip rotator, iliopsoas and adductor tone will mimic some of the bony landmark relationships associated with SI dysfunction. Sometimes it is the pelvis as a whole that is rotated, tipped or shifted in space, and that may relate to the SI imbalances. Right abductor bias (part of a right gluteal bias) will push the pelvis onto the left leg. Left adductor bias (part of a left iliopsoas bias) will pull the pelvis onto the left leg (Box 5.16).

How the pelvis is organized from there depends on what the weightbearing leg is doing. We had a question about whether you got taller or shorter when shifting weight to lift your foot and placing it up on a stool. If you get shorter, you are allowing your pelvis to sink around the weightbearing leg while the opposite side of the pelvis drops. Recall your earlier experiment on grounding your foot while standing on one leg. If you sink, you are not actively using your hip extensors and abductors.

If you get taller, you are grounding; you are using the weightbearing hip extensors and abductors to lift the opposite side of the pelvis or to prevent it from falling. There are so many factors involved in how the pelvis is organized in space in both sitting and standing that there can be no firm and fast rules about making assumptions on muscle imbalances or structural imbalances from observations of bony landmarks – sorry! This is not to claim that SI up-slips, out-flares, etc. do not exist. What I believe is that they are often part of a larger pattern of muscular and functional imbalances, and that to treat them effectively a larger view of things is very useful.

Are you spilling your guts?

Is your pelvis spilling its contents forward or back? This is a question about gluteal or iliopsoas bias. Is your pelvis turned one way or the other on top of your legs? This is a question of force couple bias. If the pelvis is turned in space to the left, it could mean that the left iliopsoas and right gluteal groups are domi-

nant. This we will call a left force couple (name it after the dominant iliopsoas and after the direction that the pelvis turns). If the pelvis is turned to the right, it could mean that the right force couple is dominant. As always, take care that you don't make these into rules – there are too many other factors and too many different ways people can move and compensate.

When stepping up with one foot on to a low stool, when doing our dynamic baseline, we asked a few questions. How smoothly does your weight shift to the right foot? This is a question of quality and ease. We want people to have a subjectively positive change. Do you get taller or shorter? This is a question of whether you actively ground with the weightbearing leg as you shift weight on to it.

Does your pelvis turn left or right as you do this? This is a question about whether a pelvic force couple is being used and about how the two sides compare – if you do it at all, which side is dominant? Do your shoulders turn left or right? This is a question of integration of upper and lower body and may give us clues about chest and ribcage mobility.

Where does your left knee end up relative to your hip? Is it to the inside or outside? This is a question about adductor/abductor balance. A very common pattern you will see with your students is one where the knee is adducted relative to the hip. This puts knee and foot at risk as the organization of the step determines the organization of the subsequent push-off. Where does your left foot end up relative to your knee? Inside or outside? Where does your left foot end up relative to the stool? Are your toes pointed inward, outward or straight forward? This is a question about knee rotation, and we will address this later on in the chapter on lower extremities.

Applications

What are we going to use this lesson for? This is a great beginning lesson in a progressive sequence of gait training for any number of neurologic and medical problems. Use lifting the unaffected leg to stimulate pressing the affected leg in stroke. Drag the long affected leg up and out on a sliding board, or progress to add weights. Facilitate ankle dorsiflexion in this pattern by timing with iliopsoas. Facilitate hip extension in the affected leg for stroke students by focusing on dragging the leg of the unaffected side up on the floor by keeping the knee down – this requires rolling of the pelvis and provides a constraint that requires using the affected/standing leg. In addition to being a basic lesson that we could use with almost all lower extremity injuries and biomechanical faults, we could use this for lumbar stabilization.

I know it's not the classic tighten-your-belly-and-stay-rigid approach, but I don't think that lumbar stability requires whole-body rigidity. What we are training our students to do is to develop an ability to control the position of the pelvis from the legs. In particular, we will tend to emphasize the pushing function of the standing leg and mobility at the lumbothoracic junction and higher. We will do more on stabilization in a later section of this chapter, where we will also do a progressive variation of this lesson called TA Leg Lifts.

Use this lesson with variations and progressions, with athletes and performance artists where accurate and powerful use of the legs is needed.

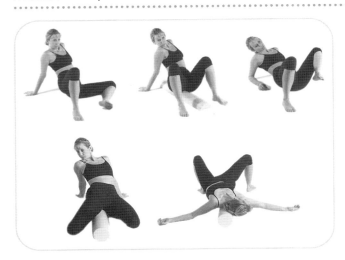

Fig. 5.51 Wishbone variations – facilitation with toys.

Variations

Positional variations for this lesson can be performed sitting on the floor and leaning back on your hands behind. Bend one leg up and draw the long leg up on the floor so the heel of that foot slides toward the hip on that side. From there, tilt that sliding leg up to stand, tilt it to the inside while the original standing foot stays centered, then tilt the original sliding leg back out again to slide it down long. Repeat this to the other side, then bend both legs up. Tilt legs alternately, pushing with the standing leg. Now keep both feet centered and both knees pointed toward the ceiling and roll your pelvis from side to side. Finish it off with the marching movement. The steps are just about identical to those of Wishbone (Fig. 5.51).

One of the advantages of this variation is that the torso, chest and shoulders are a bit freer to move. You can more easily facilitate swinging the bottom of the sternum toward the weightbearing hip with your hands in this position. This helps your students feel the advantages of integrated movement and allowing mobility through their thoracic spine.

It is also a closed kinetic chain exercise for the upper extremities that emphasizes contractions of the latissimus dorsi and lower trapezius opposite the sliding or outwardly tilting leg. The disadvantage is that bearing weight through the hands can be difficult for those with delicate or sensitive wrists. This can be ameliorated somewhat by leaning back on the elbows and forearms instead, either all the way back on the floor or leaning back on a couch, stool or similar structure.

Toys

Try this toy variation to the floor-sitting version of the Wishbone. Roll up a towel tightly. Use an 18-inch long and 1½-inch diameter semi-hard roller for this. Have a zippered sleeve sewn to cover a soft foam roller with the described dimensions, then take out the foam and stuff the cover with polyester fabric remnants. It has a great consistency: foam is too soft and closed-cell foam tends to be a bit too firm for some folk.

Use another such semi-hard roller made the same way but it is 3 inches long and 3 inches in diameter. A rolled-up towel works okay but tends to flatten out too much – try wrapping it tightly and securing it with several rubber bands or duct tape. I prefer low-tech toys because my students are much more likely to follow up with them at home.

Place the roller lengthwise under your pelvis and do any of the movements described in the sitting variation (Fig. 5.51). The advantage of using the small roller is that the pelvis can fall off it to either side. It provides a reference point and an uphill climb for the return to center. I especially like using the roller to help facilitate the last two movements: rolling the pelvis from side to side while keeping both feet centered and both knees pointed toward the ceiling, and the marching movement.

The roller helps to exaggerate lateral weight shifts, side-bending the torso and swinging the bottom of the sternum from side to side. Facilitate movement of the head and neck with this by instructing your student to roll the head opposite the direction of roll of the pelvis. Progress this to a 3-inch semi-hard or even a hard closed-cell roller. Try the rollers leaning back on elbows and forearms as well.

Lying supine on a long semi-hard 3 or 6-inch diameter closed-cell roller is one of my very favorite toy lessons. It is especially useful for facilitating the roll of the pelvis from side to side while keeping the feet centered (Fig. 5.51). Lie on the roller so head and tail are supported, both hands are on the floor and feet comfortably apart. For those students who have strong tendencies to be very narrow between their feet when standing and sitting, we can have them deliberately put their feet and knees together in this position to feel proprioceptively how it affects their ability to balance.

Putting feet and knees together makes balancing on top on the roller very difficult, and what they will often do is to tense up in a familiar place. Our cervical and shoulder girdle students might tend to default to their arms, chest, shoulders and neck. Our low back folks might co-contract their belly and back. When we then instruct them to widen their base of support and allow their legs to provide some support, they can then compare the two strategies and gain insight into how their habit of staying very narrow might contribute to their problems.

Start this variation by having them move the back of the left side of their pelvis towards the floor to their left. Some people will move like a log: head and torso move to the left along with the pelvis. Some people will try to slide their whole pelvis off the roller to the left. Some people do some bizarre contortions that are a bit difficult to explain. What we are looking for is a version of a left force couple movement.

As the left side of the pelvis drops to the left, the roller rolls along the floor a bit to the left, the torso bends to the right as part of an appropriate balance reaction and the head rolls on the roller to the right as an extension of the right side-bending torso (Fig. 5.51). We want the feet to stay centered and the knees to point to the ceiling. We also want the low back to remain more or less neutral in an AP plane.

What many people will do is to rely on their lumbar extensors to do the trunk balancing. If that is the case, direct their attention to their tendency to lift the lower back away from the roller, then have them tilt their pelvis posteriorly and lift their tailbone by pressing with their feet. This will give them a clearer sense of how they are substituting the back extensors for the hip extensors and, especially for iliopsoas-dominant folks, they will probably find using their legs to control the side-to-side fall 'off' the roller both easier and more comfortable.

After doing this movement several times in what you suspect to be their easiest direction first, reverse the direction and have them compare sides. Then alternate this movement from side to side. Then continue to alternate sides but with both hands off the floor and resting on the belly or lower ribs. Getting rid of the training wheels requires more accurate and complete balance reactions through the torso and more accurate use of the legs to control the fall. Lifting one foot from the floor is a possible progression, but realize that this will be opposite of what happened when safely ensconced on the floor, either supine or sitting.

Try this lesson with feet on the wall rather than on the floor, and progress it by sliding the roller ever farther away from the wall to progressively extend the hip joints and approximate more of a standing position. This is also a great way to challenge balance, train the use of the legs for support, and stimulate lateral balance reactions for your neurologic students.

Try air-filled plastic balls under the pelvis while supine to help facilitate the side-to-side movement of the pelvis with feet centered. Start small, say $1\frac{1}{2}$ to 2 inches diameter, and progress to larger balls, say 6 or 7 inches diameter. The advantage here is that the pelvis is again free to fall from side to side but the torso, head and shoulders remain on the floor. It will feel safer for those of your students who may have some anxiety about falling, even off a 3-inch roller. This variation blends a little bit of wobbliness with a little stability and helps your students to gain confidence that they can move.

Try a ball under one ischial tuberosity to facilitate an improvement in hip extension differentiated from back extension. Manually roll the ball under one ischium and guide the pelvis to roll diagonally up and away from that side. Facilitate an awareness of how to inhibit left lumbar extensors. Add in intention to press foot and lift ischium slightly away from ball. Progress with ball farther underneath pelvis, with hip lifted higher and with demand to use hip extensors nearer end-range.

Alternatively, place your left hand behind your head and lift your head and shoulders to reach toward the lifting right hip. This facilitates diagonal back flexion combined with unilateral hip extension. The smaller balls also work in the sitting and leaning-back variations.

With a 6-inch hard closed-cell roller, straddle it so your knees are on the floor and your feet are behind your knees on the floor. Lean back on both hands behind and do a version of the marching movement. Press with one knee and lift the other just a smidge off the floor (Fig. 5.51). Allow torso, head and shoulders to participate. This is a great quadriceps stretch on the side of the knee that presses and a great way of helping your students recognize the pelvic force couple pattern.

Lean back on your elbows and forearms to progress this. Please don't try this out on your students until you have performed it and feel comfortable with how it should be done, and don't try this with someone with acute lumbar facet irri-

tation! Come up to sitting while straddling the roller and do the same marching movement to help facilitate an understanding of the use of the legs in weight shifting and left/right balance in sitting. These are some – but not even close to all – of the possible variations of this lesson. Get on the floor, get some toys, experiment and be creative. Don't be afraid to do something different!

Much of the rest of this chapter is devoted to ways to facilitate different versions of pelvic force couples. We will explore how the two legs work together to move the pelvis in different positions, different relationships to gravity and with different functional contexts. Some of the lessons are designed to improve sitting or standing balance, some to improve bending, some to improve stepping and walking, and some to improve stability.

These designs are not mutually exclusive. Each lesson may be used to address one or more of these themes. Keep in mind that our imbalances and inefficiencies weave themselves throughout all categories of function, so improvement in one functional category can result in improvement in others. Conversely, if we leave imbalances or inefficiencies in one category, they can seep back into a function that we thought we had already addressed. The safe and sane thing to do, then, is to train pelvic force couple balance and efficiency linked to many functional categories and in gravity-neutral, belly-up and belly-down orientations.

Pelvic force couple-driven transitions

Our next lesson features a side-lying position that turns into a transitional movement to sitting. This developmentally derived lesson is an excellent vehicle for pelvic force couple training and for activating those sometimes grossly underused hip muscles, the abductors.

Recall that gait does not emerge independently of other motor functions. Other motor skills are being developed and refined at the same time. Orienting from different positions, to manipulate from upright postures and to make more complex transitional movements are learned and refined along with walking. The legs are central to all these functions and are basic Lego pieces that are present across all these functions. We will now explore pelvic force couples and how they apply to transitional movements.

Transitional movements needed by the inquisitive youngster include moving from supine to prone, supine to sit, prone to sit, prone to hands and knees, side-sit to hands and knees, hands and knees to three-and-a-half point (hands and knees but with one foot standing near hand), three-and-a-half point to squatting with hands on the floor, squatting or half-kneel to standing, and all the subvariations of moving into different sitting positions. Keep a running count of transitions as you continue through the rest of this chapter. Which transitional movements are not represented? Can you make up your own lessons around these missing movements?

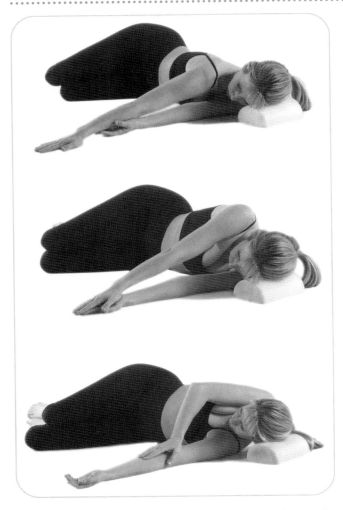

Fig. 5.52 Sliding your right knee forward and back – does the rest of your body move?

Side-lie Transitions

Variations

A. Lie on your back with your legs down long and your arms on the floor somewhere below shoulder height.

- Scan your contact against the floor. Feel differences in size; compare your perception of length of your two legs, of your two arms, of the two sides of your torso.

- Compare the ease and volume of your breath into your two sides.

- Notice if you feel rolled more to the left or the right. Is your pelvis rolled? Is your head rolled? Is your chest rolled one way or the other?

B. Turn to lie on your left side. Have your knees and feet together and knees drawn toward chest so hips and knees are bent at about 90°. Fold towels lengthwise and place

under your head for whatever support is needed, if any. Place your straight left arm in front of you and on the floor at about shoulder height. Your right hand rests either on floor in front of you or on your left arm.

- Make small movement to slide your right knee backward. Your thighs stay together but your right knee slides up the inside of your left thigh a small amount. Notice whether your pelvis, back, chest, shoulder or head move in cooperation with the sliding knee. Continue this several times.

- Reverse the direction to slide your right knee forward (Fig. 5.52). Notice whether there is cooperative movement elsewhere.

- Alternately slide your right knee forward and back. Notice ease, range and integration with/connection to other parts.

C. Turn to lie on your left side again as before.

- Lift your right knee 1–2 inches away from the left knee. Either lift the foot or keep your right foot resting on top of the left. Notice how easy/difficult it feels to lift the right knee.

- How heavy does it feel? Notice whether your pelvis rolls forward or back as you do this. Lift and lower a few times.

- Keep it lifted as you move your lifted right knee many times forward and back. Notice what else participates/cooperates. The movement is the same as in B, but with the knee lifted the whole time.

- Make sure to keep the right thigh parallel to the floor and to the left thigh. Don't raise the knee higher when moving backward or allow the knee to lower toward the floor when moving forward (Fig. 5.53). Rest fully for a while on your side.

D. Lie again on your left side as before.

- Grab hold of your right knee with your right hand. Hold the front of your knee from the outside. Pull your right knee toward your chest, but let your chest and head roll backward as if knee and chest are playing tag.

- Your right elbow stays pretty much straight (Fig. 5.54). Return to having knees together and repeat many times.

- Continue the same movement, but instead of just returning to where you started with your knees together, enlarge that direction of movement to slide your right knee down and forward toward your left foot.

- Alternate between bringing right knee up and back to roll you back, then down and forward to roll you forward.

- Continue with the same alternating movement but enlarge the movement of coming down and forward to come up on to your left elbow (Fig. 5.54). Reverse this to return to lying on your side and repeat a few times. Then enlarge the movement to come up on to your left hand (Fig. 5.54).

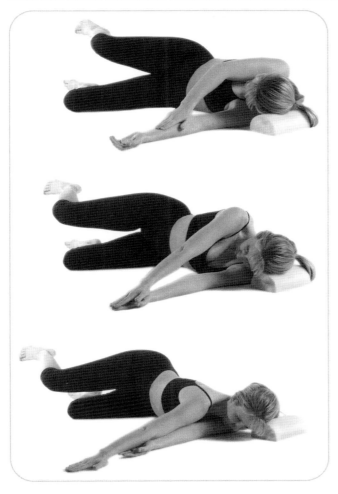

Fig. 5.53 Doing the same movement with the leg lifted.

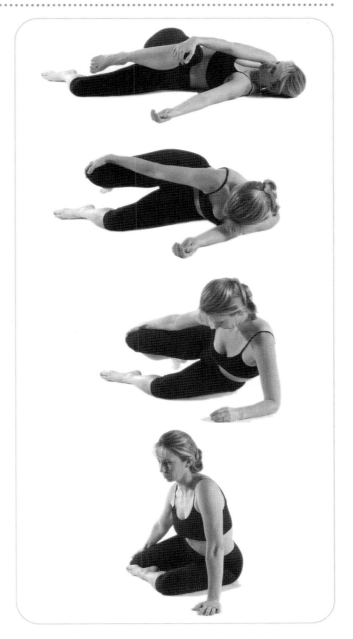

Fig. 5.54 Enlarging the pattern to transition from side-lie to sit.

- Keep your head low and bring it as close to your left knee as possible, both coming up and reversing the movement to come back down to the floor. Experiment with the placement of your left arm on the floor to find the best arrangement.

- Return once again to lie on your left side. Move your right knee forward and back. Compare this movement to when you started. How smooth is it? How integrated is it?

E. Turn to lie now on your right side in a mirror image to what you did while lying on your left side.

- Repeat the instructions above to this side.

- How does this side compare? Which leg feels lighter to lift? Toward which side do you come up to sit most easily?

F. Lie now on your back. Lift both feet from the floor and hold on to the front of your left knee with your left hand and your right knee with your right hand.

- While still holding both knees, move your left knee out to the left and roll yourself to your left side.

Reverse these movements to come back across your back to then roll yourself on to your right side.

- Repeat this rolling movement from side to side at varying speeds to further refine it. Let your head roll freely; you may even end up on your forehead or looking along the floor behind you (Fig. 5.55).

- Continue to hold your knees as you now enlarge the movement to roll through your left side to come up to sit. Reverse the movement to come back down through your back and roll up to sit to the right.

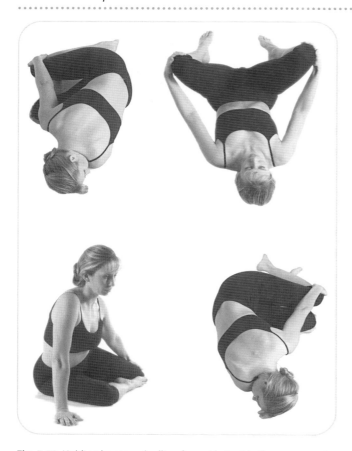

Fig. 5.55 Holding knees and rolling from side to side then come up to side-sit.

- Alternate sides and compare/contrast ease, quality and familiarity. Make wide/sweeping movements and keep your head low to the floor much of the time. Use your legs as much as possible to drive the movement.

G. Lie back on your back again with legs long and arms on the floor.

- Scan your contact against the floor. Feel differences in size; compare your perception of length of your two legs, of your two arms, of the two sides of your torso.

- Compare the ease and volume of your breath into two sides.

- Notice if you feel rolled more to the left or right. Is your pelvis rolled? Is your head rolled? Is your chest rolled one way or the other?

H. Stand up and walk around.

- How is your pelvis balanced on top of your legs while standing?

- How do your hips move as you walk?

- Does your pelvis turn in either direction in space as you walk?

Static and dynamic baselines – Side-lie Transitions

The idea of a static baseline, especially with an understanding of pelvic force couple imbalances and how they create imbalances of pelvic bony landmarks, should be pretty familiar by now. This lesson is one of those that do almost everything to one side first; this strategy tends to accentuate differences between the two sides and helps students sharpen their proprioceptive self-awareness skills.

Having a verifiable skill (coming up to sit from horizontal) tends to also bring out an awareness of differences between the two sides. The culminating movement at the end (rolling from side to side and up to sit alternately to one side then the other) tends to even out the differences a bit at the same time it allows for a back-to-back comparison. Because you already have some background on force couples, let's pick up the pace a bit.

Using the legs to roll – transitions

In variation B you lie on your left side and move your right knee backward, forward, then alternately forward and back. What is responsible for moving the right knee backward? What is happening at the hip joints? The left hip is horizontally abducting and the right hip is horizontally adducting. Are the right hip adductors in a position to pull the right side of the pelvis backward?

To a certain degree they are, but, not being connected to the floor, their ability to influence movement of the pelvis is limited. The left hip abductors, however, are in an excellent position to push the right side of the pelvis back. Could you feel them work as you did this movement? Sometimes it helps to make small movements, stop the effort and repeat several times to allow the subtle effort in the left abductors to seep into your awareness.

Should the torso, right shoulder and head roll back too? Yes indeed! Where is there effort through the torso, shoulder girdles or neck that would prevent this integrative movement? Belly or back would be possibilities. The left shoulder/arm/shoulder girdle can also act to prevent a rolling movement of the torso forward and back. This can be a good exercise in effort recognition by becoming aware of how the shoulders and head move as an extension of the pelvis and torso. With the movement of the pelvis being driven by the legs, be floppy with your arms and head.

What is responsible for moving the right knee forward? What is happening at the hip joints? The right hip is horizontally abducting and the left hip is horizontally adducting. Because the left lower extremity is connected to the ground, the left adductors may be in the best position to pull the right side of the pelvis forward. On the other hand, the right hip abductors can do this movement fully all by themselves.

If the right abductors fire, they will pull the right side of the pelvis forward because the weight and the long lever arm of the right thigh act as a counterbalance, as long as the left abductors are not contracting at the same time to prevent this from happening. This is the rub! Many people will have difficulty making this differentiation between left and right abductors.

Alternating between sliding the right knee forward and backward could be an exercise in balancing the left adductors and left abductors through reciprocal movements. It could also be an exercise in balancing the left and right abductors, which are also antagonists in this function. In fact, with force couple type movements we could say that the right and left iliopsoas are antagonists, as are the left and right piriformis, hamstrings, gluteals, adductors and so on.

I will be pointing out some of these cross-lateral antagonistic relationships as we progress through the book. Does this alternating movement remind you of another movement we have performed? It is a side-lying version of the movement at the end of the last lesson, where you were supine and rolled your pelvis left and right while keeping your feet centered (see Fig. 5.44). I warned you that you would see this movement again – and again – and again!

The movements in variation C are a version of the same rolling forward and back of the pelvis as it was in the last variation, but performed the whole time with the right leg lifted. First let's talk about what happens when you just lift the left knee.

To lift the left knee away from the right, you will have to fire the left abductors/external rotators. If this is all you do, your pelvis will fall forward as the great weight of your leg and the long lever arm of your thigh bone moves the center of mass of the pelvis/leg combination way forward of its puny base of support on the ilium and greater trochanter. This is not what most people do. They will stabilize their pelvis first.

Stability comes from the ground

To prevent the left side of the pelvis from falling forward and dragging the torso and ever-so-valuable head along with it, you will have to engage your right hip abductors/external rotators. This push of the femur into horizontal abduction prevents the pelvis from falling forward or rotating to the right. You could even take this strategy one step further and roll the left side of your pelvis backward even before lifting your right knee and thigh.

The right hip abductors/external rotators could push the right femur into the floor and roll the left side of the pelvis backward, or rotate it to the left. This last strategy may even be the best in terms of economy of movement and reduction of effort – it shortens the length of the lever arm of the left femur and reduces the subjective weight of the lifted left thigh.

In reality, all three versions are helpful. The last variation of lifting the right knee by pressing the left thigh out and rolling the pelvis back is the easiest/laziest way and can be linked to a functional context of rolling from your side to your back (as you do later in this lesson). The first variation of letting the weight of the lifting right leg roll the pelvis forward is a sneaky way of training effort recognition/reduction of the left hip abductors/external rotators.

It requires active inhibition (resetting the muscle spindle tripwire) of the left hip abductors/external rotators and it stretches your left hip pocket! If this movement is performed slowly and the left abductors/external rotators gradually pay out line in a controlled lengthening contraction, it both simu-

lates a way of bending that we will explore later in the chapter and simulates the shock absorption of the hip on heel-strike during gait.

The second version of lifting the right knee and preventing the right side of the pelvis from rolling forward is a good way to train simultaneous contraction of the abductors and external rotators of both hips. When would we use this simultaneous contraction functionally? We could use this for standing and for stabilizing the pelvis in rotational directions.

In standing, it is very common for people, especially those with an iliopsoas bias, to allow their pelvis to fall too far forward into anterior tilt. This creates a compensatory backward bend of the lumbar spine, with all those possible consequences on tissue health. We want to extend the hip joints to push the pelvis toward a more vertical position over the legs – we want to posteriorly rotate the pelvis. If we look at it as a pair of differentiated patterns, we could say that we are trying to move from an iliopsoas pattern (hip flexion and lumbar extension) to a gluteal pattern (hip extension and lumbar flexion).

In previous lessons we accomplished this push of the top of the pelvis toward vertical from a belly-up orientation by pushing the soles of the feet down into the floor or by pressing a knee into the floor, as in Side-sit Bending. What happens in standing if you have the intention to press your feet into the floor?

Pressing the feet into the ground or out on the ground?

Stand up for a moment and give your body the order to press your feet into the ground – does confusion reign? With your whole body weight pressing the soles of your feet into the floor, your CNS will think that it already is. What happens if your intention changes to one of pressing your feet outward against the floor? Imagine you are standing on a sheet of ice with your feet close together.

If you simultaneously contract the hip abductors on both sides, your feet would begin to slide away from each other. Once you get to a certain point, your body weight would take over and your feet would slide away from each other without the assistance of the abductors. Without action taken on your part, you'd be lucky to get out of that particular pickle with just a ripped pair of jeans.

Those individuals with a more highly developed sense of self-preservation will fire their adductors to arrest the disastrous splits and will pull the feet back toward each other again. Fortunately, most of us don't have to stand on ice much. The typical floor has a much higher coefficient of friction. What happens when we simultaneously contract the abductors to push the feet away from each other as if attempting to tear the carpet between the feet?

One effect could be that of posterior pelvic tilt. While we could fire off the big guns and contract the whole gluteus maximus to posteriorly tilt the pelvis, this solution lacks grace and subtlety. Try this yourself – squeeze your gluteals as if you're holding on to a quarter with your butt cheeks. Other than making you look like someone who is pinching quarters with her butt cheeks, might this not sow some chaos through your digestive tract?

Fortunately, there is a more elegant solution. Return to the intention of pressing your feet outward on the floor, as if you were trying to slide them away from each other. As you do this, use your fingertips to palpate your tensor fascia latae, gluteus medius and gluteus maximus as they attach along the top of the iliac crest. Press and release several times and feel for the firing of the superior portion of the gluteus maximus, along with the medius, probably the minimus and the tensor fascia latae. For certain, the gluteus maximus has a posterior pelvic tilt component, and I suspect from feeling it proprioceptively that the other abductors have it too.

This pressing out might also stimulate the piriformis and other short and stubbies to fire. They also have a pelvic posterior rotation component in this position. Regardless of the exact muscle breakdown, the intention to press the feet outward will result in posterior pelvic tilt unless the back extensors (or iliopsoas) fire. Palpate your lumbar extensors. Can you differentiate them from your gluteals?

This, of course, is the rub. Try it yourself many times – press out and release. Feel manually and proprioceptively for a posterior tilting of your pelvis. If you don't feel it now, keep trying it a few times each day and try it again after having performed subsequent lessons in this section. This little trick is a very valuable one to have in your toolbox; learn it well, then go forth and teach!

There are further effects on standing from this simultaneous abductor contraction. This pressing outward has another benefit: reducing knee valgus and external knee rotation. We will explore this more later in the chapter on facilitating lower extremity balance and efficiency. This abduction movement of both hips will also roll you on to the outside edges of your feet if you let it.

Try this yourself: push your feet away from each other and allow your ankles to roll outward (carefully). Activation of the abductors in standing can help reduce foot pronation – more on this later too. To counter this rolling action of the ankles into inversion ankle sprains, the peroneus longus has to fire to press the head of the first metatarsal (the big ball of your foot) into the floor. More on this later too, when discussing ankle sprains.

For now, see if you can feel this proprioceptively: press your feet out, allow your ankles to roll out, then press your metatarsal heads gently into the floor, but not so much that you roll your foot toward its inside edge and you flatten your arch. Performed elegantly, the height of your arches will raise and the length of your arches will shorten. Don't despair if you don't feel it yet. I'll describe variations of this in other positions, and we will continue with part two of this lesson later in the legs section.

Using the ground to stabilize the back

In addition to its advantage in standing, the simultaneous use of the bilateral hip abductors provides rotational stability for the pelvis and low back. Try the following: stand close to a solid vertical support (wall, doorway, post, tree) and reach forward with both arms to shoulder height. Place your hands together palm to palm and place them together against your chosen immovable object. Gradually and gently push your

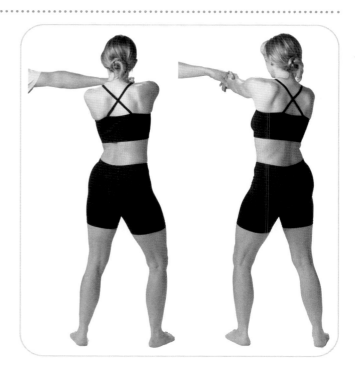

Fig. 5.56 Lateral forces acting on an unstable pelvis – then controlled through anticipation.

hands leftward against the support. What happens to your pelvis?

Try this a few times to get a sense of where your effort is – belly? Hips? Neck? Now press your feet out away from each other, press your first metatarsal heads and allow your tail to drop into posterior tilt if possible. From here, try pressing sideways against your object again. What happens with your pelvis this time? Where is your effort? What is your subjective feeling of ease?

Go back and forth between doing this lateral pushing movement both with and without grounding your feet. Which way seems more stable? What do you have to do with your abductors to prevent turning your pelvis to the right and the rotational movement this creates at your lower back? Do this experiment while pushing both to the left and to the right. Is there a difference between the two sides?

Just as was the case in lifting your top leg while side-lying, there are three main choices here. One possibility would be for your pelvis to turn in the opposite direction that you are pushing (Fig. 5.56). For instance, when pushing with both arms to the left against the support, your pelvis might turn to the right. Why? As the right internal and left external obliques work to twist the torso to the left, those same muscles exert the opposite force upon the pelvis.

The opposite internal and external obliques work both to turn the torso to the left and to turn the pelvis to the right. This particular scenario is very similar to the variation of lifting the top leg in side-lying and allowing the pelvis to roll forward. In both of these instances, the legs are not controlling the movement of the pelvis in space.

The second possibility in pushing your hands to the left is to have your pelvis stay in the same place. This is analogous to the side-lying version of lifting the top leg without rolling the pelvis either forward or back. For this to happen, the legs will have to counteract the action of the abdominals on the pelvis; they will have to resist rotation of the pelvis to the right (left hip external rotation and right hip internal rotation).

Looking at this perspective of what happens at the hip joints, we could extrapolate that the left hip internal rotators (TFL, adductors) and right hip external rotators (gluteus maximus, piriformis and other short and stubbies) would be responsible for stabilizing the pelvis on the legs in the presence of rotational forces. Because this pushing movement of the hands to the left has a component of right weight-shifting, the right hip abductors and left hip adductors also participate.

Although the left leg can be of some use in this scenario, the use of the right leg is crucial. This combination of right hip extension, external rotation and abduction is critically important for back stabilization, and we will discuss other ways of facilitating this function throughout the book. Training transversus abdominis and multifidi for intersegmental stability without linking that stability to the control of the pelvis on top of the legs is not adequate.

The third main possibility is in pushing your hands to the left as an extension of turning your pelvis to the left. This anticipatory movement of the pelvis to the left changes the movement from a reactive one to a proactive one (Fig. 5.56). This subtle preliminary turning of the pelvis to the left is accomplished by the same right hip abductors/external rotators and left hip adductors/internal rotators as in the second possibility.

The only difference is one of timing. The proactive or anticipatory use of the hips to control the movement or position of the pelvis in space kicks in a little bit earlier. This is the kind of stability many of our students with low back pain need. Try for yourself each of the three versions. Which feels most stable? Which has the perception of the least amount of effort? Which way makes you feel like an irresistible force? The immovable object?

By training our students in intentionally pressing both feet out away from each other, we are helping to facilitate this anticipatory stability. This is the difference between perching passively on the face of the earth and planting yourself to better weather life's gales. This is what allows you to take a stand. This can be learned initially, facilitated, and refined in the side-lying position.

Use this movement as an early assessment tool; have the student both press against your hands and resist your push against them. Observe their pelvis for movement and their torso for smoothness of recruitment and amount of effort. How well are they stabilizing their pelvis on top of their legs, and how well are they stabilizing their torso on top of their pelvis? Use this movement as a teaching device; once having learned this simultaneous pushing out in side-lie and other positions, bring them back to standing and press against their hands one way and then the other, then reciprocate gradually to start, then more quickly.

Have them do the same movement while their eyes are closed. This puts a premium on pressing out with both legs at the same time, as you will then be ready regardless of the direction of push. Do this with the feet and legs together to demonstrate the inherent instability of this posture. Do this with the feet very wide apart – then ask them to split the two extremes and find a reasonable distance where both stability and mobility are present. Do this with one foot forward and one foot back.

I'm not suggesting this pressing movement should be of the vein-bulging, eye-popping, split-the-earth-asunder variety. This is a subtle movement with decidedly submaximal effort. These muscles should be capable of long-duration contractions as befits their role as postural support muscles and their slow twitch muscle fiber composition. If they are accurately inhibiting the adductors, hip flexors and back extensors, the mild contractions of the abductors are easily capable of posteriorly rotating the pelvis and of pre-emptively stabilizing the pelvis on the legs.

Lacking any kind of electromyographic (EMG) evidence, I suspect that the stabilizers of the hip joints (especially the deep abductors, the superior portions of the gluteus maximus and the short and stubbies) are linked functionally to the use of the lumbar stabilizers (the transverse abdominis and multifidi). I would guess that they are linked together in a neurological loop and that they work cooperatively to stabilize the low back. Perhaps some enterprising researcher could pick up the baton and take it the next lap.

Stabilization against centrifugal forces

Let's look at this pushing-outward movement in another context. Have you thought about forces acting on the pelvis and low back when you are driving or riding in a car? When going around a corner, there is a centrifugal force that will either act to roll the pelvis left or right on the seat (weight-shift of the pelvis and side-bending movements of the lower spine) or act to roll the pelvis left or right on the seat back (turning the pelvis left and right and twisting movements of the lower back).

When going around a corner or curve in the road where you are turning right, the forces acting on the pelvis will shift weight on the pelvis to the left and/or turn the pelvis to the left. When turning left, the pelvis will shift or turn to the right. Get on a windy road or empty parking lot and alternately make sharp turns side to side – feel the slop of your pelvis from side to side and envisage the shearing stresses possible in your lower back. How could we prevent this uncontrolled movement of the pelvis and lower back? How do we stabilize the pelvis on the seat?

Depending on the set-up of the seat, doors and console in your car, you may have some options for stabilizing yourself with your legs. When going around a corner to the right, you could push outward into the driver's side door in a horizontal abduction movement to keep the pelvis from shifting and rotating to the left. My wife's car has a part of the console that I can push out against with my right thigh and knee when turning to the left.

This is not possible in my pickup, as there is nothing in the middle of the floor to push against. I use my right hand or elbow to brace against the seat or backrest to the right when turning to the left. Check it out in your own car. Find a way to brace with your left leg either against the floor or, preferably, sideways against the door, and experiment with the consequences on your back and pelvis when turning right, both with and without anticipatory bracing with your leg.

Experiment with recognizing movement stresses and counteracting them in both directions; try it in different cars if you have access to some variety. Driving and riding in a car is fundamentally different from sitting on your kitchen chair, office chair or living-room couch. A vehicle needs to be actively ridden. Manipulation of the pedals and bracing in anticipation of centrifugal forces when going around corners or curves, even long and shallow ones, makes driving much more complex and makes it deserving of some time spent on education with your students.

Working the abductors eccentrically and concentrically

The next step in variation C is to move the right knee alternately forward and back from this lifted position. The right abductors/external rotators are firing to lift the right knee, then are required to alternately shorten and lengthen while maintaining the contraction necessary to keep the right knee lifted.

The right short and stubbies contract eccentrically when moving the right knee back and concentrically when moving the right knee forward. This is the importance of keeping the knee at a steady height and the thigh parallel to the ground. It is this constraint that necessitates the quality of motor control needed to maintain a steady lift with changing muscle lengths. What is happening at the left hip? With the instruction to lift just the knee, we allowed choice by asking how your pelvis moves in space. With this variation, we are requiring that you try all three. To move the lifted right knee forward in a controlled way, the left abductors/external rotators have to do a lengthening contraction. To move the lifted right knee backward, the left hip performs a shortening contraction.

Notice the same coordination of antagonists, the same cooperative tug-of-war of opposite-hip musculature that we have seen in the described variations. Have you ever thought of the right and left piriformis as being antagonists before? They are direct antagonists in this and many other functionally relevant movements.

Adding a constraint – finding the force couples in a new venue

This next variation, D, is a more complex and multidirectional variation of the last movement of moving the lifted top knee forward and back. The first part of the instruction is to hold on to your right knee with your right hand and move your knee upward toward your chest while keeping your right elbow straight. This is a constraint that requires the right shoulder girdle and chest to roll backward, along with the head and neck.

The movement of the legs is a modified pelvic force couple, featuring left hip extension and right hip flexion. Are the left

hip extensors activated? Most people will spontaneously use their left hip extensors, but few people are actually aware of it, so we will draw their proprioceptive attention to the fact. Some people will not figure out how to use their left leg to drive this movement of bringing the right knee toward the chest. This is essentially the same marching movement we did at the end of the Wishbone lesson introducing pelvic force couples.

It even has the same movement of the pelvis on the clock: somewhere between 9 and 10.30. Think it through, or get supine and lift your right foot while pushing your left foot, then return to your side and try this movement of bringing your right knee upward toward your chest again. Can you recognize the pattern? Here again, as in our last lesson, the hip extensors, abductors and external rotators are synergistic in pushing the pelvis away.

The right hip moves into flexion with the assistance of the right iliopsoas group, though the demand on the iliopsoas is much less than while supine. The torso falls back and works with the left gluteal pattern of the pelvis to round the back into flexion. A continuation of this direction of movement would result in a transitional movement from side-lie to supine, and we end up doing just that at the end of this lesson.

What happens as you move the right knee forward and down as if sliding the right knee toward the left foot while still grasping the knee with the right hand? Let's look at what happens at the hips. The left hip flexes and horizontally adducts. The left hip flexors and adductors act to pull the pelvis toward the relatively heavier left leg. Here again, as in our last lesson, the iliopsoas and adductors are synergistic in pulling the pelvis toward the legs.

The right hip moves into extension and abduction. The right hip extensors and abductors work together to push the right side of the pelvis forward, using the hand as the ground to push against. This again makes for a pelvic force couple as the right hip extends and the left hip flexes. The continuation of this movement is a transitional movement from side-lie to side-sitting, as we do next in this section.

Whereas Wishbone was an introductory lesson for the pelvic force couple, Side-lie Transitions take your force couples out for a test drive in the real world. Whereas Wishbone is more of a simulation with few constraints and lots of wriggle room, Side-lie Transitions are the real deal and pelvic force couple strength and flexibility have to be up to snuff if they are to accomplish the task at hand.

Alternately moving the right knee up and back toward your chest and then forward and down toward your left foot trains alternating force couple balance and competence. This alternating movement also provides several spring-loading opportunities. One spring-load is using the left pushing muscles to lengthen the left pullers in the movement of bringing the right knee towards the chest and rolling back. The left iliopsoas and adductors are lengthened and the muscle spindles are stimulated.

This rolling-back movement sets the stage for the left iliopsoas and adductors to powerfully pull the right side of the pelvis forward to flex and horizontally adduct the left hip. This in turn spring-loads the left hip extensors/abductors/external rotators to either push the pelvis toward rolling back or to push the pelvis toward coming to sit, as in our very next movement.

Off the practice field and into the game – making the transition

The culmination of this variation is to extend these alternating force couples into a transitional movement of coming all the way up to side-sitting. The key here is to have the left hip sufficiently flexed and to sweep the head far enough toward your left knee to bring your center of mass close to the left thigh. A common mistake many people make is to try to come up too soon, before they have gotten close enough to the left knee for it to be of use in pushing them upright.

They have to work too hard in the arms and neck. If you make sure to keep the head close to the ground and bring it as close to your left knee as possible before trying to come upright, you will probably be more successful. If you organize your torso and legs well enough, you don't even need your hands to get yourself up! Try this for extra-extra-credit: place your hands and forearms together and keep them on your chest as you roll from supine or side-lie to side-sit.

Whereas pushing yourself upright is the responsibility of the left hip extensors, abductors and external rotators, reversing the movement to come from sitting to side-lying requires a deceleration lengthening contraction of these same muscles. To make the movement reversible, make sure you drop your head forward toward the floor in front of your left knee to start the movement back to horizontal. Note the link here to the Side-sit Bending lesson, where you were bending over and coming back upright with the intentional use of the hip extensor group. Can you see how this lesson might be a useful way of teaching some of the physical skills necessary for efficient bending? For efficient walking?

This was one of those lessons where you did everything first to one side, then contrasted the two sides when returning to your supine proprioceptive scan. What differences were you able to perceive between the two sides? What differences were you able to perceive from when you started? Were those static baseline differences from side to side evened out by the end of the exploration of the movement to the right?

How was the movement organized to this side in comparison to the other, especially the culminating movement of coming up to sit? Because most people are right-handed and because the most common right-handed patterns include a dominant left pelvic force couple (left iliopsoas and right gluteal bias), this lesson starts by going to the left. We could anticipate the left hip extensors and short and stubbies being a little longer on the left and therefore a bit easier to come up across. What did you find when you compared your ability to come up to this side with your competence and familiarity in coming up to the left (Box 5.17)?

In variation F this final variation blends, reviews and integrates everything performed in the lesson so far. It is a cumulative movement that helps the CNS in making finer distinctions, in being more aware of left/right imbalances and in reducing or ironing out those differences to some degree.

The first part of this section is to hold on to both knees while supine and roll from side to side, completing the movement in such a way as to reach with the top knee down and forward towards the bottom foot. If performed without support for your head, this results in a marvelous passive rolling

---

> **Box 5.17 Side-lie Transitions**
>
> Transitional movements from side-lie to side-sit – functional context to facilitate pelvic force couple balance and competence
>
> Large hip abduction component for both top and bottom legs – make the short and squat guys work
>
> Hip abduction for controlling lateral movement stressors – applications to low back stability, standing posterior pelvic tilt and knee and foot alignment
>
> Hip abduction for controlling neurologic/medical lateral balance and for enhancing athletic performance in skating or change-of-direction sports

---

of your head from side to side on the floor. This is a great home exercise for people with certain cervical and shoulder girdle problems, as it requires a skill in recognition and reduction of effort through the neck and shoulder girdles.

It can be performed slowly and in a controlled way with the legs providing most of the effort of the movement and the torso and head/neck going along for the ride. This builds trust on the part of your CNS that your head won't just fly off your shoulders if you let go of your neck muscles for a bit. Rolling across the weightbearing shoulder can help facilitate a softening and relaxation of shoulder girdle and upper chest musculature and can self-mobilize cervical and upper thoracic facets. Taken to its completion, one can allow one's head to roll on the floor sufficiently to see with both eyes behind you on the floor. When rolling to the left, the whole right side of your face could be on the floor. Don't force this! Just be aware of the possibility.

After having alternately rolled from side to side a few times, you then segue into rolling up to side-sitting, then back down again to your back and then up to the other side. Your torso flexes and extends. It twists and bends. Your hips bend and straighten. Your pelvic force couple muscles contract and relax. You are using one movement to stretch and strengthen a number of different muscles.

You are using pattern-specific and functionally relevant movements to help hone proprioceptive self-awareness. Who would have thought that a movement so mundane could be so complicated, so rich in detail, so pregnant with possibilities? Dr Feldenkrais seemed to have kept a special place in his heart for transitional movement lessons, and I seem to have picked up some of his ardor.

Comparing baselines and applications

The last instructions in variations G and H are for the sake of comparison. Is your static baseline different at all? Does your gait feel different? Is it smoother? Is there more mobility in or more awareness of your hip joints? Can you sense any rotational movement of your pelvis? This lesson reinforces the axiom that the pelvis turns toward the stepping or flexing hip. Did this translate into walking with you? What if it didn't? Does this make you a motor moron? No, a pelvic force couple walk can be difficult to learn and control and it's not for everyone. Keep trying it after subsequent lessons in this book and see if it gradually starts to make some sense.

Who would benefit from this lesson? It would certainly be an adjunct to Side-sit Bending when working with people with lower back pain aggravated by the way they bend. Use it to teach grounding and posterior pelvic tilt in standing for people with unstable low backs and lumbar hyperextension problems. Use it with people with iliotibial band (ITB) syndrome and trochanteric bursitis (nonacute and able to tolerate some pressure directly on the bursa).

Use it with any knee, foot or ankle injury or biomechanical fault that manifests in inefficient or insufficient push-off in gait or sport. Use it with various neck, shoulder girdle and thoracic syndromes for its ability to facilitate safe mobilization of costal, thoracic and cervical segments. Use it to stretch and strengthen the piriformis and other short and stubbies. Use it to stretch and strengthen the iliopsoas and adductors. Use it to stretch and strengthen the gluteals.

Use it to fine-tune the arthrokinematic muscles of the hip and to gain arthrokinematic control of the hip joints. Use it to reduce chronically held sympathetic tone. You can't be tense and do this movement smoothly. Your students will develop an enhanced ability to trust their bones and supporting surfaces as they roll around on them and push themselves to upright. Use it, strangely enough, to help elderly or neurologically compromised students get more easily into and out of bed!

Use it as a performance enhancement technique for a wide variety of athletes – anything that puts a premium on both powerful push off (extend and abduct) and an ability to 'absorb shock' (flex and horizontally adduct) around the hip joints in controlled or ballistic rotational movements of the pelvis.

Examples might include pitching, quarterbacking and other throwing sports, or tennis, squash, pickle ball and other racket sports. All of these, along with other asymmetrical sports such as golf and shot put, require simultaneous push-off with one leg and a deceleration or shock absorption with the other leg that involves flexion and horizontal adduction.

Sports that feature alternating force couples include all running sports, skating, cross-country skiing, swimming and cycling. There are few sports or artistic athletic performances that don't have unilateral or alternating bilateral pelvic force couples in a starring role. What better way to enhance underlying neural control and balance than by revisiting the evolution of the force couple through the developmental sequence? Stay tuned for more exciting force couple enhancing transitional lessons right after this commercial break.

Put your stroke student on her affected side and have her lift her unaffected arm. Cue to reach to the ceiling and observe for rolling back of the pelvis. Are the affected abductors working? Progress by lifting unaffected leg and cue to prevent rolling forward. The affected hip abductors and perhaps even the affected shoulder girdle adductors and arm extensors and horizontal abductors will be facilitated.

Use the lesson at face value and teach those students who need to learn to transition from lying to sitting. Think through pediatric, geriatric and neurologic applications.

Variations

Are you looking for a kick-butt alternative to the Side-sit Transitions lesson? Then try our new and improved Side-lie Transitions plus! Simply hold on to the outside edge of your foot instead of the knee of the leg you are rolling over. For instance, when rolling to the left to come up to sit, grab hold of your left foot with your left hand and straighten that left knee to the best of your ability before rolling over it and up to sit. Don't try this at home without adult supervision! Do it slowly and be reasonable with your left hamstring. If that's too easy for you, hold on to your right foot with your right hand too.

More pelvic force couple-driven transitions

Let's look next at another developmentally based transitional movement designed to facilitate pelvis force couple competence and balance. This next lesson, Cat/Camel, starts in a hands and knees position and ends up transitioning to side-sitting.

Cat/Camel

Variations

A. Lie on your back with your legs down long and your arms on the floor somewhere below shoulder height.

- Scan your contact against the floor. Feel differences in size; compare your perception of length of your two legs, of your two arms, of the two sides of your torso.

- Compare the ease and volume of your breath into two sides.

- Notice if you feel rolled more to the left or right. Is your pelvis rolled? Is your head rolled? Is your chest rolled one way or the other?

B. Come up on to your hands and knees. If your knees are sensitive to pressure, fold up a towel or blanket to protect them. If your wrists are sensitive to pressure, you can try angling your fingers in various directions, rest on your knuckles instead of your palms, or even drop down on to your elbows and forearms if need be.

- How is your weight distributed between your knees in back and your hands in front? How wide are your knees? Your hands?

- What is the shape of your back? Which parts are rounded? Which arched? Which are straight?

- Begin to alternately round and arch your back in this position (Fig. 5.57). Round your back by tucking your head and your tail, looking toward your belly button and pushing the middle of your back toward the ceiling.

- Arch your back by lifting your head and tail, looking toward the wall in front of you and pushing your belly and chest toward the floor.

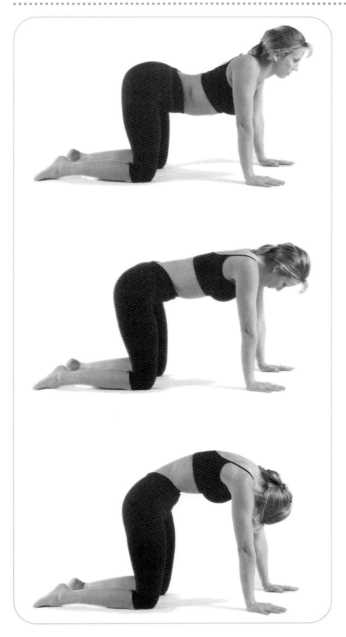

Fig. 5.57 Rounding and arching on hands and knees.

- Which direction seems easier? Most comfortable? How evenly distributed is each movement along your spine – which part arches the easiest and which part rounds the easiest?
- Is your effort primarily in your belly or in your hips and thighs as you round your back?

C. Come back up to your hands and knees and support your weight proportionally front and back (a little more weight back on your stronger and larger legs).

- Alternately round and arch your back a few times as before – use this movement to establish neutral,

a place where your back is neither rounded nor arched.

- From there, begin to sit your pelvis back toward your heels. Go slowly and gently to make sure your knees and ankles can move to accommodate this.
- Does your back tend to round or arch as you do this?
- Do this movement of sitting back toward your heels by deliberately rounding your back as you sit back and arching your back to come forward (Fig. 5.58).
- Reverse this pattern to arch to sit back and round simultaneously with coming back forward (Fig. 5.59). Which way of doing this feels best?
- Let your hands (or elbows and forearms) slide on the floor as much as they need to, but not more than what you have to do.

D. Come back to hands and knees again and establish both proportional weight front to back and a neutral spine.

- Move to look around your right shoulder toward your right foot (Fig. 5.60). Allow your torso to bend and your weight to shift toward your left knee as you do this. The right side of your pelvis actually drops a bit toward the floor and your pelvis turns to the left in space. Do this a few times to this side.
- Reverse the movement to look around your left arm toward your left foot (Fig. 5.60). How does this direction of movement compare to the other?
- Alternate from side to side a few times to compare and contrast, then rest in sitting for a moment.
- Resume looking around your right arm toward your right foot but add in a movement of sitting back toward your left heel with your pelvis (Fig. 5.61). You are combining a bending and weight-shifting movement with a movement to sink yourself back towards your left heel.
- Reverse the movement to do the same thing to the other side; look towards your left foot and sit back towards your right heel.
- Alternate from side to side a few times, then put the two halves together to make a circle. Look to your right heel, sink back to your left heel, move your pelvis across to your right heel, then back up to hands and knees. Go around in a circle several times in each direction (Fig. 5.61).

E. Come back up to your hands and knees.

- Look again towards your right foot; sit back with your pelvis towards your left heel, this time while sliding your right knee and foot backward on the floor.
- When your right leg is long behind you and you are close to sitting on your left heel, ease your left hip toward the ground to the left of your left foot (Fig. 5.62).
- You are moving to place your left hip on the floor in a side-sitting position. Reverse the movement to come back up to hands and knees. Repeat this movement several times.

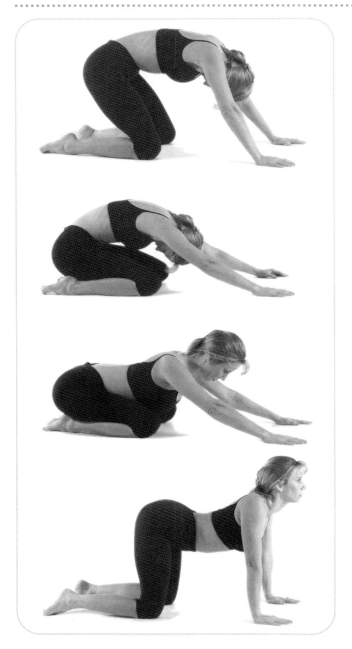

Fig. 5.58 Rounding to sit back and arching to come forward.

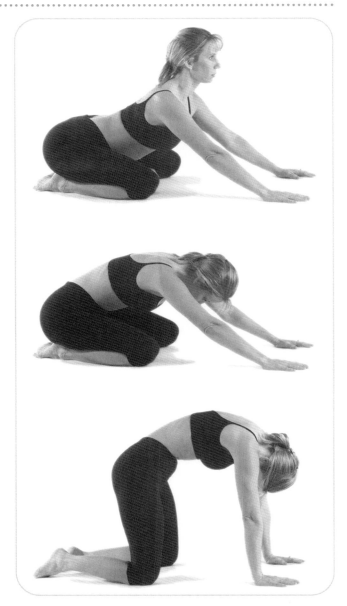

Fig. 5.59 Arching to sit back and rounding to come forward.

- Now do the same thing to the other side. Look to your left heel, sink back to your right hip as you slide your left knee and foot backward on the floor, and sit your right hip on the floor to the right of your right foot.

- Alternate from side to side a few times. How do the two sides compare? Which hip is easier to get on the floor? Which is easier to get back off again?

- Continue this alternating movement, but each time you come back up to hands and knees again move

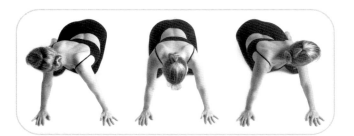

Fig. 5.60 Looking around right and left shoulders from hands and knees.

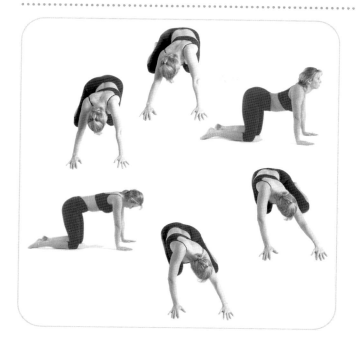

Fig. 5.61 Sitting back toward heels in circles.

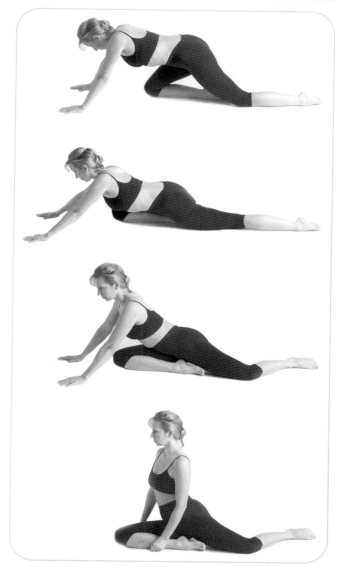

Fig. 5.62 Hands and knees – to poor man's splits – to side-sitting.

the knee of the leg that is sliding forward again off the floor and toward your forehead (Fig. 5.63).

- Round your back and drop your head to meet the ascending knee. Do your knee and forehead come close to touching? Repeat a few times.

- Enlarge the movement back to hands and knees to come instead to place your right foot on the floor just to the outside of your right hand (Fig. 5.63).

- Come back up to hands and knees again and simply round and arch your back as you did in the beginning. Is it any smoother or easier? Is the movement any more proportional through your spine? Do your legs participate more fully?

F. Lie on your back as at the beginning of the lesson.

- Scan your contact against the floor. Feel differences in size; compare your perception of length of your two legs, of your two arms, of the two sides of your torso.

- Compare the ease and volume of your breath into two sides.

- Notice if your pelvis feels rolled more to the left or right. Is your head rolled? Is your chest rolled one way or the other?

- Stand up and walk around. How do your hips move? How do your legs propel you forward? How do your ribs and shoulders move as you walk?

Static and dynamic baselines – Cat/Camel

The variation B section features both static and dynamic baselines. The static baseline while on hands and knees asks ques-

tions about how you arrange your base of support. We asked questions about distribution of weight forward and back, and about width or distance between hands and between knees. A hypothetical ideal would be a position where the hip joints are directly above the knees with the thighs vertical and the shoulder joints are directly over the hands with the arms vertical.

Some people will narrow their base of support either by having their hands too close to the knees or by having hands too close together or knees too close together. Get on the floor for a moment and try out all these deliberate errors. Feel the increased muscular effort as a result of not arranging your bones to support your weight skeletally.

What did you notice about the shape of your back initially? We could surmise that a person with an iliopsoas bias and a global torso extension pattern would be biased toward anterior tilt and global torso extension. A person with an iliopsoas bias

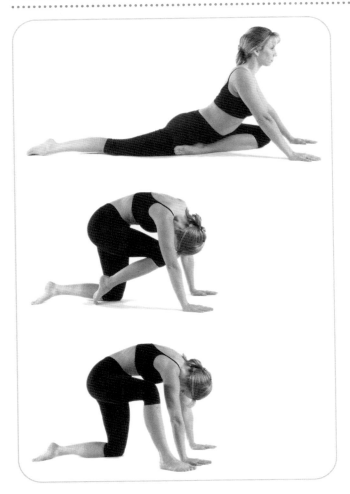

Fig. 5.63 Bringing right knee to forehead – or right foot to floor – from poor man's splits.

and a half arch type torso may be biased toward anterior pelvic tilt, lumbar extension and thoracic flexion. This is the most commonly seen organization.

A person with a gluteal bias and a global torso flexion pattern might be posteriorly tilted and flexed globally through the torso. A person with a gluteal bias and a half round type torso might be slightly arched, slightly rounded or neutral throughout their torso, but will be posteriorly rotated. This type is the easiest to miss because it can mimic other patterns. Did the shape or proportion of where you are flexing and where you are extending change at all by the end of the lesson? Can you think through the various ways each of these different scenarios might organize the head and neck?

Once you have established an adequate base of support, you then dive into the dynamic baseline portion of this section: alternately rounding and arching your back. What is the functional trigger for the rounding movement? Looking toward your belly button. Where is your effort in rounding your back? What are your choices? You could do a lot of this movement with your abdominal muscles. You could do a lot of this movement with your gluteals. You could do some of this movement

with your serratus anterior. But you can't do the complete movement without engaging all of these muscles.

Just for a giggle, try rounding your back without contracting your belly at all. Some people will be completely incapable of differentiating their belly from this movement. Although there is nothing inherently wrong with firing your abdominals to round your back in this position, it could be very beneficial to learn how to emphasize the use of your legs. Pushing both knees and hands into the ground can push you maybe three-quarters of the way away from the floor.

Can you recognize this as being a bilateral gluteal pattern? To complete the movement to end-range you'll have to bring in your abdominals and anterior intercostals. Again, in motor learning, we are emphasizing the development of choice. Conversely, if you don't use your belly at all, it would be beneficial to develop that skill. What is being stretched or inhibited? The iliopsoas, back and neck extensors, lower and middle trapezius and rhomboids, quadratus lumborum and posterior intercostals.

What is the functional trigger for arching your back? Looking forward toward the wall in front of you. Can you imagine how this would be a functional requirement for crawling? Babies are great at arching proportionally through their back in this position because they need to be able to see where they are going. Can you imagine this same pattern being useful for a cyclist? For a swimmer doing the breaststroke? For a plumber looking under the sink? For a speed skater? All these activities require an ability to orient forward while in a belly-down position and all require an ability to extend through the thoracic spine. This is one of many places to facilitate that extension.

How is arching your back accomplished? Through the lengthening contractions of belly, gluteals and hamstrings. Once again, a belly-down orientation emphasizes lengthening and strengthening the gluteal group. Once again, pattern specificity involves doing a differentiated pattern of movement featuring back extension and hip flexion. As always, doing lengthening contractions is one of the best ways to stretch muscles – in this case, the hamstrings, gluteals and piriformis, etc.

Once gravity takes this movement as far as it's going to, you can complete the movement with a shortening contraction of the iliopsoas and back extensors. Where is that transition point between letting go of effort to allow gravity to move you and a more muscularly active extension? Asking and answering questions like this is what leads to finer and finer discrimination in movement.

Watching your students move from this hands and knees position can be quite informative. The careful observer can gather information about proportion of movement through different sections of the torso, can get a sense of hamstring/gluteal/short and stubby length, get a sense of their ability to move their pelvis from their legs, and can observe for initial student understanding of head-to-tail connections and of how to bear weight skeletally. Try incorporating some functional positions and global movement patterns in your evaluation. You can pick up a lot by looking at the big picture. The rest of the lesson revolves around improving the ability to move more easily, smoothly, proportionally and completely into these two test directions.

Transitions to heel-sitting

This next variation takes a look at combining the movements of rounding and arching the back with movements of sitting back toward your heels and coming back up to hands and knees again. In variation C, we started by asking for an internal observation of tendencies. Does your back have to round as you sit back? Are the hamstrings and short and stubbies not long enough?

We deliberately mixed and matched: sit back by rounding and come back up by arching, then sit back by arching and come back up by rounding. For gluteal-biased folks we have included a constraint in intentionally arching to sit back that requires length of the gluteal group. For iliopsoas-biased folks we have included a constraint in intentionally rounding to come forward that requires strength of the gluteal group.

Try again especially these two ways of coming forward. If you come forward by arching you are keeping your hips relatively flexed and requiring primarily the quadriceps to push you back forward. The emphasis for the CNS is on straightening the knees. If you come forward by rounding, you are intentionally extending your hips with gluteal involvement to contribute to the posterior tilt aspect to intentionally rounding your back. The emphasis for the CNS is on straightening your hips.

Which way is best? Can you see that the answer to that question depends on who you are? That the easiest way for one will not be easy at all for another? That what we really want to encourage is choice? That we might actually direct people to work most on what they do the least well – their nonhabitual differentiated pattern of movement!

The movements in variation D introduce side-to-side movement, getting us out of one cardinal plane and into another. The instruction is to look first around the right arm, then the left, then alternate. Descriptive language explicitly directs a side-bending movement through the torso and a weight-shifting movement of the pelvis in space over the legs.

By the way, 'look around your shoulder' is a very specific instruction. What different movement might be triggered if the instruction were to look under your shoulder towards your foot? What if it had been to look over your shoulder? This awareness of language specificity in these and other lessons is the key to reducing confusion, both when going through the lesson yourself and when teaching it to your students.

How do you move to look around your right shoulder toward your right foot? In keeping with the spirit of the proportionality principle, we could start the movement with the biggest muscles. We could initiate this intention to look by moving the pelvis in space to the left; it is true here, as in vertical, that weight-shifting to the left would trigger a torso side-bend to the right as part of the balance response. What gets the pelvis to move to the left? What creates right hip horizontal abduction and left hip horizontal adduction?

The left adductors can pull the pelvis to the left, or the right abductors and friends can push the pelvis to the left, or they can work cooperatively in a version of a pelvic force couple. Whereas the description of the movement of the pelvis was to allow the front of the right hip to drop toward the floor and your pelvis to turn in space to the left, there is often some confusion with this.

Shift of weight with force couple movement – or by wagging the tail?

Get on the floor and try the two basic ways of shifting your weight to your left. One way is to drop your right hip and turn your pelvis to the left. The other is a sort of a wag-your-tail approach: the pelvis side-bends in space rather than rotating. This latter strategy lacks the stability and power of the former and may be indicative of restrictive hip short and stubbies.

With the weight of the pelvis falling to the left, the torso then side-bends to the right. The right abdominals and quadratus lumborum, lateral intercostals and even the latissimus dorsi work to accomplish this. The left abdominals and back extensors, lateral abdominals and latissimus dorsi are inhibited/stretched. The bottom of the sternum points to the weight-bearing hip yet again.

The head and neck can then move as an extension of the pelvis and torso to side-bend and rotate to the right to most easily and completely see the right foot. This is organizing orientation from the bottom up. Try looking toward your right foot without allowing your pelvis to move in space to the left. How successful is this in comparison?

Once looking at your right foot with your torso bent to the right and your weight over on your left hip and elongated left gluteal group, you are in fine shape to use the spring-loading effect on the left gluteals and left torso side-benders to either return you to center or continue you past center on your journey toward looking at your left foot. This is yet another example of using reciprocating movements to coordinate antagonists and maximize muscle efficiency.

Try this alternating movement with your knees and feet very close together or touching. How stable is this? Try the movement with your feet and knees very wide apart. How mobile is this? There is always a compromise between mobility and stability. If the knees are too narrow, the center of mass travels outside of its base of support and the bones are no longer in a position to effectively bear weight. If the knees are too wide apart, you have taken up too much slack in the adductors and you become stuck. Finding that compromise position requires movement, deliberately introduced choices and the self-awareness skills needed to make a judgment.

By the way, this is another place to play with the simultaneous activation of opposite-hip abductors. Try pushing out with both knees against a high-friction floor and observe the movement of your pelvis. Continue to push out with both knees, but ease off a bit with one and kick up the juice a bit in the other to allow your pelvis to move in one direction then the other. Play the abductors against each other to set up your game of catch.

Our next movement in this section is to combine the movements of weight-shifting and side-bending with the previous movements of sitting back toward the heels. When looking to the right, side-bending to the right and weight-shifting to the left, add in a movement of sitting your pelvis toward your left heel. As yet another version of a pelvic force couple, was your pelvis turned to the left and your right hip a bit closer to the floor than your left? Muscularly, the emphasis is on lengthening and strengthening of the left gluteal group, though the right adductors may be stretched depending on individual adductor tonus and distance between

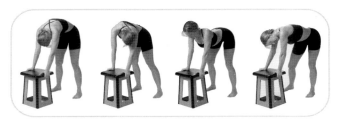

Fig. 5.64 Plantigrade version of the same basic circular movements.

Box 5.18 Cat/Camel

Transitional movements from hands and knees to side-sit –
functional context to facilitate pelvic force couple balance and
competence

Belly-down orientation emphasizes lengthening and strengthening
of the hip extensors

Links back to transitions from lie to sit and forward to transitions –
side-sit to side-sit and side-Sit to Stand

the knees. When looking to the left, did your pelvis turn to the right?

We then combined these movements into a circle. This is a good cumulative movement and we could stop the lesson here, though not this time. A nice variation for the lead-up movements and the cumulative movement so far is to do the same thing in plantigrade. Stand up and lean over a desk or counter, resting your weight on your elbows and forearms. Spread your legs and keep your knees more or less straight as you alternately round and arch, side-bend and sit your pelvis backward. Combine them into circles in each direction (Fig. 5.64).

This is a great place to lengthen hamstrings and adductors if you are specific about patterns. Anteriorly tilt your pelvis as you move your pelvis back and be sure to allow it to turn in the direction of the leg you are shifting your weight toward. Make the movements less demanding by leaning on your hands instead of elbows, or by raising the surface you lean on.

Make the movements more demanding by lowering your surface – chair seat, low stool and then floor. Make yourself less reliant on your arms for stability by doing the movements with your hands on your bent knees like a linebacker (or back yourself on to a wall in this position to enhance proprioceptive feedback or stability). All these exercises are modular; mix and match variations, positions, intentions and props, and have fun!

Poor man's splits

In variation E we continue to build on previous variations. You now modify the sitting back to one side movement by sliding your nonweightbearing leg backward on the floor. I call this movement of fully flexing one hip (but not the knee) and fully extending the other hip and knee a poor man's splits (Fig. 5.63).

The poor man's split is a good place to work on differentiated thoracic extension, as the flexed front or weightbearing hip will constrain anterior pelvic tilt and lumbar extension. Work with orientation (looking forward or up) and manipulation (reaching forward or up) functions as described previously in this chapter. It is also a good place to work on lengthening the iliopsoas. As you slide one leg backward, that hip moves into extension. The lower you can get your pubic bone to your heel and the farther back you can slide the leg, the better.

From here, press your front knee into the ground to gently posteriorly rotate your pelvis and move your lumbar spine in a flexion direction. You probably will not have a lot of wriggle room here, so don't expect a big movement. Just do it small, gently and accurately. Make sure you are doing a combination

of left hip extension with lumbar flexion without allowing your pelvis to raise away from your heel. You could further facilitate this by slowly beginning the movement of coming back forward to hands and knees with the additional intention to round your back as you do so.

From this poor man's split position, the next movement is to lower your hip to the floor to come to side-sitting. If you sink toward your left heel and slide your right leg backward, you will then move your left hip to the floor, to the left of your left heel. This again requires length and strength of the left hip gluteals, this time in greater abundance. There are many folk who have great difficulty smoothly lowering their pelvis to the floor: they bang down, and then have to use momentum to get themselves back up off the ground again to come back to hands and knees.

There are also many folk who initially have great difficulty, but as the CNS is put to work solving this problem, they learn to recognize and reduce that which is constraining them. One way to lower the bar and make this movement possible for those who struggle is to raise the floor. Put a rolled-up blanket, towels or a phone book on the floor where they will be sitting. Completing this movement of transitioning from hands and knees to sitting helps the CNS to register functional context, and often then makes it easier to progressively raise the bar again until they are able to do it with either minimal build-up or all the way to the floor (Box 5.18).

One cue that may make this movement easier for those who struggle would be to slide one hand backward on the floor to assist in taking some of the weight. Another cue would be to move their head in the opposite direction to their pelvis. For instance, when moving toward left side-sitting, as you ease your pelvis toward the floor to your left, bend your torso to the right and move your head to the right in space. Do the opposite as you come back up from here. Bend your torso and move your head to the left as you bring your pelvis back up and to the right to rest on your left heel.

Go back and forth in this small range of movement between side-sitting and poor man's splits to feel the side-bending relationships of head to tail. Alternating back and forth between transitions from hands and knees to left and right side-sitting helps to heighten awareness of differences between the two sides, and at the same time it reduces those differences and improves the overall efficiency of both force couples.

Preparation for coming to stand

Our last movement in this section involves continuing with the same transitional movement, but instead of coming just back to hands and knees, extend the movement of sliding the one leg forward to intentionally move the sliding knee and forehead toward each other. This facilitates a gluteal firing on the weightbearing hip. Do this movement 20 or 30 times in a row and feel where you experience fatigue!

What is this movement reminiscent of functionally? Think of toddlers coming up to standing. They make that transition very often from hands and knees by bringing one foot and then the other up to standing on the floor near their hands. We will pick up this lesson later in the chapter and complete the transition to stand from this three-and-a-half point position.

Baselines, applications and variations

We now return to our very first movement in this lesson to check on our dynamic baseline. As you round and arch your back in this hands and knees position, is it any smoother or more complete than it was to start with? How was your contact and balance against the floor in supine at the end of this lesson?

Who would we use this lesson for? For both pain reduction and performance enhancement, we would use this lesson with essentially the same folks that we use the Side-lie Transitions lesson for. This belly-down orientation emphasizes lengthening and strengthening of the gluteal group and is yet another way of facilitating efficient and balanced pelvic force couples, whether they are used to improve locomotion, other transitional movements, manipulation (throwing, reaching, punching, pushing or pulling) orientation or balance. We could also use this to facilitate skills needed for efficient bending. Use with neurologic, orthopedic or medical students to facilitate balance, strength and functional competence in getting up and down from the floor.

I have already described a couple of variations of this lesson: doing the circular movement in plantigrade and doing some AP movements of the pelvis in poor man's splits. A logical progression of the last variation in this lesson, coming forward from a poor man's split to bring head and knee together, would be to extend this movement to bring the sole of that foot on to the ground near the standing hand. This is a very important developmental movement, as this is how we begin our transition to standing.

Babies will bring first one and then the other foot to stand and end up in a hands-and-feet position in preparation for standing without support from furniture or parents. There is a classic lesson that does just this (Fig. 5.65). From hands and knees, bring up one foot to stand a few times, then bring the other foot to stand a few times, then alternate. Now stand up one foot and bring the other up as well.

You will be ready to do a frog hop from here. Try pressing your pelvis toward the ceiling and dropping your head toward the floor while still in quadruped. Mix and match and be creative. Later on, the toddler will want to stand up with something in one or both hands and will simply make the transition to stand from another developmentally important position: half-kneeling (Fig. 5.66).

This lesson, along with the previous two lessons, explored movements around side-sitting. The functional context of this lesson is to make transitional movements from hands and knees to side-sitting. The last lesson, Side-lie Transitions, has a context of moving from lying to sitting. Where else is there to go?

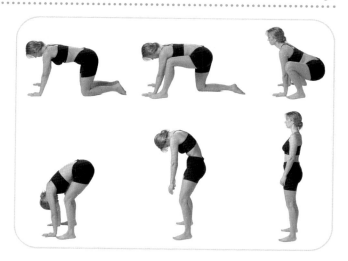

Fig. 5.65 Transitions from the hands and knees to standing, through three-and-a-half point stance.

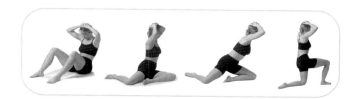

Fig. 5.66 Transitions from side-sitting to half-kneeling – progress to no upper extremity support.

Although we could design additional lessons around transitions from side-sitting to long sitting or to sole sitting or up to stand or into a three-and-a-half point stance or to kneeling or half-kneeling, it's the versatility of these positions and their potential to build developmental lessons around them that I love so much. Our final lesson in this series will explore transitional movements from right to left side-sitting.

Side-sit Transitions

Variations

A. Lie on your back with your legs down long and your arms on the floor somewhere below shoulder height.

- Scan your contact against the floor. Feel differences in size; compare your perception of length of your two legs, of your two arms, of the two sides of your torso.

- Compare the ease and volume of your breath into two sides.

- Notice if you feel rolled more to the left or right. Is your pelvis rolled? Is your head rolled? Is your chest rolled one way or the other?

B. Lie on your back with your legs bent up. Your feet are on the floor at about shoulder width and your arms are out away from your sides at about shoulder height.

- Tilt both knees slowly to the left – start small and gradually increase the size of movement without straining (Fig. 5.67).

- How easily does your pelvis roll on the floor to the left?

- How much of your back can you feel move as you do this? Do this movement several times to the left.

- Then try the same thing several times to the right.

- Alternate from side to side a few times. How does this side compare to the other?

C. Come up to sit on the floor. Place the soles of your feet on the floor at about shoulder width apart and lean on your hands behind you.

- From this position, tilt both knees toward the ground to your left (Fig. 5.67).

- How close does your left knee get to the floor? How close is your right knee? Don't force it: just notice it.

- How do your chest and shoulders move?

- Try it now tilting your knees to the right.

- Do this several times then alternate from side to side. Compare and contrast tilting knees left and right.

D. Come up to sit as before with feet standing and leaning back on hands.

- Tilt your knees to the left again, but this time add in lifting your right hand away from the floor, bringing it across your body in front and placing it on the floor somewhere near your left hand (Fig. 5.68).

- Let both of your knees come to the floor with the right knee nestled inside the sole of your left foot. This is a side-sitting position. Repeat the movement in this direction several times.

- Do the same movement to the other side. Tilt your knees to the right and reach across with your left hand to place it on the floor somewhere near your right hand. Experiment with the timing of lifting your hand. Is it easiest to lift it early on or later?

- Alternate from side to side several times. How do the two directions of movement compare? Are you gradually creeping forward as you do this? What would you have to do to not scoot forward?

E. Come up to sit again as before.

- Tilt your knees to the left and reach across to place your right hand on the floor.

- From this twisted side-sitting position, look alternately under and over your left shoulder. Use your whole body to do this. Protect your neck! Round your whole torso to look under and arch your back to look over your shoulder (Fig. 5.69).

- Tilt your knees the other way, get into the opposite side-sitting position and do the same thing. Alternately look under and over your right shoulder.

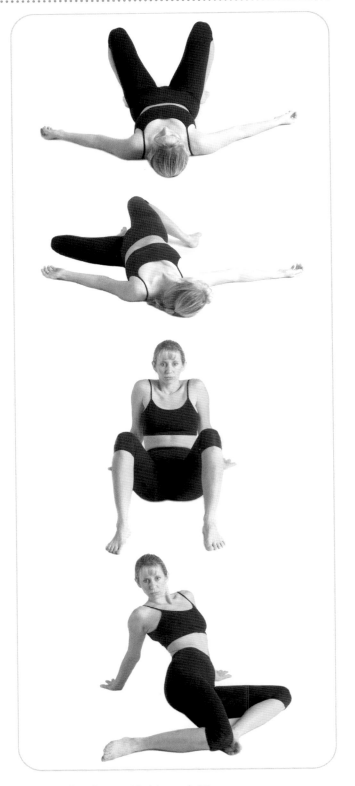

Fig. 5.67 Tilting knees while lying and sitting.

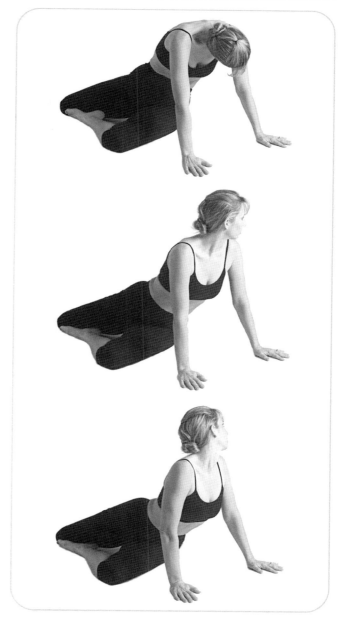

Fig. 5.69 Rounding and arching in a twisted position.

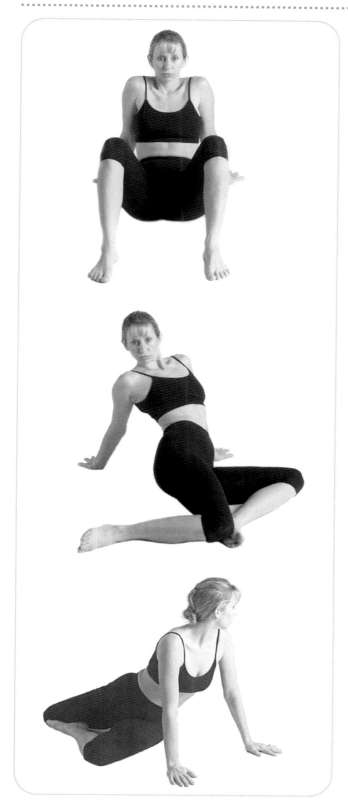

Fig. 5.68 Transition to left side-sitting – try looking over your left shoulder.

- This rounds and arches your whole back while in a twisted position. Which side is it easiest to round on? Which side is easiest to arch?

- Come back to sit with both feet on the floor and lean on both hands behind. From here, return to an earlier movement.

- Tilt your knees from side to side but keep both hands on the floor behind you. Do your knees come any closer to the ground? Is it any easier? Do your chest and shoulders participate any more?

F.   Come up to sit as before, but this time hold on to your knees with your hands rather than leaning back on them.

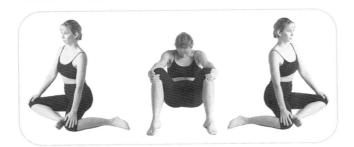

Fig. 5.70 Transition to left side-sitting without using hands.

Hold your knees so your palms cup the top of your kneecaps and your fingers point toward your feet.

- Continue to tilt your knees to the left to come to side-sitting. Both knees end up on the floor but both hands are still on your knees, though you can let your hands pivot around your knees (Fig. 5.70).

- Try this movement alternately from side to side several times. Be reasonable with yourself. There will be some who can't do this without toppling over. Straighten and get taller as you come to side-sitting and round yourself, and get shorter as you come through the middle.

- Rest for a moment leaning back on your hands.

- Now roll yourself back on to your back. You roll up along your spine toward your shoulders and let your feet and knees swing above you in the air. Use momentum to swing yourself back upright again to bring the soles of your feet to the floor (Fig. 5.71).

- Arch your back and get taller as you come upright and round yourself into a ball as you roll back on to your back. Repeat this movement of rolling back and swinging back up again.

- The next time you are on your back, instead of swinging yourself straight up to sit, swing yourself diagonally up to left side-sitting (Fig. 5.72). Your right foot will end up behind you on the floor.

- Then roll back to your back diagonally and roll yourself up to right side-sitting. Alternate from side to side several times.

- Return to holding your knees and tilting them alternately right and left. How successful is this movement now? Are you still creeping forward? If so, you are not rounding back through the middle enough.

- Continue to alternate from side to side-sitting but add in straightening your legs as you roll through the middle and bending your knees back up again as you come to side-sit. Let your hands slide up and down your thighs.

- Reach toward the ground with both the back of your knees and your lower back at the same time when rounding through the middle. Exaggerate the 'falling

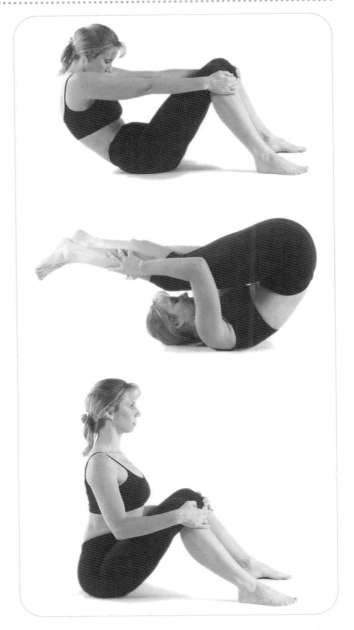

Fig. 5.71 Rolling to back and up again – use momentum to get taller.

back' as much as possible when rounding through the middle.

G. Lie on your back again.

- Scan your contact and balance from side to side in comparison to the beginning.

- Bend your knees up and tilt them together from side to side as you did at the beginning of this lesson. How does the movement compare now? Is it any easier? Larger? More inclusive of your chest and mid to upper back?

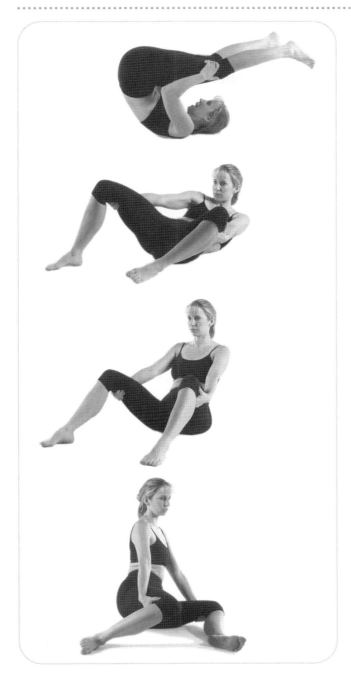

Fig. 5.72 Rolling diagonally back up to side-sit.

Static and dynamic baselines – Side-sit Transitions

What could we anticipate as being different in our static scan as a result of this lesson? Because this mostly belly-up lesson emphasizes length, strength and balance of the iliopsoas group, we might expect both a flattening of the lower back as the longer hip flexors accommodate a more posteriorly rotated pelvis and some equalization of the habitual left /right bias of

the pelvis. The legs might be wider apart or rolled into more external rotation as a result of doing alternately lengthening and shortening contractions of the adductors.

We might see a flatter thorax, a longer neck and a head resting more in neutral as a result of the thoracic extension and rotation movements that are strongly required in this lesson. The shoulder girdles might be flatter or broader against the ground, as the pectorals have been required to lengthen and the mid and lower trapezii have been working.

The upper extremities may even be rolled more into external rotation as a result of a change in thoracic and shoulder girdle bias. The observant practitioner can learn a lot from watching people move, especially watching them move in complex and demanding ways. That same practitioner can learn a lot from observing people supine, watching for anticipated changes over time and verifying anticipated results.

In variation B we come up to a hook-lying position: supine with knees bent and feet apart. Why the stipulation to have the feet fairly wide apart? One, that distance more accurately represents the distance between the feet in the side-sitting postures found later in the lesson. Two, a wider distance facilitates better stability, better control and a more optimal position from which to use the legs to control that movement of twisting and untwisting the pelvis and torso.

Mobility/stability compromise – facilitating thoracic contributions

Get on the floor and experiment with width placements of your feet in this hook-lying position. The best way to understand where your students go wrong in their organization is to try it out! Try tilting your knees alternately a few times with your feet and knees at about shoulder width apart. Do the same thing with your feet and knees together, then with your feet and knees as far apart as you can comfortably get them. This is a classic Goldilocksian/Feldenkraisian experiment. Feel for proprioceptive differences in at least three variations of the same movement.

Having your feet and knees together facilitates mobility. As the knees tilt to the left, their center of mass quickly moves outside of the left foot and the legs begin to fall to the left. The pelvis is dragged along with the legs and rolls to the left. As the pelvis rolls to the left, it pulls L5 along with it. This in turn drags along L4, then L3, and so on up the spine. This chain reaction effect is called kinematic linkage. In a perfectly organized skeleton there would be an even distribution of movement from the pelvis to the head.

All 24 vertebrae would have their contribution to make, though some contributions would be less than others. We would like to have proportionally less rotation in the lumbar vertebrae because the orientation of their facet joints is not optimal for this direction of movement and because of the shearing stresses it places on discs. We would like to have proportionally more rotation through the thoracic spine, as their facet orientation is well suited for that direction of movement.

Sadly, this is rarely the case in our clinical practice. What we often see instead is a muscular immobilization of the thoracic spine and ribcage and disproportionate rotation in the lumbar segments. You will see most of the movement occurring below the sternum. This particular violation of the good housekeeping rule is not good for most of our students with lower back pain.

Note that as the pelvis rolls to the left, L5 rotates to the right relative to the pelvis. L4 then rotates right relative to the pelvis and to L5, then L3 relative to L4, and so on. Ideally, the whole spine is rotating sequentially to the right and the head ends up rolled on the floor to the right. Because of the weight of the head, chest and shoulders, the upper body stays on the floor as the right side of the pelvis and the lower to mid back lift from the floor. We are creating a constraint that requires rotation with an extension bias.

What we are really looking for in this movement, and what we will continually facilitate throughout the rest of the lesson, is a variation of right torso extension. This combination of right rotation, right side-bending and extension of the torso is what allows the tilting knees to most easily touch the floor to the left. Try the movement again with your feet and knees touching each other. Tilt your knees and keep your chest tight, with the back of your ribcage on the floor.

Where does the movement happen? Try tilting your knees and arching/bending your back into right torso extension. Do your knees approach the floor any more easily? Think of this movement in terms of a balance reaction. As your weight shifts to the left, your torso twists and bends back and to the right in response. The head then passively rolls on the floor to the right as an extension of the movement of the torso.

Choices in tilting the knees

What controls this movement muscularly? Look at just the torso for a moment. We could say that to control the fall of the knees to the left, we need to control the movement of the torso into right extension. We could then surmise a lengthening contraction of the left abdominals and anterior intercostals in lowering the knees to the left and a shortening contraction of those same muscles in returning to the starting point. Can you feel this proprioceptively? Are your effort recognition skills acute enough yet? Do you think you can do this movement entirely with your torso? It may be possible, especially if using momentum, but it would be very difficult.

What you are probably doing is pressing the outside edge of your left foot into the floor. You are using your TFL (hip internal rotation) to lower your knees to the left, and then to push you back up again. Try this out proprioceptively – tilt your knees to the left and let them hang. Relax into this position as much as you can, then slowly and gently start to bring your knees back to center.

Try initiating the movement from the left side of your belly. Can you get all the way on to your back without pressing your left foot? Now deliberately press the outside edge of your left foot against the floor as you tilt your knees back to center – feel how much easier this is. Try pressing the inside of your right foot into the floor. What is the consequence of this?

What happens if all you do is contract your left adductors to try to lift your left knee? Your pelvis rolls to the left. What happens if all you do is contract your right abductors to lift your right knee? Your pelvis might roll more to the left. The weight of the legs and the length of their lever arm make the legs effectively heavier than the pelvis – this switches origin and insertion relationships. The abdominals and intercostals don't have anything heavy enough to anchor to (unless you are holding on to something with your arms) and are inadequate to the task of pulling the very heavy pelvis and legs uphill. The legs have to work!

Where should the legs be to be used to their fullest? Try these tilting movements again in the narrow, medium and wide-apart versions. Narrow feet enhance mobility but aren't very stable. Wide feet and knees are more stable, but having the hip joints already near end-range compromises mobility. A reasonable distance between feet and knees strikes a compromise between mobility and stability. Where that place is exactly needs to be an individual preference.

What this place does allow is a wider range that the knees can tilt before they fall to the outside of one foot while also allowing for freedom of movement of the legs. Where that place is for each individual reveals much about how they organize themselves to move, and I always make a note in my initial assessment of the width of their base of support in sitting, standing and lying.

For variety, try this tilting movement with one leg crossed all the way over the other. This further exaggerates instability, which facilitates accuracy and fine-tuning of abdominal and lower extremity control. With just one foot on the floor and that foot placed in such a way that the knees could fall equally easily left or right, the right and left abdominals are engaged in a perpetual game of miniature tug-of-war. Try this yourself. Is there a place in space for your crossed legs where there is no effort at all in legs or belly? Tilt small amounts to the left and right to feel for right and left abdominal balance.

Feel also your foot that's on the ground. Can you feel how that foot presses against the floor? If your right leg is crossed over your left and you are tilting your knees to the left and back again, you will be pressing the outside edge out against the floor with your left TFL and abductors. You can further refine this movement by simultaneously pressing your left foot back into the floor to roll your pelvis towards posterior tilt.

This has a dual benefit of stabilizing the lower back and encouraging movement at the often-stiff lumbothoracic junction (we will do a variation of this later in the segment on stabilization). If you tilt your crossed knees to the right, the inside edge of your left foot presses inward against the floor as the left hip adductors and external rotators control the movements of pelvis and torso. Notice that it is possible to control this movement entirely with one leg. Could you control this movement just from your torso if your legs were paralyzed?

Applying constraints and changing venue

The movement in variation C is really just another version of our dynamic baseline. Coming up to sit and tilting your knees from side to side is another example of our by-now-familiar change of venue. As in supine, we could experiment with distance between feet and knees, seeking that compromise between mobility and stability. As the lesson progresses, that distance becomes more defined by the requirement to get into a side-sitting position; here the distance between the feet equals the distance from the sole of the foot to the patella.

As in supine, we could ask questions about the contribution of the torso in assisting with tilting the knees. Here again, when tilting the knees to the left we are looking for an evenly distributed right torso extension. As in supine, what you will often see clinically is a tendency for your student to twist mostly below the bottom of the sternum. The chest and ribcage will often be inert, or only participating lethargically. There are some advantages to this position in tilting the knees:

- It allows for visual feedback. You can see the rolling of the pelvis and the tilting of the knees and see how close each knee comes to the floor.

- Without the constraint of the floor, the chest, shoulders and head are freer to move.

- By having your hands on the floor, your arms are now in a position to assist the unilateral extension of the torso. When tilting your knees to the left, your right torso extensors can be assisted by the right mid and lower trapezii if you push your right hand into the floor. This also facilitates a reciprocal inhibition of the pectorals, anterior intercostals and abdominals.

How would you organize your head with this movement? If balance were our only consideration, we could expect right cervical extension; the head would move back and to the right and turn some amount to the right. In this scenario, the head and neck are moving as an extension of the torso in a way reminiscent of our original sitting circles lesson. If we add in orientation to the horizon as a constraint, we could expect left cervical flexion: the head and neck would differentiate from the right extension of the torso in a way reminiscent of our original side-sitting spirals lesson. This lesson is yet another way of facilitating a high horizon.

How do you organize your legs with this movement? Do they flop around as a semi-useless appendage of your torso, or are they dynamic? Do they follow your torso or lead? Do you actively push your feet against the ground or do they passively squirm on the surface?

The rest of this lesson provides functional context (side-sitting transitions and balance reactions), constraints (hand placement and orientation) and change of venue (rolling back on to your back and up again, with some momentum) to refine and polish the cooperative use of legs and torso in this very important turning movement. How did you find your two dynamic baselines in terms of ease, organization or distribution of movement at the end of the lesson compared to the beginning? What did you learn about yourself during the lesson that resulted in that change?

Transitions from hook-sitting to side-sitting

The movements in variation D ask you to elaborate on the previous movement of simply tilting your knees by having you lift one hand and reach across to place it on the floor by the other hand. This brings you to a side-sitting position.

When tilting your knees to the left, you lift your right hand from the floor to place it back on the floor near your left hand. What is the timing of lifting that hand? Should you lift it early or late? Sit on the floor with both knees bent and both hands on the floor behind you. Without tilting your knees or rolling your pelvis to the left, just slowly lift your right hand barely away from the floor. What do you have to do to keep from falling back and to the right as you lose support from the right kickstand? Where is your effort, and how much is that effort?

You will probably notice a tendency of your pelvis to roll to the right and your torso to fall back into left flexion. This can be counteracted somewhat by pressing your right foot, but the abdominals, especially along the left side, will probably be recruited. If this is your intent in working with your students, have them lift their right hand early or simultaneously, while tilting the knees to come to left side-sitting.

On the other hand, if your intention is to reduce effort, to facilitate torso extension and to train your students to lead their movements with their legs, you might encourage them to lift the right hand late. If the movement is initiated by the tilting knees and kinematic linkage drags the pelvis and successive vertebrae along with them to the left, the right hand will lift automatically as a result of the movement of the legs, pelvis and torso. By tilting the legs first, rolling the pelvis to the left and pushing the belly and chest forward and to the left, you are shifting your center of mass to the left and over its new base of support: the left ischial tuberosity and left hand.

This shift of the center of mass reduces muscular effort as the bones can now support more weight. This is what makes this way of doing the movement subjectively easier. Try this movement again and do both versions; feel the difference between doing this with a flexion bias and doing it with an extension bias. Alternate from side to side to compare sides and to feel which version of the movement flows more naturally or smoothly.

Alternate from side to side to assess your ability to do a reversible movement as well. Do you stay on the same patch of floor or do you migrate forward? Is this a pure transitional movement or a bizarre form of locomotion? What do you have to do to not scoot forward? As you come to left side-sitting, you might notice that your pelvis rolls not straight to the left but forward and to the left. It describes a quarter-arc from 12 to 3 o'clock or 4.30.

Coming to left side-sitting encourages a right torso extension movement and is consistent with positions of the pelvis from 3 o'clock to 4.30 (left force couple to left iliopsoas organization). The mistake many people make is in not matching the rolling-forward component of the pelvis and the extension component of the torso with an equal rolling-back movement of the pelvis and an equalizing flexion of the torso. They roll forward completely to come to side-sit but don't roll back completely as they transition through the middle. Don't despair if you can't finagle a reversible movement now; there are further opportunities to figure this out later.

Subvariation to facilitate the flexion and extension components

Progressing to variation E, we are now asking for an alternate rounding and arching of your back from a twisted position. After coming to left side-sit, you then alternately look over and under your left shoulder. This detour into intentional orientation acts as a way of mobilizing the ribcage and thoracic spine; rounding and arching from a rotated position enhances the sensation of movement through the mid torso.

Although this is a reciprocating movement and both directions are important, we are particularly interested in the extension movement linked to looking over the shoulder. When instructing your students in this movement, be particularly careful about explaining even distribution of movement. Don't let them just crank away with their neck.

This section also features a recheck on one of our dynamic baselines. After doing this variation, many people will find that returning to tilting the knees from side to side from the initial sitting position and keeping both hands on the floor behind has become much easier. If their knees are coming closer to the floor, it is probably because of enhanced thoracic and chest movement; if both knees are now touching the floor, it is almost certainly because of better participation of the mid to upper torso. How was your check-up?

Look Ma, no hands!

The variation F section is a bit lengthy and includes several variations. The first is to make transitional movements from side-sit to side-sit but holding on to your knees instead of supporting yourself with your hands on the floor. The second variation has you rolling on to your back then back up again, both symmetrically and diagonally. The third variation returns you once again to Side-sit Transitions, but this time with the added complexity of straightening and bending your knees.

What is different about making side-sitting transitional movements with your hands on your knees? This version is a lot harder for most people! The balance requirements are much more stringent and necessitate much more competency in mobilizing the ribs, chest and thoracic spine to move into side-bending and extension directions. Some people are incapable of doing this without heroic effort; others couldn't do it to save their life, so be reasonable with yourself and with your students. Generally speaking, nothing is going to break; usually people just topple over sideways and land on their elbow, so don't be afraid to have some of your people try this.

One advantage of this version of the basic side-sit transitional movement is that it is a bit easier to round back through the middle to avoid creeping forward. By not leaning on your hands behind you, you are getting your shoulder girdles out of the way and can lean/fall much farther backward and can roll your pelvis farther back towards 12 o'clock than before. Another advantage of this variation is that it requires much more abdominal participation and control than when leaning on your hands and, through reciprocating movements, facilitates balance of left and right abdominal muscle tone/length.

Another advantage here is the additional requirement for iliopsoas strength. The hip flexors are required to do shortening and lengthening contractions in a mid to lengthened range to prevent falling all the way back and to bring you to side-sit. The left iliopsoas (working with the right gluteals to make a pelvic force couple) needs to contract powerfully to bring you to left side-sitting. The right iliopsoas (working with the left gluteals to make a right pelvic force couple) brings you to right side-sitting and lowers you back to center/symmetrical sitting. Holding the front of your knees still gives you some upper extremity support, but that support vanishes entirely in our last version of Side-Sitting Transitions.

Using momentum and falling to refine the transitions

The next variation of this section features a blast from the past and slight modifications of it that enhance movements performed in this lesson. Holding on to your knees and rolling all the way back on your back is a variation out of the Pelvic Tilts lesson, though in that lesson you were holding the back of your thighs near your knees. Rolling back facilitates a strong flexion movement of the torso, and coming back forward with some momentum assists in extending fully upright.

After rolling straight back and then back up again a few times to refamiliarize yourself with this earlier movement, you then segue into swinging back upright into a side-sitting position. This diagonal rolling up to sit, again using some momentum, makes getting into this side-sitting position without upper extremity support easier for most people. Once the CNS has the experience of getting into this challenging position by any means, it generally becomes easier to get into this position through other means. Did the side-sit transitional movement with hands on knees get any easier for you after having performed these change of venue rocking movements? Did anything get longer/stretched that made this easier? Did anything get activated/stronger?

Did you find this movement to be fun? Did it heighten your interest and stir your competitive juices? Did it quicken your pulse and put a sparkle in your eyes? Did it require you to focus your attention in the moment? What was your trajectory? Did you roll back then back up along your sides in a diagonal trajectory? Or did you roll up centrally along your back then move asymmetrically into side-sitting only at the end in a T-bone trajectory?

Can you do both versions and distinguish a difference? Don't underestimate the usefulness of making your home exercise programs fun and interesting. How many times have we seen students who come back to us after a relapse who have stopped doing their home exercises because of boredom?

Challenging the iliopsoas – and the abdominals

The last variation in this section makes our basic side-sitting transitional movement even more complex and demanding. Placing your hands now on the front of your thighs near your knees while doing this movement ratchets up the demand on the abdominals and iliopsoas. Straightening your knees as you come through center and bending them back up again as you come to side-sit further facilitates iliopsoas competence. Bending the knees to come to side-sit facilitates hip flexion and the powerful use of the iliopsoas.

Straightening both knees as you round through the middle facilitates hip extension and lumbar flexion and acts to lengthen and reset the muscle spindle of the hip flexors. This is a companion movement to a movement we performed earlier in the pelvic tilt lesson. In that lesson, you were falling straight back and straightening your legs then coming straight forward again and bending your legs. In this lesson you are doing the same basic thing but unilaterally and reciprocally. Try a variation of this variation where you keep your knees more or less straight the whole time as you transition from side-sit to side-sit.

Think of this approach as being modular. Look for similarities, connections, relationships, common denominators, variations off the main path, ways of building one lesson on top of another and new ways of constructing a learning environment. This trait of observing, experimenting on yourself and on students, recalling similar lessons and using your imagination not only is of great benefit to your students, it also keeps things fresh and interesting for you as a therapist. Avoid burnout or boredom by becoming curious and by giving yourself permission to try something you haven't been taught by an expert.

Baselines and applications

Come back on to your back again to finish this lesson in variation G. Bend your knees and tilt them from side to side. How far apart have you placed your feet this time? Has the movement become any easier or more complete? Are you able to more fully mobilize your chest and ribs to assist in tilting the knees in this position? How does this dynamic baseline compare to earlier attempts? How was your static baseline in comparison to the beginning?

Let's ask a variation on the question of 'What sort of folks might we use this lesson with?' What sort of upright dynamic baselines could we create for this lesson? What real-life functional movements might be influenced by this lesson? What brief thing can we have them do that might change the way they do something? And how does that brief thing we are having them do relate to their pain?

As a lesson that facilitates balanced pelvic force couples, we might reasonably expect sitting and standing left/right postural balance to be improved. We could ask our students to sit or stand and observe proprioceptively for left/right balance. More competent pelvic force couples may play out in locomotor functions. We could ask our students to walk before and after this lesson and to attend to hip and pelvic movement.

More competent pelvic force couples may play out in activities involving manipulation or orientation. We could ask our students to reach forward or to look over their shoulders from a sitting or standing position. Longer iliopsoas may result in balancing the pelvis more vertically over the legs. We could ask our students to stand up and to feel the degree of anterior/posterior tilt of their pelvis. An enhanced ability to side-bend through the ribcage may manifest in more integrated manipulation and locomotion. We could ask our students to reach overhead or to walk, and notice whether their ribs move cooperatively.

An enhanced ability to extend from pelvis to head may result in more integrated orientation and manipulation. Ask them to look or reach overhead. An enhanced ability to flex at the hip joints may result in longer hamstrings and short and stubbies. Ask them to bend over from sitting or standing as if picking something up off the floor. An enhanced ability to flex through the torso may make it easier for them to contemplate their navel. Enhanced mobility of the ribcage may improve the quality and ease of breath. Have them focus their attention on the rate, depth, location and ease of breathing before and after this lesson.

Maybe getting up from chair sitting to standing on one leg will get easier. Maybe an activated lower trapezius would improve scapular movement in reaching. Maybe an enhanced awareness of a high horizon would reduce a forward head posture. Maybe reduced adductor tone (or improved adductor/abductor balance) would result in a reduction of genu valgus, knee external rotation or foot pronation. Maybe this lesson promotes world peace. Does this sound like an every-lesson-can-be-all-things-to-all-people kind of exercise?

Getting a straight answer

This is what makes it so difficult for a Feldenkrais practitioner to answer a straightforward question. If someone asks us what we would use a particular lesson for, we could legitimately recite a long list rivaling or exceeding what you just read and give an explanation as to how that lesson related to each specific function. If someone asks us what we would do for a particular problem or diagnosis, they have really just asked the same question but in reverse.

Because knowledge of the diagnosis alone doesn't tell us what sort of movement is causing or contributing to that dysfunction, we have to rephrase the question. The question then becomes one of which lessons would we use for a particular movement impairment or dysfunction that manifests itself in a particular tissue irritation or breakdown. For instance, shearing movements may contribute to lumbar disc disease but can result from either too much flexion on bending and sitting (gluteal bias) or too much extension on standing, walking and bending (iliopsoas bias).

Neck pain could be caused by tight hamstrings (rounded posture and forward shearing at the CT junction on orientation to the horizon/computer screen/TV) or by tight iliopsoas (full arch sitting posture and forward shearing at the CT junction while looking downward to write). If we turn this question around, we could also say that the same movement dysfunctions can manifest in different areas or different diagnoses.

A strong left iliopsoas bias and strong right torso extension bias may manifest in right upper shoulder girdle pain as the right levator scapula and the right upper trapezius are being overstretched. This same left iliopsoas/right torso extension bias may manifest in left upper shoulder girdle pain as the left CT facets are being compressed and the left upper trapezius and levator are working hard in a shortened position.

It's not so much that every lesson works with every problem that every person has. What the clever movement teacher does is to ask questions and focus the attention of each person on that person's basic movement and postural patterns, and how those particular patterns manifest themselves in that particular person's particular problem. This approach de-emphasizes the memorization of minutiae and stuffing yourself with studies while emphasizing cooperative problem solving. It also encourages a strong knowledge of movement, how to recognize it and how to influence it in others.

If we work with someone who has degenerative disc disease from flexion stresses, we might emphasize stronger hip flexors and longer hamstrings and might have an impressive array of lessons to help facilitate this and bring it into real-life function. If we work with someone with CT shearing effects from slumped sitting, we might use many of the same lessons but with a different focus. We might ask slightly different questions or link the lessons to different functional categories. We would direct our student's attention differently whether the focus was on low back pain or neck pain, but the same basic movement lessons could be used.

This is why it is important to have some meaningful functional context in mind when starting a lesson with someone. What you do with them before the lesson starts (what movements you ask them to do, what aspects of themselves are you asking them to pay attention to) sets the tone for the rest of the lesson and sets up a later comparison that makes it clear to your student the benefit of doing the particular exercises you have prescribed.

Variations

1. While in left side-sitting and alternately looking over and under your left shoulder, have your left leg spread wide to the left and the left knee approaching being straight (be reasonable) to coax a little length out of those hamstrings.

2. Do the first part of the lesson while leaning back on your elbows and forearms instead of leaning on your hands.

3. Do Side-Sitting Transitions by deliberately walking yourself forward (easier) and by deliberately walking yourself backward (harder). Vary this by keeping your feet and legs lifted away from the floor the whole time or by blending it into a movement transitioning into poor man's splits.

4. Do Side-Sitting Transitions while holding on to your feet.

5. Do Side-Sitting Transitions with your feet off the ground.

6. Do Side-Sitting Transitions holding on to your feet and holding them both off the ground.

7. Do Side-Sitting Transitions with your legs long and spread the whole time (knees don't have to stay locked, but allow them to bend minimally).

8. Do Side-Sitting Transitions with your legs long and spread and off the ground (this is a belly buster). Do Side-Sitting Transitions with your legs long and spread and off the ground while holding on to your feet (mostly in our dreams).

9. Do Side-Sitting Transitions and expand to a transition to half-kneeling with your hands interlaced and on top of or behind your head. No putting your hand on the ground, and do it really slowly to fully appreciate the balance, flexibility and strength this movement requires.

10. Do Side-sit Transitions with your hands interlaced and on top of or behind your head (makes you more top-heavy). Go back through each of these described variations and mentally design a four- to seven-variation lesson that gets you there.

Think back to the developmental progression of the book so far. We have proprioceptively explored falling from vertical, lifting the head to orient from supine, prone and side-lie, rolling from back to belly and across the floor, coming up to side-sit from lying, coming up to hands and knees from side-sit, and coming from hands and knees or side-sit to half-kneeling.

An adult transition – into and out of a chair

The next logical lesson would be from half kneeling to standing, but we are going to skip that step for the moment and come back to it later. Our next lesson is a bit more adult. We will be exploring transitions from chair sitting to standing and will use the lesson to improve sitting posture, standing posture and bending/lifting organization.

Sit to Stand

Variations

A. Sit near the front edge of a kitchen-style chair or stool. It should be firm enough to feel your sitting bones, but padded enough to be comfortable. Have your feet on the floor at least shoulder width apart, with your knees over your feet.

- Scan the contact of your pelvis and its position on the chair. Is there more weight forward or back on your pelvis? Is there more weight to the left or to the right?

- Feel the shape of your back. Is it rounded? Arched? Rounded in some places and arched in others?

B. Still sitting in your chair –

- Stand up, then sit back down a few times. Does this seem like a lot of effort to you?

- Do you have to move your feet on the floor before you can get up? Do you have to use momentum, or can you do this slowly and in a controlled way?

- Do you tend to use your arms to help you? Do you come up favoring one leg over the other?

C. Still sitting in the chair –

- Begin to roll your pelvis forward and backward on the chair.

- Notice how you coordinate your head with your pelvis and the timing of your breath.

- Feel how your pelvis bones change their contact on seat: rolling forward brings the weight more toward the pubic bone and rolling back brings the contact more toward the tailbone.

- Continue rolling forward and back and add in looking up and down in coordination (Fig. 5.73). Find center: where your sitting bones are neutral and your eyes are on the horizon.

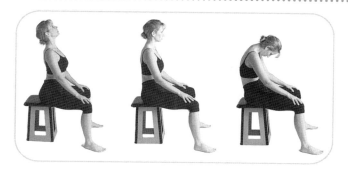

Fig. 5.73 Looking up and down in sitting – rolling your pelvis forward and back on the seat.

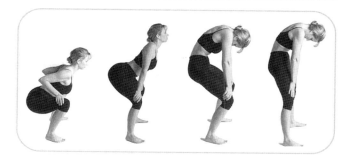

Fig. 5.75 Same movement in a linebacker pose – combine with raising and lowering pelvis.

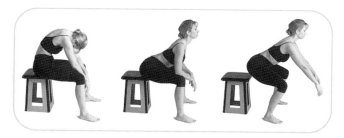

Fig. 5.74 Rounding and arching in other positions – segue into lifting pelvis off seat.

D. Sit on a chair with your feet wide and your knees over your feet. Lean your elbows and forearms on your knees.

- Feel the weight of your feet on the floor and make any adjustments necessary to relax the soles, toes and calves of your legs. If you move your feet back a bit or even under your seat, you will feel the weight on your toes and some effort in your calves.

- Once there, push with your feet into floor to roll your pelvis backward (Fig. 5.74). Roll your pelvis backward on the seat and round your back as you look down towards your belly button. Push with your hips and keep your toes and calves relaxed. Release the push to come back to neutral. Repeat.

- Be sure to push your feet straight down into the ground (you will feel effort in the back of your thighs) rather than forward along the ground (where you will feel effort in the front of your thighs).

- Now from neutral look forward and upward while pushing your belly and chest toward the floor between your thighs (Fig. 5.74) Be careful with your neck. Move head and neck in proportion to your ability to arch your upper back.

- Alternate rounding and arching your back – rolling your pelvis forward and back on the seat and looking up and down. Intentionally use your legs to control this movement. Can you round your back without tightening your belly?

E. Sit on a chair, feet wide on the floor as before. Lean forward so your arms dangle down between your knees and your hands hang towards or even touch the floor.

- Slowly swing your arms forward and back – drag your knuckles on the ground if possible. Round your back as you swing your arms back and arch your back as you swing your arms forward.

- Move your head and eyes to assist. Alternate a few times, then the next time you swing your arms forward and arch your back –

- Lift your pelvis off the seat 1–2 inches (Fig. 5.74). Lower your pelvis softly to the seat as you swing your arms back again. Repeat this movement of lifting and lowering your pelvis in a controlled way several times.

- Do your feet stay centered on the floor? Do your toes press or grip the floor? Try moving your feet forward a little. Do your toes lift from the floor? Try moving your feet back a little.

- Can you get your center of mass far enough forward over your feet to lift your pelvis very slowly? You'll have to bend a lot at your hips and straighten your back; having your arms out in front also helps.

F. Stand with your feet a bit wider than shoulder width apart with the chair seat just behind you. Lean with your hands on the front of your thighs near your knees, like a linebacker. Knees are bent but elbows are straight. Give the weight of your arms and upper body to your thighs – lean heavily with your hands on your knees.

- Alternately look up and down, rounding and arching your back (Fig. 5.75). Repeat the same basic movement you did in sitting while in this position. Keep leaning heavily with your hands on your knees; support most of your upper body weight with your arms.

- Initiate the movement of rounding your back and 'tucking your tail' by pressing with your feet, as in sitting. How much can you round your back without tightening your abdominal muscles?

- Let go of the push to allow your back to arch, then push your belly and chest forward toward the floor to lift your head to look forward toward the horizon.

211

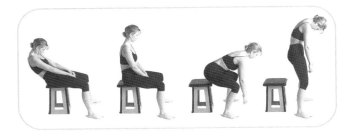

Fig. 5.76 From falling back – to sit – to stand.

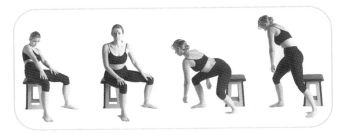

Fig. 5.77 Diagonal fall back – to diagonal up to stand.

Box 5.19 Side-sit Transitions

Transitional movements from side-sit to side-sit – functional context to facilitate pelvic force couple balance and competence

Belly-up orientation emphasizes length and strength of hip flexors – links to previous transitions

Orientation and reaching requirements are applied constraints – coordinating the chest and upper body with the legs and pelvis

---

- Continue arching and rounding, but begin to bend your knees and lower your pelvis as you arch and straighten your knees and raise your pelvis as you round (Fig. 5.75). Allow your elbows to bend and straighten, but always keep your hands glued to your thighs near your knees.

- Gradually lower your pelvis all the way to barely brush your chair seat, then come back up again. Combine to move from sitting (while leaned forward) to almost standing. How close can you push your pelvis toward vertical and how much can you tuck your tail while still keeping your hands on your thighs?

G. Come back down to sit on your chair again near the front edge.

- Roll your pelvis back on the chair and lean way back. Round your back and drop your head toward your chest as you do this.

- From here, come back forward again by rolling your pelvis forward on the seat and arching your back. Lean way forward or even swing your arms forward if you need to.

- Lift your pelvis in a controlled way off the seat and slowly press yourself to standing (Fig. 5.76). Push your pelvis toward vertical first and let your back follow. Repeat several times, then rest.

- As a diagonal variation, instead of rounding straight back and coming straight back forward again and up to standing, fall back and to the right then come back forward and up to stand diagonally over your left foot.

- Do the same movement to the other side: lean and round back and to the left, then come back forward and up over your right foot (Fig. 5.77). Which side is easier?

- Return to our original movement: simply stand up from a chair then sit back down again, as we did at the beginning of this lesson. Is this movement easier or organized any differently than it was to begin?

Static and dynamic baselines – Sit to Stand

As a physical therapist, I was taught that proper sitting could be measured with a protractor. The ankles, knees and hips are bent at 90°. The hip, shoulder and ear line up vertically. The midline of the face, sternum and pubic symphysis line up vertically. The eyes, shoulders and iliac crests are level on the horizontal plane. These are quantitative criteria. They are objective. They are measurable. They are handy for documentation purposes. But they are rarely seen in the wild.

Real human beings don't have the geometrical perfection of machines. Attempting to achieve that level of perfection through bony or soft tissue manipulation or through exercise is a chimera. Asking your students to strive for geometrical symmetry when they have neither an internal sense of how they habitually organize themselves nor the proprioceptive or motor skills needed to get to where they are supposed to be is an exercise in futility.

As much as we might like it to, it's just not going to happen! Our students might be better off if we as practitioners started looking more at dynamic and proprioceptive criteria rather than just static and geometrical criteria in determining proper sitting posture. How well could she move from that position versus how perfectly balanced is she in a three-dimensional grid? Let's first review some of our static proprioceptive cues for easy and balanced posture.

One of the proprioceptive static criterions we have already discussed in the sitting circles lesson is that of balancing the weightbearing pressure on the ischial tuberosities. Forward and back balance brings the pelvis to vertical in a frontal plane and sets the tone for balancing the shoulders and ears in a skeletal weightbearing fashion over the pelvis. Left-to-right balance across the ischia brings the pelvis to vertical in the sagittal plane and sets the tone for balancing the sternum and facial midline in a skeletal weightbearing fashion over the pelvis. Ischial pressure against a weightbearing surface is a subjective criterion that students can find and reproduce with their eyes closed.

Another proprioceptive static criterion we have discussed is that of achieving a high horizon. This also tends to require that the pelvis be close to vertical and that the thoracic spine be extended. This also gives people who fully round or who half arch an internal and reproducible way of improving their posture that is independent of mirrors or plumb lines.

Dynamic criteria for ideal sitting posture

In terms of dynamic criteria, we have discussed how an ability to fall as easily backward as forward and as easily to the left as to the right might be used as an active way of finding a neutral zone of posture. Review for a moment the role the four cornerstone muscles of the pelvis have on preventing falls forward/back, left/right or any of the other 356 directions.

Recall how we can extrapolate cornerstone muscle imbalances (iliopsoas and gluteal bias and left or right force couple bias) from an observation of postural imbalances and how we can reduce those imbalances by gaining competence in moving in all of those 360 directions.

Another dynamic criterion we have discussed is being able to orient all around ourselves in a 360° sphere equally easily in all directions. This also tends to balance the cornerstones and the cylindrical torso. We could also use more complex dynamic criteria for ideal sitting, the ability to make transitions and to manipulate.

Reaching from a sitting position is a bit more complex than it may seem to be at first. Whether reaching forward, overhead or out to the side, there could be integration with and subsequent movement of the pelvis on the seat. These connections between reaching and weight-shifting of the pelvis will be further explored in Section 4.

One direction you might take a moment to explore is down and to the right and down and to the left; I call this the tip test. This test illustrates the dynamic criteria in organizing the legs in sitting. How far apart should your knees be? Where should your feet be on the floor? Where should your feet be in relation to your knees? The tip test addresses the first question: how far apart should your feet and knees be?

The tip test

To do the tip test, first sit toward the front edge of a stable chair. Place your feet and knees together so they touch each other. Slowly begin to reach with your right hand toward the floor directly down and to the right. Make sure you are bending straight to the side and not leaning or bending forward at all (Fig. 5.78). How close can you reach to the floor before you

feel in danger of tipping over? Do this movement a few times to the right, then switch to the left. How stable do you feel in that direction?

Now spread your feet and knees to approximately shoulder width apart and do the same thing. Reach directly down and to each side a few times and compare stability, ease and range of movement to what it was like when your feet and knees were together. Now spread your feet and knees as wide as you can go; do the same thing here. Where is the compromise between mobility and stability? The tip test illustrates the role the legs play in side-to-side mobility and stability in sitting, but does it really matter how far apart your knees are when you are just sitting down to write a letter or surf the net? I would say yes!

Having knees and feet close together (as many people do) in sitting has several disadvantages:

- It is unnecessary effort. The adductors are working hard to maintain a position that has little to do with function and much to do with maintaining modesty or with attaining an artificial aesthetic.

- Through constant excitation of the adductors, there is a simultaneous inhibition of the abductors and probably the gluteals. Those muscles that help us to ground ourselves into the floor are shut off, and we are left to precariously perch on our ischia like a worm standing on his tail. The legs participate minimally in balance and require the lumbar or abdominal (or both) musculature to work much harder than they need to.

- It is difficult to move efficiently from this position. The chronically firing adductors lock the pelvis in place and can necessitate too much lumbar or SI movement, leading in turn to joint or disc instability or degenerative changes.

- It compromises left-to-right mobility. Reaching left and right (and even reaching forward, as we'll find in Section 4) and spiraling to look left and right becomes constrained and compartmentalized because the pelvis is not able to participate fully. This can contribute to neck and glenohumeral dysfunction.

- Holding the knees together often goes along with a systemic pattern of pulling in that can be indicative of generalized high tone and sympathetic dominance.

- Try a simple manual assessment. Have your student sit at the front edge of a chair with feet and knees touching. Press gently through the right knee, longitudinally along the femur. Observe and feel for give and a rotation of the pelvis. Do the same to the other side. Then do the same thing with knees fallen apart to relax adductors; bring feet wider and underneath knees. Feel how much looser and more responsive the hips and pelvis are!

Demure – yet deadly!

How far apart to have your knees is a function of the length of your adductors. What we will often do with people is to get them to recognize the effort in the adductors then to have them deliberately sit like Barbie, knees and feet properly clamped together. If they can recognize and reduce effort of the adductors in sitting, they can allow their knees to fall away from each other just by surrendering to gravity.

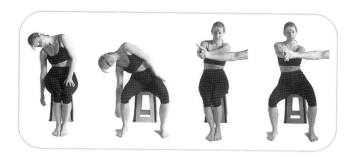

Fig. 5.78 The tip test and the twist test.

After determining the distance between the knees by this method, I'll have them bring their feet underneath their knees and do the tip test, both here and in Barbie sitting. As a variation on the tip test, you can have your students put both hands together and out in front at about shoulder height. Push sideways on their hands as if trying to twist them right and left, and have them feel for stability with knees apart and with knees together – the twist test (Fig. 5.78). This is a variation of the standing stability testing we did in Side-Lying Transitions, again testing the ability to ground with the gluteal/abductor family.

In addition to the many folks who sit with their knees very close together, you have no doubt noticed that there are also a significant number of people who sit with their knees very wide apart. Whereas this could be perfectly legitimate for people whose adductors are sufficiently long and whose feet are sufficiently flat on the floor to still permit easy movement of the pelvis in balance orientation and manipulation, this is not most often the case. What many people will do is to let their knees fall way out as a reflection of a strong gluteal/external rotator bias and of simultaneous adductor inhibition.

They will then either put their feet on the floor under their chair (tiptoe weightbearing and short hamstrings) or frog-legged and resting on their outside edges with the soles of their feet facing each other. Neither variation fulfills our dynamic criterion of being able to move equally easily in all directions – try the tip test, the resisted rotation test, or getting up from sitting to standing without moving your feet from these positions!

Observing your students in sitting can yield valuable clues. Where the pelvis is on the clock may tell you a lot about cornerstone bias and left/right imbalance. Observing their legs and feet may tell you a lot about likely directions of mobility and restriction, and gives you some initial clues as to how they do or don't use their legs to control the movement and position of the pelvis in space. Observing horizon height will give you clues about probable distribution of movement of the spine in orientation. Just keep in mind the importance of the legs in sitting, the relationship between 'static' posture and dynamic movement, and the importance of developing proprioceptive criteria for efficient sitting.

Some legs to stand on

Stand up from your chair then sit back down a few times. Does this seem like a lot of effort to you? Do you have to move your feet on the floor before you can get up? Do you have to use momentum, or can you do this slowly and in a controlled way? Do you tend to use your arms to help you? Do you come up favoring one leg over the other? In variation B these questions address the main focus of this lesson: getting up from sitting to standing.

We could say that one of our criteria for proper sitting would be that place from which you could move from sitting to standing without having to make any preparatory postural adjustments, such as moving the feet somewhere else on the floor or using your hands to push. We could say that one of our criteria for proper standing posture would be that place from which you could move from standing to sitting without engaging in similar extraneous movements. These questions set up the dynamic baseline of this lesson. Did you answer these questions any differently at the end of the lesson?

The meat of the lesson is designed to help sharpen the physical and proprioceptive awareness skills necessary to reduce effort and enhance your subjective feeling of ease, to reduce the need to use momentum or to push with your arms, and to balance the two sides. The physical and proprioceptive skills learned in this lesson are useful when working with someone on sitting posture, standing posture and proper bending/lifting technique.

Looking up and down – falling forward and back in sitting

The initial movement in variation C of this lesson, of rolling the pelvis forward and back in the seat and coordinating it with torso movements, orientation and breathing, is a review/overlap with the beginning of the sitting circles lesson. Everything is the same in terms of muscular breakdown, use of the legs in each direction, and so on.

The next movement in variation D starts in a position of leaning forward with your elbows and forearms on your thighs near your knees. The instructions are to first place your feet according to proprioceptive criteria and then to push your feet into the floor to roll your pelvis backward and look towards your belly button.

To stand up from sitting, your feet can be neither too far forward nor too far back. If too far forward, you will have difficulty getting your center of mass far enough forward over your feet to be able to stand. If placed too far back, you will topple over forward. There is a zone of possibilities that will work. How do we fine-tune what works best?

By discovering that placement of the feet on the floor where there is no effort in the calves or soles of the feet (ankle and toe plantarflexors), you are arranging yourself to bear weight skeletally. By leaning the weight of your upper body on your knees, you are balancing extra weight on top of the tibias. If the top of the tibia is angled forward (the feet are too far back), the additional weight of the upper body will tend to topple the tibia further forward and necessitate active ankle plantarflexion.

To feel this proprioceptively, you will probably have to try all three versions. If the top of the tibia is angled too far backward (the feet are too far forward), that will get washed out when coming up to stand. An ideal position for the feet might be that place where your feet are as far underneath you as possible without feeling effort in calves or toes.

Pressing the feet into the floor from this position results in rolling back the pelvis on the seat, if you inhibit the antagonistic musculature sufficiently. This belly-down orientation features a shortening contraction of the hamstrings, gluteals and short and stubbies when rolling back/looking down. There is a lengthening contraction of those same muscles to return to neutral. By placing the feet in relation to the knees in such a way that the calves and feet are turned off, we are further refining the ability to push the feet with the powerful proximal hip extensors. Are you able to roll your pelvis back and round your back without using your abdominal muscles in this position? Useful motor skill or mere party trick? You be the judge.

Engaging the iliopsoas and back extensors to roll the pelvis forward, arch the back and lift the head to look forward is the next movement in this section. We want to encourage a full hip hinge to allow the pelvis to roll far enough forward to bring your center of mass over your base of support. Arching the back and engaging the iliopsoas inhibits the hamstrings and gluteals and facilitates this ability to flex fully at the hip joints.

Alternating back and forth between rounding and arching is yet another example of using reciprocating movement to balance antagonists or antagonistic directions of movement. This is also another excellent position to work on differentiation of the thoracic and lumbar spine, using extreme hip flexion to again limit lumbar extension while using an antigravity movement of looking forward to facilitate thoracic extension.

The next movement is really just a continuation of the last. In variation E you are still rolling your pelvis alternately forward and back on the seat, but instead of leaning on your elbows and forearms you are dangling your arms between your knees and swinging them forward and back in time with the rolling of your pelvis.

One difference is that your arms are no longer supporting the weight of your upper body. The legs have to work much harder to hold up your weight; this is a degree of difficulty progression. Another difference is the change of venue: intentional movement of the arms (manipulation) rather than the eyes (orientation). Why dangle the arms between the knees? Why not dangle them to the outside? Because we will usually want to encourage a wider rather than a narrower base of support.

Especially when we are using this lesson to teach bending skills, we want to be pattern specific. When bending from a standing position, a wide spread between the feet simultaneously lowers your center of mass and increases your stability, and it's easier to get your hands to the floor inside your feet than it is to do so from the outside.

Transition from Sit to Stand – focusing on the initial lift

We then segue this arm-swinging movement into a movement of barely lifting your pelvis away from the seat. This is the critical moment of transition. You are going from sitting to standing here within a very narrow range. Initially, it's okay to use some momentum. Gradually, you may be able to clean things up to where you could do this movement very slowly, or stop and reverse it at any time. This is another proprioceptive criterion we often use to find efficient and well-balanced movement.

The finer and finer the distinctions you can make in a lesson, the more precise the moment of transition and the more controlled/slow/reversible you can make the movement, the better. Another proprioceptive criterion built into this lesson is the question about what your toes do. Do they lift from the floor? Are the dorsiflexors being recruited because you are close to toppling backward?

Your feet may be too far forward to get your center of mass far enough forward. Or you could reach your arms forward to help bring your center of mass farther forward. Do your toes press into the floor or hammer? Your weight is too far forward; try moving your feet forward. Have you noticed how closely this position of just starting to lift your pelvis off the seat with

your hands near the ground resembles the postures of weightlifters and sumo wrestlers?

Use this lesson to teach principles of bending and lifting. This lesson encourages a wide base of support, an awareness of front-to-back balance and an ability to get your hands on or near the floor while maintaining a neutral back. It emphasizes the full bending of the hips and powerful use of the legs in both decelerating the bend forward and accelerating the push-up to standing.

Reversing field – transition from stand to sit

We have a change of venue in variation F. Stand with your feet a bit more than shoulder width apart, with the chair seat just behind you. Lean with your hands on the front of your thighs near your knees, like a linebacker. Give the weight of your arms and upper body to your thighs. Lean heavily with your hands on your knees.

This linebacker position is a great one to work from, either as a standalone or when leaning with your pelvis against a wall. It is a little like a hands and knees position in that you are getting upper extremity support for your upper body. This position is also a mirror image of some of the positions you used in Pelvic Tilts. This is a belly-up variation of sitting on the floor with knees bent and placing your palms on the front of your thighs near your knees.

The movement of alternately rounding and arching is also identical. The difference is orientation to gravity. The pelvic tilt version emphasized lengthening and strengthening the iliopsoas. The linebacker position emphasizes the length and strength of the gluteals/hamstrings.

Movements of alternately rounding and arching here feature differentiated patterns of lumbar flexion with hip extension and back extension with hip flexion. The instruction to deliberately push with the feet into the floor and relax your belly is to facilitate the mindful use of the legs in pushing away from the floor.

Recall one of the main errors people make in bending and lifting: the tendency to pull their torso to vertical with their back extensors instead of pushing their pelvis to vertical first then following with the torso. People with iliopsoas bias tend to do this more, so this gluteal strengthening aspect of the lesson is very useful with them.

The next instruction in this section asks you to continue the same basic flexion/extension movement but to now bend your knees and elbows and lower your pelvis as you arch, then straighten your knees and elbows and raise your pelvis as you round. Your elbows can bend and straighten but always keep your hands glued to your thighs near your knees (Box 5.20).

This association of the basic flexion/extension movement with raising and lowering your pelvis helps to encourage fuller

---

Box 5.20 Sit to Stand

Transitional movements from sitting to standing – functional context to facilitate pelvic force couple balance and competence

Belly-down orientation emphasizes length and strength of hip extensors

Facilitates competence in sitting, bending and standing

hip flexion and extension. Keeping your hands glued to your thighs when pushing your pelvis toward vertical is a constraint that makes you flex your back when pushing up to stand. This is something that is very foreign to many people. For these folks, coming up from sitting to standing is performed much like bending over. When bending, they allow their pelvis to fall too far forward on their legs and need to catch the fall with the lumbar extensors.

Coming back upright, they again pull themselves up with their back rather than pushing with their legs. Remember when you tell your students to lift with their legs that they may have no real proprioceptive idea what you are talking about. They may just interpret it to mean that if they just bend their knees a little, or come down to a squat, they are doing what you ask. When someone comes to you with back pain aggravated by bending/lifting, assume they don't know how to do it, figure out what their mistake or invariance is and lead them step by step to the promised land.

Generic or one-size-fits-all body mechanics advice is about as useful as generic stock market advice (buy low, sell high). One of the nice things about doing reciprocating movements is that it does have something for everyone. Iliopsoas- and gluteal-biased folks both benefit from this lesson, but will need the tone and emphasis to be different.

Think again back to the variation in Pelvic Tilts where you were sitting on the floor with your hands on your thighs near your knees. In one of the last variations of that lesson, you were rolling back at the same time you were sliding your heels away from yourself and straightening your knees.

This is again a mirror image of the movement of pushing your pelvis upward and toward vertical, but in another orientation to gravity. Both directions of movement emphasize iliopsoas length. Did you feel a tug or stretch on the front of your hips with this movement of pushing to vertical? Can you recognize the basic underlying pattern in the two positions?

Can you think of any other belly-up orientation versions of the same movement? (Rolling back while seated in a chair, rolling back while sitting on your feet, etc.) Can you think of any other belly-down orientation versions of the same movement? (Hands and knees, side-sitting and leaning forward, plantigrade, sitting on your heels and leaning forward, etc.) This approach is actually quite simple. Look for patterns, then teach them in a number of different positions and in a number of different functional contexts.

Putting the pieces together – rocketing out of your seat

Our last section in this lesson is a cumulative movement. In variation G you put the whole thing together by rolling back while sitting, using the initial lengthening of the iliopsoas to spring-load a movement into anterior pelvic tilt and back extension. This movement in turn leans you forward and spring-loads the gluteals and hamstrings to push you to standing.

You are then encouraged to draw outside the cardinal lines by rolling back and then coming back up in a diagonal. You could add some detail here by sliding both hands alternately down one shin, then up again, then up along the thigh to the belly. What might be some of the benefits of doing this move-

ment of coming up to stand primarily on one leg and then the other?

- It is a reciprocating movement, and as such helps to balance right and left pelvic force couple musculature.
- It is a degree of difficulty progression and further refines accuracy, balance, strength and flexibility. Try crossing one leg over the other and coming up from sitting to standing in this diagonal.

Return now to our original movement, our dynamic baseline. Simply stand up from a chair and sit back down again, as we did at the beginning of this lesson. Is this movement easier or organized any differently than it was to begin? What did you learn about center of mass and base of support? Did any of your physical skills improve? Balance? Strength? Flexibility? Which of these skills would be useful for bending and lifting? Which of these skills would be useful for improving standing and sitting posture? Could you distinguish which particular skills are needed by which particular person and their own particular pattern biases?

Applications and variations

Being a cumulative lesson for this segment on pelvic force couples and bending, all the benefits of previous lessons accrue to this one. Besides the obvious applications to geriatrics and neurologic rehabilitation, there are ample opportunities to work with knee and ankle rehabilitation here. We will revisit this lesson with toy variations in the last chapter, on legs.

Variations on this lesson include simply raising or lowering the height of the seat to make the movements either easier or more challenging. This is a nice way to segue into teaching squatting skills. There are even some people who can take this movement to its logical conclusion and lower all the way past squatting to sitting on the floor!

An effective variation is to get them into a linebacker pose with their pelvis leaning back against a wall. The wall makes a handy proprioceptive reference point. Roll the pelvis up and down on the wall and round and arch the back. Progress this lesson by sliding the hands up and down the thighs and shins, either coordinating it with flexion/extension movements of the torso or finding a neutral spine and sliding up and down with purely hip flexion and extension.

Vary this lesson by sliding the hands diagonally up and down thigh and shin, again either coordinating the movement with unilateral torso flexion/extension movements or finding a neutral spine and keeping it. Connect the dots and make a circle. Try it both leaning with your hands on your knee, introducing an upper extremity closed kinetic chain movement and consequent mobilization of ribs, thoracic spine and shoulder girdles, and by allowing your arms to dangle passively between your knees. This requires more lower extremity power and precision and is an opportunity to recognize and reduce effort in the scapular musculature, differentiating rhomboids and mid-low trapezius from the thoracic extensors and posterior intercostals.

Vary this sequence by placing your feet very far away from the wall or very far away from each other. This is an excellent way to encourage longer hamstrings and adductors. Progress this lesson by coming away from the wall and doing the flexion/extension, diagonal and circular movements here, both with coordinated spinal movement and with a neutral spine. Mix and match and be creative.

Both the Sit to Stand movements and the linebacker movements lend themselves very well to the placement of rollers under the feet. This will be explored in more depth in the segment on the legs and knees.

Now that we have explored the ways in which the legs act to control the pelvis and back, let's turn our focus to a specific clinical problem. Let's talk about lumbar/SI stabilization.

References

1. Cailliet R. Low back pain syndrome. Philadelphia: FA Davis, 1977.
2. Sahrmann S. Diagnosis and treatment of movement impairment syndromes. St. Louis, MO: Mosby; 2002: 103–7.
3. Irvin RE. Suboptimal posture: the origin of the majority of idiopathic pain of the musculoskeletal system. In: Vleeming A, Mooney V, Dorman T, eds. Movement, stability and low back pain. Edinburgh: Churchill Livingstone; 1997: 133–55.
4. Farfan HF. Mechanical disorders of the low back. Philadelphia: Lea & Febiger; 1973.
5. Janda V. Muscles, central nervous motor regulation and back problems. In: Korr IM, ed. The neurobiological mechanisms in manipulative therapy. New York: Plenum Press: 1978; 27–41.
6. Cailliet R. Neck and arm pain. Philadelphia: FA Davis, 1976.
7. Cailliet R. Shoulder pain. Philadelphia: FA Davis, 1977.
8. Burkart S. The shoulder: examination and rehabilitation. Course Manual: NE Seminars, p. 42.
9. Sahrmann S. Diagnosis and treatment of movement impairment syndromes. St. Louis, MO: Mosby; 2002: 193–263.
10. Downs JR. Treating the TMJ dysfunction. Osteopathic Physician 1976;43:106–13.
11. Jull GA. Cervical headache: a review. In: Boyling J, Palastanga N. Modern manual therapy of the vertebral column. Edinburgh: Churchill Livingstone; 1996: 333–47.
12. Grieve G. Common vertebral joint problems. New York: Churchill Livingstone; 1988.
13. Beckwith CG. Headache. Journal of the American Orthopedic Associations 1988;48:385–90.
14. Jull GA. Headaches of cervical origin. In: Grant R. Physical therapy of the cervical and thoracic spine, 2nd edn. New York: Churchill Livingstone; 1994: 261–85.
15. Richardson CA, Jull GA. Concepts of assessment and rehabilitation for active spinal stability. In: Boyling J, Palastanga N, eds. Modern manual therapy of the vertebral column. Edinburgh: Churchill Livingstone; 1994: 705–20.
16. Sahrmann S. Diagnosis and treatment of movement impairment syndromes. St. Louis, MO: Mosby; 2002: 88–93.
17. Mooney V, Robertson J. Facet syndrome. Clinical Orthopedics Related Research 1976;115:149–56.
18. Dolan P, Adams MA, Hutton WC. Commonly adopted postures and their effect on the lumbar spine. Spine 1988;13:197–201.
19. During J, Goudfrooij H, Keessen W, Beeker Th W, Crowe A. Towards standards for posture: postural characteristics of the lower back system in normal and pathologic conditions. Spine 1985;10: 83–7.
20. Beck A, Killius J. Normal posture of the spine, determined by mathematical and statistical methods. Aerospace Medicine 1973;49:1277–81.
21. Sahrmann S. Diagnosis and treatment of movement impairment syndromes. St. Louis, MO: Mosby; 2002: 52–7.
22. Kotsias J. Tai-chi tao for physical therapists: applications and interventions. Caledonia, MN: American Tai-Chi Tao; 1996.
23. Nachemson A. Toward a better understanding of low back pain: a review of the mechanics of the lumbar disc. Rheumatologicals Rehabilitation 1975;14:129.
24. Brinckmann P. Stress and strain of human lumbar discs. Clinical Biomechanics 1988;3:232–5.
25. Jacobsen F. Medical exercise therapy. Fysioterapeuten 1992;59: 19–22.
26. Dolan P, Adams MA, Hutton WC. Commonly adopted postures and their effect on the lumbar spine. Spine 1988;13:201.
27. Horst M, Brinkmann P. Measurement of the distribution of axial stress on the endplate of the vertebral body. Spine 1981;6:217–32.
28. Fahrni WH, Trueman GE. Comparative radiological study of the spines of a primitive population with North Americans and North Europeans. Journal of Bone and Joint Surgery 1965;47B: 1105–27.
29. Pearsall DJ, Reid JG. Line of gravity relative to upright vertebral posture. Clinical Biomechanics 1992;7:80.
30. Weiselfish S. A contemporary clinical analysis of biomechanical dysfunction. Manual therapy with muscle energy technique for the pelvis, sacrum, cervical, thoracic, and lumbar spine, pp. 42–45.
31. Kahle W, Leonhardt H, Platzer W. Color atlas/text of human anatomy. Vol. 1 The locomotor system. New York: Thieme; 1992.
32. Sahrmann S. Diagnosis and treatment of movement impairment syndromes. St. Louis, MO: Mosby; 2002: 58–61.
33. Nachemson A. The possible importance of the psoas muscle for stabilization of the lumbar spine. Acta Orthopedica Scandinavica 1968;39:47–57.
34. Mooney V, Pozos R, Vleeming A, Gulic J, Swenski D. Coupled motion of contralateral latissimus dorsi and gluteus maximus: its role in sacroiliac stabilization. In: Vleeming A, Mooney V, Dorman T, eds. Movement, stability and low back pain. Edinburgh: Churchill Livingstone; 1997: 115–23.
35. Lee D. Treatment of pelvic instability. In: Vleeming A, Mooney V, Dorman T, eds. Movement, stability and low back pain. Edinburgh: Churchill Livingstone; 1997: 445–60.
36. Kotsias J. Tai-chi tao for physical therapists: applications and interventions. Caledonia, MN: American Tai-Chi Tao; 1996: 10–11.
37. Dychtwald K. Bodymind. New York: Jove; 1978.
38. Johnson J. The multifidus back pain solution. Oakland, CA: New Harbinger Publications; 2002.

CHAPTER SIX

Outsmarting lower back pain

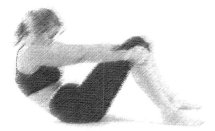

Chapter outline

Layers of stability

1. Intersegmental stability – controlling arthrokinematic movement of vertebrae relative to each other.

2. Torso stability – controlling the movements of the chest and upper body relative to the pelvis.

3. Pelvic stability – controlling the movements of the pelvis relative to the legs.

Stressors of the lower back

1. Flexion stressors. Postural – sitting, squatting. Movement – bending, pulling, lifting, sit-ups. Weak back extensors and hip flexors. Tight hip extensors and abdominals.

2. Extension stressors. Postural – sitting, standing, lie supine or prone. Movement – two-handed push or pull, lean or bend/return to upright, carry/weight in front, locomotion (shock absorb, incomplete hip extension, use of iliopsoas of stepping leg), global extension (push-ups, back bends, certain yoga postures). Weak abdominals and hip extensors. Tight hip flexors and back extensors.

3. Multidirectional instabilities. The worst of both worlds – combination of flexion and extension instabilities. All hip musculature is short, lower torso co-contractions, probable thoracic stiffness.

4. Lateral/rotational stresses. Postural – asymmetrical sitting, standing, lying. Movement – centrifugal forces, locomo-

tion, push objects laterally (right/left), one handed push or pull, acceleration/deceleration/controlling ballistic movements (swing golf club, baseball bat). Particularly nasty when in combination with extension bias – extension/rotation especially is on our least wanted list.

Intersegmental stability

1. Arthrokinematic control of movements of joint surfaces relative to each other.

2. Hodges' research on correlation between back pain and recruitment strength, sequence and differentiation of the transverse abdominis (TA) and multifidi.

   - Correlation between the early activation of the arthrokinematic muscles and the absence of back pain.

   - Correlation between a delay in the activation of these muscles and people with back pain.

   - Arthrokinematic stabilization ideally precedes gross skeletal movement.

   - Both TA and multifidi kick in with both flexion and extension stressors.

   - Neither TA nor multifidi have flexion or extension effects on spine.

3. Lesson 1: *TA Facilitation*.

   - Facilitation of transverse abdominis with directed movements of pelvic floor.

   - Reciprocating movements – open and close pelvic floor/pull in and push out TA. Going in both directions to facilitate awareness, control and balance.

- Timing TA/pelvic floor piece with breathing. Way to help in differentiating TA from obliques and rectus abdominis. Exhaling with TA contraction to train for short duration/higher intensity stressor. Breathing independently with TA contraction for longer duration/lower intensity stressor.

- Anterior and posterior tilt of the pelvis coordinated with TA/floor piece – coordinating in both directions so arthrokinematic stability is independent of direction of movement of spine/pelvis.

- Coordinating arthrokinematic stabilizers with both iliopsoas group (for the gluteal biased/flexion stress susceptible) and with the gluteal group (for the iliopsoas biased/extension stress susceptible).

4. Lesson 2: *TA Diagonals*.
   - Blending intersegmental and pelvic stability.
   - Sitting and supine exploration of unilateral TA contraction with diagonal movements of the pelvis. Using gluteals to stabilize pelvis from rolling into anterior tilt when lifting opposite foot. Using iliopsoas to stabilize the pelvis from falling back into posterior tilt. Balancing left and right TA.

5. Lesson 3: *TA Leg Lifts*.
   - Companion/continuation of the TA series. Long lifted leg to increase demand on pelvic and intersegmental stability.
   - Crossover swing of lifted leg to coordinate standing leg gluteals and adductors and to encourage lumbothoracic junction and thoracic mobility in extension/rotation.

Stability in standing and bending

1. Lesson 4: *Half-kneel Bending*.
   - Blending intersegmental stability with gross movements of pelvis and back, in belly-down orientation, relating to bending.
   - Disallowing flexion at the low back when bending lengthens the gluteals and hamstrings and strengthens the back.
   - Using reciprocating movements to find spinal neutral and staying there on bending and return to upright movements.
   - Descriptions of kneeling and squatting possibilities – substitutes for bending, especially if prolonged (over 10 seconds).
   - Disallowing extension at the low back when pushing pelvis to vertical lengthens the hip flexors and strengthens the hamstrings and gluteals in context of reducing lumbar lordosis in standing.
   - Contralateral and homolateral bending strategies and upper extremity support.
   - Manual resistance of movements of the pole simulating control of rotational stresses in one-hand pushing and pulling.

- Manual resistance of movements of the pole simulating weight-in-front stresses – or substitute with medicine ball, jug of milk or other weighty object.

- Manual resistance of movements of the pole simulating two-handed pushing and pulling stresses – mimic a vacuum or push broom – simulate shoveling or lifting something else with a long lever arm. Resist two-handed pushing and pulling of a horizontal pole.

2. Lesson 5: *Split Stance Bending*.
   - Identical twin to Half-kneel Bending, only taller.
   - Training control of anterior pelvic tilt in standing through split stance or foot up on chair, stool, etc.
   - Training control of weight in front stresses with a medicine ball or manual resistance of pole. Other manual resistance as in Half-kneel Bending applicable.
   - Flamboyant postures and grandiose movements may make some people self-conscious – they want to be able to change the result of their movements/postures (pain) without actually changing their movements/posture. Model behavior and make clear choice between comfort and familiarity/conformity.

Stability in gait

1. Types of gait stressor.
   - Rotational – waddle walk.
   - Lateral shear – swish walk.
   - Extension stresses – lumbar extension as shock absorber, inadequate hip extension, weight in front stress created by iliopsoas of lifting leg.
   - Jarring stressors – not enough adduction/internal rotation (IR), hybrid movement of hip joint with bend of knee.
   - Stability through rigidity – the doll body walk.
   - The cure for the locomotor blues is a competent force couple gait featuring full hip extension and complete push-off.

2. Lesson 6: *Knee Walking*.
   - Blending locomotor function with intersegmental stability.
   - Dancing the Charleston – the pelvic force couple two-step. Use music to reinforce.
   - Reciprocating simulated shock absorption and push-off – on one leg – from kneeling or split stance – from half-kneeling – and up to standing split stance.

3. Lesson 7: *Steppin' Out*.
   - Companion lesson to Knee Walking – same advantages and applications regarding gait; use music again.
   - Very important movement variation of lifting the front leg high – plus variations. Falling back of pelvis on legs great skill for iliopsoas biased – control of postural and weight in front extension stresses.

Lateral/rotational stability

1. Control relationship of chest/shoulder girdles to pelvis with obliques – blend/coordinate with intersegmental stabilizers.

2. Control rotational relationship of pelvis/low back to legs with hip abductors (and adductors).

3. Categories of lateral stress include centrifugal forces, locomotion, acceleration or deceleration of ballistic turns, pushing or pulling laterally, or pushing forward or pulling back with one hand.

4. Lesson 8: *Dead Bug Roll*.

   • Facilitates pushing outward with the legs to stabilize the pelvis, blending this pelvic stabilization with intersegmental stability and control of gross torso-on-pelvis movement – coordinating all three layers.

   • Train relationship of chest to pelvis in log rolling. Relate to transitions, orientation, manipulation.

   • Strong and accurate use of the hip abductors and short and stubbies in transitional movement – train to use in car for control of centrifugal forces.

   • Simultaneous abductor engagement, along with a slight weight shift backward is the ultimate in pushing the pelvis toward vertical on the legs – very useful for controlling postural anterior tilt.

   • Train abductors to both stabilize pelvis in space to resist lateral movements and to move pelvis laterally in space to push an object laterally in space.

   • Pole facilitation – recognition and control of lateral/rotational forces – being either an immovable object or an irresistible force – swinging quicker to simulate control of ballistic movements.

   • Advanced lumbopelvic stability lessons forthcoming in legs chapter.

Lumbothoracic differentiation

1. Necessity for half-archers and multisegmental unstables – thoracic extension with lumbar flexion (half-archers) or with a neutral low back (multisegmental unstables).

2. Lesson 9: Differentiated Back Bends

   • Belly-up use of ball or roller mobilizes the thorax into extension.

   • Importance of using legs to posteriorly rotate pelvis – don't use the abdominals.

   • Belly-down hamstring constraint strengthens the thoracic extensors without going into lumbar extension.

   • Ball under low back lift head/shoulders to create nonhabitual differentiated pattern for the half round types.

3. Movement model for treating low back pain.

   • Misuse of equipment – taking responsibility for their pain and taking credit for their improvement.

   • Identification of categories of movement and postural stressors – what hurts?

• Identification of nonhabitual movement and postural patterns – what feels good – what to use for first aid?

• Learning to control movement and postural stresses – development of proprioceptive/pattern recognition skills.

• Learning to control movement and postural stresses – development of physical skills (gross skeletal flexibility and strength; ability to stabilize in all three layers).

• Low back kata – a possible home exercise program.

Layers of stability

What do we mean when we say we want to stabilize the lower back? The purpose of this chapter is to explore lumbopelvic stability and how to influence it in our students. We can think of stability as being necessary on three levels. We need intersegmental stability: the ability to micromanage the relationships between or the arthrokinematic movement (amount and direction of roll and slide) of each vertebra relative to another. We need torso stability: the gross ability to stabilize the torso/chest in relation to the pelvis. We need pelvic stability: the gross ability to stabilize the pelvis on top of the legs.

How do we facilitate stability at each layer? How do we blend the three levels together? How do we get our students to utilize stabilization strategies in real life? Is there really a magic button muscle that, if we can get it stronger, will make all our spinal problems disappear? Let's start our discussion of stabilization with a definition of stability and a review of the section one schematic on antagonist coordination.

For a simple definition, we can say that stabilization is the ability to keep movement at a joint inside its physiological limits using muscular control rather than relying on connective tissue constraints. Recall our schematic representation of antagonist coordination in Chapter 1. Muscle A is the agonist that contracts to pull the disc leftward on the page and Muscle B is the antagonist that lengthens to accommodate the movement (Fig. 6.1).

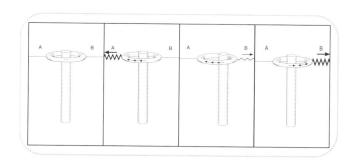

Fig. 6.1 Schematic representation of normal coordination of antagonists – reciprocal inhibition.

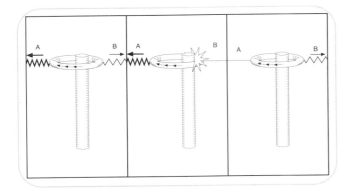

Fig. 6.2 Schematic representation of co-contractions – hypermobilities – hypomobilities.

In a well-organized system excitation of Muscle A inhibits Muscle B. This is called reciprocal inhibition. Muscle A keeps contracting until the edge of the disc approaches the post, then stops contracting as Muscle B fires to decelerate and stop the ring from striking the post. Muscle B then becomes the agonist and contracts to pull the ring to the right on the page, whereas Muscle A is now antagonistic and needs to be inhibited and lengthened to accommodate the movement in this direction. This is how things should work. The antagonists work cooperatively in this schematic to move the bone fully within its physiological limits, but not beyond it.

Let's say now that Muscle A really prefers the on switch to the off switch, and it doesn't stop contracting when the disc nears the post. Because Muscle A likes the on switch, that will mean that Muscle B habitually hits the off switch (aided by reciprocal inhibition) and may be slow or completely negligent in decelerating the ring. We get a train wreck as the bone violates its physiological limit (Fig. 6.2). Ligaments stretch and are damaged. Joint capsules strain to contain the runaway bone. Joint surfaces collide and cartilage is mashed. We call this joint hypermobility or instability.

Taken to extremes, we get joint subluxation or even dislocation. Whoever is in charge of the on and off switches is not paying attention. If we make Muscle B lift weights to get stronger, will that stop movement past the physiological limit? Maybe – but Muscle B also needs directions on when to apply that strength, and Muscle A needs directions on when to stop pulling. For that to happen, someone needs to be cognizant of where one bone is in relation to another. Instability, then, is an inability of the CNS to recognize physiological limits and an inability of the antagonists to control movement in certain directions.

If we take our schematic idea a little further and look at the relationship of the part to the whole, we could say that individual joint instabilities very often arise from repeated violation of the good housekeeping rule: the distribution of movement for a particular function is not even. Something moves too much because something else doesn't move enough – there is a hypomobility or co-contraction going on elsewhere (Fig. 6.2). These hypermobility/hypomobility pairs are very common clinically, in both spinal and extremity joints. We

could even say that part of stabilization is the art of finding somewhere else to move.

Because we all have both anterior/posterior and left/right imbalances, we might anticipate many instabilities to be unidirectional. Start with an awareness of flexion/extension bias. Generally speaking, we'll want to recognize and avoid habitual directions of movement and seek out and gain competence in nonhabitual movements. Continue with an awareness of right/left bias. Generally speaking, we'll want to use our nonhabitual diagonal (right flexion, left extension, etc.) for first aid and give our habitual diagonal a wide berth.

Sometimes, instabilities are multidirectional. Either through traumatic incident or through long-standing habit, movement of the back into any direction is unrestrained by antagonist control. These types are a bit trickier to work with and require a slightly different approach. Whereas many of the lessons from earlier in this section are appropriate for people with unidirectional instabilities (emphasizing nonhabitual directions), these are sometimes too much for folks who slosh uncontrollably around their lower back. The lessons in this chapter can be used with instabilities of all types.

Knowing when to use the umbrella

Let there be no illusions about what we are up against. Helping someone recognize how the way they are moving their back contributes to their back pain and guiding them toward moving in fundamentally different ways in this intersegmental part of their bodies is not a task for the impatient or the faint of heart. The CNS has a certain inertia to it: once a certain movement or postural pattern is set into motion, it takes a powerful force (pain can be a great motivator) to effect a change of direction.

When we talk to students about maintaining a neutral spine, their idea of neutral is going to be different from yours. Their calibration of neutral and calibration of physiological limit will be set inaccurately. The hypomobile partner in the hypermobility/hypomobility pair keeps movement funneled toward the path of least resistance – the poor over-worked hypermobile segment.

Their proprioceptive awareness is probably going to be less than acute as well as less than accurate. And even if you can get them to find true neutral in your office, getting them to recognize how to constantly monitor themselves and maintain that neutral as they go about their daily activities is a difficult task. Fortunately, there are some effective ways of leading your horse to water that usually result in that horse drinking.

We as physical therapists cannot stabilize someone's back for them. Stabilization is a perceptual/motor skill that everyone needs to learn through experimentation and personal discovery. Imagine a person living in a rainy climate such as Seattle. She likes to walk outdoors but hates to get wet, so she never goes out. That should present no problem – that's what umbrellas are for.

Asking her why she doesn't just use an umbrella and still go out for walks, she replies that she has never heard of one. Being the kindly sort, let's give her an umbrella. She replies that she doesn't know how to operate one, so we instruct her. Later, we see her out walking in the rain with her umbrella, but she isn't using it.

On further inquiry, we discover that not only doesn't she know how to use an umbrella, but that short of a torrential downpour she really can't perceive rain either. She only knows that she is soaked by the time she gets home. Being the kindly sort, we help her with the last bit of information she needs to walk in the rain without getting wet: the ability to perceive the rain.

Although this analogy may seem silly, it is not far from the truth when talking about lower back instability and pain. The umbrella is analogous to having access to intrinsic and extrinsic spinal stabilization muscles, such as transverse abdominis or multifidi. By itself, training someone in the acquisition and use of these stabilization tools is not enough. With rain being a metaphor for postural and movement stressors of the lower back, we also need to instruct them on recognizing those stressors: they need to know when it's raining so they can deploy their umbrella.

Before we explore those ways of facilitating lumbar stability and how/when to use it in daily life, let's take a look at various stressors of the low back.

Flexion stresses

Flexion stresses are situations in which the antagonists are allowing too much movement into lumbar flexion and posterior pelvic tilt. These stresses might result in posterior lumbar and sacroiliac (SI) ligament overstretching, disc shearing stresses/degeneration/blowout and muscular and fascial overstretching. The muscles responsible for checking too much movement into lumbar flexion are the spinal extensors and the hip flexors/pelvic anterior tilters. These muscles are too weak.

The muscles responsible for pulling the lumbar spine into too much flexion are the abdominal and hip extensor/pelvic posterior tilters. These muscles are too tight. This simultaneous torso and hip muscular antagonist imbalance illustrates again the importance of training our students with differentiated patterns of movement.

Postural stresses

Postural stresses are mainly sitting and squatting. For those of us who sit in their car an hour a day, work at a desk, sit down to meals, then flop on the couch to watch a little TV at the end of the day, sitting poorly can have major cumulative effects. When sitting, the gluteal biased among us tend to roll their pelvis back into posterior tilt. This results in lumbar flexion, whether the torso pattern is full round or half round (Fig. 6.3).

We could say that they are falling backward – they are in a belly-up orientation. We could surmise shortness of the hamstrings/gluteals and chronically engaged abdominal muscles. We could anticipate weakness of the iliopsoas/hip flexors. We might expect soft or deep couches or chairs, recliners, bucket seats in cars and planes and sitting on the floor to exaggerate the posterior rotation/flexion. They might do better with straight-backed chairs, perhaps some lumbar support into lordosis, or even one of the kneeling chairs. The forward slant of

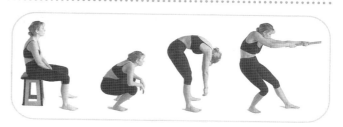

Fig. 6.3 Flexion stresses – sitting, squatting, bending and pulling.

the seats on these chairs more easily allows the pelvis to fall forward, with the desired effect of stimulating the back extensors.

The caveat with this chair is that you have to use your legs a lot to brace against this tendency to fall forward. This may get uncomfortable or tiring for some. Also, when dispensing advice about what kind of chair to sit in, keep in mind that no chair can make you sit correctly. The determined habitualist can still posteriorly rotate and flex the lower back even in one of these chairs. These folks rarely sit on the floor, and look pretty awkward when they do.

Squatting is something we encourage people with back pain to do instead of bending over. Although this is great advice for most people most of the time, for some people this position still encourages unstable directions of movement for their lower back. Because of the likely lack of full hip flexion, they will still round their backs when they squat. They need considerable hamstring/gluteal/short and stubby length to have a chance of getting to a neutral spine position (Fig. 6.3).

Have you ever heard the term plumber's butt – aka carpenter's butt or back with a crack? Gluteal-biased individuals in bending-intensive occupations often show a bit of natal cleavage when squatting. This position is a nice functional assessment tool to assess pelvic bias, though I wouldn't suggest using 'plumber's butt' as a diagnostic code.

Standing doesn't tend to stress the lower back into flexion with very many people: it is fairly rare to see someone in lumbar flexion in standing. Lying supine or prone is generally fairly comfortable and doesn't tend to contribute to flexion stresses, though sleeping on the side in a fetal position (and resultant prolonged lumbar flexion) would be in character for these folks.

Movement stresses

Activities that tend to produce flexion stresses on the lower back include bending, pulling, and certain vegetative functions. In most cases, these movement stresses are predictable from observations of postural stresses. Bending over or leaning forward produces flexion stresses on the low back when the hip joints cannot flex enough (Fig. 6.3). The legs are not allowing the pelvis to fall far enough forward, and additional flexion movement is required in the lower back. Muscles that constrain the ability of the hips to flex are the hip extensors: gluteals, hamstrings and the short and stubbies.

Think of how many times we bend or lean forward during the day. We bend or lean forward to pick up things

> **Box 6.1 Flexion stressors**
>
> Postural stresses – sitting and squatting
> Movement stresses – bending, pulling, lifting and vegetation
> Correlated with habitual gluteal/abdominal bias and habitual psoas and back extensor weakness
> Antidote is back extension and hip flexion – the nonhabitual differentiated pattern

(manipulation). We bend/lean to eat or drink something (vegetative). We bend to get up and down from sitting to standing and from lying to sitting (transitional movements). We bend to look more closely at something (orientation). We lean forward when climbing a steep slope or when biking (locomotion). We bend to punctuate conversation with body language (communication). We bend to prevent ourselves from falling over (balance) (Box 6.1).

What you can assume as a clinician is that your gluteal-biased students will be doing proportionally more of their bending with lumbar flexion, and that this inertia of the CNS weaves its way into every nook and cranny of function. What you can also assume is that these same students will have no idea they are bending so often or for such a multiplicity of reasons. It might be that the only time they think of themselves as bending, and direct some of their attention to what their back is doing, is when they are lifting something substantial from the floor.

Whereas the deep-bending-with-added-weight is a common storyline from people with low back pain, the incident that precipitated the visit to your office will not be an isolated one. The more frequent but less dramatic bending movements that we do so much of in our daily activities is analogous to the steady beating of waves against a rock – wearing down tissue a little bit at a time. The traumatic incident is the storm-driven wave – the straw that breaks the camel's back.

This is why it is important not to just teach classic bending and lifting ergonomics, but to also help them to become aware of these more frequent stresses. Train them in proprioceptive self-awareness and pattern recognition so that the new habits of spinal neutral and nonhabitual differentiated patterns are counterwoven throughout the CNS. Control the smaller and more frequent stressors as training for the main events of life.

Pulling is another activity that may result in flexion stresses. Pulling requires a movement or a shift of weight backward. The gluteal-biased person will be more likely to push with her legs and to roll her pelvis into posterior tilt (Fig. 6.3). Her under-utilized back extensors will probably allow a segment or segments of her back to move beyond its physiological limit into flexion and strain passive elements around those joints.

The most notorious of pulling stresses is lifting something on or close to the ground: here the direction of pull is vertical. Horizontal pulling stresses might include pulling on a rope to drag a boat out of the water, dragging a heavy object toward you across a shelf or counter (scooting your computer a little closer), pulling a heavy wheeled cart or even a grocery cart toward you, pulling open a door (some of which can be quite heavy), and water skiing.

Many pulling stresses are a hybrid of horizontal and vertical directions: pulling while bent over. Pull-starting a lawn mower, yanking up a stout weed or tenacious seedling, moving furniture or dragging other heavy objects across the ground, or fighting a frantic fish at the end of your line are some examples. Pulling is also an activity that may result in an extension stress – more on this in a bit.

Certain vegetative functions can also be implicated as flexion stressors. Defecating involves both sitting (or squatting) and abdominal contractions (Valsalva). Depending on positioning, the forward thrust of copulation can create repetitive and, depending on enthusiasm levels, vigorous movements into lumbar flexion. Although I wouldn't suggest you attempt to assess these functions firsthand, I think you can safely guess how they would do it based on other observations, and that you could discreetly direct them to be aware of their back even while in the grasp of their reptilian brain.

Predictable imbalances, specific skills needed and evaluation

To summarize, people who are unidirectionally unstable into flexion have predictable hyper-/hypomobility pairs and require specific functional and physical skills. The primary hyper-/hypomobility pair should be obvious: not enough flexion at the hip joints requires too much flexion of the lumbar and/or SI joints. Secondarily, a chronically flexed and rigid thoracic kyphosis contributes to the falling-back bias and to a general difficulty in coming upright or extending through the spine. Here is a chicken-and-egg question for you. Did the chronically flexed thoracic spine cause the posterior pelvic tilt or did it result from it? Perhaps this is a false choice: maybe they developed in parallel, hand in glove?

Specific functional skills that these people need are to stabilize vertebral segments relative to each other, to stabilize the torso on the pelvis and to stabilize the pelvis on the legs. They need to learn to pull their pelvis forward from a falling-back position in sitting. They need to learn to allow their pelvis to fall forward more completely on their legs when bending/lifting/leaning.

Physical skills needed include transverse abdominis and multifidus control, an ability to differentiate these from the obliques and rectus, and an ability to utilize these intersegmental stabilizers independently of the direction of stress. They need to learn to lengthen/inhibit the hamstrings, gluteals and hip external rotators. They need to learn to strengthen and use both appropriately and at the proper time their iliopsoas and other hip flexors and their erector spinae/quadratus lumborum. Proprioceptive skills include pattern recognition skills, recognition of how to move into the nonhabitual differentiated patterns of hip flexion and back extension, and how to find and recalibrate spinal neutral.

On initial evaluation you can glean valuable clues about what is going on in someone with back pain by asking certain questions when taking a history. What hurts and what feels good? With unidirectional flexion instability, they may relate pain on sitting, bending, lifting or pulling activities. They generally feel better lying prone or doing lumbar extension movements in a variety of positions. As always when working with complex organic–emotional entities (people), this is not an exact science.

Some people have very limited proprioceptive self-awareness and are poor historians. Some repetitive or prolonged sub-maximal stresses may not manifest themselves immediately. The cumulative effects result in pain, but many people are unable to make that connection. Use the history to form initial impressions and use the time to discreetly observe (while they are unaware that they are being observed) any postural or movement patterns that the person may be exhibiting.

You could start a more formal objective evaluation of people with lower back pain in sitting. Observe from the side for the position of the pelvis on the seat and for clues to direction and strength of the gluteal/iliopsoas bias. Take note of the position of their legs. The gluteal-biased person may sit with knees and feet wide apart (consistent with gluteal and short/stubby shortness) or may tuck her feet under the chair (consistent with hamstring shortness). To assist her in feeling the shape of her back, run a straight edge along her spine (foam roller or foam pad, a short dowel, whatever).

Ask her to assess the front-to-back balance of her ischial tuberosities on the seat and correlate that with the shape/direction of movement of her back. Start teaching and directing your student's attention to certain key things at the same time as you are assessing. In a motor learning approach, what good does it do for just the practitioner to have the information while the student remains ignorant?

Ask your students to reach for their feet from sitting to get a sense of their strategy for bending. The gluteal-biased person will probably be round along their whole back. Run a straight edge along their spine again to assist them with pattern/shape recognition again. Differentiate a global flexion pattern (full round) from a kyphotic thoracic spine but extended lumbar spine (half arch) through observation of the position of the pelvis in sitting relative to vertical, and observation of distribution of flexion along the spine while bending.

The half arch features a more anteriorly tilted pelvis in sitting and a much flatter lumbar spine in bending, relative to the flexing thorax. Use these criteria to spot out the elusive half round – they will flex more in the lower spine on bending and appear to be upright and erect in sitting while the pelvis is subtly falling backward.

Observe in sitting from the back and front for left/right imbalances. Is there more weight on one side of the pelvis, or is the pelvis turned left or right? If the pelvis is rolled straight back, we could surmise a bilaterally symmetrical gluteal bias. If the pelvis is rolled back and to the left, we could surmise a right gluteal bias. Higher tone in the right gluteal group would result in right hip extension, external rotation and abduction – if the leg were freer to move than the pelvis.

Because this is not usually the case in sitting, the pelvis would roll into posterior tilt, left rotation and weight-shift to the left. We could say that this person is gluteal biased with a left pelvic force couple dominance, which results in a right torso flexion pattern. The direction of first aid, the nonhabitual direction, would be into right anterior tilt and left torso extension. Watch for asymmetries and match to observed length and strength differences in the hip musculature. Be prepared to make your assessments flexible.

Have them stand up and observe the balance of the pelvis on the legs in standing. Is it organized consistently with unidirectional flexion instability (pelvis close to vertical or in a ski-jumper pose) or is it excessively anteriorly tilting (possible multidirectional instability)? Observe bending from a standing position or, if they are too acute for that, have them lean with their elbows and forearms on a desk in a modified plantigrade position and see if they can bring their pelvis to horizontal and their back to neutral, or past neutral into extension. The additional length required from the hamstrings in this position may make this difficult for the gluteal-biased person.

Ask them to sit cross-legged on the floor and then to progress to long sitting. Their ability to sit upright in these positions tells us a lot about iliopsoas strength and hip extensor length, and illustrates for them the consistency of their flexion bias. This might be a good place to educate them briefly on the tissue consequences of repetitive flexion stresses. Blend gross observations with segmental mobility testing, palpation, neurologic testing and any other favorite evaluation methods. How do the trees relate to the forest?

Extension stresses

Extension stresses are situations in which the antagonists are allowing too much movement into lumbar extension and too much movement into anterior pelvic tilt. These stresses might result in anterior lumbar and SI ligament overstretching, disc shearing stresses/degeneration/blowout, muscular and fascial compression, facet joint compression/closed pack and eventual degenerative joint disease. Spondylolisthesis would also be aggravated by extension stresses.

The muscles responsible for checking too much movement into lumbar extension are the abdominals and the hip extensors/posterior pelvic tilters; these muscles are too weak. The muscles responsible for pulling the lumbar spine into too much extension are the erector spinae/quadratus lumborum and the hip flexors/anterior pelvic tilters; these muscles are too tight.

Postural stresses

Postural stresses might include: sitting in anterior pelvic tilt (full arch or half arch), standing in anterior pelvic tilt (full arch or half arch), lying supine with legs long or lying prone (Fig. 6.4). Sitting with anterior tilt is probably a function of an over-reliance on the back extensors and a faulty calibration of neutral; the other postures add in the factor of short hip flexors. Whereas sitting with anterior tilt can be fairly easily corrected through recalibration of neutral, anterior tilt in standing and other postures that require full hip extension can be more difficult to change. There are some tricky physical skills they will have to learn.

Although sitting by itself doesn't have to be an extension stressor, sitting for a long period can allow for a gradual shortening of hip flexors and can make subsequent standing and walking more difficult.

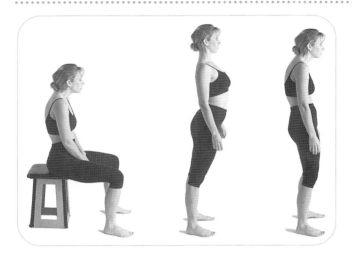

Fig. 6.4 Postural extension stresses – sit half arch and stand full arch with anterior tilt – stand with posterior tilt bias but lumbar extension.

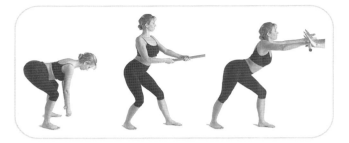

Fig. 6.5 Bending with too much extension – pulling – and pushing with the back.

To make things even more complex, gluteal-biased people will sometimes be susceptible to extension stresses. They will shift their weight far forward on to their toes and hang on their anterior hip ligaments. This is a version of posterior tilt, but because of the extreme shift of the center of mass forward, the nearly always kyphotic chest will collapse and fall backward (Fig. 6.4). This creates a long kyphosis and a short and compressed lordosis; gluteal-biased people can create extension stresses in standing.

Movement stresses

Movement stressors into extension are sometimes subtle and sometimes blatant, and there are a lot of them! The blatant ones might include lying prone and lifting legs, arms or head, or standing and reaching or looking up. These are examples of global extension movements and are best avoided by those of us who are unstable into lumbar extension. These global extension movements are very common throughout many different exercise systems. Yoga has a lot of postures/asanas that combine hip and back extension. Pilates also has several global extension exercises in it, as does Feldenkrais. Think back to the very early worm lessons: London Bridges, Xs and Os and Baby Rolls. These types of exercises are inappropriate for your students who are unstable into extension.

Other stressors include forward bending, pulling, pushing, carrying, stepping, and certain vegetative functions (the withdrawal phase of copulation, standing urination). Unlike the flexion stresses produced on bending by the insufficient hip flexion of the gluteal-biased organization, extension stresses are created in forward bending through a failure of the legs to control the fall of the pelvis forward. The hips flex too much, the pelvis falls too far forward and the worm is forced to extend too much (Fig. 6.5). The erector spinae are asked to do more than the manual recommends, the lumbar joints are in a compressed/close-packed position and the capsules and ligaments are straining to try to maintain some intersegmental stability.

With this particular error in bending being performed mostly by people with an iliopsoas bias, we might anticipate a weakness of the abdominals and a loss of anterior torso support. This abdominal weakness in a belly-down orientation leads to forward shearing strains of one vertebra on another, thereby contributing to the early stages of extension hypermobility or to a frank L5 on S1 spondylolisthesis.

When a gluteal-biased person leans slightly forward to pick out oranges in the grocery store, pick up a magazine off a table, pet the dog, change the station on a car radio, reach into the bottom drawer of the desk, or an infinite number of other reasons for leaning forward, the flexion stress on her low back is comparatively minimal. She probably hasn't bent enough yet for hip flexion to be constrained by the hip extensors. When an iliopsoas-biased person leans over, however, there is often an immediate strain: we get a Tinkerbell pose as the tailbone lifts and the back arches.

The same propensity to allow the pelvis to fall too far forward in standing postures and bending movements is present when leaning over. Although leaning forward may not have the same intensity of stress as a full bend, it can make up for it in volume and duration. We lean over far more often to fill our coffee cup and to turn on the TV than we do to bend over fully to tie our shoes or pick a penny up off the floor.

We also lean forward and stay there: standing at the sink to wash dishes, standing in the kitchen to stir the noodles, standing in the laundry room to iron clothes, and standing at the bathroom mirror while shaving or putting on makeup. Assembly-line work, sewing, writing and watch repair – we could go on forever. How many common activities do you lean forward for during the day? How often do you lean forward and stay there for more than 10 seconds? How much more often are you leaning and bending forward than you are leaning and bending back?

In reversing a bending or leaning movement to come back upright to sit or stand, there is another opportunity for the iliopsoas-biased person to create extension stresses. Rather than using her legs to initiate a posterior tilting movement of the pelvis toward vertical, then having her back follow her pelvis, the iliopsoas-biased person will commonly extend her back to initiate or complete the movement of coming back upright, then follow with the pelvis.

The difference is a fundamental one. In the first instance the legs are pushing her pelvis and torso toward vertical; in the

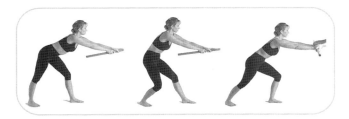

Fig. 6.6 Pulling and pushing from the legs reduces extension stresses on the lower back.

second, the back is pulling the torso toward vertical. Think back to the other explorations of bending you have performed in Cat/Camel, Side-sit Bending and Sit to Stand. You will have an opportunity to feel this distinction again proprioceptively in subsequent lessons in this chapter.

Pulling from the back or pushing from the legs?

The mechanism of strain for pulling movements is very similar to that for coming upright from a bent or leaned-over position – overuse of the back extensors to pull and not Using the Legs to push (Fig. 6.5). Pulling movements can actually be a good way to train the iliopsoas-biased person to use her legs better and to stabilize her torso on her pelvis, and can be a preferred way of wheeling/sliding/dragging heavy objects across the floor (it's fairly easy to flex the lumbar spine while pulling, in comparison to pushing) (Fig. 6.6).

Pushing can very easily be an extension strain. Pushing a lawnmower or a grocery cart, pushing a door open, pushing your couch back to your wife's preferred location, sliding a box toward the back of the closet shelf, pushing the Sheetrock on to the wall, or pushing the guy with the basketball out of the key might be performed in too vertical a position.

When applying that horizontal pushing force from a vertical or slightly leaned position, the effect is usually to extend the lumbar spine and co-contract the muscles of the lower torso (Fig. 6.5). On the other hand, if you bend over to bring your pelvis and torso close to horizontal, you can reduce that extension stress and put yourself in a better position to apply the power of your legs (Fig. 6.6).

The stealth stressor – weight-in-front

Lifting or carrying a weight with your arms out in front of you is a somewhat stealthy extension stress. Although the weight of the arms alone is enough to trigger the following chain of events, we'll analyze what happens when we lift a 20-pound weight with straightened arms just off a shelf at shoulder height. As you might recall from physics class, the long lever arm created by lifting the weight far away from your body magnifies the 20 pounds several times over.

This is one reason why we instruct our students to lift things only after having them somehow close in to their bodies. There are two things to keep in mind here. One is that even light

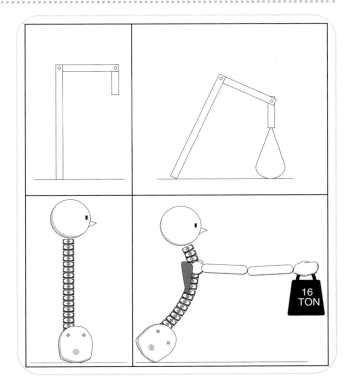

Fig. 6.7 Schematic and worm variations of weight in front – creating an extension stress.

objects held or picked up at arms length can be stressful. Two: even when holding objects in close to your body, they are still in front of you. This still creates a lever arm and an extension stress, especially with heavy objects (a box of books) or prolonged holding or carrying (e.g. an infant).

Lifting your garbage can up on to the curb, folding your sheets or towels, lifting your child out of a crib, putting a stack of dishes away into the top cupboard, moving a ladder, putting a pot of water on the stove to boil, using a posthole digger, passing the big platter of vegetables over to your Uncle Bill, putting the bag of grapefruit up on the scale at the grocery store, changing a tire – need I go on?

How does lifting or carrying something in your arms create extension stresses? As you take on the weight of the object, this shifts your center of mass forward (Fig. 6.7). To keep you from completely falling over forward, your back extensors kick in. This happens regardless of what you do at your pelvis. But what happens at your pelvis is critical in determining the amount of extension stress these functional activities generate. If you are a worm with arms, you fall over forward (Fig. 6.7).

For the Tyrannosaurus with arms, it is possible to stay upright. If the Tyrannosaurus is iliopsoas biased and if the pelvis is not stabilized on the legs (Fig. 6.8), if the pelvis is allowed to fall into anterior tilt, if the hip joints are allowed to flex too much, the back has no choice but to arch – joint compression, foraminal narrowing, muscular tension and the rest

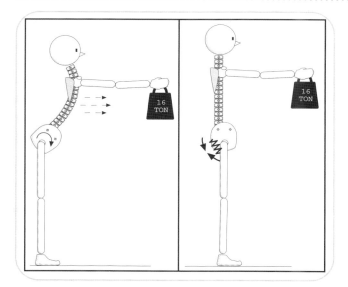

Fig. 6.8 Tyrannosaurus versions of weight in front – pelvis falls forward on the legs – then stabilized with the gluteals.

Just say no to weight-in-front stresses

Proactively, we could train our students to recognize and preplan for weight-in-front stressors by shifting the weight back on the feet, bending the knees a bit and rolling the pelvis under, controlling weight in front by directing the pelvis to 'fall back.' We will explore this experientially later in the chapter. Although it is possible to train much enhanced stability in the presence of weight-in-front stresses, the best way to control those stresses is to not subject yourself to them when there are other options available.

A hand truck or dolly is something everybody with a twitchy back should have around the house and something they should use at every opportunity. Wheeling things around instead of carrying them in front of you will make your back dance the jig and thank you profusely. Having a sturdy box or crate around that fits nicely on to your hand truck is a good idea as well. Carry groceries in it, put your laundry in it, bring in the firewood, etc. Put the crate on your hand truck to move around or, alternatively, carry the box around on your backside.

Observe people in other parts of the world where they routinely carry heavy objects repeatedly or over long distances, and you will notice that weight is either borne vertically (slung over a shoulder or placed on top of the head) or posteriorly. Start experimenting with carrying things in front, then switch and figure out how to arrange your arms to carry things in back.

Try this experiment. Load up a basket or small box with 10–15 pounds and place it on your kitchen counter. First face the box and pick it up in front of you. Step away from the counter a little to exaggerate the lever arm, and slowly pick up the box. Feel for effort in your back and for any subtle falling forward of your pelvis on your legs. Carry the box around your dwelling or out to your car to assess comfort, ease or strain on your back.

Bring the box back to your kitchen counter again, put it down, turn around and pick up the box by reaching back with your hands behind you. Hold on to the bottom of the box or to the handles (very useful) and rest its weight on the back of your sacrum. Walk around with the load in back this time and compare strain or ease to your front-loaded carry. Experiment with suitcases, kitchen chairs and bags of compost – be creative and find out how many things can go behind!

of it follows. If the pelvis is stabilized (the Tyrannosaurus discovers her gluteals), the back can stay neutral and the legs can contribute much more to resisting the forces dragging your torso down and forward (Fig. 6.8).

Try the following experiment with a student or colleague. Have her lie on her back with her legs down long. Have her reach both hands forward toward the ceiling and place her palms together; hold hands there. Sit on the floor above your partner's head and place one of your hands on top of her hands. Gently and slowly push her hands down towards her feet. Observe visually and have your student observe proprioceptively for activation of the lumbar extensors and an arching of the lower back away from the floor. Repeat this movement several times to help your student recognize the effect of this simulated weight-in-front stress on her lower back and pelvis.

After doing this several times with her legs down long, have her bend her knees up and place her feet flat on the floor. Cue her to press her feet into the floor to roll her pelvis into posterior tilt, as we did in Pelvic Tilts. Press into the top of her hands from this position. Observe visually and have your student observe proprioceptively the enhanced stability of the lower back and pelvis. With the legs in a position to stabilize the pelvis, cue her to recognize the advantages of controlling weight-in-front stresses with the hip extensors.

You can do this experiment by yourself by lying on your back, holding a long pole horizontally with its top end placed against a wall or heavy piece of furniture. Press the pole upward into the wall both with legs long and with legs straight. Appreciate the enhanced stability gained by Using the Legs. Contrast pelvic stabilization from the legs with straight intersegmental stabilization (not a snowball's chance in Panama), or even with classic belly-driven pelvic tilt. We will progress this idea of recognition and control of weight-in-front stresses later when we work with forward bending.

Extension stresses in gait

Stepping, as part of either locomotor or transitional movements, is another common extension stressor. Actually, there are three potential stressors in stepping. One is heel-strike. How do you absorb shock and what is the orientation of your pelvis and the shape of your lower back on impact? The second potential stressor is a short hip flexor on the push-off leg. Another potential stressor in stepping is the act of lifting the stepping leg and firing that hip flexor.

On heel-strike there is a certain amount of force generated up through your skeleton. There are several possible candidates for shock absorbers along the way. It is possible for the foot and ankle to absorb some shock, though with those tiny little springs I wouldn't recommend that the bulk of the shock be

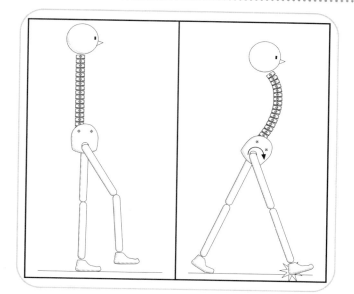

Fig. 6.9 Gait extension stressor – heel-strike.

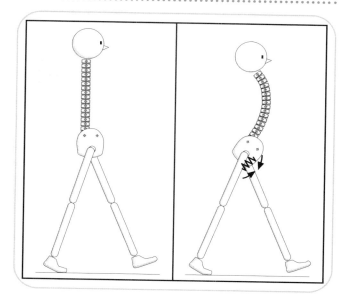

Fig. 6.10 Gait extension stressor – hip flexor of push-off leg too tight – necessitates completion of push-off through lumbar extension.

absorbed there. The knee is in a good position to absorb shock because it is bent at the moment of impact.

The hip joint would definitely be one of my choices, though it depends on how the pelvis is oriented on heel-strike and how the pelvis is allowed to move on the newly weightbearing leg. If the pelvis is already in anterior tilt when the foot hits the ground, there is a good possibility that the confused-about-physiological-limits-into-extension CNS will not control even more movement of the pelvis into anterior tilt.

Shock is absorbed by the rotational movement forward of the pelvis and a deepening of lumbar lordosis (Fig. 6.9). Alternately or simultaneously, if the pelvis is in anterior tilt on heel-strike and the abductors (part of the gluteal family and likely to be chronically inhibited by the iliopsoas dominant) are asleep at the wheel, the pelvis can translate excessively laterally and create lateral shearing forces in the lumbopelvic region. This is actually a lateral stressor and should be covered in the next segment, but it tends to go along with extension stresses, so I mention it here as well.

How could shock be absorbed safely by the hip joint? By allowing the pelvis to turn and the newly non-weightbearing side to drop a little. This is part of a force couple walk. In stepping forward with the left leg, for instance, the right hip extends to push off and the left hip flexes to step. As you discovered in the last chapter, this simultaneous use of opposite iliopsoas and gluteal groups has the effect of turning the pelvis toward the stepping leg: the iliopsoas pulls the pelvis toward and the gluteal pushes the pelvis away from.

The left hip on impact would then be flexed and (modified) horizontally adducted. It is the horizontal adduction component that makes for a good shock absorber. The abductors and the smaller arthrokinematic muscles act as springs by catching the pelvis through lengthening contractions. As a fringe benefit, those same springs are then stretch reflex primed to push off into the next step. Isn't this is an incredibly efficient and elegant system?

What happens if the hip joint doesn't move to absorb shock? The next thing in line is the lower back. If already in any degree of anterior tilt and lumbar lordosis and without the hip joint softening the blow, each heel-strike can be a jarring event to close-packed joints. What is another thing that happens if the hip joint doesn't yield on impact? The health of the hip joint is affected. Invariant loading creates focal compression areas on the articular cartilage, and inadequate movement of the joint surfaces sliding on each other compromises lubrication and nutrition delivery. Is this a recipe for eventual hip joint replacement? Is it coincidental that most hip degenerative changes are a result of too little movement, and that most lower back problems are a result of too much movement?

The ribcage and thoracic spine, as well as the shoulder girdles and neck, also have a roll to play in shock absorption, but we will leave discussion of these to the chapter on the head and shoulder girdles. The one thing that should be mentioned here is that if we are going to encourage a moderate amount of side-bending of the pelvis in walking and encourage some hip joint softness, there is going to have to be some amount of side-bending movement through the ribcage as well. You will have an opportunity to feel this proprioceptively a bit later.

The next stepping stressor after heel-strike is the ability of the push-off hip joint to fully extend. When pushing off with the right leg behind you, if the muscle spindles of the right hip flexors are not set at a long enough tripwire to allow full right hip extension, the tight hip flexors will pull the pelvis forward into anterior tilt and the push-off is completed not through the hip but through lower back extension (Fig. 6.10). This is fairly typical of iliopsoas-dominant people, who have difficulty differentiating hip extension from back extension.

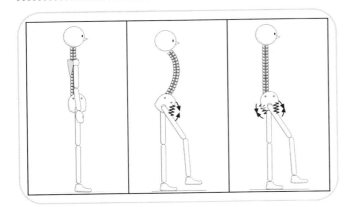

Box 6.2 Extension stressors

Postural stresses – standing, lying supine with legs long, lying prone, possibly sitting

Movement stresses – bending backward, gait, up from bend/chair, lifting, pushing or pulling from extended position

Weight in front stresses – avoid with wheels or carrying behind. Control with intersegmental stability and use of hip extensors

Gait stressors – shock absorption, too-short psoas necessitating completion of push-off by lumbar extension and contracting of psoas of stepping leg

Fig. 6.11 Gait extension stressor – activation of psoas of stepping leg pulls pelvis down and forward, then stabilized by the opposite gluteals.

Another major extension stressor linked to stepping is simply the act of lifting and moving forward the stepping leg, through the contraction of the iliopsoas. We already know through our explorations on the floor and in a chair that contraction of the hip flexors pulls the pelvis into anterior tilt and the lower back into extension. When standing, if you lift your left leg by engaging your left iliopsoas only, your pelvis will roll into anterior tilt and your lower back will lordose (Fig. 6.11).

To prevent this, you could either tighten your belly or extend your right hip (Fig. 6.11). I am suggesting that we train people to stabilize their pelvis in space primarily through their legs, with the superficial abdominal muscles playing more of a supporting role.

Imbalances, needed skills and evaluation

Note that there are extension stressors in balance, orientation, locomotion, manipulation, vegetative and transition functions. They are everywhere, and for most people are more prevalent than flexion stresses. Note that so many of these extension stressors have to do with shifting your center of mass forward – bending forward, reaching forward, leaning forward, carrying something in front of you and stepping forward.

How much more often do we do these than bend backward, reach back, lean back, carry something behind you or step back? It's not that we never do these things, but we spend the majority of our lives orienting towards and manipulating the environment in front of us. It wouldn't be surprising if there were more people with back pain as a result of extension stresses than with back pain as a result of flexion stresses.

Does the sheer volume of stressors intimidate you? Am I going to have to remember all this? How am I ever going to teach this to my students? The task seems – and probably is – impossible if you approach this from the standpoint of trying to teach a huge list of 'dos and don'ts'. What I would suggest you do is to teach physical skills, movement principles, proprioceptive awareness skills and recognition of categories of stresses, along with certain examples to help them get the idea, then send them home with homework that includes

them making up their own list of their own common stressors (Box 6.2).

This puts the ball in their court by making them more active problem-solving participants. Recognition of categories of stressors helps them anticipate and preplan certain movements, keeps them on their toes proprioceptively and helps them to become better self-regulators.

The physical skills needed by people who are unstable into extension are:

- Proprioceptive recognition of extension stressors;
- Longer hip flexors and back extensors;
- Stronger hip extensors and abdominals;
- Intersegmental control through the transverse abdominis and the multifidi that is independent of direction of movement or stress;
- Recognition of how to move more into nonhabitual differentiated patterns of hip extension and back flexion and finding spinal neutral, or even biasing slightly toward back flexion with selected activities.

The functional skills needed by these folks include the ability to stabilize the torso relative to pelvis and the ability to push the pelvis backward toward vertical from an anterior tilt position, and to prevent the pelvis from falling too far forward when bending/leaning, lifting/carrying or stepping. The hypermobility/hypomobility pairs are too much movement into lumbar extension, not enough movement into hip extension and/or not enough movement into thoracic extension.

On evaluation, the following subjective complaints are typical. They often experience pain on lying supine or prone, standing and sometimes sitting (if sitting with lordosis). Pain may be present on bending, or even more probably on a return to upright. Carrying and lifting probably hurt. Leaning over for longer periods (dishes, ironing, woodworking, etc.) will hurt.

Often their pain is not felt immediately with the activity or stressor: it is often felt hours or a day/days later. This makes it more difficult to establish the relationship between self-use and pain for the student. It usually feels better to lie supine with the legs bent up or supported by a large bolster, to squat, to lean back against a wall or to bring a knee to the chest.

Objective clues might include the presence of lordosis in sitting and almost certainly in standing. There will probably be a large space between the lower back and the floor while supine with legs long, which reduces significantly when the knees are bent up. On bending, their lower back may stay straight or even arched a bit, and they may come back upright by deepening their lordosis and pulling up with their lumbar spine.

You'll have to watch carefully for this. Watch for this phenomenon when your student moves from sitting to standing as well. Other evaluation techniques for extension stability, access to intersegmental stabilizers, ability to differentiate back extensors from hip extensors and lumbar extensors from thoracic extensors and hip flexor length will be presented later in the chapter.

Multidirectional instabilities

Multidirectional instabilities are really just a nasty combination of the flexion and extension instability syndromes. The legs have such a tight grip on the pelvis that it is constrained from moving freely in any direction. The gluteals, hamstrings, short and stubbies, hip flexors, adductors and abductors are all on a short leash, and assessing hip movement manually is like trying to bathe a cat. No matter which way you direct them to move with your hands, you encounter resistance.

With these multidirectional pelvic hypomobilities and with a continuing requirement to function in the real world, the lower back finds itself between anvil and hammer. These folks use their lower back for everything. This is where they both initiate movement and move the most. There tends to be co-contraction tendencies throughout the musculature of the lower torso that complement the co-contractions around the hip joints. One result of this organization type is to increase compression forces acting on the lumbopelvic region.

Another fringe detriment is that not only are the antagonists allowing too much movement, they are arguing with each other the whole time. The CNS is driving with the brakes on. To make matters even worse, they are usually restricted in thoracic and costal mobility, which takes away another movement option and greases further the slippery slope into lumbar hypermobility. These types of people can be difficult to work with because of a lack of safe direction to move into. It is hard to constrain a sloppy lower back while mobilizing fossilized hips and ribs.

Posturally, the person with multidirectional instability most often sits with posterior pelvic tilt and lumbar flexion, and stands with anterior pelvic tilt and lumbar lordosis. This lordosis is usually of the half arch rather than the full arch type; the thoracic kyphosis tends to be invariant (Box 6.3). Another type of multidirectional instability occurs with generalized hypotonus and systemic joint hypermobility – the entire skeleton is sloppy.

What movements hurt for these people? Everything. What positions are comfortable? None for very long. These people are wriggle worms. They need to change positions or activities frequently. They go from sitting to standing, shift their weight around when standing, change stances, lean against the wall, take a few steps around, sit back down, lean forward for a while, then recline back in the chair, etc. They may not be comfortable at night and wake frequently to change positions. Understandably, they might look a little desperate when they come in to see you.

Box 6.3 Multidirectional instabilities

Worst of both worlds – too flexed in sitting and bending and too extended in standing, bending and controlling weight-in-front stresses

Legs have a death grip on the pelvis and won't allow full hip extension or full hip flexion or full rotation of pelvis on legs – the lower back has to do it all

Thoracic spine and ribcage usually pretty dense too – yet more responsibility for the lower back

No safe direction to move – train in neutral spine, lots of intersegmental stabilization, mobilize the hips and train in avoidance strategies and use of upper extremities for weightbearing and control of bending/leaning/weight in front stresses

---

These people need a lot of work with intersegmental stabilization and a lot of detailed work on finding spinal neutral. They need to gain mobility in the hips and thorax without further compromising the lower back. Work more diligently in helping them to find and maintain a vertical pelvis and torso, and put a lot of focus on using their legs to initiate movements.

Train them in upper extremity weightbearing and strategies to use their arms to assist and support bending and some transitional movements. Go even more slowly with both individual movements and pace of the curriculum, and talk with them extensively about preplanning movements and alteration of lifestyle. Then cross your fingers and hope for the best.

Lateral/rotational stresses

Lateral or rotational stresses are situations in which the antagonists are allowing too much movement into side-bending or rotational directions. We can think of lateral stresses as being adjuncts to the flexion and extension stresses. Figure out flexion or extension bias then look for the left/right balance. There will always be some blending of the two cardinal plane imbalances.

Postural stresses

The pelvis might be posteriorly rotated and turned to the right or anteriorly rotated and turned to the left. Review if need be from earlier chapters and look for diagonal patterns in your students: right and left torso flexion and right and left torso extension. Correlate the torso patterns to position of the pelvis and see if you can sleuth out the various muscle imbalances through the hip joints and lower torso.

We get lateral stresses with both gluteal- and iliopsoas-biased people. These flexion/rotation and extension/rotation stresses (because rotational and side-bending movements in the spine are related, I'm using 'rotation' to denote a side-bending/rotation combination) both create shearing and compressive strain on discs and joint surfaces, and can contribute to eventual degenerative changes in the discs or joint surfaces of the lumbar spine or SI joints. Symptomatically, emphasize more the awareness of imbalance and the control of lateral stresses in someone who complains of one-sided lower back pain, but still work with the flexion/extension bias first.

What might be driving this left/right asymmetry? One likely candidate is pelvic force couple imbalance. Another probability is a hip adductor/abductor imbalance. The adductors and abductors coordinate with each other in a kind of secondary pelvic force couple arrangement to initiate or resist rotational and lateral weight-shifting movements. We will be exploring this relationship proprioceptively and developing strategies to assess and facilitate lateral stability in subsequent lessons.

Movement stresses

Lateral movement stresses include centrifugal forces, locomotion, acceleration or deceleration of ballistic turns, pushing or pulling laterally, or pushing forward or pulling back with just one hand. Centrifugal forces include riding in a car or other vehicle that is going around a corner or a curve in the road, or riding on a roller coaster or other carnival rides. Which way would your pelvis roll on the seat if you were negotiating a left-hand turn?

It would either roll to the right and create more of a side-bending movement to the left, or would turn to the right and create more of a rotational movement of the pelvis to the right underneath the torso (left spinal rotation). Lateral locomotion stresses are generally of the too-much-rotation or the too-much-lateral-shear of the pelvis variety. We'll use a couple of the upcoming lessons to facilitate a more stable low back during gait.

Examples of acceleration or deceleration of ballistic turns includes swinging a tennis racket, baseball bat or golf club. Throwing a ball or Frisbee, catching a rambunctious 4-year-old boy as he's running past you and kicking a soccer ball are other examples (Box 6.4).

Examples of pushing or pulling laterally include pulling open a van door, getting pulled around by a rambunctious dog on a leash, or closing/opening a curtain or sticky window. Other examples include sliding several coats/hangers one way and the other on closet dowel, paddling a kayak, raking/sweeping laterally, moving a piano or couch away from the wall, turning a corner while pushing a lawnmower or grocery cart, or chopping down a tree.

Box 6.4 Lateral stressors

Postural stresses – habitual rotation or side-bend of pelvis creating rotation or side-bend of lower back in opposite direction

Movement stresses – centrifugal forces, acceleration or deceleration of ballistic turns, pushing laterally and pushing or pulling forward or back with one arm

Gait stresses – waddle walk and swish walk

Antidote is – balancing pelvic force couples to reduce postural strain, training hip abductors to control lateral and rotational movement of the pelvis and training abdominal obliques to control relationship of torso to pelvis

---

Examples of pushing or even just reaching straight forward or pulling straight back with one hand include pushing open/pulling open a convenience store door, reaching for a bottle of wine, shoveling snow or pushing a broom or vacuum, bowling, paddling a canoe or pull-starting a weed-whacker.

Examples of rotational locomotion or transitional stresses includes the waddle walking introduced in the last chapter, getting in and out of a car or a booth at a restaurant, not twisting the pelvis to match the twisting of the shoulders, head and chest to breathe in swimming, rolling over in bed, or sharply changing the direction of your walk or run. Note the presence of rotational stressors throughout different functional categories.

Intersegmental stability

Intersegmental stabilization is the ability of the muscular system to control the movement of vertebrae in relation to each other. Stabilization can mean keeping the joints from exceeding their physiological limits. Stabilization can also mean maintaining the desirable arthokinematic movement of the joints. Arthrokinematic movement refers to the unseen sliding and rolling of joint surfaces relative to each other that accompanies the gross movement of the bone that we can observe, called osteokinematics. As an example, let's look at a movement into shoulder abduction. This ball and socket joint features the movement of the humerus (the ball) on the glenoid fossa (the socket).

For the humerus to abduct without the ball rolling upward and completely out of the glenoid fossa, the ball has to slide downward in the socket (Fig. 6.12). This combination of roll

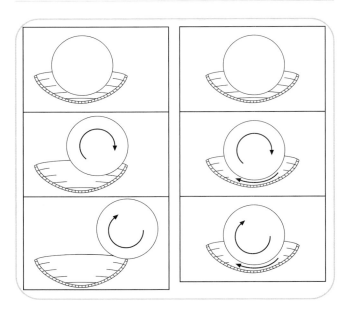

Fig. 6.12 Rolling and sliding movements of convex on concave surface.

and slide is very important for the health of the joint. If proper arthrokinematic movement is not present in a joint during movement, there will be uneven compressive forces on the articular cartilage and uneven tensile stresses on the joint capsule and intra-articular ligaments.

This is true for the ball and socket joints of the shoulders and hips, the wrench-like elbow (radiohumeral) joints, the double-egg shaped joints in the knees or the relatively flat spinal joints. They all require mechanisms to control the way the joint surfaces move relative to each other. In the shoulder, a group of four muscles called the rotator cuff provides this mechanism. In the hip joints, it is the short and stubbies. In the spine, the transverse abdominis, multifidi and perhaps the iliopsoas seem to serve this purpose.

Intersegmental spinal stabilizers

The transverse abdominis is oriented horizontally, arising laterally by six slips from the inner surface of the cartilage of ribs 7–12, from a deep layer of the lumbothoracic fascia, from the inner lip of the iliac crest and ASIS and from the inguinal ligament. The transverse abdominis then attaches via its aponeurosis to the linea alba. It is deep to the external and internal obliques, runs a transverse course from origin to insertion and runs just about from xiphoid to pubis. It is not found just in the lower belly.[1]

The multifidi are the deepest layer of the wad of muscles that runs along the spine. They arise laterally from the sacrum, from the mamillary processes of the lumbar spine, from the lateral processes of the thoracic spine and from the articular processes of the seventh to the fourth cervical vertebrae. The muscle bundles cross two to four vertebrae, diagonally up and in and insert on the spinous process of higher vertebrae. They are like the rotator cuff and the hip external rotators: short, squat, and in very close proximity to the joint.

The psoas major originates from the lateral surfaces of T12 through L4, from their discs and from the costal processes of L1 through L5. The psoas major then joins the iliacus and proceeds as the iliopsoas across the iliopubic eminence through the muscular lacuna to insert on the lesser trochanter of the femur. The iliacus fills the iliac fossa and originates from there and from the region of the anterior inferior iliac spine.[2]

A group of Australian researchers did extensive ultrasound imaging and surface EMG readings for the muscles of the lower torso and came to some interesting conclusions. Paul Hodges, along with CA Richardson, GA Jull and JA Hides, has written multiple articles concerning the relationships between these muscles and low back pain. The following material about intersegmental stability is from these materials, plus a continuing education course I attended in 2000 in which Mr Hodges was a presenter.[2-16] The name of this course was 'Science of Stability: Clinical Application to Assessment and Treatment of Segmental Spinal Stabilization for Low Back Pain.'

Following is a synopsis of some of their findings:

- For people without back pain, excitation of both transverse abdominis and multifidi precedes that of other torso musculature in the presence of a movement stressor. The muscles that control the movement of the joint surfaces relative to each other kick in before the obliques, rectus abdominis and erector spinae do. There is a preparatory presetting of the arthrokinematic muscles before gross movement occurs – this is a good thing.

- For people with low back pain, excitation of both transverse abdominis and multifidi is delayed. There is no preparatory presetting of the stabilizers.

- For people with low back pain and lagging TA and multifidi, once they improve their ability to recruit those muscles, low back pain diminishes.

- Both TA and multifidi work in the presence of both flexion and extension stressors, another sign that the stabilizers seem to work somewhat independently of the gross motor system.

- TA can't flex the lumbar spine or posteriorly tilt the pelvis. Multifidi can't extend the spine or anteriorly tilt the pelvis – another sign that the stabilizers seem to work as a somewhat independent system.

- TA and multifidi usually contract and can be facilitated together. It appears that the CNS controls the stabilization system separately from the movement system. There is an arthrokinematic and a gross motor system. This tonic and phasic split is just another manifestation of the inner and outer layers of the onion – separate but connected.

- The TA is thought to assist in lumbar intersegmental stabilization through its attachment to the lumbothoracic fascia. TA contraction helps make the torso a rigid cylinder, it creates intervertebral compression, and it may posteriorly glide the lumbar vertebrae.

- The TA is thought to assist in lumbar intersegmental stabilization through intra-abdominal pressure and the hydraulic mechanism that creates to stabilize the vertebrae anteriorly.

- The TA is thought to assist in sacroiliac joint stabilization through the force closure of the SI joints and the pubic symphysis support gained through pulling the ASISs closer towards each other.

- The multifidus is thought to assist in lumbopelvic stability through segmental compression, through segmental control of shearing movements, through fascial tension and through sacral nutation.

Can itty-bitty muscles really stabilize the huge and all-powerful pelvis?

It is my suspicion that this arthrokinematic system has corollaries elsewhere throughout the body. If the lumbar spine is to be stable, the pelvis needs to be stable on the femurs, the tibia needs to be stable on the femur, the tibia needs to be stable on the talus and the foot needs to be stable on the floor.

Although the work of Hodges et al. is a great start in rethinking our whole approach to low back pain, we need to expand our concept of intersegmental stabilization to include the chest and thoracic spine, the feet and knees, and most especially the hip joints. The short and stubby muscles of the hip joint are prime suspects as being accomplices with the intersegmental stabilizers. They may even turn out to be the masterminds of the whole stabilization operation!

As you proceed through this chapter, what you will be learning are ways to:

- facilitate proprioceptive self-awareness of habitual movement and postural patterns specific individual;
- facilitate proprioceptive self-awareness of categories of movement and postural stresses specific to that individual;
- facilitate increasingly refined motor control over the intersegmental stabilizers through various facilitation techniques and the application of constraints;
- facilitate an ability to control and direct the movement and position of the pelvis in space from the legs;
- facilitate an ability to blend spinal intersegmental control with control of the pelvis (mobility and stability) directed from the legs; and
- facilitate an ability on the part of your student to blend physical skills with proprioceptive self-awareness skills and apply those skills to real-life activities.

In teaching the participants in these studies to gain spinal intersegmental control, Hodges and his associates have described facilitation techniques and passed on some clinical tips. The initial directive language, 'pull in your belly button, tighten your lower belly, staple your belly button to your back-bone, bulge the muscles in very close to your lower spine,' the use of a pressure-sensitive air bladder as a form of biofeedback and the use of pelvic floor contractions to facilitate TA contractions can be attributed to his group. A nod here should also go to Joseph Pilates, who created many exercises designed to facilitate core strength.[17]

In this chapter, we will be attempting to expand upon and facilitate a deeper refinement of TA and multifidi activation and differentiation through the directed global and differentiated coordination of breath, intersegmental contractions and pelvic floor. We will also be exploring ways to blend the tonic with the phasic by simultaneously stabilizing and moving the rest of your skeleton freely in functional, everyday movement.

Clinically, I've found TA Facilitation to be successful with most people. On the other hand, I've found trying to teach multifidus contraction differentiated from the erector spinae to be very difficult. The verbal commands suggested by Hodges (gently bulge or tense the muscles of your lower back, or push my fingers away from these bones) are a tough sell. I can't even figure out how to do it, nor have most of the physical therapists I have discussed this with.

Digging deep for the multifidi

Jim Johnson, in his book on the multifidus, advocates a series of exercises to strengthen this muscle.[18] There is a hands-and-knees leg lift, a hands-and-knees arm lift and a hands-and-knees leg and arm lift. Instructions are to find spinal neutral and stay there without allowing your back to move. Hold, repeat and progress repetitions and weight. There is another exercise done prone. Lift a leg or an arm, keep spinal neutral, and so on. The last exercise is a standing TA activation.

How do you get the CNS to contract a muscle that isn't associated with making some sort of bony or expressive move-

Box 6.5 Intersegmental research

Intersegmental stabilizers preceding gross movement equals less low back pain and vice versa
Train intersegmental stabilizers and back pain diminishes
Stabilizers don't contribute to lumbar flexion/extension or pelvic tilt
TA and multifidi wired and facilitated together
Both stabilizers work independently of the direction of stress

ment? With TA excitation although there is not an intention to move a bone, at least there is an intention to move the belly button or the pelvic tubing. Because movement into lumbar extension or anterior pelvic tilt is not desirable because of the activation of the erector spinae, there isn't an intention for the CNS to latch on to when teaching multifidus contractions (Box 6.5).

Lifting a leg on hands and knees or prone would normally move the back unless it were stabilized or prevented from moving. Ergo, if we can't get the multifidus to fire with back extension or anterior pelvic tilt movements, then just about any movement of the limbs lacking back motion should do the trick. Consequently, many of our current crop of lumbar stabilization exercises have movement of a leg as an ingredient.

A very popular current exercise is a supine leg lift, progressing to straightening the lifted leg and progressing to double leg lifts. Standing stabilization exercises require maintenance of a neutral back, standing on one leg and reaching the opposite foot alternately forward, backward and sideways on the floor. This is an ingenious idea! We will explore qualitative exercise versions of these types of exercise in this chapter.

Johnson also used a prone orientation for his multifidus facilitation. Probably a wise choice, but can you spot the fly in the soup? Lifting a leg from a prone position is a global pattern of movement. The hip extensors fire and the back extensors almost surely fire as well. There are probably only a couple of hundred people in this whole country who could pull this off without firing their erector spinae!

If you are able to keep your pelvis from tilting anteriorly and your back from arching, it's not because you contracted your multifidi. You are probably doing something with your belly, chest and arms or with the opposite leg to stay stable. Global extension patterns are not how we want to teach lumbar stabilization skills. The hands-and-knees position is a better one, but the devil again is in the details.

Most people will be tempted to arch their back while lifting a leg behind, reverting to childhood for a moment with a global extension pattern. Even if you do prevent your back from arching and your pelvis from rolling into anterior tilt, you are probably controlling that movement in part from your superficial abdominals and in part from your weightbearing hip. And if that is the case, we might as well admit that we should be training our students in that very skill!

Hodges suggests using a pressure-sensitive cuff while supine: hook-lie and bulge your lower back into the cuff without rolling into posterior tilt. You could try side-lying and making ghost movements (have an intention to lift your tailbone without moving your pelvis, or to slide your head back without moving your head). The hip abduction movement from a side-lie position, again without letting the pelvis or back move, is another suggestion. This again begs the question of what really is stabilizing the pelvis; it's not the multifidi. Recall our breakdown of lifting a leg in side-lie during Side-lie Transitions. It is the grounded leg that controls what happens to the pelvis. Again, why not just admit that the legs stabilize the pelvis and start teaching this skill to our students?

Work with facilitating the TA, palpate the multifidi to ensure they are wired in with the TA, and then trust that they develop and coordinate together. According to Hodges, the TA and multifidi usually contract and can be facilitated together, so there are associative linkages between the two. In the end, what is important to our students is not whether they can contract the multifidi independently of the longissimus, but that they have an enhanced subjective sensation of stability, they can recognize a proprioceptive difference between what they were doing and what you are teaching them to do, there is a reduction of symptoms and they are able to function at a higher level at work and play.

A belly-down orientation is a good one in which to facilitate the multifidus. Perhaps if we facilitated TA and cultivated an ability to distinguish true from habitual spinal neutral, we could use bending, leaning or holding weight in front as contexts for strengthening the multifidi. We could train the TA and then go back to Cat/Camel, Side-sit Bending or Sit to Stand and use them to train recognition of spinal neutral in a belly-down orientation. We could train the TA and go forward to TA Leg Lifts, Half-kneel Bending, Split Stance Bending, Knee Walking, Steppin' Out or Peerless Pivots to do the same. Why not train the three layers of stability all at the same time?

Now, on to the main event: how do we go about teaching intersegmental control and blending it with phasic control? How do we get our students to recognize postural and movement stressors? How do we get our students to change lifelong habits that have resulted in unstable joints?

TA Facilitation

Variations

A. Stand for a moment. Have your weight equally distributed between your two feet and arms hanging down at your sides.

- Notice how wide apart your feet are. How stable are you when you gently sway from side to side?

- Notice how your weight is distributed front to back on your feet. How stable are you when you gently sway forward and back? Which direction of sway feels most stable, side-to-side or front to back?

- Notice how your pelvis is balanced on your legs. Is it vertical? Or is it tipping or spilling forward or backward? Is it turned in space left or right? Is one side of your pelvis farther forward than the other?

- Slowly lift your left foot a little away from the floor, just enough to clear your toes off the floor. Return your foot slowly back to the floor; shift your weight

back on to that foot so that you again have equal weight on both feet.

- Pause for a moment, then repeat lifting and lowering your left foot several times. How stable are you standing on one foot?

- Does your pelvis turn left or right? Does your pelvis spill or tip forward or back? Does your lower back change its shape? What do you do with your belly?

- Do the same lifting and lowering movement, this time with your right foot.

- How stable you are standing on this foot? Does your pelvis turn left or right? Does your pelvis spill or tip forward or back? Does your lower back change its shape? What do you do with your belly?

B. Lie on your back with your legs down long and your arms somewhere on the floor below shoulder height.

- Notice the contact you make against the floor.

- Feel the position of your pelvis. Is your tailbone pressing into the floor or lifting away? Is it rolled left or right?

- Feel how your weight is distributed along your spine. Which parts press into the floor and which are lifted from the floor? Feel in particular your lower back. Is it lifted from the floor? How much? How comfortable is it?

C. Continue to lie on your back with both arms on the floor, but now bend up both your knees and place the soles of your feet on the floor. Experiment a little with the placement of your feet on the floor and the width between your knees so that your legs are easily balanced and able to fall equally easily inside or out.

1. Begin to make a small movement of pulling in your belly button. Pull your belly button gently in toward your backbone. This is a contraction of your lower and deeper belly only.

- Place your fingers on your lower belly just above and to the right and left of your pubic bone. Cough and feel if this gets those muscles to contract.

- Do that a few times, then try to pull in your lower belly again without coughing. See whether there is a contraction or a tightening of the muscles of the lower belly (Fig. 6.13).

- Is it possible to tighten your lower belly to pull in your belly button without contracting your upper belly?

- Place your fingers under the front margins of your ribs to monitor for whether this area tightens. Try to make this as soft as possible as you do the movement.

- How smooth and controlled does this movement feel? How strong does it feel?

- Does pulling your belly button toward your backbone feel symmetrical? Or does your belly button pull off to the right or left?

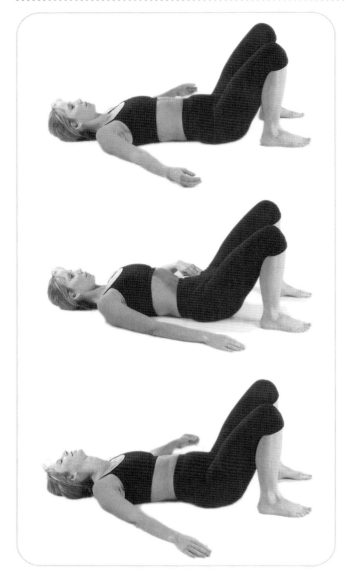

Fig. 6.13 Pulling in the lower belly, not the upper.

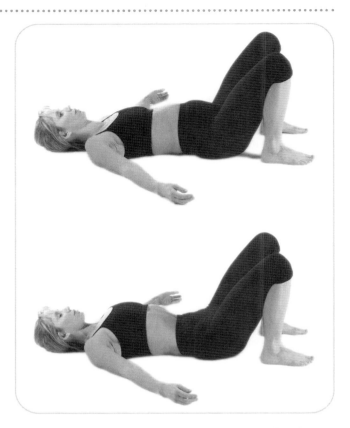

Fig. 6.14 Seesaw breath – move held breath between belly and chest.

D. Continue to lie on your back with your knees bent.

- Continue with this movement of pulling in your lower belly, but now begin to add in a pulling up and in of your pelvic floor. There are three openings in your pelvic floor.

- The back opening in your pelvic floor is your anus. The front opening is your urethra (stops and starts your flow of urine). The middle opening depends on whether you are female (vagina) or male (pull up your testicles).

- Combine pulling in your belly button with pulling up and squeezing the pelvic floor. Try tightening your front opening but not the backside. Repeat this movement many times.

E. Resume lying on your back with your legs bent up.

- Take a breath and hold it, then move your held breath back and forth between your belly and your chest. This is a seesaw breath (Fig. 6.14).

- Expand your belly and push your belly button forward toward the ceiling as you push your breath down. Collapse your chest so your breastbone sinks back toward the floor.

- Expand your chest and push your chest forward toward the ceiling as you pull your held breath up. Let your belly suck in as if tacking your belly button back on to your spine.

- Alternate back and forth with your held breath but do empty your lungs periodically, cycle through a few breaths to reoxygenate, then resume this same movement of moving your held breath back and forth between belly and chest.

- After familiarizing yourself with this movement, add in tightening of your lower belly and pulling up/in your (front and middle) pelvic floor as you move your air into your chest.

- Then relax and push down or bulge out your lower belly and pelvic floor openings as you move your air down into your belly.

- Alternately tighten your lower belly and pelvic floor and relax/push out your lower belly and pelvic floor in time with the movement of your breath into your chest and into your belly.

- Add in rolling your pelvis gently up and down on the floor in time with your breath, belly and pelvic floor.

- Roll your pelvis upward on the floor and flatten your lower back as you pull your breath into your chest and pull in your lower belly/pelvic floor (Fig. 6.15).

- Roll your pelvis downward on the floor and lift your back slightly from the floor as you push your breath into your belly and push out your lower belly/pelvic floor (Fig. 6.15). Alternate back and forth several times.

- Continue to coordinate breath/belly/pelvic floor but roll your pelvis in the opposite direction to the one you were just doing. Roll your pelvis upward and flatten your back as you push out your belly/pelvic floor and move your breath into your belly.

- Roll your pelvis upward as you pull your belly/pelvic floor in and move your breath into your chest.

- Go back to coordinating your pelvis with your breath/belly/pelvic floor in the original way. Which way of organizing your pelvis with this basic movement seems most natural?

- Go back to your original movement of simply pulling in your lower belly. How does it compare now in terms of smoothness, strength and familiarity to when you started?

F. Lie on your back again with your knees bent up and your arms on the floor.

- Do the seesaw breath again a few times by holding your breath and moving it back and forth between belly and chest. Now continue with the same alternate expansion and constriction of belly and chest, but now instead of doing it while holding your breath, take a breath into your belly and exhale by expanding your chest.

- As you breathe in, expand your belly and collapse your chest. As you exhale, expand and lift your chest in such a way that you could fit your fingers under the front margins of your rib cage. Alternate back and forth several times.

- Now add in the pulling in/up of your belly button/pelvic floor when you breathe out and lift/expand your chest. Add in the pushing out/down of your belly button/pelvic floor when you breathe into and expand your whole belly. Alternate coordinating breath, belly and pelvic floor.

- Add in rolling your pelvis alternately up and down on the floor. Initially, roll your pelvis upward and flatten your back as you exhale/pull in belly and floor/lift and expand your chest, then roll your pelvis down and lift slightly your back as you inhale/push your belly and floor out/collapse your chest. Alternate several times.

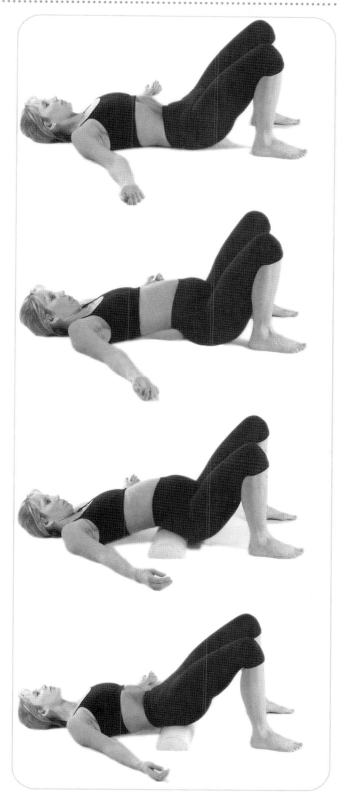

Fig. 6.15 Coordinating the movement of pelvis with lower belly and pelvic floor – with a helpful toy.

- Reverse the coordination. Roll your pelvis in the opposite direction you just did. Alternate and determine which way of coordinating your pelvis/breath/belly/pelvic floor works best.

G. Lie on your back as before, knees bent.

- Go back to doing a seesaw breath. Move your held breath back and forth between your belly and chest. Coordinate with belly/pelvic floor and with rolling your pelvis.

- Now move your breath into your chest, pull in your lower belly and floor and stay in this position of having your chest lifted/expanded and your lower belly held in.

- From here, breathe in and out several times. Keep your chest lifted and your belly in as you breathe. Can you expand your breath out into your lower ribs or even forward into your upper belly while keeping your lower belly in? Let go of everything, then repeat this same thing several times. How easily can you breathe while maintaining lower belly/pelvic floor tension?

- Go back to our original movement: simply pull your belly button back toward your backbone. How does this movement compare to when you first tried it?

- Straighten your legs and lie flat on your back for a moment. How is your contact against the floor and how is your pelvis and back balanced from side to side now?

H. Stand up.

- Notice how wide apart your feet are. How stable are you when you gently sway from side to side?

- Notice how your weight is distributed front to back on your feet – how stable are you when you gently sway forward and back? Which direction of sway feels most stable, side to side or front to back?

- Notice how your pelvis is balanced on your legs. Is it vertical? Or is it tipping or spilling forward or backward? Is it turned in space left or right – is one side of your pelvis farther forward than the other?

- Try gently pulling in your lower belly and floor and breathing freely in this position. How does it compare to lying down?

Static and dynamic baselines – TA Facilitation

For our initial scan, stand for a moment with your weight equally divided between your two feet and arms hanging down at your sides. Notice width of feet, weight distribution front to back and balance of pelvis on legs. This static scan is similar to others. Standing gives you an opportunity to assess flexion/extension and right/left bias. Lift one foot then the other off the floor slightly. The dynamic baselines are concerned with gross standing stability: to shift weight from side to side and from heels to toes and to lift one foot. In addition

to assessing gross stability, how steady are you in moving from side to side with your feet close together?

We can start to get a sense of how someone manages this stepping movement, this extension stressor in terms of lumbopelvic stability. How is the position of the pelvis controlled in space? Without activation of the right gluteal group when lifting the left foot, the left side of the pelvis would drop and the pelvis as a whole would fall into anterior tilt as the left iliopsoas pulls the pelvis toward the left leg at 4.30. During assessment, watch from the side and from the front for changes in the position of the pelvis in space and the shape of the lower back.

You could also watch for a general shortening effect. Watch the top of the head relative to the background for whether they get shorter (less active abductors and hip extensors) or taller (pushing actively into the floor with the weightbearing side). Watch also for a turn of the pelvis left or right. Does the pelvis turn equally toward the stepping leg in each direction? Does it turn in the opposite direction of the stepping leg? Does it turn in one direction but not the other? Does it have a habitual bias and stay turned to that side?

In variation B, lie on your back with your legs down long and your arms somewhere on the floor below shoulder height. Here we do a typical supine scan, with emphasis on the relationships of the pelvis and lower back to the floor and to comfort/discomfort in the lower back. Is this position uncomfortable? Is it any better when you bend your legs up? What might this tell you?

Continue to lie on your back with both arms on the floor in variation C, but now bend up both your knees. Make a small initial movement of pulling in your belly button. This would be accomplished by the transverse abdominis. This is another dynamic baseline. How accessible is it? How balanced is it left to right? How differentiated is it from the upper belly?

There are instructions here to pull in your belly button and to palpate just medial to the ASISs. Does this mean that the TA is only in the lower belly? No, we know that it extends up to the level of the seventh rib. The lower belly is a place where only the internal obliques and the TA are present, though. The external obliques are missing from this section. This makes the lower belly easier to palpate and gives some proprioceptive focus to our students. Keep in mind that it isn't really the upper and lower belly you are differentiating, but the deep and the superficial.

What is the importance of differentiating the lower from the upper belly? Contraction of the upper belly inhibits the diaphragm and full and easy breathing. People who are chronically contracted in their upper belly tend to default the movement of their breath to their upper chest and tend to engage their scalenes and other anterior cervical musculature to increase the vertical dimension of the chest cavity. Chronic holding of the upper belly constrains the movement of the lower ribs, mid to lower thoracic spine and lumbothoracic junction and contributes to funneling movement stresses down to the lower back. According to Hodges, chronic holding of the superficial abdominal musculature also seems to have an inhibitory effect on the intersegmental lower belly musculature.

Facilitating TA with the pelvic floor and breathing

Now that we've focused our attention on and established some static and dynamic baselines, the rest of this lesson is designed to help someone get a better sense of how to do this intersegmental movement smoothly and accurately and in a way that differentiates the intersegmental stabilizers from the superficial lower torso musculature.

Continue to lie on your back with your knees bent in variation D. Resume with this movement of pulling in your lower belly, but now add in pulling up and in your pelvic floor. These pelvic floor movements, reminiscent of Kegel exercises, are extremely helpful, with nearly everyone getting an associative contraction of the transverse abdominis. There is a description of the three openings and an emphasis on contracting the front openings rather than the back. This particular differentiation is difficult for most people to do, so be sure to allow for approximations.

Let them contract the whole pelvic floor initially and hope that with practice and refinement they can separate the anal sphincter from the anterior floor musculature. What is the relevance? What associative havoc are we wreaking on the lower digestive tract if we ask people to keep their anus squeezed shut constantly? Is the clamping down of the anal sphincter associated with anxious emotional states? Should any muscle in your body be constantly contracting, or are we designed to reciprocate relaxation and contraction, to volley back and forth between rest and work cycles?

Resume lying on your back with your legs bent up in variation E. Take a breath and hold it, then move your held breath back and forth between your belly and your chest. This is a seesaw breath. In addition to using the pelvic floor to help facilitate transverse abdominis contractions, we can also use directed breath. We are using these reciprocating movements of the breath to facilitate reciprocating movements of the pelvic floor and transverse abdominis. Achieving motor control over the intersegmental stabilizing muscles is not just about contracting: it is also about letting go. It is this contrast between contraction and relaxation that helps the CNS recognize more clearly what is happening; exaggerating differences clarifies those differences.

Pushing your held breath down into your lower belly necessitates relaxing the TA and suggests a bulging down and out of the pelvic floor muscles. Pulling your breath up into your chest serves the dual purpose of facilitating a TA contraction (as the belly button naturally pulls back toward the spine) and inhibiting the superficial abdominals (lifting and expanding the chest is very hard to do with the obliques and the rectus contracting). This basic seesaw breath is yet another piece to add to our Lego project.

After familiarizing yourself with this movement, add in tightening of your lower belly and pulling up/in your (front and middle) pelvic floor as you move your air into your chest, then relaxing and pushing down or bulging out your lower belly and pelvic floor openings as you move your air down into your belly. Alternately tighten your lower belly and pelvic floor and relax/push out your lower belly and pelvic floor in time with the movement of your breath into your chest and belly.

Do these movements all seem to fit together? Try organizing your breath and lower belly/pelvic floor contractions the opposite way – differentiate them. Do these movements seem to fit together with the same ease? We've linked three Lego pieces so far. Let's add another one.

Adding osteokinematic movement to arthrokinematic stabilization

As you continue with the movement of coordinating your seesaw breath with simultaneous TA and pelvic floor contractions, add in rolling your pelvis gently up and down on the floor. Roll your pelvis upward on the floor and flatten your lower back as you pull your breath up into your chest and pull in your lower belly/pelvic floor. Roll your pelvis downward on the floor and lift your back slightly from the floor as you push your breath into your belly and push out your lower belly/pelvic floor.

Alternate back and forth several times. We are coordinating intersegmental muscle contraction with mild posterior tilt and lumbar flexion, then coordinating a relaxation/inhibition of these same muscles with anterior tilt and lumbar extension. TA contracts with the gluteals and relaxes with the iliopsoas.

Why are we moving the pelvis and lower back at all if what we are looking for is stability? Almost by definition, our students with lumbar instability don't know where spinal neutral is: their calibration of middle of the range is skewed. We are using small reciprocating movements, as we have throughout this book, to clarify through experience where a truer neutral is and how it compares to habitual neutral (Box 6.6).

We are also asking for movement because we want to use the floor as a reference point. When the back is lifted from the floor, the back is extending. When the tailbone is lifted, the back is flexing. Neutral is where lower back and tailbone are both (more or less) on the floor. Link the external reference point (contact with the floor) with internal reference points (proprioceptive awareness of where bones are in relation to each other). The third reason we want to introduce some phasic movement here is to begin to coordinate the ability to use the spinal stabilizers with the muscles that control the movement, position and stabilization of the pelvis in space. We want to link the intersegmental stabilizers with the four cornerstone muscles of the pelvis, which should also be considered to be intersegmental muscles.

The next ingredient we add to the pot is a differentiation of the direction of movement of the pelvis from the contractions of the TA and pelvic floor. Here, we are asking the intersegmental muscles to contract in time, not with the gluteals as

---

Box 6.6 TA Facilitation

Facilitating TA contraction through directed breath and pelvic floor

Differentiating TA contraction from abdominal obliques with breathing constraint

Coordinating and differentiating TA contractions with Pelvic Tilts

Facilitating awareness of how to maintain intersegmental stability and breathe independently with diaphragm

we did in the last variation, but with the iliopsoas. This will be a more difficult differentiation for most people. Which way of coordinating intersegmental relaxation and contraction with the two directions of movement of the pelvis might make more sense for the iliopsoas-dominant student who suffers from extension stresses? Which way would make sense for the gluteal-dominant student?

Using half a foam roller or a rolled-up towel or blanket, placed crosswise underneath the pelvis, can further facilitate this rolling of the pelvis into anterior and posterior tilt. The roller enables the pelvis to fall more easily in each direction and provides another reference point upon which to move and change points of contact. It can also make much clearer the instructions you might make to direct these rolling movements of the pelvis from the legs. A very slight activation of the hip flexors with the intention to lighten the feet will have an immediate effect on the balance of the pelvis on the roller: it will fall downward towards the feet.

The last instructions in this section are to backtrack to previous movements for the purpose of an intermission comparison. Go back to coordinating your pelvis with your breath/belly/pelvic floor in the original way (another opportunity for a Goldilocks comparison). Go back to your original movement of pulling in your lower belly. How does it compare to when you began? Has the addition of more balls to juggle helped to refine and strengthen your ability to recruit your transverse abdominis?

Directing your breath to apply a constraint

Lie on your back again with your knees bent up and your arms on the floor in variation F. Do the seesaw breath again a few times. Then switch from holding your breath to breathing a particular way: inhale into your belly and exhale by lifting and expanding your chest. This movement is similar to the seesaw breath. Your TA and pelvic floor bulge out and relax now as you breathe into your belly, then pull in and up as you breathe out by expanding your chest.

Lifting the chest requires a lengthening and an inhibition of the superficial abdominal muscles. We are finding ways to differentiate the obliques and rectus from the transverse abdominis. Functionally, this is obviously a big step up from holding your breath: now your students can practice their intersegmental stabilization without turning purple. We can even train some of our students to time the effort of doing a shorter duration/higher intensity stressful movement with an exhalation. Once this piece is assembled, it is attached in turn to all the other pieces we have performed so far. We add in pulling in the belly button and pelvic floor and then rolling the pelvis as we did in the previous variation.

Because we are mixing and matching pieces so much, we might as well use the next instruction to differentiate your breathing from the movements of your intersegmentals and pelvis. Or we could use it to differentiate the movement of your intersegmentals from your breath and pelvis. How many different combinations are possible by using TA, pelvic floor, breath and pelvis?

Variation G is designed to help make the movement of the breath independent of the contraction of the intersegmental

muscles. There are many movement stressors that we can complete in the cycle of the breath and where the strategy of exhaling and combining that with the activation of your intersegmental musculature would work. There are also many movement stressors that last much longer and require a sustained contraction of the TA and multifidi. In this situation, we would still like to be able to breathe freely without having to resort to gasping with our scalenes.

This coordination of constant TA contraction with relaxed upper abdominals and freely moving breath will be present throughout the rest of this stabilization series of lessons. The relaxation of the upper/superficial abdominals makes it possible to breathe using the diaphragm, both forward into the upper belly and out laterally into the lower ribs. This has the twin benefits of not requiring scalene breathing and of helping the CNS to further differentiate the upper from the lower, the superficial and the stabilizing abdominal muscles.

Comparing baselines

Now at the end of the lesson, we go back once again to our baselines. How are you pulling in your belly button now? How strong, how differentiated from the upper belly? How are you contacting the floor now? Did the attention to and intentional movement of your intersegmental tonic muscles have any effect on the tone or balance of your phasic torso and pelvic muscles and how they allow your bones to contact the ground?

Finally, you come back up to standing again. Notice the width of your feet. Sway gently left and right, then forward and back. How stable do you feel on your feet? Try gently pulling in your lower belly and pelvic floor and breathing freely in this position. How does it compare to lying down? Try lifting first one then the other foot. Do this both with and without pulling in your belly and pelvic floor. Which gives you a better subjective feeling of stability? Could you walk around and maintain this intersegmental support? Can you do it without squeezing your anus shut?

Blending intersegmental and pelvic stability

This last lesson, TA Facilitation, is a chunk of movement we can build a variety of lessons around. Try going back through previous lessons to figure out how this piece could be coordinated with any of the earlier lessons of this Tyrannosaurus section, or even with the earlier worm lessons. Do just that when working with unidirectional instabilities. We want our students to find out how good that nonhabitual differentiated pattern can feel, and that they have a safe direction they can move into at the same time as we teach intersegmental stability. Then progress both unidirectional types to the remaining lessons in this chapter.

With multidirectional instabilities, we might start with the following lessons or very easy and small variations of them, and emphasize much more finding and maintaining spinal neutral. The next lesson picks up where TA Facilitations left off. We will review briefly then continue the movements of coordinating the intersegmental stabilizers: the breath and the pelvis. We will deviate from the cardinal lines and begin to explore left to right TA balance, and will further coordinate the intersegmental stabilizers with the pelvic stabilizers (the legs).

TA Diagonals

Variations

A. Stand for a moment, weight equally divided between your two feet and arms hanging down at your sides.

- Notice how wide apart your feet are. How stable are you when you gently sway from side to side?

- Notice how your weight is distributed front to back on your feet. How stable are you when you gently sway forward and back? Which direction of sway feels most stable, side to side or front to back?

- Notice how your pelvis is balanced on your legs. Is it vertical? Or is it tipping or spilling forward or backward? Is it turned in space left or right? Is one side of your pelvis farther forward than the other?

- Slowly lift your left foot a little away from the floor – just enough to clear your toes off the floor. Return your foot slowly back to the floor and shift your weight back on to that foot so that you again have equal weight on both feet.

- Pause for a moment, then repeat lifting and lowering your left foot several times. How stable are you standing on one foot?

- Does your pelvis turn left or right? Does your pelvis spill or tip forward or back? What do you do with your belly?

- Do the same lifting and lowering movement, this time with your right foot. How stable are you standing on this foot?

- Does your pelvis turn left or right? Does your pelvis spill or tip forward or back? What do you do with your belly?

B. Lie on your back with your legs down long and your arms somewhere on the floor below shoulder height.

- Notice the contact you make against the floor.

- Feel the position of your pelvis. Is your tailbone pressing into the floor or lifting away? Is it rolled left or right?

- Feel how your weight is distributed along your spine. What parts press into the floor and which parts are lifted from the floor? Feel in particular your lower back. Is it lifted from the floor? How much? How comfortable is it?

C. Continue to lie on your back with both arms on the floor, but now bend up both your knees and place the soles of your feet on the floor. Experiment a little with the placement of your feet on the floor and the width between your

knees so that your legs are easily balanced and able to fall equally easily inside or out.

- Begin to make a small movement of pulling in your belly button. Pull your belly button gently in toward your backbone. This is a contraction of your lower belly only.

- Place your fingers on your lower belly just above and to the right and left of your pubic bone. Feel whether there is a contraction or a tightening of the muscles of the lower belly.

- Is it possible to tighten your lower belly to pull in your belly button without contracting your upper belly?

- Place your fingers under the margins of your ribs to monitor for whether this area tightens. Try to make this as soft as possible as you do the movement.

- How smooth and controlled does this movement feel? How strong does it feel?

- Does pulling your belly button toward your backbone feel symmetrical? Or does your belly button pull off to the right or left?

- Deliberately pull your belly button back and to the left. How successful are you in this direction? Pull your belly button back and to the right. How successful are you in this direction? Does one direction seem easier than the other?

D. Come up to sit on the floor. Bend your knees and place the soles of your feet on the floor in that same balanced manner you found when lying on your back. Lean back on both hands behind you. Let your arms support your weight and let your whole back sink and round backward (Fig. 6.16). If you have discomfort in your hands or wrists, try leaning back on your elbows and forearms or against a couch or chair.

- Gently pull in your belly button toward your backbone, pull up/in your (preferably front and middle) pelvic floor openings and roll your pelvis slightly backward on the floor. This results in further rounding your back. Repeat several times. How smooth and controlled is the movement here?

- Do a seesaw breath as you continue this movement; coordinate as before by pulling your belly/pelvic floor in as you move your breath into your chest and roll your pelvis back, then push your belly/pelvic floor out as you move your breath into your belly. Alternate several times.

- Then try pulling your belly button back and to the left. Pull your belly button back and in a diagonal to the left. Which side of your lower belly contracts to do this? Exhale and expand/lift your chest as you do this. Inhale into your belly as you bring your belly button back to center.

- How might you coordinate your pelvis with this diagonal movement of your belly button? Try rolling your pelvis back and to the left on the floor. You can gently press your right foot into the floor to accomplish this

(Fig. 6.16). Repeat several times, coordinating breath out/chest up, belly button back and to the left, rolling your pelvis back and to the left. Pause for a moment.

- Then resume this same movement of pulling your belly back and left and rolling your pelvis back and to the left. Add in slowly and gently lifting your left foot off the floor. (Fig. 6.16).

- Make sure your pelvis still rolls back and to the left. Your right foot will have to press into the floor to assist with this. Continue to coordinate with breath/belly/pelvic floor.

- This movement results in turning your pelvis to the left. Allow your shoulders to turn to the left the same amount as your pelvis. Your back can round a bit and bend a bit (left side of waist and ribcage gets longer and right side gets shorter) but don't twist. Move shoulders and hips the same amount.

- Now lift your left foot as before and stay there, left foot lifted, pelvis and shoulders turned to the left.

- From there, breathe into your belly/push out your belly and floor; exhale by lifting your chest and pulling in your belly and pelvic floor. Stay in this same exact position but alternate inhaling/relaxing belly and floor and exhaling/tightening lower belly and floor. Can you achieve stability independent of your lower belly?

E. Come back to sit again as before, knees bent and leaning back on hands.

- Go through the same sequence of movements as in D, but to the other side.

- Pull your belly button back and to the right, roll your pelvis back and to the right, pull in your belly/pelvic floor and expand/lift your chest.

- Add in the movement of lifting your right foot and allow your pelvis and shoulders to turn to the right. Allow the right side of your waist and ribcage to get longer. How does this side compare to the other?

- Try the movement of lifting your right foot, allowing your pelvis and chest to turn to the right and staying there while you breathe into your belly and exhale with an expansion/lifting of your chest. Pause for a moment.

- Then alternate the movement of lifting one foot then the other (Fig. 6.17). Exhale and pull in your lower belly/pelvic floor as you lift, inhale and push out your belly and pelvic floor as you return that foot to the floor, and exhale/pull in again as you lift the other foot. Alternate from side to side and appreciate your ability to move your belly button diagonally in each direction.

- Return to sitting with both feet on the floor. Try simply pulling your belly button back and to the left, then back and to the right. How do these movements compare to when we began?

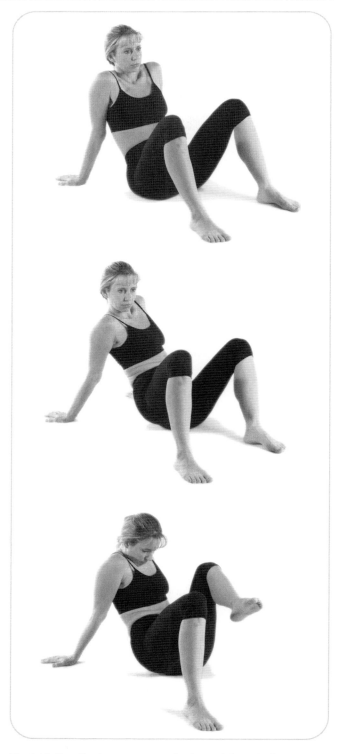

Fig. 6.16 Coordinating movement of pelvis with lower belly and pelvic floor in a diagonal direction.

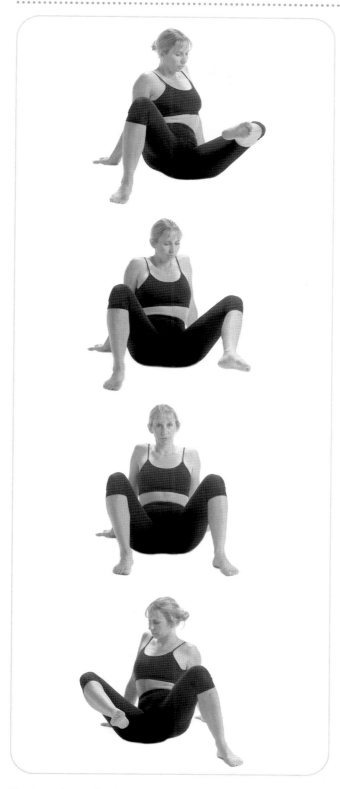

Fig. 6.17 Alternately lifting left and right foot while pressing with the opposite – keep intersegmental stability.

- Lie on your back with your knees bent and simply pull your belly button straight back to your backbone. How is the coordination of this movement going? Pull back and to the left, then to the right. How is this going?

- For extra credit, or if you are more comfortable lying on your back than sitting up, try this same series of movements while lying on your back with both legs bent up.

F.   Stand again for a moment. Have your weight equally divided between your two feet and arms hanging down at your sides.

- Notice how wide apart your feet are. How stable are you when you gently sway from side to side?

- Notice how your weight is distributed front to back on your feet. How stable are you when you gently sway forward and back?

- Notice how your pelvis is balanced on your legs. Is it vertical? Is it turned in space left or right? Is one side of your pelvis farther forward than the other?

- Slowly lift your left foot a little away from the floor. Return your foot slowly back to the floor then repeat lifting and lowering your left foot several times.

- As you do this, notice how stable are you standing on one foot. Does your pelvis turn left or right? Does your pelvis spill or tip forward or back? What do you do with your belly?

- Try letting your pelvis and shoulders turn a bit to the left, pull up lower belly/pelvic floor, push your pelvis back toward vertical.

- Do the same lifting and lowering movement, but this time with your right foot.

- Notice again how stable you are standing on one foot. Allow your pelvis and shoulders to turn to the right and pull belly/pelvic floor up and in.

Baselines – TA Diagonals

Because this lesson so closely approximates the last one, we won't review this one in a step-by-step manner. We'll just point out a few salient features. The whole static and dynamic baselines in standing and lying supine were identical to the first lesson except for one fiendish little variation: the instruction to pull your belly button back and to the left and then back and to the right. It is a good strategy to overlap lessons: start one lesson by reviewing the end of the previous one. This helps students to recognize the progression and enables them to draw on past experience.

You probably perceived differences in your ability to move your belly button diagonally to each side. They will be present; the only question is the degree of imbalance and the acuity of your proprioceptive sense in recognizing it. The TA imbalance will also probably be correlated with pelvic and torso imbalances. For instance, if you can more easily pull your belly button back and to the left, you are able to more easily engage the right TA. Consistent with right TA bias would be some element of shortening along the right side of the torso, perhaps from a left iliopsoas or right gluteal (or left force couple) bias. Check this out with yourself, colleagues and students.

Taking the TA out for a test drive

We break new ground with this lesson when we come up to sit, leaning back on hands behind. We start again with a review of the basic anterior/posterior movement of the pelvis coordinated with floor, TA and variations of directed breath (held and seesaw, reciprocal intersegmental movements timed with the breath, and constantly held intersegmental stability with independent breath).

We continue from there into diagonal pelvic movements coordinated with diagonal TA movements. The right gluteal pushes the pelvis back and to the left, the belly button is assisted in moving in that direction, and the right TA is encouraged to boost the movement of the belly button in that same back and to the left direction. There is a turning movement of the pelvis, which is encouraged in this lesson, along with encouragement to allow the chest and shoulders to turn in the same direction and for the same amount as the pelvis. This ensures minimal rotational shearing at the lower back. We are allowing a movement slightly to moderately into right lumbar flexion, depending on the type of instability. Most of the time, even people with multidirectional instabilities can learn to do this with minimal flexion or rotational stresses.

Additionally, for the most common of directional instabilities (extension), this position and direction of movement is just the ticket. This belly-up orientation is much safer for unstable extenders: gravity is assisting in rolling the pelvis and back into posterior tilt and lumbar flexion. Pushing the foot into the floor, which engages the gluteals and moves the pelvis away from its unstable direction, is just what the doctor ordered.

The next movement added is lifting the left foot when rolling the pelvis and pulling the belly button back and to the left. Recall similar movements in the Wishbone lesson. This stepping movement, which is an extension stressor for most people, is more easily controlled in this position. The weight-bearing leg is required to push into the floor to counteract the tendency of the pelvis to be dragged forward and to the left towards the lifting left leg. This is particularly true if you are truly inhibiting your obliques and rectus abdominis as you lift the leg.

By pulling up and expanding the chest on exhalation, or pulling up and staying there while breathing independently, you are still asking for a differentiation of the lower from the upper belly. Without the obliques and rectus to stabilize the pelvis from rolling into anterior tilt, the weightbearing leg is your only remaining option. This is another example of the progressive application of constraints funneling someone's movement options down to the one you want him or her to learn.

Putting the whole thing together and alternating from side to side is a great way to help your student become aware of and to reduce right/left TA and pelvic imbalances.

As in the previous lesson, a half foam roller or rolled towel can be a nice adjunct here. Place the roller lengthwise along the sacrum and allow the pelvis to fall off to the left and right.

Use ingrained balance reactions to facilitate asymmetrical lower torso and TA movements.

As in the previous lesson, you could experiment with coordinating and differentiating your TA, pelvic floor, pelvis and breath in different ways. Did you try pulling your belly button back and to the left as you rolled your pelvis back and to the right? As a variation for those with sensitive wrists, more acute back pain or a general inability to be comfortable on the floor, try doing this lesson in a chair or stable stool.

Rigidity vs stabilization

Notice that we are encouraging movement of the pelvis and trunk in this lesson. We may encourage movement into flexion if comfortable, and will encourage a side-bend component to this lesson with everyone but those with the most extreme instabilities. What we don't want to see much of is rotation. Just be sure to turn pelvis and shoulders the same amount.

Contrast this with a doll body approach to stabilization. Current stabilization protocols seem to encourage a cardinal plane rigidity that Barbie herself would be proud of. We ask our students to lift one leg in supine (or prone, side-lie or stand) and allow for zero pelvic and torso movement. We ask for a constantly maintained neutral spine in all three planes and for a level pelvis in gait. We are helping to immobilize the chest and ribcage, just the place most of our folks need to have more movement and where they may be unintentionally encouraging a fear of movement.

Try this movement of lifting one leg away from the ground again in hook-sitting, while leaning back on your elbows and while lying on your back. Try it both with the lifting leg bent and the lifting leg down long. Try it both by allowing your pelvis to roll on the floor toward your lifting leg and by keeping your pelvis immobile on the floor. What you will find is that it is much more effort to keep your pelvis from moving. The abdominals and the arms have to brace.

Contrast that sensation with the relative ease of lifting the leg and allowing your pelvis to move. TA and multifidus contractions will be more easily felt when the rest of the belly and back are not adding their voices to the choir. It is easier to feel the way the weightbearing leg works to encourage a rotational movement of the pelvis and to discourage a movement of the pelvis into anterior tilt. It is easier to allow your shoulders to turn and your torso to side-bend; let it get a little longer on the side of the lifting leg (Box 6.7).

Doesn't the movement of the pelvis on the floor and the side-bending of the torso mean I have lost stability? Why does easier mean better? My opinion only: easier is better because of the lazy tendencies of the CNS. Local stabilization when needed is a lot easier sell than a rigidity and effort that goes

---

Box 6.7 TA Diagonals

Facilitating TA balance right to left

Blending unilateral TA contractions with pelvic force couples

Lifting a leg to increase need for stability of pelvis from weightbearing leg

into nothing but self-compression and isometric work. For the vast majority of your students you don't need a straitjacket, you need a corset.

By allowing the movement of the pelvis around the legs, we are facilitating an awareness of how to move around the hip joints and how to control extension stresses from the legs. By allowing a pelvic force couple movement we are laying the groundwork for maintaining intersegmental stability while turning the pelvis from the legs. By allowing a pelvic force couple movement we are laying the groundwork for maintaining intersegmental stability while walking with a pelvic force couple gait. Just say yes to intersegmental stability, specific directional stability of the pelvis and lower back, and free and fluid movement elsewhere through the skeleton!

Alternatives – plan B

As another way of facilitating TA contractions, try both straight back and diagonal falling backward movements while sitting in a chair or sitting cross-legged, long-legged or side-sitting on the floor: palpate lower belly for initial activation of TA and lift the chest or breathe into the upper belly to differentiate from obliques and rectus. Begin to roll your pelvis backward on the floor, but don't let your spine round in a balancing reaction. Feel for the contraction of the TA almost immediately upon leaning back. Keep the obliques and rectus semi-inactive by disallowing torso flexion. Try straight-on versions to start with, then progress to diagonal leans.

Alternatively, lie supine with your legs in the air and a ball under the middle of your sacrum and play with diagonal directions of movement without your legs being in a position to assist; coordinate the second and third layers of the onion (Fig. 6.18). Balance supine on the floor with a ball under your pelvis. Lift both legs toward the ceiling and feel for the direction of fall of your pelvis off the ball. If it falls to the left, feel for and intentionally engage the right TA along with the appropriate obliques. Do to the other side and compare the two.

For your students who are unstable into flexion, your emphasis in TA Facilitation will be on intersegmental stabilization linked to iliopsoas contraction and anterior pelvic tilt (Fig. 6.19). Link pulling up and in of pelvic floor and TA with rolling pelvis straight or diagonally forward to link intersegmental stability with the iliopsoas. Enlarge upon this theme in floor or chair sitting; lead the movement of coming back upright from a falling-back position with the pelvis/iliopsoas. Do this initially by leaning back on hands behind, then progress to no hands to functionally strengthen the iliopsoas.

Although this lesson is written as being performed from a sitting-up position, it could just as easily be performed from supine. Some people are more comfortable here, and it is a bit easier to feel the movement of the pelvis and the shape of the back relative to the floor. Try both ways and use what you like, or mix and match!

This next lesson completes this series of belly-up TA Facilitation lessons. It again starts where we left off in the last lesson, and breaks new ground through lengthening the lifted leg and changes of position during the lesson.

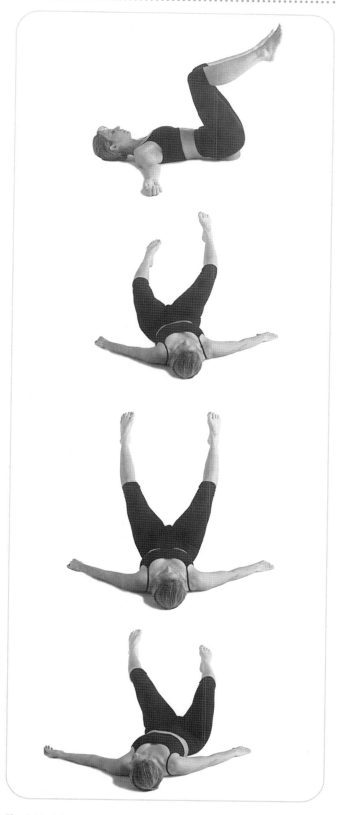

Fig. 6.18 Balancing pelvis on ball helps balance left and right TA – and helps define neutral.

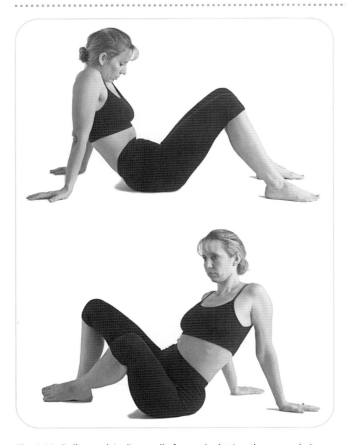

Fig. 6.19 Rolling pelvis diagonally forward – letting the psoas do its work – emphasize for people with flexion hypermobilities.

TA Leg Lifts

Variations

A.   Lie on your back with your legs long and your arms somewhere on the floor below shoulder height.

- Scan your contact against the floor as before. How fully supported are you by the floor? How balanced are you from side to side?

- Make a few movements in this position of pulling in your lower belly and your pelvic floor.

- Do a few seesaw breaths in this position (moving held breath back and forth between belly and chest) and coordinate with pulling in/up and pushing down/out the lower belly/pelvic floor.

- Continue the same basic coordination but breathe continually – breathe into belly and push out lower belly/pelvic floor – exhale by expanding/lifting your chest and pulling in belly/pelvic floor. Pause for a moment.

- Then differentiate your breath from your belly/pelvic floor. Breathe out and relax your belly and floor and breathe in while you pull your belly in. Try this a few times, then pause.

- See if it is possible to pull in your lower belly while pushing out your pelvic floor. Relax your openings as you tighten your lower belly. You will probably find this difficult. The next time you are urinating, try pulling in your lower belly while keeping your urine flow uninterrupted. Pause.

- Go back to the original movement of pulling in your belly and floor together in time with your breath. How coordinated and how strong does this movement feel now?

- Pull your belly button back and to the left a few times, then back and to the right a few times, then alternate. How are your diagonals doing?

B.   Come up to sit on the floor. Lean back on both hands behind you and place the soles of both feet on the floor in front of you.

- Pull your belly button back and to the left, roll your pelvis back and to the left and lift your left foot off the floor (Fig. 6.20).

- Refamiliarize yourself with this movement a few times, then do the same thing but to the other side. Compare and contrast movements in each direction.

- Alternate from side to side. Pause for a moment with both feet on the floor.

- The next time you roll your pelvis and pull your belly button back and to the left, stay in that position a moment with your left leg lifted. From here, breathe into your belly/exhale with lifted chest several times. Your pelvic floor and lower belly pull in and push out in coordination with your breath.

- Repeat this same movement to the other side.

C.   Come up to sit on the floor as before. If you can, lean back on your elbows and forearms instead of leaning on your hands. If this position is not feasible, stay on your hands.

- Lift your left foot from the floor as before, roll your pelvis, pull in your belly/pelvic floor and time with an exhalation and lifting/expansion of your chest. This time, instead of placing your left foot back on the floor, continue to keep your left leg lifted as you tilt your left leg out to the left as if you wanted to place your left knee on the floor (Fig. 6.20).

- You have to roll your pelvis to the left and press with your right foot into the floor to do this.

- As you bring your lifted left leg back to center, continue the movement of your left leg now to the right, as if you were going to cross your left leg over your right (Fig. 6.20). This rolls your pelvis across the floor to the right. Your right foot remains centered, with your right knee over your right foot.

- Alternate back and forth between tilting your left leg out to the left and over to the right. The right foot stays centered the whole time. The pelvis moves around a stationary right leg.

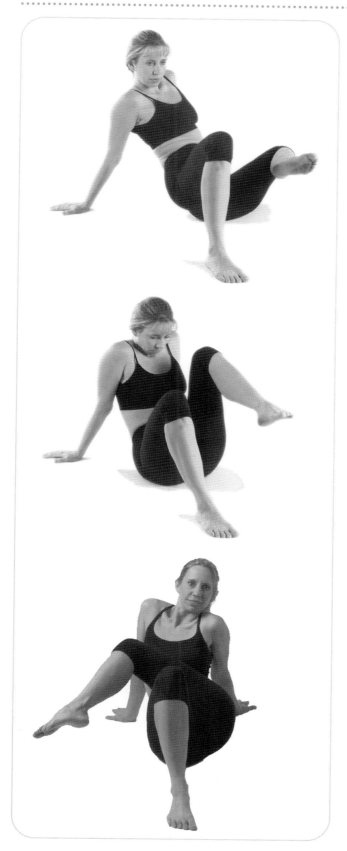

Fig. 6.20 Lifting the leg and swinging it left and right – rolling pelvis left and right.

- Pause at the end-range of each movement and belly breathe. See if your ability to keep yourself stable can be independent of a tight lower belly.

- Rest in sitting for a moment, then resume the position of leaning back on hand or your elbows and forearms. Repeat this same sequence of movements to the other side. Compare and contrast your two sides.

D. Come back up to sitting on the floor, leaning back on your elbows and forearms if possible. Your knees are bent and the soles of both feet are on the floor.

- Coordinate lifting your left foot with your belly/pelvic floor/stabilization and with a chest lifting exhalation and stay there for a moment.

- Instead of putting your foot back on the floor this time, extend your left leg down long (Fig. 6.21). This is a movement as if you were going to straighten and rest your left leg down on the floor but keeping the leg just slightly lifted away from the floor. Reverse the movement to bend your left leg back up again and repeat.

- Keep some part of your lower back close to or on the ground as you do this. As you lift your left leg and roll your pelvis to the left, the left side of your low back will press toward the floor.

- As you extend your lifted left leg down long, the center or even the right side of your lower back presses into the floor.

- Initially, keep your lower belly/pelvic floor pulled in and find a way to breathe independently of your stabilization. Breathe into your upper belly or out into your lower ribs.

- Then try extending your lifted left leg down long and holding it there with some part of your lower back against the floor. Can you release your lower belly and pelvic floor contractions while still staying stable? Can you breathe freely?

- Repeat this same sequence of movements to the other side. Compare and contrast.

E. Come up to sitting, lean back on your elbows and forearms.

- Lift your left leg with breath/belly/pelvic floor coordination, extend the lifted leg down long, then reverse the movement to come back through center and to swing the left leg over to the right, as if crossing your left leg over your right.

- Put the whole thing together: the lifted left leg tilts out to the left, extends down long, comes back to being tilted out to the left again, then swings across to the right. Reverse and repeat.

- If you like, try this movement with your left leg more or less straight the whole time (Fig. 6.22).

- Try this same thing to the other side.

F. Lie on your back with both knees bent and both feet on the floor.

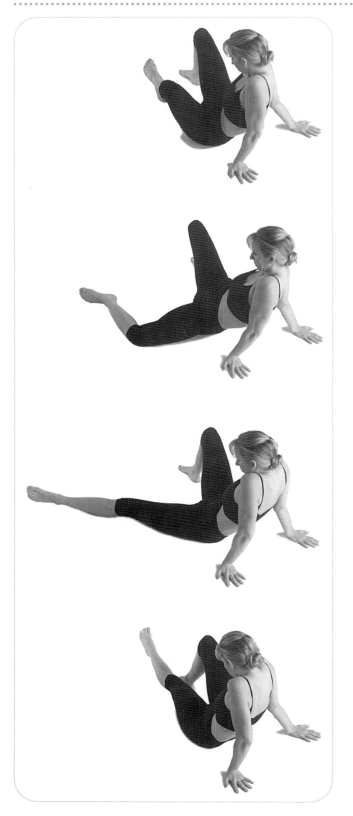

Fig. 6.21 Extending the lifted leg down long – keep some part of your lower back rounded back and keep upper belly soft.

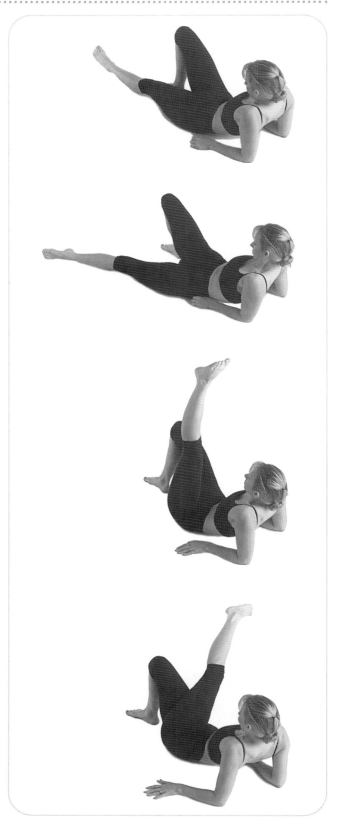

Fig. 6.22 Same thing in a different position – try with lifted leg straight the whole time for extra credit.

- Do the same thing here while lying on your back, as you just did when leaning back on your elbows and forearms.

- This is the same movement of your leg and pelvis, but a somewhat more difficult position in which to keep some part of your lower back on the ground, especially when trying to do it without tightening your upper belly.

- Do the same movements to the opposite side and compare.

- Go back to an earlier movement. Pull your belly button back and to the left, back and to the right, and straight back. What is the quality and control of this movement like now?

G. Stand up. Walk around.

- Pull up/in your lower belly and pelvic floor as you walk.

- Push down/out your lower belly and pelvic floor as you walk – compare the two.

- Can you breathe into your upper belly as you walk and hold in your lower belly? Chew gum at the same time?

Baselines – TA Leg Lifts

Predictably, this lesson starts with some static and dynamic baselines while supine. How is your contact? How is it to pull in your belly button? How about pulling your belly button in and to the right? To the left? Review your seesaw breath and coordinate with belly and floor. Differentiate direction of breath from belly and floor.

Differentiate TA from pelvic floor. This one is pretty hard, but worth the effort, not that it's likely to become a popular party trick, but because of the attempt at finer and finer discrimination there is considerable CNS reorganization that can occur even when the movement is not completely accurate. Try pulling in your TA without stopping your flow of urine.

Come up to sit on the floor in variation B. Lean back on both hands behind you and place the soles of both feet on the floor in front of you. Review from the last lesson the movements of pulling in your belly button, exploring the diagonals and adding in the lifting one foot to create a pelvic force couple. Refamiliarize yourself with this movement a few times, then try a new path.

To hold or to let go?

The next time you roll your pelvis and pull your belly button back and to the left, stay in that position a moment with your left leg lifted. From here, breathe into your belly and exhale with lifted chest several times with your pelvic floor and lower belly pulled in and pushed out in coordination with your breath. How stable does your back feel here with your leg lifted and your belly and floor pushed out and down? Is it possible to be stable without contracting the superficial or even the deep abdominals?

Practitioners of the martial art of tai chi believe so and consciously practice the ability to soften their lower belly while doing complex and demanding movements. Other martial arts and meditation disciplines, as well as the traditional teaching of the Feldenkrais Method, hold this same view. I believe this emphasis on relaxation of the lower belly in these systems is not contradictory to what we have learned about back pain from recent studies.

The ability to relax the entire belly and still be stable is contingent upon a somewhat advanced ability to use the legs to firmly control the movement and position of the pelvis. On one hand the contraction of the TA, even if completely differentiated from the superficial abdominals, still constrains free diaphragmatic breathing. On the other hand, both research and proprioceptive research support the concept of using the TA to stabilize the lower back.

Perhaps there is a compromise on this issue. When resting or in a well-supported position, we could recommend that our students rest their intersegmental stabilizers. Then, when they recognize the presence of a stressor, to contract them. Using them when needed requires your students to be alert to movement and postural stresses and to act accordingly. Relaxing them when not needed allows for a needed rest cycle and keeps the TA/multifidus contraction from becoming habituated and turning gradually into background noise that eventually fades from consciousness altogether.

The corkscrew

Come up to sit on the floor again in variation C. Lean back on your elbows and forearms if possible. Lift your left foot from the floor as before, roll your pelvis back and to the left, pull in your belly/pelvic floor, and time with exhaling and lifting/expanding your chest. This time, instead of placing your left foot back on the floor, continue to keep your left leg lifted as you tilt it out to the left.

You have to roll your pelvis to the left and press with your right foot into the floor to do this. This is a version of a force couple movement that enlarges the turning movement of the pelvis. Intersegmental stabilization stays on and breath is independent. You will probably recognize this movement from previous lessons: TA Diagonals and Wishbone.

Continue the movement of coming back through center to cross your left leg over your right. This movement rolls the pelvis to the right and an odd corkscrew movement through the back at the lumbothoracic junction. The right leg is simultaneously pressing the right foot into the floor with the gluteals and hamstrings and pulling the pelvis across to the right with the right adductors and/or right iliopsoas. Note the shifting of allegiances. The gluteals and adductors/iliopsoas switch from being antagonists to being synergists.

The benefit in this movement at the pelvis is to further enhance and refine the control of the pelvis through the legs. The benefit of this movement at the back is through its ability to mobilize the lumbothoracic junction and thoracic spine without stressing the lower back into extension/rotation patterns. This is possible as long as the pelvis is biased slightly towards posterior tilt and the lower back is near to or on the ground. The resultant flexion movement at the lumbar

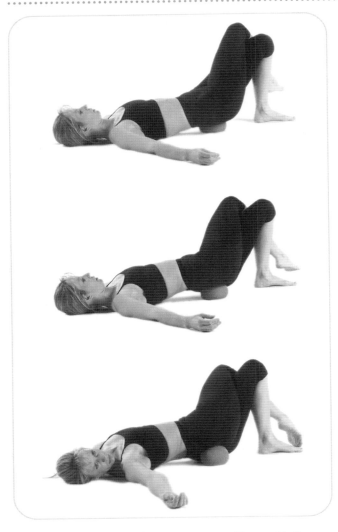

Fig. 6.23 Facilitating the corkscrew movement with a small ball on one side of the pelvis.

segments provides us with a facet locking technique and funnels the rotational movement farther up to the upper lumbar and lower to mid thoracic segments.

This can sometimes be an elusive movement to find; try using a ball to facilitate it. Lie on your back and place a small to medium-sized soft rubber ball between your sacrum and the floor. Cross your right leg over your left and keep your left foot centered on the floor as you roll your pelvis towards the floor to the left (Fig. 6.23). The resultant balance response closely mimics the movement of the pelvis and back, and can be used to facilitate awareness of how both to allow this unusual movement through the spine and to train the legs to control the movement.

Do this to both sides and compare/contrast movements to right and left. Coordinate with TA, floor and breath. Small movements with legs crossed on this ball are excellent ways of

training proprioceptive sensitivity to directions of fall and recognition of effort throughout the lower torso and hips. The half-roller or rolled-up towel or blanket can be used here as well, but not as elegantly.

As you come back to the movements of tilting the lifted leg alternately from side to side, pause at the extreme of each movement to reciprocate your breath with your TA and floor contraction/relaxation. This is another opportunity to test your stability independent of tightened obliques and rectus. Doing the same thing to the other side provides contrast and further opportunities to enhance tonic and phasic control.

Stabilization leg lifts – with a qualitative twist

Come back up to sitting on the floor again in variation D, but leaning back on your elbows and forearms if possible. If this position is difficult, do from supine. Continue with the same movement, but this time instead of just tilting your lifted left leg toward the floor to the outside, keep the leg lifted as you extend your left leg down long. This is a movement as if you were going to straighten and rest your left leg down on the floor but keep the leg just slightly lifted away from the floor. This requires a lengthening contraction of the hip flexors on that side and can be a great iliopsoas stretch if performed accurately.

Keeping some part of your lower back on or near the ground as you do this protects your back from extension or rotational stresses. As you lift your left leg and roll your pelvis to the left, the left side of your lower back should press to the floor. As you extend your lifted left leg down long, the center or even the right side of your lower back presses into the floor. This movement of straightening the left leg and swinging it to the right to come to midline is analogous to what we did by crossing one leg over the other. It triggers that same rolling of the pelvis to the right.

With the lifted leg long, the right leg has to work even harder and more accurately to keep the pelvis from rolling into anterior tilt. There are probably fewer of you at this point who can extend your leg down long, flatten your lower back and keep the superficial abdominal muscles inhibited. Don't let this stop you from trying: hope springs eternal and even the attempt at doing this can be very rewarding.

Contrast this way of doing leg lifts to more traditional ways. This lesson emphasizes pelvic stabilization through use of the legs and de-emphasizes use of the superficial abdominals. With traditional leg lifts, the belly is the focus of the stability and the whole torso is held rigidly. All I can suggest is that you learn both, make proprioceptive comparisons, then decide. Which way of stabilizing your pelvis seems to be the most effortless? Does it make sense, then, to progress someone to lifting and straightening both legs at the same time (Box 6.8)?

Without the floor, you are probably doomed. The weight of the legs added to the pelvis is way too much for the belly to control short of all-out eye-popping effort. Most situations in which you are likely to find yourself confronted by movement or postural strains are times when at least one leg or foot are on the ground; use the ground as a reliable partner that allows

---

Box 6.8 TA Leg Lifts

Continuation of TA Diagnoals – pick up where we left off

Straightening the lifted leg to increase need for stability and to lengthen hip flexor

Doing the corkscrew movement to facilitate lumbothoracic and thoracic mobility and to coordinate same-side gluteals and adductors

Summary movement for the stabilization series

---

your legs to assist you in stabilizing your pelvis and lower back. Train your students to recognize and use the floor as a partner in stability. Restrain yourself next time you have a desire to have your students do double leg lifts. Let them – nay, encourage them to – use the floor.

Summing up the stabilization series

Come up to sitting again in variation E, leaning back again on your elbows and forearms. Put the whole thing together: the lifted left leg tilts out to the left with breath/belly/pelvic floor coordination, extends down long, comes back to being tilted out to the left again, then swings across to cross over the right leg. Reverse and repeat. This is a movement that wraps up the whole stabilization series: TA Facilitation, TA Diagnoals and TA Leg Lifts.

It is a nice summary or cumulative movement for this whole series and will end up in the low back kata described at the end of the chapter. It blends intersegmental stabilization with advanced pelvic stabilization via the legs. It lengthens the hip flexors and strengthens the hip extensors. It lends itself well to modifications for your gluteal-biased folks; just allow the hip flexors to do their job of rolling the pelvis forward.

If you'd like an extra credit assignment, try this movement with your left leg more or less straight the whole time. In particular, try keeping the knee of the lifted leg extended as you bring it up and out in the basic 'Wishbone' movement. This is a great hamstring lengthener. Stop periodically to do seesaw breaths. Try this same thing to the other side.

Try the same movements while lying on your back. This demands more length from the iliopsoas (a great way to stretch the hip flexors) and more strength/control from the gluteals. Are you still able to coordinate floor and belly with these more demanding movements? Be sure to keep some part of your lower back in contact with the floor and try to soften/inhibit your superficial abdominals; apply and remove TA and pelvic floor contractions as you will. Time movements with your breath and breathe independently. Do the whole movement keeping the knee of the lifted leg straight.

At the end of the lesson, lie on your back again with both knees bent and both feet on the floor. Go back to an earlier movement: pull your belly button back and to the left, back and to the right, and straight back. What is the quality and control of this movement like now? Did you experience walking or standing differently?

Stability in standing and bending

Now that you are getting a better sense of how to control and coordinate your intersegmental stabilizers with the movement of your pelvis using stepping as a functional context, let's change our venue. We will now be exploring movements and facilitating intersegmental stability in belly down and vertical orientations. How can we facilitate an ability to push the pelvis to vertical and the lower spine to neutral in upright postures? How can we facilitate stable bending?

These next couple of lessons are performed with toys: a long pole and a half-roller or tightly rolled towel or blanket. The pole is basically a wooden dowel or even a broom handle that is long enough (five to six feet unless you are pretty tall) and strong enough to support some of your weight without breaking. The pole is used to assist if needed with balance and to assist if desired with supporting some body weight when bending forward. It is also used as a reference point for directions of movement.

A wall would do as a substitute in a pinch. The half-roller is optional but nice in terms of protecting your patella and in terms of being able to get the metatarsal heads to touch the floor. Be reasonable with yourself; many people are unable to kneel for very long. Protect yourself. Let's play!

Half-kneel Bending

Variations

A. Stand on your knees for a moment. Kneel on the floor.

- Notice how steadily you are balancing. Is there much sway forward/back or left/right?

- How is your pelvis balanced on top of your legs? Is your pelvis spilling or falling forward? Is your pubic bone closer to the ground than your tailbone?

- Is your pelvis turned right or left? Place your index fingers on the two prominent bones on the front of your pelvis – the ASISs. Look down to visualize their relative positions. Is one bone farther forward than the other?

- Come back to your personal middle and stay there. From there, exhale, lift your chest and pull in your lower belly/pelvic floor. Repeat a few times to familiarize yourself with this movement in this position.

- Add in making very small movements to round and arch your back; roll your pelvis slightly forward and back (Fig. 6.24).

- Slowly and gently turn your pelvis/torso/shoulders together alternately right and left. Observe how first one bone and then the other comes farther forward as the other bone goes back (Fig. 6.24). Which direction of movement is easier?

- Are these basic movement combinations easier in this position or when lying down on your back?

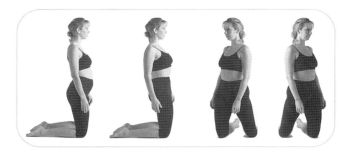

Fig. 6.24 Finding neutral and stabilizing, then turning pelvis side to side.

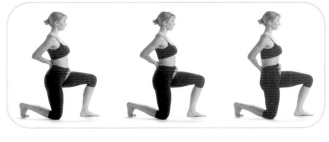

Fig. 6.25 Spilling pelvis forward and pushing it back in half-kneeling – monitor movement with hands – push pelvis close to vertical and stay there.

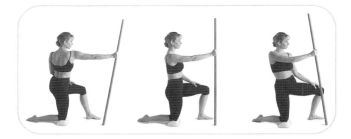

Fig. 6.26 Moving the top of the pole forward and back – rotating pelvis around the standing hip. Keep pelvis as vertical as possible.

- Rest for a moment off your knees. Sit, lie, stand, whatever you'd prefer.

B. Come now to a half-kneeling position. Your right knee is on the floor (or on a half-roller) and your left foot is forward on the floor. Both the right thigh and the left lower leg are vertical; your right hip joint is over your right knee and your left knee is directly over your left heel. If your right knee is on the floor, have your right foot flat. The top of your foot and your toenails are touching the floor. If your right knee is on a half-roller, you could place the toes of your right foot as if in a starting-block position: the pads of your toes and the balls of your right foot are on the floor.

- Place your right hand back on your sacrum and your left hand forward on your lower belly (Fig. 6.25). Roll your pelvis forward so the hand on the lower belly drops and the hand on your sacrum lifts.

- Then roll your pelvis back so the lower belly hand rises and the hand on your sacrum drops; this points your tailbone toward the floor (Fig. 6.25).

- As you tilt your pelvis backward toward vertical, your lower back rounds or flattens a bit and you may start to feel a little pull or stretch in the front of your right hip or thigh. This is desirable as long as it's not done too aggressively. Repeat this movement several times.

- Exhale, lift your chest and pull in your lower belly/pelvic floor. Inhale to collapse your chest and push out your lower belly/pelvic floor. Repeat a few times to familiarize yourself with this basic intersegmental stabilization movement in this position.

- Now coordinate your pelvis with these movements. Tilt your pelvis back and drop your tailbone toward the floor as you exhale and pull in your belly/pelvic floor; get taller.

- Tilt your pelvis forward and make a small movement lift your tailbone out behind you as you inhale and push out your belly/pelvic floor; get shorter. You are mildly rounding and arching your back (Fig. 6.25). Find a place where your back is neither rounded nor arched, but neutral. Stay there for a bit.

C. Come back to half-kneeling again, this time to the opposite side. Your left knee is on the floor or half-roller and your right foot is forward.

- Repeat the instructions of B to the opposite side.

- Compare the two sides. Does one side feel better coordinated? Does the front of your hip and thigh feel a little tighter on one side?

D. Come to right half-kneeling with the right knee on the floor and hold on to a pole with your right hand. The 5- or 6-foot-long pole is for balance and to use as a reference point. You could use a chair or wall instead. Have your right elbow straight and the pole straight out in front of you.

- Pull in your lower belly/pelvic floor, find your neutral spine and stay there while breathing independently.

- From there, move the top end of the pole forward a little bit (Fig. 6.26). Do this by turning your pelvis and shoulders to the left. Reverse and repeat this movement a few times.

- Then move the top of the pole backward a bit (Fig. 6.26). Keep your elbow straight and turn your pelvis and shoulders to the right. Do this a few times.

- Then alternately move the top of the pole forward and back. Make sure to maintain the pull in/up of your belly/pelvic floor and the neutral position of your back. Where can you breathe freely with your lower belly held in?

E. Come to left half-kneeling and hold on to the pole with your left hand.

- Repeat the instructions of D to the opposite side. Compare sides.

- Lie on your back and take a full rest. Feel the contact you make against the floor, especially through your legs, pelvis and lower back.

F. Come to right half-kneeling and hold about three-quarters up the pole with your left hand and near the middle of the pole with your right hand. Point the fingers of your right hand toward the ground.

- Pull in your lower belly/pelvic floor, tilt your pelvis back and organize your breath to be independent. Find that place where your back is neutral and keep this going.

- Then begin a small movement of sliding your right hand down the pole toward the floor (Fig. 6.27). Make it small to start with! Do not go all the way to the floor!

- As you begin to slide your right hand down the pole, lean yourself over slightly by bending at your hip. Keep your back the same exact neutral shape as it was when you were upright, but allow your pelvis to turn a bit to the left.

- This is just a continuation of what you were doing previously when you were moving the top of the pole forward and back. You start the movement by turning your pelvis and shoulders to the left, then continue by leaning forward.

- Let the top end of the pole swing out to the left a bit.

- Push yourself back upright by pushing your left foot into the floor – remember that your back stays the same shape the whole time, and that you are still maintaining your lower belly stabilization.

- Repeat this movement many times. Start small and gradually increase the size. Don't make touching the ground your goal. Make the movement accurate through the whole range. Enlarge the movement to your satisfaction (Fig. 6.27).

G. Come to left half-kneeling, holding on to the top of the pole with your right hand and the middle of the pole with your left hand.

- Repeat instructions F to the opposite side. Compare and contrast sides.

- Lie on your back to rest.

H. Come to right half-kneeling and hold the top three-quarters of the pole with your right hand and the middle of the pole with your left.

- Pull in belly and pelvic floor and find spinal neutral – breathe independently.

- Begin a small movement to slide your left hand down the pole. Allow your pelvis to turn to the right and the top of the pole to swing a bit out to the right and backward. You could either shift your weight forward or back as you do this, but I'd recommend shifting back.

- Gradually enlarge the movement. Recognize how you use your legs to control your bend forward and to power your return to upright half-kneeling (feel the stretch on the front of your hip) (Fig. 6.28).

- Alternate back and forth between sliding your right hand down the pole while holding near the top with your left hand then sliding your left hand down the pole while holding near the top with your right hand. You will turn your pelvis and torso alternately left and right while bending (Fig. 6.29).

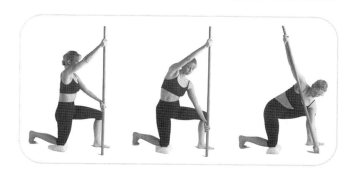

Fig. 6.28 Homolateral bending – same hand reaching to same foot. Stay stable and neutral.

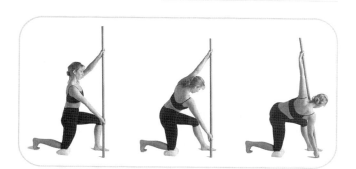

Fig. 6.27 Contralateral bending – opposite hand to opposite foot. Keep intersegmental stability and low back flat/neutral.

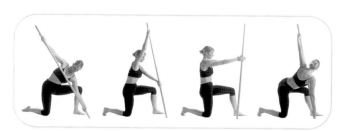

Fig. 6.29 Alternately slide one hand then the other toward the ground.

I. Come to left half-kneeling, holding the top of the pole with your left hand and the middle of the pole with your right.

- Repeat instructions H to the opposite side. Compare and contrast sides.

- Lie on your back to rest.

J. Stand on both knees again for a moment.

- Notice how steadily you are balancing now in comparison to when you started.

- How is your pelvis balanced on top of your legs? Is your pelvis spilling or falling forward? How does this compare to when you started?

- Place your index fingers on the two prominent bones on the front of your pelvis – the ASISs. Look down to visualize their relative positions. Is one bone further forward than the other?

- Slowly and gently turn your pelvis/torso/shoulders together alternately right and left. Observe how first one bone and then the other comes further forward as the other bone goes back. Which direction of movement is easier?

- Come back to your personal middle and stay there. From there, exhale, lift your chest and pull in your lower belly/pelvic floor. How is this coordination going?

- Stand up on your feet and repeat instructions J in this position.

The kneeling family tree

The baselines in this lesson are in a somewhat unusual position: turning from a kneeling position. Why kneeling? Because the kneeling family of postures and their cousins, the squatting family, are extremely valuable tools for someone who is unstable in either direction with bending, pushing or pulling stresses. The kneeling family includes kneeling, half-kneeling, squat kneeling, half-squat kneeling, sit kneeling and half-sit kneeling (Fig. 6.30). Squat kneeling allows you to sit on your heels and rest some of your weight skeletally through your vertical foot. Sit kneeling is the same except for how you distribute your weight along your shin and the top of your foot.

The kneeling family has several advantages. The first thing to recommend it is the fact that it dramatically lowers your center of mass, lowers your horizon, and lowers the zone in which you can reach and manipulate objects with your hands without having to bend. Moving into these positions instead of bending or leaning over allows the legs to do more of the work and the pelvis and back to remain in a more vertical orientation. This is particularly valuable if you need to hold the position for a while.

Another advantage of these positions is that they increase your stability by greatly enlarging your base of support. Standing on your feet gives you a relatively small base of support surface area and a relatively narrow range of front-to-back stability. The ratio of surface area to height of the center of mass makes standing the most unstable of postures. The advantage of standing lies in its great freedom of movement.

Another advantage, especially with the lower to the ground versions, is that kneeling postures bend the hips enough to provide a hamstring constraint. By constraining the ability of the pelvis to fall into anterior tilt, we are protecting the back from postural extension stresses and from weight-in-front extension stresses. Suggest some of these positions to your students as places to lift from or to hold on to some amount of weight in front.

Kneeling on two knees certainly gives you a greater surface area of your base of support, but the position of the center of mass way forward within the base is less than ideal for the iliopsoas biased among us. This position gives you good stability against falling back but is poorly designed for controlling extension stresses (falling forward/bending, reaching, pulling, carrying/weight-in-front, stepping).

In addition, if you are iliopsoas biased and are susceptible to anterior tilt postural stresses, this position will probably challenge your hip flexor length and spill you more into lumbar extension. Whereas we would rarely recommend full kneeling to people as a commonly used position, we could use it as an assessment tool, as a position in exploratory exercise, and a place from which to push or pull objects over some distance (Knee Walking).

Half-kneeling gives us much greater stability. Its base of support has a relatively large surface area, even though it is an odd tripod shape. With a very long front-to-back length and with the center of mass located around the mid-point, half-kneeling gives us tremendous anterior/posterior stability. This position is a great alternative for prolonged bending or leaning and is an excellent substitute for sitting, in that it provides an opportunity to be strengthening the hip extensors on the forward leg while stretching the hip flexors on the standing leg.

This position, then, is especially useful for those suffering from extension stresses. The forward leg is in a great position to resist forces that want to pull the back into extension and the pelvis into anterior tilt (shifting the center of mass forward by lifting, bending, carrying, etc.). On the other hand, this position doesn't have a very broad base of support from side to side: it lacks lateral stability. Often, even just being in this position is challenging. People will sway around and put out their arms, will even sometimes require something to hold on to. This is unacceptable with the nonelderly back pain sufferer: they need to have good enough balance to be stable in this position. Although this position is great for holding postures for a while and for some bending, lifting or holding a weight, there are better postures for pushing, pulling and controlling lateral stresses.

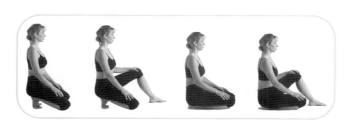

Fig. 6.30 Getting your center of mass closer to the ground enhances stability – full and half-squat kneeling – full and half-sit kneeling.

Squat kneeling brings us back to a four-point base of support, lowers our center of mass farther and perches our center of mass toward the back of the base. This is an easier place to balance your pelvis vertically and to bring your lower back to neutral. There is no requirement for long hip flexors as there was in kneeling and half-kneeling. This is also a good place to control weight-in-front stresses.

Both knees are forward and in a good position to push to counteract the anterior tilt of the pelvis. The center of mass is already back and acts to automatically cancel out weight-in-front stresses. The more or less equal length and width of the base of support of this position makes this a good compromise for controlling both moderate lateral stresses and moderate extension stresses. This is also a nice gateway for access to the squatting family.

Half-squat kneeling can give us both greater front-to-back and better lateral stability, depending on how far forward and how far out to the side you place your foot. This is another position where it is relatively easy to balance your pelvis vertically and to bring your lower back to neutral. This is a nice position for controlling pushing and pulling stresses.

When pulling, you have out in front of you the leg that is pushing your body backward. Control the position of the pelvis and the lower back depending on direction of instability; bias toward nonhabitual direction if unidirectionally unstable. In pushing, you can get down low and bend over to bring the line of your torso to a position consistent with the line of push.

The forward leg controls the fall forward of the pelvis and is in a position to support you when the object you are pushing moves. The back leg is in a good position to push you and your object forward. The same basic thing is performed when pushing laterally: widen your base by bringing the standing foot out farther. Half-squat kneeling is a stable/mobile position. You can be stable while sliding or rolling heavy objects. Granted, you can't slide or roll something very far, but you can do a number of these movements in sequence and take something as far as you want to go. Better to take more time and be more stable than to drag or push something heavy from a standing and bending over position.

Sit kneeling requires a degree of foot and ankle mobility that not everyone possesses. This is a pity, as sit kneeling is a very comfortable place to rest and is very stable with a wide and long base of support, with the center of mass toward the back of the base and with an even lower center of mass. Base of support size and shape are roughly analogous to the squat kneeling variations. The difference is that in sit kneeling, more bone is on the floor. This is again a good position for controlling extension stresses and has decent lateral stability as well. Mostly, though, this is a rest posture.

Half-sit kneeling is analogous to half-squat kneeling. It has the same basic features and advantages, but with half-sit kneeling you can get your center of mass even lower (if your hamstrings or adductors allow it) and get even more bone on the floor.

The squatting family tree

Related to the kneeling family by marriage is the squatting family. Because the knees aren't on the ground, however, these

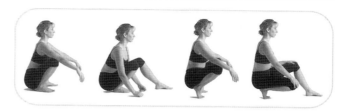

Fig. 6.31 Getting your center of mass closer to the ground enhances stability – full and half heel squatting – full and half metatarsal squatting.

postures are more unstable. Depending on whether you are squatting with the metatarsal heads or the whole sole of the foot is bearing weight, the surface area of the base of support can be even smaller than in standing. On the other hand, the center of mass is still much lower than in standing and can help reduce bending or leaning stresses on the lower back.

The hip flexors don't have to be long for the pelvis to be vertical and the back to be neutral, though the gluteals and short and stubbies do have to be long enough to avoid creating flexion stresses. Heel squatting requires a considerable ankle dorsiflexion range of motion that, although common in some parts of the world, is not very common in cultures that use chairs a lot (Fig. 6.31). The center of mass is way back relative to the base of support, sometimes even necessitating ankle dorsiflexion contractions to keep from falling over backward.

This can be a very nice position for the iliopsoas-biased person to use but is probably poison for the gluteal dominant or someone with multidirectional instability. Half-heel squatting just brings one foot out in front or to the side. It is analogous to half-squat kneeling or half-sit kneeling (Fig. 6.31). If by some miracle you can get into this position, you could use it for many of the same things.

Perhaps more practical, and certainly more doable for most of us, is metatarsal squatting (Fig. 6.31). This features an extremely small base of support, but again with a low center of mass and with a decent chance for both iliopsoas- and gluteal-biased folks to bring their pelvis to vertical and their back to neutral. Rather than use this as a resting position or one form which to perform a protracted task, use this to lower yourself down for a moment then come back upright again.

It is a fairly easy transitional movement for those with adequate knees. You can also lift from here, though you will have to bend forward somewhat to get your hands all the way to the floor. Once in upright squatting, though, you can keep your pelvis close to vertical and your spine neutral all the way up to standing.

Another nice position to lift from is half metatarsal squatting (Fig. 6.31). This gives you a larger and longer front-to-back base of support dimension and allows the whole sole of one foot to be on the ground, rather than being perched up on the toes of both feet. Having the one leg forward can control any bending or leaning movement, and is in a good position to power your load back up to vertical in preparation for coming up to standing. This is also a nice resting position (if you are someplace where you don't want to kneel or sit and get your clothes dirty) if you alternate left and right half metatarsal squatting.

A variation of half metatarsal squatting is long half metatarsal squatting. Place the forward foot way out in front or to your side, but keep the sole of that foot flat on the floor (requires plantarflexion and inversion mobility). Use in exercise to lengthen hamstrings and adductors. Make transitions from side to side to facilitate and provide functional context. Use functionally when walking in a low tunnel, ducking under a downed tree on a hiking trail, chasing your kid under the monkey bars, or other duck and move activities.

Use the arms for support

All of these low stances can become even more stable with the addition of some upper extremity support. Have the student use one hand on the floor, furniture, the wall or other firm object, and use one hand instead of two when performing a prolonged task while low to the ground. We'll go through a couple of lessons later around squatting and how to make it more accessible for someone.

One way of using the arms for support is to facilitate an ability to move around in squatting positions. You need something to grab hold of that won't move: a door frame, rope or kitchen counter will do in a pinch, but something like a ballet bar is perfect. You rely on your arms to prevent you from falling back and to bring you back forward again. This is a pulling function of the arms. Use the arms this way to train the legs and feet.

Another way of using the arms for support is when bending, lifting or engaging in weight-in-front stresses. You'll need something you can lean on that won't move: wall, furniture, car, etc. You rely on your arms to prevent you from using your back so much under described conditions. Lean on your kitchen counter as you unload the dishwasher. Lean on your washing machine as you unload the dryer. Lean on the wall as you pick up your kids' toys and your husbands' socks.

Lean on the freezer door as you bend to get the lettuce out of the crisper. Lean on your chopping block as you bend to pick up and stack your firewood. Lean on your own knee as you bend to pull up your sock. Let your patients know and run them through a few drills to give them the opportunity to feel proprioceptively that the upper extremities are valuable allies to your legs and intersegmental stabilizers in the epic battle against low back pain.

Aren't these exercises a bit hard?

Do some of these described positions and movements seem a little athletic for your typical 50-year-old mother of three with chronic lower back pain? Some of them may be and will forever remain so. Some of them will be initially, but can be something she can work toward. Some of them might be borderline initially, but she can be taught to refine, use and love them. She might even surprise you and be capable of some of them on her own. How do you know unless you try? I would suggest that getting into these positions and doing some of these movements is precisely the type of athleticism these people need.

I would suggest that their time is better spent on the floor learning to move and refine movement options than it is resting on a heating pad. I would suggest that their time is better spent on the floor moving in unfamiliar and complex ways than it is in a gym doing cardio machines and isolated and cardinal plane weight training (though that would be something to add later after new movement skills are learned and can be incorporated into exercise).

I would suggest that unusual positions and movements are good for our students precisely because they are unusual. This introduction of variable movement into their invariable lives is very often just what they need! The clever practitioner can take the concepts learned in these lessons and modify them to fit each individual.

Much as I would like to explore more fully the squatting and kneeling families and how to develop lessons around these positions and transitional movements among these positions, I am disinclined to go into that sort of detail in this book. Be bold. Take the initiative. Explore and create lessons on your own around these positions. At the very least, familiarize yourself proprioceptively with these positions and use them yourself as substitutes for bending, sitting, pushing, pulling and holding, so you can authoritatively dispense this valuable information to your students. Model these behaviors at work, where your students can see that you are walking the walk.

Baselines – Half-kneel Bending

Let's come back now to our discussion of the lesson itself and of the initial static and dynamic baselines. The kneeling position is going to be difficult with hip flexor restrictions, which are extremely common and which will drag the pelvis into anterior tilt. Observe for a turn of the pelvis right or left. Is this a clue to a possible pelvic force couple imbalance or some cosmic fluke?

Observing your students turn alternately left and right gives you an opportunity to assess both the ability of the pelvis to turn freely on the legs and the amount of rotation of the torso on the pelvis. Watch for proportion of movement and balance of movement. Proportionally, we might expect that the pelvis would be limited in its ability to rotate in comparison to the twisting movement of the torso on the pelvis if that person has an unstable back. This is another example of a hyper-/hypomobility pair.

Tight right adductors and hip flexors will constrain the turning and shifting of weight of the pelvis to the left. This would probably result in too much left rotation happening in the lower spine and lead to eventual instability. A tight left piriformis will also constrain the turning and shifting of weight of the pelvis to the left and set up the same instability scenario. What is a manual therapist to do when she detects L5 instability to the left but doesn't know where its hypomobile partner is? Follow the pattern!

The balance of this turning movement from side to side and the position of habitual center give us clues about pelvic force couple imbalances and about probable rotational or lateral instabilities. As a general rule of thumb, if the pelvis twists more easily toward and is positioned to the left, the lumbar spine will move too much into right rotation. Both postural and movement adjustments are probably to be made here. If someone has unilateral low back pain partly because of imbalanced lateral stresses, how do we know if the pain is coming from the compression of the joint on the side the rotation happens towards, or from the gapping and overstretching of the joint on the side the rotation happens away from? Follow the pattern!

Blending gross movement with stabilizers – now belly down

Variations B and C feature a half-kneeling position. This would take a lengthy verbal instruction and a picture is worth a thousand words, so look back at the illustration (Fig. 6.25). Place your hands front and back on your pelvis and use them to guide/monitor the movements of your pelvis into anterior and posterior tilt. Use this reciprocating movement to establish a (close to) vertical position for your pelvis.

From this vertical position, add in the previously learned pieces of pelvic floor and TA activation, timing and independence of your breath and mild anterior and posterior tilt. For most people, you will be emphasizing the posterior tilt of the pelvis and the sensation associated with lengthening the hip flexors.

Come to half-kneeling again in variations C and D and hold on to the pole with your hand. Pull in your lower belly/pelvic floor, tilt your pelvis back toward vertical and extend the top of your head tall toward the ceiling, and stay there while breathing independently. Moving the top of the pole alternately forward and back (while maintaining intersegmental stability and a high horizon) provides the functional context for turning the pelvis and torso together from side to side while in this position.

Try guiding your student to be aware of how to rotate the pelvis around the hips, rather than the torso around the pelvis. Do not twist at the waist! Think of turning your whole torso as in a log roll. Which direction does your pelvis rotate most easily? When turning the pelvis to the left while in right half-kneeling (right knee on the floor), there is a horizontal adduction movement (and maybe some flexion) of the left hip joint and an external rotation and extension movement of the right hip.

Therefore, rotation of the pelvis to the left in this position would be constrained by the left gluteals and short and stubbies and by the right adductors and hip flexors. Therefore, rotation of the pelvis to the left in this position is accomplished by the contraction of the left hip internal rotators (and perhaps the left iliopsoas) and by the right gluteals and hip external rotators.

Therefore, this would be a good position and a good movement to stretch those muscles that constrain and strengthen the muscles that power this movement. When turning the pelvis to the right while in right half-kneeling, there is a horizontal abduction movement of the left hip (perhaps some extension) and an internal rotation movement of the right hip (probably with some flexion).

Therefore, rotation of the pelvis to the right in this position would be constrained by the left adductors and by the right short and stubbies. Therefore, rotation of the pelvis to the right would be powered by the left hip extensors/abductors/external rotators and by the right hip flexors and internal rotators. Therefore, this would also be a good position and a good

movement to stretch those muscles that constrain and strengthen the muscles that power this movement.

Partner simulation of pushing and pulling stresses

What are we going to use these movements for? Pushing and pulling with one hand. Try the following manual resistance technique: find a partner so you can practice the roles of both mover and resister. From this right half-kneeling position and still holding the vertical pole with the right hand, the resister gets into a split stance position in front of the pole and resists the pushing forward of the top of the pole and the movement of the pelvis into left rotation (Fig. 6.32).

Initially, this can be an evaluation technique. This is a lateral stressor that would create a left rotational stress at the low back if the pelvis were not stabilized from twisting to the right by the contracting obliques. Observe the right side of the pelvis carefully as you gradually apply a minimal to moderate amount of resistance. Does the right side of the pelvis waver back just a bit? Or is the movement of pushing the top of the pole forward with your right hand initiated from the pelvis and powered by the legs?

Is the right side of the pelvis coming forward? Are your students maintaining intersegmental stability? Are they still able to breathe? The complexity and the subtlety of this movement is why you go slowly and gradually. Let your students recognize what is going on and what they have to do to create that subjective feeling of stability. Don't make this a test of wills!

Do the same basic thing for pulling, except resist the movement of the top of the pole backward. Do they initiate this movement with a turn of their pelvis to the right and by pushing their left foot into the ground? Resist reciprocating movements of the top of the pole forward and back, or have them hold the pole steady while you try to move it in one direction, then the other, then alternately. Vary by holding pole horizontally . . . resist push and pull both eccentrically and concentrically. Progress from slight or mild resistance to moderate and heavier resistance, but avoid a full-on test of strength with your students.

Make sure you as the resister are in a good stable position and are practicing what you preach about intersegmental stability. Progress to a home program with resistant tubing or bands if desired. The devil here is in the detail, so make sure

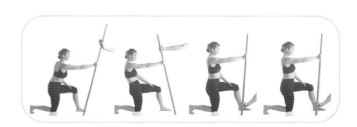

Fig. 6.32 Manual facilitation of push and pull stresses – initiate turn from the pelvis. Simulation of weight in front – preparatory posterior tilt of pelvis/push with front leg.

they have an understanding of the use of their legs, the movements of their pelvis, and the ability to maintain intersegmental stability before you turn them loose without adult supervision.

Bending over – we're going down!

Come to half-kneeling again in variations F and G and hold near the top of the pole with your right hand this time and near the middle of the pole with your left hand; point the fingers of your left hand toward the ground. Pull in your lower belly/pelvic floor, tilt your pelvis back and get tall, and organize your breath to be independent. Keep this going as you do a small movement of sliding your left hand down the pole toward the floor.

This is our first foray into a belly-down position during this stabilization series. This is a big destabilizer for a lot of people, so make the first several movements very small and very slow. The idea is very similar to what we did in Side-sit Bending. We moved slightly into anterior/posterior tilt and lumbar extension/flexion to proprioceptively find neutral, then continued to focus awareness of the shape of the lower back as we started to fall forward. We used the forward leg to control the fall of the pelvis forward, to push the pelvis back to neutral, and to thereby assist in maintaining spinal neutral in a side-sitting position. We are doing the same thing here in a different venue – making sure the legs control the movement of the pelvis so the back can remain neutral (Fig. 6.33).

Sliding one hand down the pole as the other stays near the top is a constraint, a reference point and a form of training wheels. Whereas the pole enhances your feeling of balance and is able to support some of your weight, it also suggests that your chest and shoulders turn to the left. Facilitate this turn by cueing to look towards the top of the pole initially.

This in turn invites the pelvis to participate by also turning to the left, which is what we would like to see with asymmetrical bending (reaching down with one hand). If the shoulders, chest and pelvis turn the same amount, and if the bending happens at the hip joint instead of the back, the back is theoretically not moving (or at least not moving much) and should be stable.

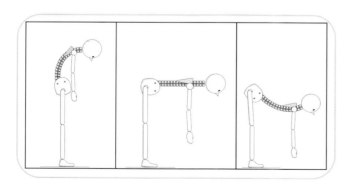

Fig. 6.33 Bending without enough fall forward of the pelvis – with neutral back – with too much fall of pelvis forward.

Stop periodically at different points in the movement to do a seesaw breath timed with intersegmental contraction and relaxation. Can you be stable even without holding in your lower belly? Most people are able to manage at least a deep lean or a moderate bend with this movement, but some people with more extreme multidirectional instabilities, or someone in an acute stage, might have difficulties.

Try going slowly and make tiny movements; they are going to be bending and leaning and twisting much more just by going through their daily routine over the next hour or so than they will get from tiny leaning movements, so at some point they will need to learn to negotiate relationships to gravity other than horizontal and vertical. With your more stable, advanced or athletic students, do this movement deeply and quickly for several minutes. Keep your form and your intersegmental stability and stand by with the sweat towel.

Contralateral and homolateral bending

The movement of sliding the right hand down the pole with the left foot forward is contralateral bending: the opposite hand reaches for the ground near the opposite foot. Note the similarity of the position to sports activities such as bowling and tennis, and to previous movements in Side-sit Bending, Side-sit Transitions and Sit to Stand. The next variation in this lesson works with homolateral bending: reaching the same-side hand toward the same-side foot.

Come to right half-kneeling in variations H and I and hold on to the top of the pole with your right hand and the middle of the pole with your left. Pull in belly and pelvic floor and tilt your pelvis back and stay tall while breathing independently. Begin a small movement to slide your left hand down the pole. Allow your pelvis to turn to the right and the top of the pole to swing a bit out to the right and backward.

Here we use swinging the pole out to the right and back and placing the right hand near the top of the pole while sliding the left hand down as constraints that suggest the pelvis turn to the right, this time while bending. You might also discover the advantages in shifting your weight backward toward your right knee/leg, though it is possible to do this movement with a shift of weight forward as well. Try both versions and compare for subjective feeling of stability. This is homolateral bending, reaching a hand toward the ground near the same side foot.

Try placing the pole differently to facilitate a shift of weight back with the homolateral bend. With the left foot forward on the floor and the right knee on the ground, place the bottom end of the pole on the ground back near the right foot. Hold the pole to the right of your body with your left hand and point the top of the pole forward and upward about 45°. Slide your right hand down the pole toward your right foot.

Homolateral bending is actually one of the more stable ways of bending if you have the adductor length and the balance for it. By turning your pelvis nearly sideways and bending over, you have changed the orientation of the back to gravity. Instead of having to work so much to control flexion and extension stresses, you now are balancing the pelvis sideways and can use your lateral torso musculature more. When standing, lifting the back leg behind you acts as a counterweight to your forward-

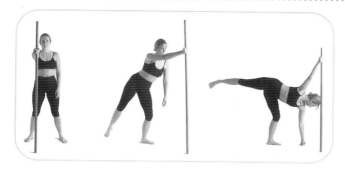

Fig. 6.34 Facilitating ipsilateral bending – use with a wall or with furniture to create a very stable bend.

bending torso, arranging torso and leg in a line like the cross-piece on a capital T.

Try the following movement in standing. Stand with both feet parallel and hold the vertical pole with your right hand. Imagine a stick running through your body from your right heel to your head. Simultaneously lift your right leg toward horizontal behind you and lean your torso forward toward horizontal. As you do this, turn your whole pelvis and torso to face toward the wall to your right and reach a bit with your left hand toward the floor (Fig. 6.34).

Repeat this teeter-totter movement many times to refine timing, coordination and balance, then try it faster to make it feel more automatic. You could also bend over into this T position and stay there as you then reach the opposite hand toward the ceiling and toward the floor to create a rotation of your pelvis and torso together around the standing hip. This is horizontal adduction and abduction of the flexed hip and is a great way to wake up dormant short and stubbies (Fig. 6.35).

Another bending drill to try illustrates the advantages of using some upper extremity support to reduce stress on the low back. Stand facing a wall at about arm's length distance. Place your left hand on the wall at about shoulder height and imagine a stick running from your left heel, up through your left leg and up through your spine to your head. Start bending forward to reach your right hand toward the floor. As you do this, lift your left leg behind you to maintain your imaginary stick from heel to head.

Allow your pelvis and chest to turn to the left so the left side of your torso faces the ceiling. This is a homolateral bend. Reverse this by swinging your left leg back toward the ground and your torso back upright. You are pivoting around your left hip in both directions. Your left hip flexes and externally rotates to bend, then extends and derotates to come back upright. The hand provides another point of support and helps to reduce bending and weight-in-front stresses. Do the movement small and slowly to start with, then faster and larger. Do both sides and compare/contrast left and right. Train your students in this bending strategy and suggest examples for home use.

Fringe benefits

With all these movements of bending and coming back upright again, make sure to complete the movement of your pelvis to

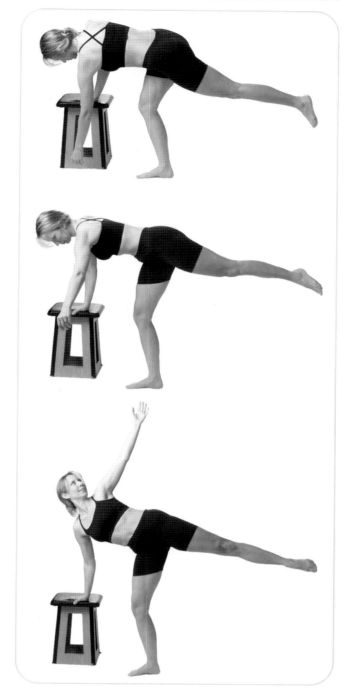

Fig. 6.35 A quick and dirty bun buster.

vertical. Create and revel in the sensations of lengthening hip flexors! This half-kneel position is a great one for stretching the rectus femoris and iliopsoas. Contrast to standing, bending one knee completely backward and grabbing that foot with the hand on the same side. This exercise is very difficult to do without creating a global pattern of hip extension and lumbar extension. Its functional relevance is also questionable because that leg doesn't complete a closed kinetic chain.

Be careful of look-alikes and accept no substitutes. There is another common way of lengthening the hip flexors that is also done from this half-kneeling position. Lunging forward to move the hip into extension, rather than keeping the thigh vertical and posteriorly tilting the pelvis is the way this exercise is commonly performed. The common version of a hip flexor stretch has disadvantages relative to a qualitative version:

- With the lunging version, there is an exquisite temptation to allow the pelvis to anteriorly tilt and the lumbar spine to extend in a global pattern of movement.
- With the lunging version, there is no reciprocation of movement. Pushing the front leg when coming up from a bending position in this lesson lends itself well to the intention to push.
- This results in a more intentional movement of the pelvis and back and a more specific CNS requirement to inhibit the opposite hip flexors.
- With the lunging version, there is a lack of specific functional context. The hip flexor lengthening is not related to upright standing.
- Most people will agree that it doesn't *feel* as effective as the qualitative version.

This is also a good position to facilitate multifidus strength. Leaning forward with a neutral spine in a belly-down orientation accrues the benefits of multifidus strengthening from Johnson's hands-and-knees and prone positions, with none of the drawbacks. We can make it pattern specific, cue to neutral back specific to the student, and link it with the hip arthrokinematic muscles in a meaningful functional context.

Combine homolateral bending with upper extremity support

To make this movement usable, teach this movement next to a wall so students can use their nonreaching hand by leaning against the wall to assist with balance and support their weight. This use of upper extremity support in bending and leaning would be a valuable tool for many people with low back pain and instability. It is particularly useful around the house: picking up the kids' toys, grabbing your shoes out of the closet, getting the cereal box out of the bottom drawer of your kitchen, etc.

There are usually lots of counters, furniture, walls, railings, tables or chairs around to assist. You might even hesitate to mention this idea to your students because it seems so obvious, but habit is a powerful thing that can blind us to even the most obvious of solutions. Tell them they aren't violating any ergonomics laws if they use their upper extremities to help protect their back (Box 6.9).

Use an arm for support in bending over and coming back up, or for support while remaining in a bent-over position. Lean over to unload your clothes washer, but keep one hand weightbearing and use the other to manipulate the clothes. This instruction to slow tasks down a bit and to use just one hand when possible to manipulate while in a prolonged bent position might be another pearl of wisdom your students will thank you for (while marveling that they hadn't thought of the same thing before).

Box 6.9 Half-kneel Bending

Blending intersegmental stabilizers with ability to control anterior tilt of pelvis

Great hip flexor stretch – great hamstring and short and stubby length and strength

Train for bending with neutral spine and standing with reduced lumbar lordosis

Use for multifidus strengthening – belly-down orientation and neutral spine

---

Coming back to the lesson, use the movement in this segment to emphasize again to your students the proprioceptive sensation of using their legs to control the fall forward and to power the return to vertical. Make sure they complete that movement to vertical when coming up, and have them use the sensation of hip flexor lengthening as their cue that they are there. Try this deeply, quickly and repetitively for several minutes if stable enough to do so. Does anyone else enjoy that rubbery feeling in the legs and the gyroscope feeling of the pelvis on the legs after this lesson as much as I do?

Use manual resistance techniques again to resist the movements of coming up to vertical from a leaned-over or bent-over position. Go slowly and move in a close to vertical range to start, so they can feel the initiation at their pelvis and the additional pressure of their forward foot on the floor. Progress to deeper bends and stiffer resistance. Do both contralateral and homolateral variations.

Simulating weight in front stressors – cue to control from legs

Once they have a good sense of the use of the front leg in counteracting forward/extension stresses, have your students place the pole vertically in front of them again. Place the pole fairly far away so their elbow (or elbows, if you have them hold on with both hands) is straight. Have them lift the bottom of the pole off the floor a slight amount, simulating a carry or hold stress. Alternately, use a medicine ball or weight.

Have them recognize how to preplan this movement by pushing their forward foot into the ground and pushing their pelvis toward vertical/posterior tilt in anticipation of forces acting to pull the pelvis into anterior tilt (Fig. 6.32). Cue to push foot to control forward fall of pelvis and to reduce effort or strain in the lower back.

Precede this drill with a similar exercise in supine. Have your student lie supine with legs long. Hold a pole longitudinally in front of her and have her hold the pole with both hands. Cue her to resist movement of the pole down towards her feet and direct her attention to the stability of her pelvis. By pushing downward, we are simulating a weight-in-front stress. Pushing upwards in response requires your student to fire the back extensors, which will anteriorly tilt the pelvis. Here she has a choice.

The psoas addict will probably give in to the inevitable and let her back arch. The student trained in abdominal-based stabilization will contract rectus, obliques and anterior intercostals in a desperate attempt to stabilize. The clever student will press her heels into the floor and try to stabilize with her legs, with some success. Have your various students bend up their knees and cue them to press feet into floor and roll pelvis into posterior tilt. Have them compare and contrast different stabilization strategies: the legs option, the belly option and the let it hang loose option.

Resist pushing and pulling stresses another way by having them place the end of the pole way out in front, holding it like a vacuum or push broom and pushing and dragging it across the floor in front (Fig. 6.36). Resist manually, or think of a way to affix some weight to it, then progress to a home program. From this same position, have them lift the end of the pole away from the floor with both hands, as if simulating shoveling or lifting something else with a long lever arm (Fig. 6.36).

Resist manually and cue to use the front leg to push, or resist with weights and progress to home program. Resist two-handed pushing and pulling of a horizontal pole (Fig. 6.36). Do the whole lesson over again but with a change of venue. Stand and have one foot up on a chair seat or bench.

Suggest to your students using this half-kneel position as a substitute for sitting. It will put you at about the same height as sitting, but has some advantages. It imposes a functional demand to lengthen the hip flexors and fascia. It requires active use of the forward leg. It gives the person who sits all day an opportunity to extend the hip joints. Suggest using this position as a substitute for prolonged or repetitive bending: unload the dishwasher and put the dishes up on the kitchen counter from half-kneeling, then stand up to distribute dishes upward from there.

Positional variations of this lesson are legion. We already did one, Side-sit Bending. Try it in sit kneeling, half-sit kneeling, half-squat kneeling, half-squat, chair-sit, stand and lean back against a wall, and linebacker pose. Look back to the described variations in Chapter 2, where you rounded and arched your back in a progression of positions from three-and-a-half point stance to half-kneeling (Figs 2.30 to 2.33). Try it in a split stance position, which is where our next lesson is learned.

Use this lesson and the half-kneel position judiciously with your neurologic patients. Challenge balance and facilitate hip extensor competence. Reconnect manipulation functions to movements of the pelvis and torso.

The next lesson, Split Stance Bending, is a very close companion to the last one. I will include the written description and illustrations for it, but because so much of it is the same as in Half-kneel Bending, we will just make a few observations instead of going through a full analysis. This lesson, like the last, works with controlling weight-forward stressors and facilitating a vertical pelvis and neutral spine while upright.

Split Stance Bending

Variations

A. Stand for a moment on both feet.

- How grounded are your feet to the floor? How is your pelvis being supported in space by your legs?

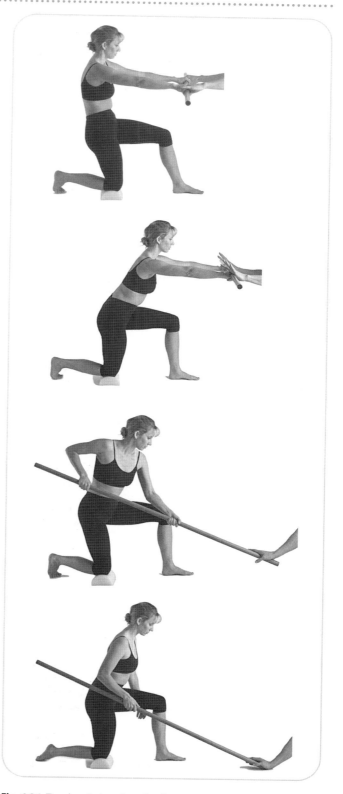

Fig. 6.36 Two-handed push and pull. Simulated extension stress – shoveling or sweeping.

- Reach your right hand toward the ground near your left foot – reach a bit diagonally down and to the left. How do you organize this movement?

- Does your back move relative to your pelvis? How did your pelvis move relative to your legs? Did you move one or both feet before you bent over?

B. Stand in a split stance: put your left foot quite a bit forward on the floor with your right foot behind you. Place your right heel on the half-roller if you have one, otherwise you could either have your heel on the ground or your heel lifted from the floor so you are on the balls of your feet.

- Place your right hand back on your sacrum and your left hand forward on your lower belly (Fig. 6.37). Roll your pelvis forward so the hand on the lower belly drops and the hand on the sacrum lifts.

- Then roll your pelvis back so the lower belly hand rises and the hand on your sacrum drops. This points your tailbone toward the floor (Fig. 6.37).

- As you tilt your pelvis backward toward vertical, your lower back rounds or flattens a bit and you may start to feel a little pull or stretch in the front of your right hip or thigh. This is desirable as long as it's not done too aggressively. Repeat this movement several times.

- Exhale, lift your chest and pull in your lower belly/pelvic floor. Inhale to collapse your chest and push out your lower belly/pelvic floor. Repeat a few times to familiarize yourself with this basic intersegmental stabilization movement in this position.

- Now coordinate your pelvis with these movements; tilt your pelvis back and drop your tailbone toward the floor as you exhale and pull in your belly/pelvic floor; get taller.

- Tilt your pelvis forward and make a small movement to lift your tailbone out behind you as you inhale and push out your belly/pelvic floor; get shorter. You are mildly rounding and arching your back.

- Find a place where your back is neither rounded nor arched, but neutral.

C. Come back to this split stance position again, this time to the opposite side. Your left foot is behind you, heel up on the half-roller if you have one. Your right foot is now on the floor in front.

- Repeat the instructions of B to the opposite side.

- Compare the two sides. Does one side feel better coordinated? Does the front of your hip and thigh feel a little tighter on one side?

D. Come to right split stance (right foot behind on the floor) and hold on to a pole with your right hand (Fig. 6.38). The 5- or 6-foot long pole is for balance and to use as a reference point. You could use a chair or wall instead. Have your right elbow straight and the pole straight out in front of you.

- Pull in your lower belly/pelvic floor to stabilize your back, tilt your pelvis back to bring your back to neutral, push your head tall and stay there.

- From there, move the top end of the pole forward a little bit (Fig. 6.38) Do this by turning your pelvis and shoulders to the left. Reverse and repeat this movement a few times.

- Then move the top of the pole backward a bit (Fig. 6.38). Keep your elbow straight and turn your pelvis and shoulders to the right. Do this a few times.

- Then alternate moving the top of the pole forward and back. Make sure to maintain the pull in/up of your belly/pelvic floor and the neutral position of your back. Can you still breathe freely with your lower belly held in?

- Feel how you have to move around your hips to keep your feet centered (not allowing them to roll to their inside or outside edges) and parallel to each other.

E. Come to left split stance and hold on to the pole with your left hand.

- Repeat the instructions of D to the opposite side. Compare sides.

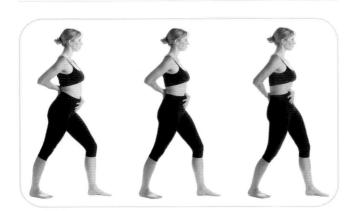

Fig. 6.37 Spilling pelvis forward and back in split stance – monitor movement with hands.

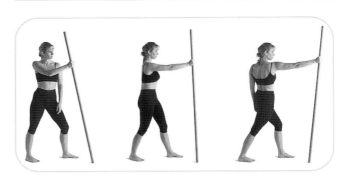

Fig. 6.38 Turning pelvis left and right – top of pole goes forward and back. Keep your pelvis as vertical as possible.

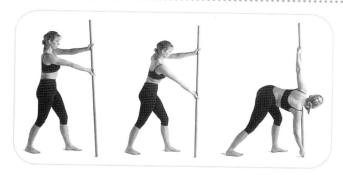

Fig. 6.39 Contralateral bending – opposite hand reaching to opposite foot. Keep intersegmental stability and neutral back.

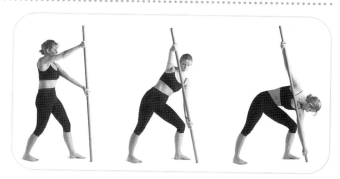

Fig. 6.40 Homolateral bending – same hand reaching to same foot. Stay stable and neutral.

- Lie on your back and take a full rest. Feel the contact you make against the floor, especially through your legs, pelvis and lower back.

F. Come to right split stance and hold near the top of the pole with your left hand and near the middle of the pole with your right hand – point the fingers of your right hand towards the ground.

- Stabilize, neutralize your back and organize your breath to be independent. Keep this going as you begin a small movement of sliding your right hand down the pole towards the floor (Fig. 6.39). Make it small to start with; do not go all the way to the floor.

- As you begin to slide your right hand down the pole, lean yourself over by bending at your hip. Keep your back the same exact shape, but allow your pelvis to turn a bit to the left. This is just a continuation of what you were doing previously when you were moving the top of the pole forward and back.

- You start the movement by turning your pelvis and shoulders to the left, then continue by leaning forward. Let the top end of the pole swing out to the left a bit.

- Push yourself back upright by pushing your left foot into the floor. Remember that your back stays its same shape the whole time and that you are still maintaining your intersegmental stabilization.

- Repeat this movement many times; start small and gradually increase the size (Fig. 6.39). Don't make touching the ground your goal. Make the movement accurate through the whole range.

G. Come to left split stance, holding on to the top of the pole with your right hand and the middle of the pole with your left hand.

- Repeat instructions F to the opposite side. Compare and contrast sides.

- Lie on your back to rest.

H. Come to right split stance and hold on to the top of the pole with your right hand and the middle of the pole with your left.

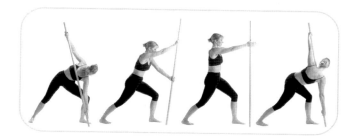

Fig. 6.41 Alternating sliding one hand then the other toward the ground.

- Pull in belly and pelvic floor and tilt your pelvis back; breathe independently.

- Begin a small movement to slide your left hand down the pole. Allow your pelvis to turn to the right and the top of the pole to swing a bit out to the right and backward (Fig. 6.40).

- Try shifting weight back to your right leg. Gradually enlarge the movement; recognize how you use your legs to control your bend forward and to power your return to upright split stance (feel the stretch on the front of your hip).

- Alternate back and forth between sliding your left hand down the pole while holding near the top with your right hand, and sliding your right hand down the pole while holding near the top with your left hand. Your pelvis and torso will turn alternately left and right as you bend (Fig. 6.41).

I. Come to left split stance, holding the top of the pole with your left hand and the middle of the pole with your right.

- Repeat instructions H to the opposite side. Compare and contrast sides.

- Lie on your back to rest.

J. Stand normally again, balanced side to side on both feet.

- How are you grounded? How are you supporting your pelvis?

- Reach toward the ground near your left foot with your right hand. How are you organizing this movement in comparison to when you started?

- Walk around – feel the movement of your hips, legs and pelvis.

Baselines – Split Stance Bending

The initial baselines are not much different than in Half-kneel Bending, except for the unilateral reaching toward the ground from a standing position. Is there some resemblance to contralateral bending here? The two versions of contralateral bending possible here are either to leave your feet where they are and allow your pelvis to turn to the left around your pelvis as you reach across and down to the left (made easier by widening your stance and bending your knees some amount), or to slide the right leg backward or the left leg forward on the floor.

They are both contralateral bends from a split stance position. Where did you do your twisting as you made this asymmetrical bending movement? Did you rotate your pelvis around your legs or your torso around your pelvis? Did you even entertain the possibility of either moving your feet into a split stance or widening into a horse stance (feet wider than shoulders and parallel, knees bent and pelvis vertical) in preparation for bending?

Like the half-kneeling stance, the split stance has much greater front-to-back stability and is very good for controlling flexion and particularly extension stresses. The same shift-of-the-weight-forward extension stresses that we worked with in half-kneeling are handled in this position by the same forward leg.

Applications, considerations, and variations

I have my students with hip flexor tightness who are susceptible to extension stresses get into and out of this position frequently during the day, and encourage them to use modifications of this split stance as a substitute for parallel standing and as a way to handle forward weight stresses. They are simultaneously giving first aid to their back by moving into a non-habitual differentiated direction, stretching the hip flexors, strengthening the hip extensors and reinforcing the neurological pathway in the CNS.

One of the problems you might run into when teaching people new postural and movement possibilities is some resistance to change. They are worried about what other people will think of them and fear they look silly doing something different. This is particularly true with some of the more (to them) flamboyant postures, such as half-kneeling or split stance standing, and of the more flamboyant ways of bending, such as split stance or wide (horse) stance bending.

Culture and set emotional beliefs and associations make a powerful current to fight against, but there are many who would gladly forgo convention for increased comfort and stability. Give them a choice and let them decide for themselves. This is all you can really ever do with your students anyway. One of the big differences between the split stance and the half-kneeling position is that both feet are now on the floor. This

increases your choices in movement considerably because you've added possible movement in the knee, ankle and foot of the back leg of the stance.

This also increases your chances for error. How you organize your feet on the floor is important for lumbar stabilization, so we toyed with using the half-roller under the back heel in this stance, but will defer discussion about the feet and about using toys to the chapter on working with knee, ankle and foot dysfunction. Suffice it to say for now that a person with buns of steel and feet of clay is still unstable. Some of what you learn about how to engage the feet to the floor in that next chapter will be applicable to lumbopelvic stabilization – the adventure continues.

The meat of the lesson review, in this new and inherently less stable position, is the same coordination of contralateral and homolateral bending with intersegmental stabilization and finding and maintaining a neutral back. Muscle breakdowns, advantages and points of emphasis are essentially the same as with Half-kneel Bending. Try the manual resistance stuff you learned in the last lesson. Resist pushing and pulling movement of the vertical pole (held at shoulder height) and the horizontal pole (held at hip height). Resist lifting the bottom of the vertical pole from the floor and progress to lifting the distal tip of the horizontal pole away from the floor shovel style. Resist a two-handed push and pull of a horizontal pole.

One difference between Split Stance Bending and Half-kneel Bending is the increased requirement this places on the hamstrings, requirements for both length and strength. This is a great lesson to progress your gluteal-biased and flexion-unstable folks because of the need for hamstring length. Train your gluteal folks to use these movements in real life to impose functional demand on the hamstrings to lengthen many times over the course of the day (Box 6.10).

This is also a great lesson to progress your iliopsoas-biased and extension-unstable folks to because of the need to push the pelvis to vertical from the front leg. Train your students in using split stance positions to control anterior pelvic tilt bias in standing and to control weight-in-front stresses in standing.

This split stance position is a more difficult one to facilitate hip flexor length, but is well worth teaching your students; teach this skill in standing and they can do it anywhere. The key to lengthening the hip flexors of the back leg in standing is to be pattern specific. Get up for a moment and get into a split stance. Keep your weight centered between front and back leg and roll your pelvis into posterior tilt.

What most of you will do is to bend the knee of the back leg so the hip joint doesn't need to extend. Try tilting your pelvis posteriorly, let your knee bend as it wants and stay there. Keeping your pelvis vertical, slowly straighten your back knee to push your back heel toward the floor. Feel for anterior hip

---

Box 6.10 Split Stance Bending

Twin of Half-kneel Bending, only taller

Great hamstring stretch – train for bending with neutral spine and standing with reduced lumbar lordosis

Hip flexor stretch details – be pattern specific then straighten the back knee

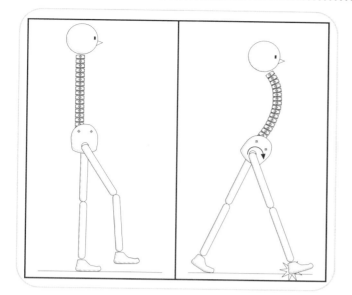

Fig. 6.42 Gait extension stressor – heel-strike.

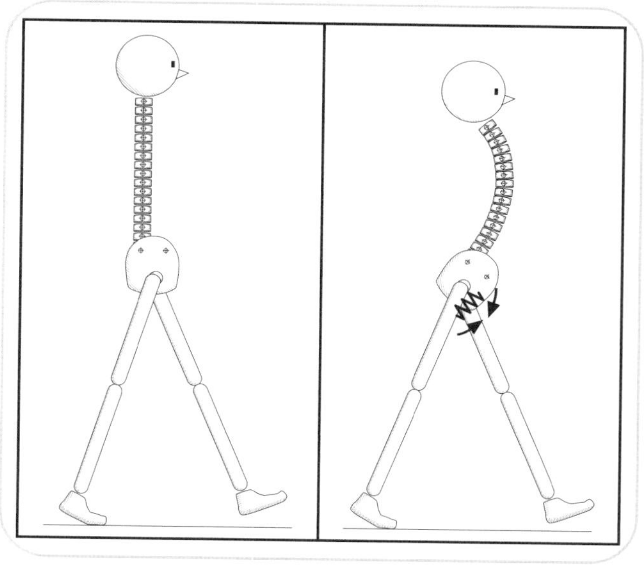

Fig. 6.43 Gait extension stressor – hip flexor too tight.

and thigh stretch. Cue to push the front foot from the hamstrings to maintain or increase posterior pelvic tilt.

Stability in gait

Let's review some of the common stressors of walking, some of the physical skills people with unstable backs might need when walking, then go on to exploring ways of facilitating a more stable walk.

Common gait-related stressors for the lower back include how you absorb shock on heel-strike, how completely you extend your hip in push-off and how you support the weight shift of the center of mass forward when lifting the stepping leg (Figs 6.42 to 6.44). These are *extension* stresses for the low back. All these are most likely to happen with the iliopsoas biased because of inadequate gluteal recruitment and inadequate hip flexor length.

Other gait stressors include rotational and lateral shear stresses. The pelvis might rotate or laterally shear under the torso. The pelvis may turn in one or both directions while walking. If the pelvis turns to the left when stepping forward with the right leg, when one side of the pelvis turns in the direction of the push-off leg (Fig. 6.45), there will probably be a right rotation movement at the lower back. Because the torso is highly unlikely to rotate to the left along with the pelvis (try this yourself to see why), it will either rotate mildly to the right or will stay more or less stationary.

Contrast the *rotation* at the low back that occurs with this waddling type of gait with the rotation of the pelvis on the legs that occurs with a force couple gait (Fig. 6.46). This style of gait accommodates the contralateral relationship between the

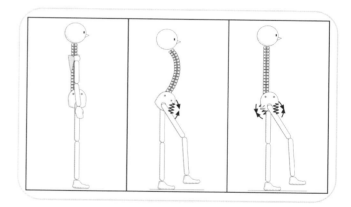

Fig. 6.44 Gait extension stressor – activation of psoas needs to be stabilized by opposite gluteals.

swinging arms and the scissoring legs while allowing the chest, shoulders and pelvis to turn all in the same direction. The force couple gait facilitates stability of the lower back without sacrificing fluidity elsewhere. The doll body walk is another way of reducing lateral and rotational stresses in gait; this is stability through rigidity (Fig. 6.47). A possible irritant of the low back with this type of gait is a *jarring* stress. With no give in the hip joint of the stepping leg into flexion and our horizontal adduction hybrid and no side-bending movement of the torso, the low back is subject to repeated hard landings just walking out to the mailbox.

The pelvis could also *laterally shear* under the pelvis. This lateral movement of the pelvis is made possible by the inattention to the hip abductors (Fig. 6.48). The torso can also twist or shift laterally on the pelvis if the pelvis is unable to turn or side-bend on the hip joints. Walking is so complex, with so

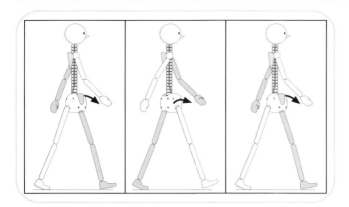

Fig. 6.45 Rotational gait stresses – the waddle walk.

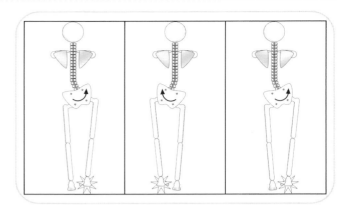

Fig. 6.48 Lateral shear gait stresses – the swish walk.

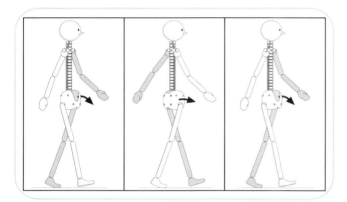

Fig. 6.46 Control rotational and lateral stresses through integrated movement – the force couple walk.

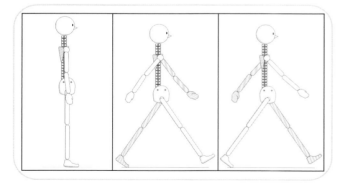

Fig. 6.47 Control rotational and lateral stresses through rigidity – the doll body walk.

many possibilities for errors or imbalances, that it is a wonder we get around at all.

Rather than try to figure out every nuance of imbalances and inefficiencies, get a general impression of proportion of movement, blend in what you know about other postural and movement imbalances, train them in intersegmental stabilization, and train them in pelvic force couple competence and balance.

The next couple of lessons can help you add on what you have already taught your students about controlling the shift of weight forward when lifting the stepping leg, completing push-off with full hip extension, maintaining intersegmental stability and spinal neutral and coordinating the force couple musculature to turn the pelvis. These next two closely related lessons are really just continuations of the last two. We will be exploring transitions from half-kneeling and split stances that closely resemble gait.

Knee Walking

Variations

A. Stand on your knees; kneel with arms at sides and knees around shoulder width apart. Pad them with towels or blankets if needed.

- Feel how you are standing. How is your weight distributed between your two knees?

- Are you experiencing any feelings of strain, effort or discomfort? If you had to stand here for an hour, what would start to protest?

- How is your pelvis balanced on your legs? Is it vertical or spilling forward? Is your pelvis turned right or left?

- Take a very small step forward with your left knee. How well is this movement organized? How smooth is it? How do you organize your pelvis to step forward? To step back? Reciprocate this movement

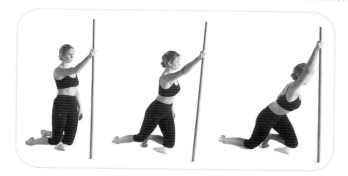

Fig. 6.49 Dangling your right knee, then dropping it a little, then sliding it backward. Spinal neutral and core stability.

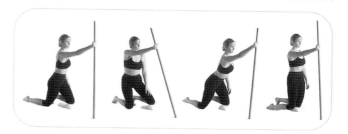

Fig. 6.50 Shift weight back on to your right knee, then power back forward again to dangle knee.

and repeat it a few times, then take a few small steps forward with your right knee. How does this side compare?

B. Kneel again, but only on one leg. Place your left knee on the foam half-roller (or tightly rolled blanket or towels) and let your right knee dangle off the end of the roller to the right. Hold a pole vertically in your right hand (approximately 5–6 feet long, half an inch diameter wooden dowel: broomstick/mop handle/closet dowel /martial arts bo) with the end of the pole on the ground and out a bit to the right (Fig. 6.49).

- As you balance here for a moment, pull in your lower belly and pelvic floor as you exhale and expand your chest. Keep this segmental stabilization going and breathe independently.

- Roll your pelvis forward and back a few times to find where your spine is neutral. Keep your back in neutral and keep your back stabilized with your lower belly.

- Then slowly and gently lower your right knee toward the floor. Just move a bit in that direction – don't worry about touching your knee to the floor (Fig. 6.49). Lift back up again and repeat this small movement many times.

- Can you do this movement and keep your back from arching or rounding? Which direction do you turn your pelvis? Try allowing your pelvis and chest to turn to the left, bending and twisting around your left hip joint.

- Add in sliding your right foot and knee backward on the floor (Fig. 6.49).

- You will have to lean forward a bit to accommodate the movement of your whole right leg backward. Let your pelvis turn to the left but keep holding on to the vertical pole with your right hand.

- Reverse to return; bring your torso back upright as you slide your right leg forward and twist pelvis and chest to the right to come back to center. Repeat several times, then lie on your back to rest.

C. Kneel this time with your right knee on the half-roller and your left knee dangling off the left edge.

- Repeat as above to the opposite side.

- Compare strength, flexibility, familiarity and coordination between the two sides.

D. Kneel again on your left knee with your right knee dangling, holding the pole with your right hand as before. Stabilize your back by pulling in your lower belly and pelvic floor. Lift and expand your chest to keep your upper belly soft and breathe independently as you maintain lumbar stability.

- Drop your right knee, turn your pelvis and chest to the left, lean forward and slide your right foot/leg backward a little bit on the ground behind (Fig. 6.50). Slide your leg about halfway back and stay there.

- From there, shift your weight back on to the right knee and turn your pelvis and chest to the right (Fig. 6.50). Keep leaning a bit forward as you do this, but keep your back neutral and stabilized.

- Come back forward again by shifting your weight forward on to your left knee while bringing your torso more upright and turning your pelvis to the left.

- Alternate between shifting your weight back on to your right knee and sticking your right hip out, then coming back forward by straightening your right hip, turning your pelvis to the left and squeezing/contracting your right cheek.

- Enlarge this movement to lift your right knee off the floor again to come to your starting position, balancing on one knee with the right knee dangling off the edge (Fig. 6.50).

- Combine the two movements to again slide your right knee back, shift your weight back on to it, shift back forward again to lift your right knee from the floor and return to the start. Pause for a moment and rest in this position.

- Resume this same basic movement, but this time as you shift your weight forward on to the left knee and turn your pelvis to the left, continue now to take a large step forward with your right foot.

- Place the sole of your right foot on the floor so that your hip and knee are both bent at about 90° and

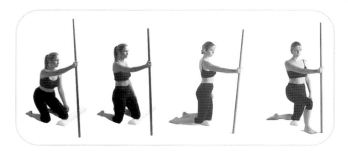

Fig. 6.51 Alternating steps to half-kneeling – turn twice coming forward and twice moving back.

your knee is directly over your foot. This is a half-kneeling position (Fig. 6.51). Complete the movement by fully straightening your left hip and contracting your left gluteals.

- Reverse this movement to slide your right leg back, shift your weight back on to and turn toward the right leg, and then reverse the movement again to come back forward to half-kneeling. Repeat several times.

- Try allowing your pelvis and chest to turn to the right as you come forward to half-kneel in a counterpoint to the turning to the left of your pelvis and torso as you slide your leg back. Remember to squeeze your left cheek.

E.   Kneel this time with your right knee on the half-roller and your left knee dangling off the left edge.

- Repeat as D above to the opposite side.

- Compare and contrast the two sides.

F.   Come back to place your left knee on the roller, but this time put your right foot forward on the floor in the half-kneeling position.

- Make the same basic turning and shifting movement you were just doing, but now in this position.

- Shift your weight forward and turn your pelvis and chest to the right, then shift your weight back on to your left knee and turn to the left (Fig. 6.52). Lean over a bit when coming back on to your left knee.

- Stick your left hip out and bend forward a bit. Come more upright when coming back forward; squeeze your left cheek. Repeat several times.

- Enlarge this movement by shifting your weight forward on to your right foot, lifting your left knee from the roller and coming up to stand or to the seat of a chair or step (Fig. 6.52).

- Reverse the movement to bring your left knee back to the roller and shift your weight back on to the left knee again. Repeat several times.

G.   Repeat instructions as above to opposite side.

H.   Stand on both knees again, no pole.

- Feel how you are organized now compared to when you started.

- Take a step forward with your left knee, then step back, then forward and then back. Do the 'Charleston.'

- Do the same thing with your right knee.

- Walk forward on your knees. How does your pelvis turn? What do you have to do to keep your lower back from arching and your tail from lifting?

- Walk backward on your knees.

- Stand up and walk around; what do you notice?

Baselines – Knee Walking

The establishment of proprioceptive baselines this time involves stepping. Stepping forward from kneeling is challenging for someone susceptible to extension strains. Be careful about how far forward you go: it should be able to be performed slowly, small and reversibly. This might be a bit much for grumpy knees too; use your judgment. How was your balance? How were your force couples coordinating? Did your pelvis turn in the direction of your stepping knee? Could you feel your gluteals kick in?

Stepping back mimics shock absorption around the hip

Kneel again, but only on one leg in variations B and C. Place your one knee on the foam half-roller and let the other knee dangle off the end of the roller to the outside. One-legged stances are characteristic of walking and running: you knew we would get to one before the book was finished. After reviewing the TA Facilitation and the coordination with breath, pushing the pelvis to vertical and establishing a neutral spine, we start to explore a movement of dropping your dangling knee toward the floor then coming back up again.

This movement asks for alternate lengthening and shortening contractions of the hip abductors on the weightbearing side. This dropping of the hip mimics the shock absorption that should be happening in the abductors on heel-strike. Raising the knee again and shortening the abductors mimic a part of push-off. When you played Goldilocks and tried various ways of organizing your pelvis to do this, what did you discover? Is a cardinal plane side-bend your best choice?

For most people, there will be a turn of the pelvis away from the dropping leg. This flexion and modified horizontal adduction of the weightbearing leg even more closely approximates shock absorption in walking and running, and adds more meat (gluteals and short and stubbies) to the mix. When reversing the movement to come back up again, we might expect to see an unwinding of this twist.

This is created as the contracting abductors, gluteals and short and stubbies act to turn the pelvis away from the push-off leg (and toward what will become the stepping leg). Much of the rest of the lesson is to facilitate an awareness of lumbopelvic movement in gait and to develop the physical skills needed to refine and balance this alternating shock absorption and push-off movement around the hips.

Sliding the leg backward while leaning forward and toward the weightbearing leg is designed to further clarify and enlarge

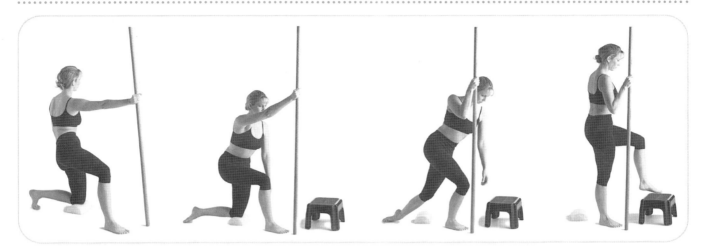

Fig. 6.52 Alternating steps to standing – turn twice again in each direction.

upon this theme. Note the similarities between this position and the contralateral reaching you were doing in Half-kneel Bending, or the transition from hands and knees to side-sitting you did in Cat/Camel. Just keep adding in pieces – this is a modular system.

Shifting weight from a split kneeling position

We now add a little wrinkle in variations D and E. Shifting the weight back and turning the pelvis and chest in the direction of the back leg is reminiscent of the homolateral bending movements we did in half-kneel and Split Stance Bending. The movement of the pelvis and torso and the adjustments that have to be made around the hip joints are very similar to the homolateral reaching you did in previous lessons.

The hip joint of the front leg has to move into horizontal abduction to keep the knee over the floor (adductor length), and the hip joint on the back leg has to twist into internal rotation and flexion (short and stubby length). This can be a difficult movement for many people and is pretty quadriceps intensive. Why bother?

One reason is that it represents the opposing swing of the pendulum in walking. If we want to train someone to move forward and turn towards the stepping side as they walk, we can facilitate an awareness of movement into that direction by starting from the opposite extreme. Move back and turn away from the stepping leg to load the springs that propel you forward and turn you towards the stepping leg. This functionally strengthens the gluteals, hamstrings and short and stubbies of the back leg and helps to associate them with gait. Do this alternating movement quickly for several minutes and observe where you perceive muscle effort and eventual fatigue.

A different interpretation

There are a couple of ways of doing this movement. The way that works best for mimicking shock absorption and push-off is to stick out your hip and lean yourself over a bit, as in homo-

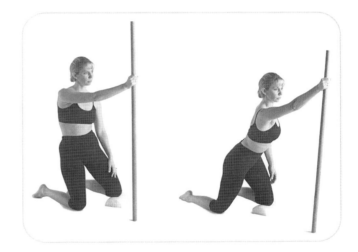

Fig. 6.53 Shifting back and posteriorly tilting pelvis, then coming forward and bending – this is reversed from the lesson.

lateral bending. This is the variation we will emphasize when facilitating change in gait patterns.

Another way of doing this movement is useful because it can be a great stabilization tool for people who don't handle extension stresses well. We could ask our students to weight-shift backward in this position and suggest a falling-back movement of the pelvis and torso, rather than leaning forward and anteriorly tilting. This version creates posterior tilt of the pelvis and a flattening and lordosis reduction of the lower back (Fig. 6.53).

The first variation has you flexing and internally rotating the back hip and leaning your torso forward as you come back, then extending the back hip and bringing the torso upright when you come back forward. The second version has you extending your back hip, tilting your pelvis posteriorly and coming upright as you sit back, then bending over to come forward. Try both variations to appreciate the distinction.

Notice the demand this variation puts on your quadriceps. In a normal balance reaction the torso leans forward as the pelvis moves back, the center of mass stays fairly balanced between the two feet, and movement and effort are provided by the hip joint. In this variation, the whole center of mass moves backward and the only thing preventing you from falling back is knee extension and a soon-to-be-quivering-if-you-keep-this-up-for-long quadriceps. We will see a variation of this movement again in the next chapter on legs, and will discuss the quadriceps in a bit more detail.

Psoas addicts who like this simulation of falling back can also benefit from wearing a backpack that hangs low on the sacrum and that has a thick, wide waist belt. The shift of the center of mass backward and the push the weight of the back-pack gives the sacrum can make backpacking an enjoyable activity for people who habitually extend. Sometimes even folding your hands and putting them behind your back 'professor style' can shift your center of mass backward enough to make standing more comfortable.

This can also be a great ergonomic tool for these same folks. You can use variations of this movement in standing for one-handed pulling and can manually resist that movement by holding the pole lance-style. You can use this movement to lower your center of mass and get your hands closer to the ground, and it can be a substitute for leaning, prolonged leaning and some shallow bending.

You can use this movement in anticipation of loading some weight in your hands. The falling back of the pelvis counteracts the shift of weight forward as you load your arms. Recall that load amounts depend on both amount of weight lifted and the length of the lever arm, so picking up a bag of oranges at arm's length can be a significant strain.

You can use this to lift something from waist height and to hold heavier weights in front of you. You can even walk with this bias of falling back and dropping your tail when carrying heavier things from place to place: moving boxes, moving your garbage can, carrying your kitchen chair into the next room, etc. However, using a hand truck or carrying things on your backside is an even better bet. We will be seeing this movement again in the next lesson and in the legs chapter; there are some pretty dandy foot, ankle and knee applications.

Putting a couple of steps together

The variations in F and G modify and mimic the forward and back shift of weight of the previous variation but in a different position: half-kneeling. This again facilitates the push-off action of the back leg and the shock absorption action of the front leg. It again mimics a stepping movement and segues into a subsequent movement of transitioning to standing. Alternatively, this could segue into yet another step if you place a stool or other step in front.

You could even combine this variation with the last one to make a series of connected movements from being back on one leg, to being forward on one leg, to coming to half-kneeling, to shifting back to the back leg again, to shifting forward, then coming up to stand. How many turns of the pelvis can you count here? You could even blend this with previous lessons and transition to poor man's splits, floor sitting, Side-sit Transitions and down to supine (Box 6.11).

Box 6.11 Knee Walking

Reciprocating push-off and shock absorption movements at each hip

Training pelvic force couple organization to reduce rotational, lateral and extension gait stresses

Sequencing multiple steps together and reciprocating between stepping forward and stepping back

Variation of shifting weight back – staying upright and tucking the tail to control weight-in-front stresses and standing postural extension stresses

---

In the final section of this lesson, stand on both knees again with no pole. Return once again to our baselines and check for differences from when you started. Stepping forward and back with one knee is like an old dance step called the 'Charleston.' Step forward and turn your pelvis to the stepping leg, then step back and turn your pelvis to the weightbearing leg. Once your students have learned and are somewhat competent in the various movements of this lesson, try having them do some of the reciprocating movements, in either standing or kneeling, in time to music.

Start with slower music and let them get a sense of timing. Progress to peppier tunes to make them go a little faster. This repetition reinforces the pattern in the CNS and improves the physical skills (strength and flexibility) needed for the movements. It's also a lot more fun than being on your hands and knees and doing two sets of opposite leg and arm lifts 20 times each side. Timing the movements to music triggers associations with dancing and tends to disinhibit people from shaking their pelvis around.

Many of the movements in our standing lessons can be facilitated by music; put on some Rolling Stones to work on your quick pivots, some classical to work on your controlled stepping, and some Elvis to work on your pelvic anterior and posterior tilt in standing. It might even get people to turn off the TV and get off their duffs. Maybe they will get off the couch, practice some lesson movements in time with the music and like it enough to keep doing it – anything to get people to be generally more active.

Pole play

Knee Walking is a nice gait facilitator: the feet and knee joints are removed as degrees of freedom, and the hips and pelvis have to play a more prominent role. Facilitate a force couple gait by placing the pole horizontally across either the front (ASIS to ASIS) or the back of your pelvis (across the middle of your sacrum). Keep the pole exactly where it is relative to your body and move the right end of the pole forward as you take a step forward with your left knee (Fig. 6.54).

Move the left end of the pole forward as you step with your right knee. The pole acts as a lateral extension of your pelvis and magnifies the direction of turn. It also provides a reference point for the movement of your pelvis. Do first one side, then the other, then take sequential steps. Move the right end of the pole backward when you step back with your left leg. Do the mirror image to the other side. Use the pole this way to facili-

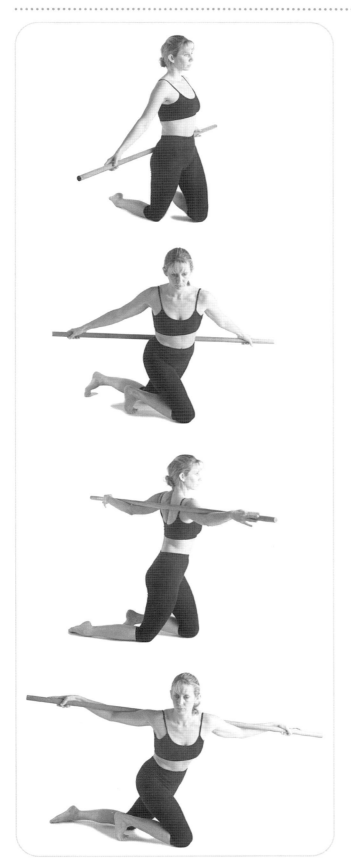

Fig. 6.54 Using the pole to facilitate pelvic force couple steps.

tate student awareness of the position and movement of the pelvis with any of the previous variations of this lesson.

You can approximate this same thing without a pole by placing your hands on the tops of your iliac crests and pointing your elbows out to your sides. Use the intention to move the opposite elbow forward with the stepping leg. Probably you will actually do this sequence in standing rather than kneeling when working with your students. Progress this idea by holding the pole horizontally across your upper back with your hands out wide to hold the pole near the ends.

Move the right end of the pole forward when you step forward with your left knee, etc. The pole across the shoulders helps coordinate upper body rotation in the same direction of pelvic rotation and helps minimize rotational and lateral stresses at the low back. You could get really fancy and manually resist Knee Walking by having your student hold a pole lance-style in each hand and resisting her martial advance across the room.

One word of caution here. Knees, both skin and joint tissues, can get a bit sensitive with high volumes of movement. Some of the repetitive practice might be better performed while on your feet. Try using Knee Walking or this combination of a turn and shift of weight movement functionally to push or pull low, heavy objects.

Steppin' Out

Variations

A. Stand with feet comfortably spread and with your arms hanging at your sides.

- Feel how you are standing. How is your weight distributed between your two feet? How is your weight distributed front to back on your feet?

- Are you experiencing any feelings of strain, effort or discomfort? If you had to stand here for an hour, what would start to protest?

- Slowly pick up your left foot as if you were going to put it up on a low stool. As you do this, notice how steady your balance is.

- Does your pelvis turn left or right? Where in your standing leg can you feel additional effort?

- What are you doing with your stabilizers. What are your lower belly and pelvic floor doing?

- Do the same thing with the right foot. Pick it up to place or as if to place the right foot on a stool. How does this side compare to the other in terms of balance, movement of the pelvis or effort in the standing leg?

B. Stand with your left foot on a half-roller and hold on to a long pole with your right hand (approximately 5–6 foot-long half-inch dowel). Hold onto the pole with your right hand in front of you and out a bit to the right. Place your left foot on the half-roller (or tightly rolled blanket, towels or phone book) lengthwise so that the middle of your heel and the spot between the first and second balls of

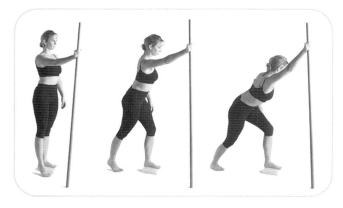

Fig. 6.55 Dangling your right foot, dropping it a little, then sliding it backward. Keep back neutral and maintain intersegmental stability.

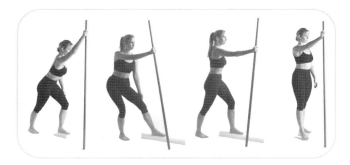

Fig. 6.56 Step back and shift weight on to your right foot, then power back forward again to dangle foot.

your left foot are on the top of the curve of the roller. Let your right foot dangle off the right edge of the roller (Fig. 6.55).

- Find your stabilizers; combine breath, pelvic floor and lower belly with mild front/back rocking movement of your pelvis as before. After doing this already familiar movement several times in this position and establishing a vertical pelvis and neutral spine, find your corset/stabilization and keep it there, breathing independently.

- Keep this stabilization steady as you slowly lower your right foot toward the ground (Fig. 6.55). Make it a small movement and don't worry about touching the ground.

- Can you do this movement and keep your back from arching? Which direction do you turn your pelvis? Try turning deliberately to the left with your pelvis and shoulders – bend and twist around your left hip.

- Repeat several times, then add in sliding your right foot backward on the floor (Fig. 6.55).

- You will have to lean forward a bit to accommodate this movement of sliding the right foot behind you to keep your back neutral. Let your pelvis turn to the left but keep holding on to the pole with your right hand.

- Reverse to return, bringing your torso back upright as you slide your right foot forward and twist pelvis and chest back to the right. This brings you back to where you started with your right foot dangling (Fig. 6.55).

- Repeat several times, then lie on your back to rest. Compare your two sides, especially your legs, pelvis and back.

C. Stand this time with your right foot on the half-roller and your left foot dangling off the left edge. Hold on to the pole with your left hand.

- Repeat B as above to the opposite side.
- Compare strength, flexibility, familiarity and coordination between the two sides.

D. Stand again with your left foot lengthwise on the roller and with your right foot dangling, holding the pole with your right hand as before. Stabilize your back by pulling in your lower belly and pelvic floor. Lift and expand your chest to keep your upper belly soft; breathe independently as you maintain lumbar stability.

- Drop your right foot toward the floor, turn your pelvis and chest to the left, lean forward a bit, and slide your right foot backward a little bit on the ground behind. Repeat this several times, then slide your leg about halfway back and stay there.

- From there, shift your weight back on to your right foot and turn your pelvis and chest to the right (Fig. 6.56). Continue to let your torso lean forward and stick out your right hip back and to the right.

- Come back forward again by shifting your weight forward on to your left foot while bringing your torso more upright and turning your pelvis to the left. Complete straightening your right hip by pinching your right cheek/contracting your right gluteals.

- Alternate between shifting your weight back on to your right foot and sticking your right hip out, then coming back forward by straightening your right hip, turning your pelvis to the left and squeezing/contracting your right cheek. Alternate between shifting your weight forward on to your left foot while coming upright and shifting your weight back on to your right foot while leaning over.

- Enlarge this movement to lift your right foot off the floor again to come to your starting position, balancing on one foot with the right foot dangling off the edge. Combine the two movements to again slide your right foot back, shift weight back on to it, shift back forward again to lift your right foot, and return to the start. Pause for a moment and rest in this position.

- Resume this same basic movement, but this time as you shift your weight forward on to the left foot and

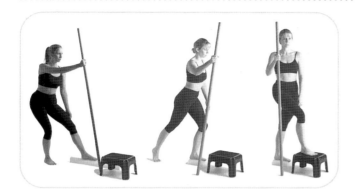

Fig. 6.57 Alternating steps to half standing – turn twice both coming forward and moving back.

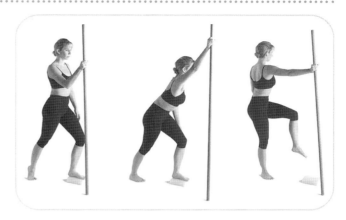

Fig. 6.58 Lifting the front leg, spilling your pelvis backward and straightening your standing knee to push taller.

turn your pelvis to the left, continue now to take a step up on to something (chair, stair, bench, table) with your right foot (Fig. 6.57).

- Place the sole of your right foot on the step so that your knee is directly over your foot. This is a half-standing position. Complete the movement of straightening your left hip by pinching your left cheek.

- Reverse this movement to slide your right foot back, shift your weight back on to and turn toward that right foot, and then reverse the movement again to come back forward to step up on a stool or chair seat. Repeat several times.

- Try allowing your pelvis and chest to turn to the right as you come forward to half-stand in a counterpoint to the turning to the left of your pelvis and torso as you slide your foot back.

E. Stand this time with your right foot on the half-roller and your left foot dangling off the left edge.
- Repeat D above to the opposite side.
- Compare and contrast the two sides.

F. Come back to place your left foot on the roller again with your right foot dangling off the edge.
- Drop and slide your right foot back on the floor about halfway and stay there.
- Shift your weight back on to the right foot and turn your pelvis and chest to the right.
- Stay in this position as you alternately lift and lower your left foot slightly away from the roller several times (Fig. 6.58).
- This time, you are sitting back and putting all your weight into your right leg. Make sure your right knee is still above your knee.
- Bring your torso and pelvis upright as you lift your foot and get taller, then lean your torso forward a bit and get shorter as you place your foot back down. Repeat this several times, then rest.

- Enlarge this movement of lifting your left foot to slide the sole of your left foot up the pole toward your right hand (Fig. 6.58). Try pushing your pelvis to vertical or even a bit rolled back/tuck your tail as you straighten your right knee to get taller.

G. Repeat instructions as above to opposite side.

H. Stand on both feet again, no pole.
- Feel how you are organized now in comparison to when you started.
- Take a step forward with your left foot, then step back, then forward and then back. Do the 'Charleston.'
- Do the same thing with your right foot.
- Walk forward. How does your pelvis turn? What do you have to do to keep your lower back from arching and your tail from lifting? Take long steps and allow yourself to lean forward.
- Walk backward. Take long steps and allow yourself to lean forward.
- Take shorter steps walking backward by shifting your weight back and 'sitting' back on one leg then the other. Try walking forward this way; lead with your pelvis and stay back on your heels.

Quick comments – Steppin' Out

This lesson is just a twin of the previous lesson, only taller. The movements of the pelvis, the muscular breakdown, the applications and the pole facilitation techniques are the same. The main differences are that the feet are now on the floor instead of the knees, and there is a surprise ending to the lesson.

Whereas we completed the last lesson with a step forward, lifting the back leg to move forward, in this lesson we finish with a high lifting of the front leg and balancing on the back leg (Fig. 6.58). In moving forward and lifting the back leg, we are arresting ourselves from falling forward with our front leg. When moving back and lifting the front leg, we are arresting

Box 6.12 Steppin' Out

Reciprocating push-off and shock absorption movements at each hip

Training pelvic force couple organization to reduce rotational, lateral and extension gait stresses

Sequencing multiple steps together and reciprocating between stepping forward and stepping back

Variation of shifting weight back and lifting front leg – staying upright and tucking the tail to control weight in front stresses and standing postural extension stresses

ourselves from falling backward with our back leg. The first movement might be of particular benefit to the gluteal-biased person. The second movement might be of particular benefit to the iliopsoas-biased person (Box 6.12).

Lifting the front leg high triggers a shift of weight backward and suggests posterior tilt of the pelvis and bending of that knee. This movement is analogous to the described variation in Knee Walking, where you shift weight back and tuck your tail rather than lean forward. This movement is also a literal progression of some of the variations in Wishbone. In this position, the hip and knee are bent a bit and the short iliopsoas shouldn't be as much of an impediment to posterior tilt.

From here, the intention to lift the foot high by sliding it up the pole serves three purposes.

- It both facilitates and makes more difficult the posterior tilt of the pelvis and the powerful contraction of the weightbearing gluteals.

- The intention to slide the foot up high may trigger straightening of the weightbearing knee and create a situation in which the hip flexors are required to lengthen further and the hip joint is required to more fully extend.

- Lifting the front leg high stimulates transverse abdominis contraction – palpate this on yourself and your students. You are again coordinating the ever-so-desirable coordination of intersegmental stabilizers with the hip extensors and abductors.

This movement can also be taught by getting into this falling-back position with the front leg slightly lifted, emphasizing posterior tilt and alternately straightening and bending your knee. If balancing on one leg is a problem, let your students use their hands to assist – pole, wall, chair, whatever. This is also a common tai chi stance and one we will be coming back to again in the next chapter. Try standing with one foot up on a chair seat and the other on the floor (half-standing). Shift your weight back on your standing heel, bend your standing knee 15–20° and tuck your pelvis under (extreme posterior tilt).

Keep your pelvis rolled back relative to vertical and slowly push taller by straightening your standing knee. This demands considerable hip extension range and hip extensor strength. Push the other foot into the stool and use the hip extensors/hamstrings on that side to assist in keeping the pelvis rolled back from vertical. These are great variations and movements we should encourage our iliopsoas-biased students to do little bits of many times a day.

Blend Charleston movements into steps. Use pole across sacrum or hands on hips as described in Knee Walking. Do sequential marching steps across the floor; bring the knee up high to facilitate full push-off from the push-off leg, and let your pelvis turn in the direction of your stepping leg. Do sequential skating movements across the floor; reach opposite hand toward opposite knee or lower leg and bend around the front hip to simulate shock absorption. Combine the two if desired. Use Knee Walking and Steppin' Out with neurologic and medical students. Use with strokes, total knee or hip replacements or below-knee amputees to re-establish force couple balance and competence.

Kendo steps

I learned a great gait facilitator when I took a kendo class a few years back. Kendo is a Japanese sword-fighting style – you've probably seen the guys with armor and helmets whacking each other with long bamboo swords. Try the following drills. Stand with your feet about hip width apart and with your hands on your hips. Keeping both feet flat on the ground (don't lift your heels!) and slide your left foot forward on the floor. As you slide your foot forward, move your right elbow forward to guide the rotation of your pelvis to the left – in the direction of your stepping leg.

Keep your heels and toes on the floor and make sure you keep your right knee straight. Only slide your foot forward about a half step, just so the heel of your left foot is even with the toes of your right. Emphasize straightening your right hip (pinch your right gluteal) and keeping your pelvis as close to vertical as possible; keep your tailbone pointed to the floor! You should be feeling a stretch in your right hip flexors. This movement emphasizes rotating your pelvis around your legs and extending your back hip to prevent anterior pelvic tilt. This reduces extension and rotation stresses on the low back.

Do this movement of sliding your left foot forward several times, and then do the same thing with the right. Compare and contrast the two sides – which hip extends most easily and which way does your pelvis turn most easily? Then, slide one foot forward, come back to where you started, then slide the other foot forward; alternate from side to side. Then, slide one foot forward and then the other; glide across the floor. Practice your kendo walking in the privacy of your own home, then tone it down a bit as you go out into public and work with your more competent force couple gait.

Try kendo walking backward, again sliding the whole sole of the foot and coordinating stepping the foot back and moving the opposite elbow back at the same time. Try introducing a lateral component to this movement: slide one foot forward and outward at the same time, as in a skating movement. This can be done backward as well.

The one-legged standing blues – and the antidote

Lifting one leg is good for people who subject themselves to lumbar extension stresses by standing with a one-legged collapse. This is where you shift your weight to one leg and drop the opposite side of your pelvis by allowing the weightbearing leg to sag into a flexion/horizontal adduction/internal rotation hybrid (Fig. 6.59). It is very common in psoas addicts as

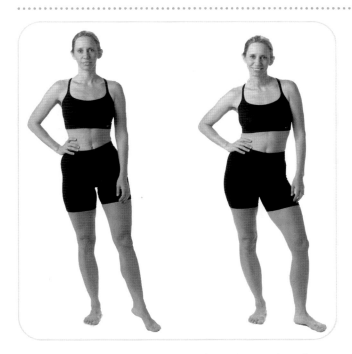

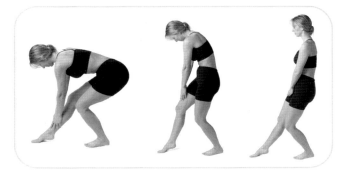

Fig. 6.60 Bending from a split stance position – front leg is empty. Work your gluteals and hamstrings!

Fig. 6.59 Start from upright one leg standing – then one leg collapse standing.

it allows the gluteal group to lounge around instead of working. If shifting to the right leg, the pelvis falls into anterior tilt and the left side of the pelvis drops. The lumbar spine adjusts by bending back and to the right. This applies compression stresses to the right side of the lower back.

Try the following variation of this lifting of the foot variation. Have your left foot in front and your right foot back, then sink yourself back on to your right foot and lift just the heel of your left foot so just your left toes are on the ground and 80% of your weight is on your back/right foot. From here, slide both hands down your left leg toward your left foot (Fig. 6.60). Be sure to keep your weight back on your right leg and your left toes just touching the floor.

Keep your back neutral and maintain your intersegmental stability as you slide your hands repetitively up and down your left leg. This puts a premium on your right hip extensors and hip rotators and is great for teaching bending ergonomics, the push-off function in gait, and for keeping the knee over the foot. Try both sides and compare range, strength and familiarity. Use these types of positions and movements to control weight-in-front stresses, to reach down a slight to moderate amount without needing to bend forward, and to reach for and pick up objects out to the sides in a way that reduces weight-in-front stresses.

This movement of 'sitting back' on to the back leg is a very useful one for controlling weight-in-front stresses and should be an important part of every physical therapist's repertoire. This movement both counterbalances the weight in front by shifting weight back and puts the pelvis into neutral or slight posterior tilt in anticipation, to prevent the pelvis from rolling forward and the lower back from arching. This same strategy can be used from the horse stance position.

Use the pushing-taller aspect of this movement as well. Counsel your psoas students to engage in active one-legged standing as frequently as possible during the day. It trains fuller hip extension and reduces habitual antagonist imbalance. With higher leg lifts, it stimulates transverse abdominis contraction (palpate this for yourself and train your students to palpate as well), links intersegmental stabilization with pelvic stabilization and trains competent pelvic force couples. Cue to standing more on the nonhabitual weightbearing side, pushing the foot into the floor to lengthen the habitually compressed side of the torso. Advise those with leg length discrepancies on the advantages of one-legged standing in allowing for a more balanced pelvis and spine in standing.

This completes our section on stabilizing the lower back in gait. We will now focus our attention more on lateral stresses and how to blend intersegmental stability with lateral pelvic control.

Lateral stability

Rotational or lateral shearing stresses on the lower back are created by rotational or lateral shearing movements of the pelvis under a relatively more immobile torso, or by rotational or lateral shearing movements of the torso on top of a relatively more immobile pelvis. In either case, with lateral movements of the pelvis or torso in space, or with turning or rotational movements of the pelvis or torso in space, we would like the pelvis and torso to move laterally or to rotate together.

Log rolling movements can be a nice way to initially train students with lateral instability to move their pelvis and chest/thorax/shoulders together and train their abdominal obliques in maintaining that log-like relationship. Of course, logs can't initiate their own roll, so we'll have to train the extremities, especially the legs, to initiate and provide the power for turning and lateral shifting movements. The legs will also have to be sufficiently differentiated from the pelvis to allow sufficient movement of the pelvis in space as to not require too much movement at the lower back.

Review of lateral stresses

To review, some categories of lateral stress include centrifugal forces, locomotion, acceleration or deceleration of ballistic turns, pushing or pulling laterally, or pushing forward or pulling back with one hand.

- Centrifugal forces – riding in a car or other vehicle that is going around a corner or a curve in the road, or riding on a roller coaster or other carnival ride.

- Lateral locomotion stresses – generally of the too-much-rotation or the too-much-lateral-shear of the pelvis in gait. Also changing directions or pivoting.

- Acceleration or deceleration of ballistic turns – includes swinging a tennis racket, baseball bat or golf club. Throwing a ball or a Frisbee, catching a rambunctious 4-year-old boy as he's running past you, or sharply changing the direction of your walk or run are other examples. Even turning to look over your shoulder or reaching out to the side or across in front of you are lateral stressors. These are rotational movements initiated from the floor, and the core needs to stabilize while the abdominal obliques need to work to maintain a stable relationship between the pelvis and chest.

- Pushing or pulling laterally – examples include pushing open a door, closing/opening a curtain, sliding open a sticky window, sliding several coats/hangers one way and the other on closet dowel, paddling a kayak, raking/sweeping laterally, moving a piano away from the wall, walking a rambunctious dog on a leash, turning a corner while pushing a lawnmower or grocery cart, or chopping down a tree. These are rotational movements usually initiated from the arms and upper body. The core again needs to maintain intersegmental stability while the obliques again work to maintain the chest to pelvis relationship.

- Pushing or even just reaching straight forward or pulling straight back with one hand. Examples include pushing open/pulling open a door, reaching for a bottle of wine, shoveling snow or pushing a broom or vacuum, bowling, paddling a canoe or pull-starting a weed-whacker.

- Making transitional movements such as getting in and out of a car or rolling over in bed.

The transverse abdominis and the multifidi need to work to maintain intersegmental stability. The internal and external abdominal obliques and internal and external intercostal obliques need to work to maintain the relationship of chest to pelvis and prevent twisting the pelvis under the torso or the torso on top of the pelvis. What works to move and therefore to stabilize your pelvis in space during rotational and lateral movements? This would be an assignment for the hip abductors and external rotators, with an occasional assist from the adductors.

Dead Bug Roll

Variations

A. Stand for a moment with your weight equally divided between your two feet and arms hanging down at your sides.

- Stand near a doorway or wall corner and reach forward to place your right hand against the inside of the doorway.

- Gently press your hand sideways into the doorway. You will be pushing against an immovable object as if you wanted to push it to the left. Pretend you are widening your doorway (Fig. 6.61).

- Does your pelvis move in space as you do this? Does it turn left or right?

- Try the same thing with the left hand pushing against the opposite side of the doorway; left hand pushing to the right. How does this side compare? What happens at your back with this movement?

B. Lie on your left side. Bend your hips and knees to about 90° and have adequate support underneath your head (try a short stack of towels).

- Place your straight left arm out in front of you on the floor and place your right hand on top of your left palm.

- From there, lift your right hand a little bit away from your left hand. Lift only 6–7 inches – your hands shouldn't be wider apart than your shoulders. Lower back down and repeat (Fig. 6.62).

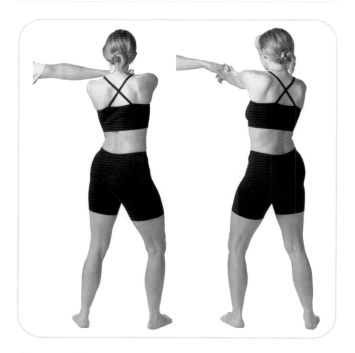

Fig. 6.61 Pushing out laterally – which way does your pelvis turn?

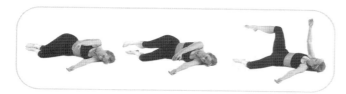

Fig. 6.62 Lift right arm – lift right arm and leg – lift both and open 'book' to ceiling.

- How heavy does your arm feel? How does the rest of your body, especially your pelvis and lower back, respond to this movement? Pause for a moment.

- Then take a breath and hold it, then move your held breath back and forth between your belly and your chest. This is a seesaw breath.

- Expand your belly; push your belly button forward as you push your breath down. Collapse your chest so your breastbone sinks back.

- Expand your chest; push your chest forward as you pull your held breath up. Let your belly 'suck in' as if tacking your belly button back on to your spine.

- Alternate back and forth with your held breath but do empty your lungs periodically, cycle through a few breaths to reoxygenate, then resume this same movement of moving your held breath back and forth between belly and chest.

- After familiarizing yourself with this movement, add in tightening your lower belly and pulling up/in your (front and middle) pelvic floor as you move your air into your chest.

- Then relax and push down or bulge out your lower belly and pelvic floor openings as you move your air down into your belly. Alternately tighten your lower belly and pelvic floor and relax/push out your lower belly and pelvic floor in time with the movement of your breath into your chest and into your belly.

- Pull in your lower belly and pelvic floor as you exhale and expand your chest. Keep this segmental stabilization going and breathe independently.

- Then simultaneously lift your right arm, right knee and right lower leg and foot off the left side (Fig. 6.62). Lift again only 6–7 inches. Lower simultaneously and repeat. Imagine that your arms and legs make up the binding of a book.

- You are opening the book just a crack and closing it back down again. Do this very slowly and in a controlled way.

- Try thinking about pushing out into the floor with your left thigh and knee. You are pushing your knees away from each other. Keep your lower belly and pelvic floor pulled up and in, but breathe freely into your upper belly or lateral ribs.

- Gradually enlarge the movement to open the 'book' wider (Fig. 6.62). How close can your right thigh and right arm come to vertical without your left knee lifting away from the floor?

- Repeat this slowly many times and appreciate the work it takes in the outsides of both hips and the concentration required to move your thigh and arm precisely together in such a way that there is no twist through your torso. You are log rolling.

C. Lie on your right side with knees and hips bent up. Arrange your arms as above.

- Go through the same sequence of movements here as you did on the other side.

- Coordinate belly, pelvic floor and breath.

- Hold belly and floor steady and breathe independently.

- Lift left arm and left leg gradually farther away. Open and close the book several times on this side. Compare this side to the other.

D. Lie again on your left side as before.

- Stabilize your back; pull in belly and pelvic floor, and breathe independently.

- Lift your right arm and right leg so that your arm and leg are parallel to the floor. Knees are hip width apart and hands are shoulder width apart. Keep this distance and keep both arm and leg lifted.

- Then move your right hand and right knee alternately forward and back (Fig. 6.63). This is a rolling movement. You will roll your pelvis, torso, shoulders and head forward and back on the floor, but the leg and arm stay lifted and parallel to the floor.

- Imagine you are rolling a ball between your upper arm bones and between your thigh bones. Do this slowly, make sure you don't drop or raise your leg or arm, and keep your stabilization with a lifted chest and relaxed upper belly.

E. Lie on your right side again.

- Repeat as D to opposite side. Compare the two sides.

F. Lie on your left side again.

- Stabilize, and then lift your right arm and leg. Reach your right hand and right knee forward, stay there, and try opening your book from here. Can you stay rolled forward and open your book easily? Pause for a moment.

- Then move your lifted right hand and right knee backward and combine this backward rolling movement with opening your book. How easy is this in comparison to rolling forward?

- Stabilize, lift arm and leg, roll back and open your book. Continue this movement by rolling far enough toward your back to be able to lift your left leg and arm. Roll yourself on to your back with legs and arms still lifted, feet and elbows off the ground.

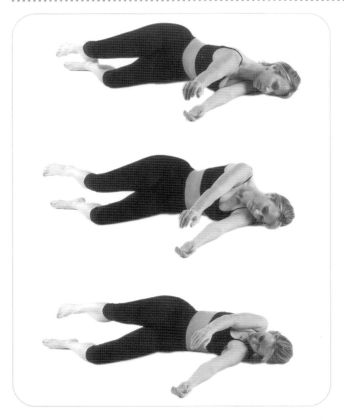

Fig. 6.63 Lift arm and leg together and move them forward and back.

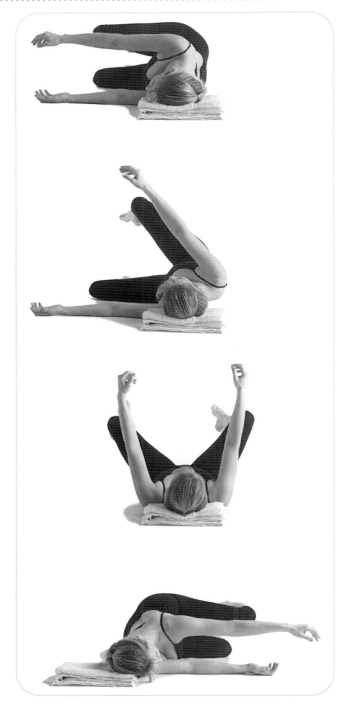

- Complete the movement of rolling to your back by closing the book again – bring your left arm and left knee to touch your right knee and arm. You are on your back with legs and arms lifted, like a dead bug.
- Reverse the movement to come back on to your left side. Feel how you 'catch' yourself with your left arm and leg. Repeat several times.

G. Lie on your right side once again.
- Repeat F to the opposite side.
- Alternate rolling from side to side by alternately opening and closing your book (Fig. 6.64). Your torso rolls like a log, your legs do most of the work of moving you, and your lower belly/pelvic floor/ stabilization stays constant. Breathe freely.

H. Stand up again.
- Push laterally (sideways) against an immovable object again with your right hand.
- How does this movement compare to before? Do you have a clearer sense of how to use your legs to stabilize your pelvis in space?
- Try initiating the movement of pushing leftward with your right hand from your legs and pelvis as if turning your pelvis to the left, slightly preceding your hand push.

Fig. 6.64 Log rolling from side to side.

- Do the same thing pushing rightward with your left hand. How do you organize your pelvis to push sideways? Try this with your feet close together and your knees straight. How powerful or stable does this feel?
- Try this with your feet wider apart, with your knees softly bent, with your tailbone pointed toward the

ground and with your lower belly and pelvic floor engaged in stabilizing your back on top of your pelvis. How powerful or stable does this feel?

- Try this from a split stance and from half-kneeling.
- Stand sideways to a wall and push your shoulder into it. Push sideways and feel how you can use your legs to initiate and power this movement.

Dead Bug Roll – pushing laterally to assess static pelvic stability

Because we already have a sense of what kinds of activity might create lateral stresses, let's explore for a moment ways of clinically assessing and ways of facilitating lateral stability and the awareness needed to identify lateral stresses.

The initial dynamic baseline in this lesson is to push laterally against an immovable object with the pushing hand at shoulder height. This is a nice self-assessment tool. In the office, you can simulate this movement by having your sitting or standing student place the palms of her hands together and extend her arms forward at shoulder height. From here, you can press laterally against her hands and have her resist. It's going to be hard to assess multifidus contractions from here, but you might be able to manage a transverse abdominis palpation.

What you might also do is to observe visually for movement of the pelvis in space, even if the movement is small or fleeting. If the pelvis is not stabilized on the legs, the likelihood is that the intersegmental stabilizers are not fully engaged either. The arthrokinematic spinal and hip musculatures are both likely to be wired into this tonic stabilization loop of the CNS – excitation and inhibition patterns are probably intertwined.

If you are pushing against her hands from her left, she needs to push to the left. If all she does is pushes with her arms without torso or pelvic stabilization, her whole pelvis and torso turns to the right (activation of the shoulder horizontal abductors). If she adds in her right internal and her left internal obliques to assist in turning her torso to the left but doesn't stabilize her pelvis on her legs, her pelvis will twist to the right and a left rotation stress is created at the lower back. Something has to stabilize the pelvis in space; it might as well be the legs, because they are attached to the floor.

Clinically, you can assess this lateral push in standing on feet or knees, any of the squatting or kneeling families, floor or chair sitting, or lying down. In standing, have your students compare stability with feet close together and knees straight to having feet wide apart and knees bent. Have them stand with their pelvis and back on a wall and push; use the wall as a proprioceptive reference point. Do this same thing in sitting, or even have them cross one leg over the other to help clarify to them the importance of Using the Legs to control lateral stresses even in sitting.

In supine, have your student resist lateral movement (push against one or both hands held at shoulder height, or have them hold the pole crosswise in front at shoulder height) with legs long and again with legs bent. With legs long, they are not in a good position to resist rotational movement of the pelvis. When pushing her hands leftward against resistance, we can expect her pelvis to roll or twist on the floor to the right as a result of the action of the opposite-side internal and external abdominal obliques. If the legs are not in a good position to stabilize the pelvis, the back twists.

Do again with legs bent and cue to push feet into floor to stabilize. Cue to push feet into the floor or to push the right foot *outward* on the floor to counteract this twist. This is analogous to the supine facilitation of weight-in-front stressors we did as an experiment earlier in the chapter. Contrast by trying this with your legs bent and with your feet off the floor to further appreciate the role the legs play in lateral stabilization of the lower back – work your multifidi as much as you like and see how far it gets you in this position!

Use this as a home stabilization drill by having them press their pole or push one hand out laterally against wall, heavy furniture or a doorframe. Coordinate intersegmental stabilizers, hip abductors and abdominal obliques with upper extremities and a manipulation function to achieve the three levels of stabilization: arthrokinematic stability, stabilization of the pelvis on the legs and stabilization of the torso on the pelvis. Cue proprioceptive awareness of muscle effort of the three muscle systems, bring to upright positions as described below, and suggest specific applications to daily life.

These types of isometric stability drill simulate situations in which you are resisting movement imposed on you through external forces. Centrifugal forces (going around a corner in a car), resisting being pushed (stand in a flowing river, maintaining your territory under the basketball rim, resisting the impatient tug of your daughter's hand) and pushing against an immovable object (using a screwdriver to bore into the wall) are examples of static rotational stability. However, we also need to consider dynamic rotational stability.

Moving laterally to assess dynamic pelvic stability

Pushing laterally to move an object laterally in space is very different from holding your position against an outside source. Although the stabilization strategies are similar in that they blend the intersegmental, pelvic and torso stabilizing musculatures, there is an important difference.

When pushing laterally to move an object, engagement of the transverse abdominis/multifidi and the abdominal obliques is the same: they still stabilize the vertebrae relative to each other and the chest relative to the pelvis. What is different is what happens at the hip joints. When moving laterally, we want the pelvis to be able to move laterally in the direction we are pushing. This is needed to reduce rotational strains on the lower back. Let's get on the floor to illustrate this.

Lie on your back on the floor, bend your knees up to place your feet on the floor and reach both hands forward toward the ceiling. With your arms at shoulder height, place the palms of your hands together. This arrangement of your arms creates a long, skinny triangle. Keep your palms and fingertips precisely together and don't allow your elbows to bend as you tilt your triangle to the left. What most people will do is to twist their shoulders and upper body to the left and keep their pelvis where it is on the floor. Use as an assessment tool with students, observing whether this intention to move distally (hands) elicits a proximal response (rolling the pelvis on the floor in the same direction as the tilting triangle).

Let them have at it a few times, direct their attention to how they are doing it and how it feels, then direct them to use their legs. Cue to roll pelvis on the floor to the left, rolling the torso like a log that matches the amount the chest and shoulders roll to what the pelvis can do. Make sure knees stay pointed to the ceiling and feet stay flat on the floor; don't allow the knees to tilt in and out. This movement requires rotational movement of the pelvis on top of stable legs and is just the movement we need in standing to push an object laterally.

Repeat the movement of rolling the pelvis and torso like a log and tilting the triangle to the left several times, then switch to tilting the triangle to the right. Compare and contrast the two sides. Next, replace your triangle with your pole. While still lying on your back with knees bent up, hold the pole with both hands straight out in front of you. The pole is vertical and one hand is farther up the pole than the other. Tilt the pole to the left, slowly, and appreciate the enhanced awareness of lateral stability this provides. This constraint of tilting a relatively heavy object with a long lever arm to the side in this position requires the coordination of all three layers of stability.

Repeat several times to the left, and then switch to tilting the pole and rolling like a log to the right. Compare and contrast the two sides, then alternate. Increase speed if control and safety are demonstrated. Substitute dumbbells or other dense object for the pole, or substitute a large ball or an imaginary beach ball hugged to the chest for triangle. This is a great position to start training your students in how to recognize and control dynamic rotational stresses. Progress to vertical orientations.

Create a link to upright postures by moving your supine student close to a wall. Put them up close to the wall so the outside of one knee and thigh can be against the wall. Cue to press out into the wall with the hip abductors on that side, and use descriptive language to bring the student's attention to the three layers of stability. Cue to press out against you with the pole or triangle arms, both isometrically and by allowing movement of the pole or arms in space.

Next, have your student sit in a chair without armrests that is pushed up against a wall. Have her sit in the chair so the outside of her right thigh and right knee are against the wall. Tuck a pole under her left arm and have her hold it with both hands shotgun style, or use triangle arms.

Cue her to push hands or the end of the pole against you to the left. Have her hold while you push, the cue to move hands or pole in space against your resistance. Resist in same direction, coming back to simulate pushing laterally to control movement of an object laterally (think eccentric/lengthening contractions). Or, resist movement in opposite direction (Fig. 6.65). Progress by moving away from the wall and performing the same drill.

What is different about being away from the wall? The wall can't provide a stable place for the knee and thigh to press out against any more. We just added another two degrees of freedom and another two degrees of complexity to pushing an object laterally. The knees and feet now need to be stabilized. In particular, the stabilizing presence of the hamstrings and peroneus longus is needed. We will defer discussion of facilita-

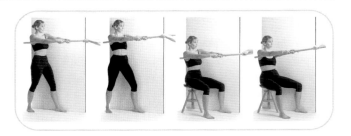

Fig. 6.65 Simulation of lateral stressor – facilitation of lateral stability through hip abductor activation. Progress by moving away from the wall.

tion techniques for foot and knee stability until the next chapter. In particular, look to the Rolling the Foot and Horsing Around lessons for exploration of hip, knee and foot coordination in lateral movements or lateral stability. Have the student practice this movement at home with an assistant or pushing against a doorframe, heavy couch, etc.

Use the pole in a similar way in standing. Stand in a split stance with left leg forward and right leg back (right split stance) and with the outside of the left thigh and knee against a wall. Use triangle arms or hold pole shotgun style under right arm with both hands and resist movement to the right. Use variations as described with sitting (Fig. 6.65). Progress by moving away from the wall as before.

Another great place to initially assess and train lateral stability initially is in side-lying. The first movement of the next variation of this lesson asks you to lie on your side and lift the top arm. Make glaringly obvious to your students the advantages of using the bottom leg to push out into the floor by adding manual resistance to the lifting arm. Cue them to push both the bottom leg and the bottom arm into the floor to assist with stability.

Observe for their ability to differentiate hip abductors from back extensors. Start a home program by having them do this while holding a weight out with this long lever arm. The rest of the lesson is designed to facilitate this pushing outward with the legs to stabilize the pelvis and to blend this pelvic stabilization with intersegmental stability and control of gross torso-on-pelvis movement. Be sure to train your student to be both immovable object and irresistible force.

Opening the book

In variations B and C, lie on your side and lift one arm. This is another dynamic baseline that should become easier and clearer as the lesson progresses. The review of breath and pelvic floor facilitation of intersegmental stabilizer muscles is performed here in yet another position, another relationship to gravity.

Where this so far simple movement gets a bit more complex is when you have to start coordinating lifting your arm with lifting the top leg. The metaphor of opening a book can be a good one here in terms of getting simultaneous torso log rolling and extremity differentiation. Cue the simultaneous pushing out of both knees: the weightbearing leg pushes out into the floor and the lifting leg pushes outward toward the ceiling. This is a very important Lego piece.

Simultaneous abductor engagement gives you the ultimate in control over frequently alternating or unpredictable lateral stresses. It is very useful for lumbopelvic stability. Simultaneous abductor engagement, along with a slight weight-shift backward (simulation of falling back) and a differentiation/inhibition of the lower back extensors, is the ultimate in pushing the pelvis towards vertical on the legs. It is very useful for controlling postural anterior tilt.

This involves the use of the upper gluteus maximus, the gluteus medius and minimus and the tensor fascia latae. Simultaneous abductor engagement also has many beneficial effects on the knees and feet, which we will explore in the next chapter. This is a skill well worth learning and using and it is a skill rarely found in the general population.

As we progress from this stabilization chapter to the next chapter on legs, we will be following the trail of the hip abductors and the control of the feet on the floor. The first few lessons in that chapter will work on coordinating the hip abductors with the peroneals to stabilize the feet on the floor; these can be thought of as additional lumbar stabilization lessons.

Rolling an imaginary ball between arms and thighs

Lie again on your left side as before in variations D and E, stabilize your back and lift your right arm and right leg so that they are parallel to the floor. Keep this distance and keep both arm and leg lifted as you simultaneously move your right hand and right knee alternately forward and back.

This rolling of your pelvis, torso, shoulders and head forward and back on the floor with the leg and arm lifted and parallel to the floor encourages log rolling and lumbar stability along with extremity differentiation. Imagine rolling a ball back and forth between your arms to direct movements of chest and upper back, and imagine rolling a ball back and forth between your thighs to direct movements of your pelvis and lower back. Have we seen this movement before?

Review variation C in Side-lie Transitions for muscular analysis. The top leg abductors are doing shortening and lengthening contractions, and these reciprocal movements are stretching and strengthening the same muscle. If the top leg was resting its weight on the bottom leg, the bottom leg abductors would be doing shortening contractions to roll back and the bottom leg adductors would be doing shortening contractions to roll forward. These reciprocal movements would also coordinate the antagonists.

Because the top leg is lifted, the weight of the front leg shifts the center of mass far enough forward to create a rolling-forward movement all the way through the range of movement. In this scenario, the bottom leg abductors also do alternating shortening and lengthening contractions that mirror the shortening and lengthening contractions of the top leg. Think of a dance or a cooperative tug of war. Both abductors are constantly engaged, but as one shortens the other one lengthens.

What would happen if this particular coordination of the abductors were to occur in supine? Lie supine with legs bent up and with palms together in front at shoulder height to make a triangle. This time, instead of keeping your triangle precisely intact, slide your right hand past your left hand and toward the ceiling. Did you push your right foot into the floor and lift your right hip? Use as an assessment tool with your student. Did she reach forward by pushing from the legs or by rotating her spine?

Cue to roll pelvis to the left and move torso like a log. Repeat with right hand reaching several times, switch to the left and alternate. Progress this lessonette by doing the same movement with a dumbbell in one hand, then the other. Use two weights and alternate. Blend with unilateral 'bench press' by bending and straightening elbows. Use a pole in one hand and push toward the ceiling with the same log-rolling movement of pelvis and torso, making sure to keep knees upright and feet centered on the floor. Manually resist movement of pole toward ceiling to simulate one-handed push. Manually resist movement of pole away from the ceiling to simulate one-handed pull. Cue awareness of accurate use of legs to move pelvis and of accurate recruitment of obliques, transverse abdominis and multifidi to stabilize torso and vertebrae.

Bring to standing and repeat this process of simulated one-handed pushing and pulling with back and pelvis against a wall and feet a foot or more away from the wall. Cue to press feet to roll pelvis and low back to neutral, then to log roll pelvis and torso on the wall in coordination with one hand reaching forward. Progress this lessonette with manual resistance, pulleys or elastics, and by moving away from the wall. Blend with similar drills from half-kneel and Split Stance Bending lessons.

Instruct your students in recognition and control of rotational stresses, but counsel them to abstain from said stresses if possible. You are almost always going to be better off pushing or pulling straight forward or back than you are going to be pushing or pulling laterally. You are almost always going to be better off pushing or pulling with two hands rather than with one. Motor planning sometimes means figuring out a way to avoid something.

Pushing out to tear the carpet

Stand up for a moment. Put your feet slightly wider than your shoulders and bend your knees, then rock your weight backward on your feet to sit back in a high horse stance. Imagine you are simultaneously straddling a horse, standing on a sheet of ice and wanting to slide your feet away from each other. If you did this on ice, you would do the splits (an unfortunate event for most of us).

Because you are presumably standing on a surface with some friction, your feet won't slide away from each other. Think of trying to push your feet away from each other as if trying to tear the carpet between your feet. Your hip abductors will kick in and cancel each other out in terms of lateral movement. Palpate your upper gluteals along and just below the rim of the iliac crest and your TFL for activation.

This is analogous to lying on your side and lifting the top leg without allowing the pelvis to roll either forward or back. While standing and doing this simultaneous pushing-out movement, notice if there is any posterior tilting movement of your pelvis. This is what will happen if you are able to differentiate the hip abductors (especially the upper gluteals, along with an ability to differentiate upper from mid and lower gluteals) from the back extensors; this is easier said than done for most people.

Palpate lower back extensors as you do this, or whip out your biofeedback machine to facilitate an awareness of how to accomplish these differentiations. Go back to side-lying and lift the top leg several times without allowing yourself to roll forward or back. Is there any element of posterior tilt here? Are the back extensors quiet? Palpate or hook up to biofeedback. Try this movement in side-lying with your legs long. Lift the top leg and allow your pelvis to posteriorly rotate if you can.

Don't force it to happen through abdominal contraction. With both of these side-lying movements, try pressing back (not out into the floor) with the bottom leg before lifting. This is like doing a side-lying pelvic tilt with your gluteals and hamstrings, using the friction of the floor against the outside of the weightbearing leg as a substitute for having the sole of the foot on the floor.

Come back to standing in a high horse stance again. Push out with both feet. Can you allow your pelvis to rotate posteriorly? Keep your abductors engaged and pushing against each other as you turn your pelvis alternately right and left. Allow your weight to shift a bit in the direction you are turning. This movement is analogous to lying on your side with your leg lifted and rolling forward and back with your lifted leg parallel to the ground. Anticipate more information on this movement in the next chapter (Box 6.13).

These are simultaneous mirrored abductor contractions: your legs are tossing your pelvis from side to side. This is a version of driving with your brakes on, but in this case it is a good thing. This is what martial artists are doing when they say they are grounding or rooting themselves. It is very stable, very dynamic, and very satisfying at a very deep and primitive level.

Rolling like a log to your back

Lie on your left side again in variations F and G. Lift your arm and leg again and experiment with lifting the leg and arm higher toward the ceiling, both with rolling your pelvis and with torso rolled forward and rolling back. Lifting your leg while rolled forward facilitates end-range horizontal abduction of the lifted leg and a fuller shortening of those muscles.

It is also harder because of this, and because of shifting your center of mass forward. Lifting your leg while rolling back facilitates separating your legs and lengthening the adductors. The adductor of the bottom leg in particular is lengthened through

the action of rolling the pelvis back on the weightbearing leg, by the reciprocal inhibition effect of firing the abductors on that side, and by using those bottom leg adductors in a lengthening contraction to decelerate your fall backward.

If you can lift the top leg close enough to vertical to shift your center of mass in back of your fulcrum, you have created a situation in which you have first a lengthening contraction of the adductors to keep from rolling all the way on to your back and then a shortening contraction to start your roll back on to your side. Once your center of mass has shifted back in front of the bottom hip again, your bottom leg abductors take over to decelerate your fall back forward in a lengthening contraction. This is analogous to what happens when swinging a baseball bat or doing some other ballistic turning movement.

The abductors of the side towards which you are turning do lengthening contractions to slow then stop the movement of the pelvis. You have to simultaneously use your opposite internal and external obliques to keep your torso from continuing to rotate on your pelvis and your intersegmental stabilizers to maintain intersegmental stabilization. We might as well train them to all work together.

Putting the whole thing together to roll from your side all the way to your back with your arms and legs lifted (the Dead Bug), then back to your side, then alternating from side to side, completes the lesson. This allows for back-to-back comparison and weak side correction, and for association with a real-life functional context.

At the end of the lesson, stand up again and repeat your dynamic baselines. Were you able to translate what you learned in side-lie to standing and pushing sideways? Push laterally against an immovable object again with your right hand with your feet close together and your knees straight. How powerful or stable does this feel?

Try this with your feet wider apart, with your knees softly bent, with your tailbone pointed toward the ground, with a high horizon and with your lower belly and pelvic floor engaged in stabilizing your back on top of your pelvis. How powerful or stable does this feel? Try this in sitting, half-kneel, etc. Sustain this for a few minutes – clarify which muscles are engaged and how competent they are by working to some level of fatigue.

Drill it in – facilitating awareness of lateral stresses and control

We have already described ways of using a pole to facilitate awareness and control of rotational stresses in supine, side-lie, half-kneel and split stances. Further variations include using the pole in other ways while standing. Place the pole horizontally across your upper back, holding it with both hands yoke style. Have your student stand with both feet together, knees straight or locked, tail lifted, lower belly soft – however many details you want to put into it. Stand at one end of the pole and push that end forward, backward or alternating (Fig. 6.66).

Observe for, and have her feel proprioceptively, the stability of her pelvis on her legs and of her torso on her pelvis. Repeat the test in a horse stance: feet wide, knees soft, pelvis near vertical, intersegmental stabilizers engaged, etc. Use variations of isometric, eccentric, concentric and alternating resist-

---

Box 6.13 Dead Bug Roll

Training the obliques to control movement of trunk on pelvis – training the hip abductors to control pelvis on the legs
Facilitating proprioceptive awareness of lateral stresses
Manual simulation of lateral stresses – cue to control all three layers of stability

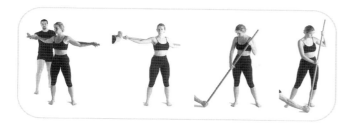

Fig. 6.66 More simulation of lateral stressors – facilitating an awareness of three layers of stability.

ance here. Instruct in a home program pushing against an assistant or an immovable object.

Simulate ballistic movements by more rapidly swinging the yoke from side to side. Be very careful here: it's very easy to allow too much movement. Start with small and slow movements and progress to faster but still small. Progressively widen her feet to come to low horse stance. Cue her on attention to sensory information from legs, feet and belly. Blend into walking.

Stand in a horse stance and hold the pole vertically with both hands broom style. With her left hand on top and her right hand below, push the bottom of the broom to the left and resist manually against a heavy or immovable object or by friction against the floor (Fig. 6.66). Observe for initiation or initial stabilization of the pelvis in space. Does she organize this movement from the ground up or from the top down?

Relate functionally to raking and sweeping and have her use these activities, with focused proprioceptive awareness, as part of her home exercise assignments. Use vacuuming in a similar fashion after having trained her in one-hand pushing and pulling stabilization with a pole in half-kneeling and split stance postures. Design lessons around bending and rotating movements such as bowling, pushing a heavy box laterally on the floor, or pulling out a low, heavy drawer. Start by teaching the patterns, then add in resistance with pole, weights or elastics.

Lumbothoracic differentiation

So far we have discussed mainly the relationships between the legs, pelvis and lower back. There is another very important relationship for the lower back, and that is its relationship to the chest/ribs/thoracic spine. For most full arch types this ability to differentiate the lumbar from the thoracic spine is perhaps less crucial than for other types. For full-archers, rolling the pelvis posteriorly and flexing the torso will probably resonate throughout the whole spine.

We will be doing mostly global torso flexion with these folks (with differentiating hip extension). For the full-rounds, we'll probably emphasize global torso extension (with differentiating hip flexion). A word of caution here: many full-rounders in sitting also overextend in standing and may be closet multisegmental unstables. Make an accurate determination as to whether your student is also unstable into extension. If so, then treat more like a half-archer.

Half arch folk present a very common problem. Global torso flexion movements initially are great (in conjunction with differentiating hip extension), but we can't just leave it at that.

- The chronically flexed thoracic spine plays havoc with the health of the neck, shoulder girdles and glenohumeral joints. If we try global extension movements to reduce postural and movement strains on the neck and shoulders, your half-archers will extend at the places of least resistance – the neck and low back.

- Once these folks with upper body movement impairments and tissue strain are upright again they will default back to lumbar and cervical extension for postural support, and will default back to lumbar extension when trying to integrate looking and reaching upward movements with the rest of the torso. They will need to learn differentiated thoracic extension (from both lumbar and cervical areas).

- The chronically flexed thoracic spine violates the good housekeeping rule. Any movements requiring torso extension will happen disproportionately at the lumbar and cervical spine.

- The chronically flexed thoracic spine violates the skeletal weightbearing rule. When asking your half arch folk to roll their pelvis posteriorly toward neutral in a sitting position, as their pelvis comes to vertical and their lumbar spine comes to neutral they are going to feel that they are slumping (which they are). These folks like to think they are sitting or standing upright, but what they are really doing is to let the chest fall backward then compensate for that by rolling the pelvis way forward. The lumbar spine is extending more because the thoracic spine can't.

- These folks very commonly have problems in both the low back (extension related) and in the neck and shoulder girdles (thoracic flexion related). If you don't want Peter to have to pay for Paul's mistake, you'll have to learn how to facilitate the skill of a differentiated spine.

Coincidentally, I happen to have some ideas on how you might accomplish this.

Differentiated Back Bends

Variations

A. Lie on your back on the floor with your legs down long and your arms resting on the ground somewhere below shoulder height.

- Notice how your hips, back and shoulders contact the ground.

- What parts of your spine touch the floor and what parts are lifted away from the floor? How many of your vertebrae are on the floor?

- How flat is your pelvis on the floor? How is it balanced from side to side?

- How flat are your shoulders and neck? What part of your head is on the ground? Is that contact point

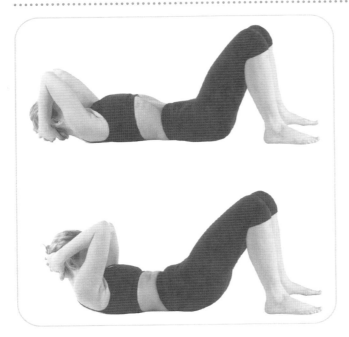

Fig. 6.67 Lifting then lowering head and tailbone – lift both ends of the spine to flex globally.

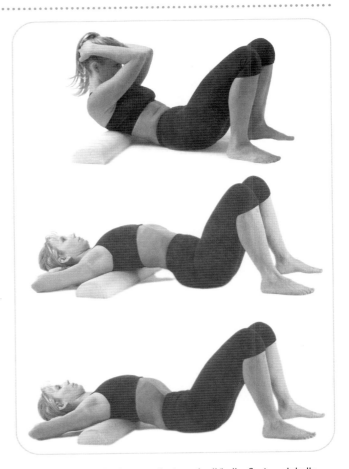

Fig. 6.68 Lying on back over roller/towel roll/ball – flexing globally – extending globally – then rolling pelvis upward to flatten lower back only.

closer to the top of your head or closer to the base of your spine?

B. Lie on your back with your knees bent up. Have your feet about shoulder width apart. Interlace your fingers and put both hands behind your head (Fig. 6.67).

- Begin to make a small movement to lift simultaneously your tailbone and the top of your head away from the floor – lift your head and tail. Return both head and tail to the floor and repeat several times (Fig. 6.67).

- Gradually enlarge the movement – make sure head and pelvis lift the same amount. Try to lift from both ends in such a way that the vertebrae in your spine both lift and lower back down again sequentially.

- Lift and lower one vertebra at a time, as if lifting and lowering individual links in a chain.

- You could imagine a puppeteer holding strings attached to the top of your head and the tip of your tailbone. Imagine lifting both ends high enough to place all your weight on one vertebra exactly in the middle of your spine.

C. Lie on your back again with your knees bent up and your hands interlaced behind your head. This time, place a half foam roller (or small ball, rolled up towel or blanket) under the vertebrae in the middle of your spine (Fig. 6.68).

- Keep your pelvis on the floor this time as you again lift your tailbone to roll your pelvis upward on the floor as you lift your head farther away from the floor. This is the same movement as before, except that you keep your pelvis on the ground.

- As you lower head and tail back down again, let your back arch backward and roll your pelvis downward a bit on the floor as if moving to press your tailbone toward the ground (Fig. 6.68).

- Alternate back and forth between lifting head and tail to round all along your back, then lowering your head and tail to arch all along your back. Repeat this several times.

- Now lower your head and tail toward the floor and stay there. Keep your head and shoulders where they are and gently roll your pelvis upward on the floor; gently lift your tailbone (Fig. 6.68).

- This is a movement that asks you to stay arched or backward bent through your mid back while you simultaneously round or flatten your lower back to the floor. Make sure you do this rolling movement of your pelvis on the floor by pressing your feet and using your legs.

- Don't tighten your belly to flatten your back! Do this several times with the roller (or ball, towels, etc.) across your middle vertebrae.

- Change the position of the roller on your back and do the same thing. Move the roller farther up your back and pivot around a different section of your spine.

- Do the same basic movements in this position – move the roller farther up again and repeat, and so on. Try this sequence of movements at several places along your spine.

- Come off the roller and lie flat on your back again. How are you contacting the floor in comparison to when you started? How flat? How long? How wide? How balanced from side to side?

- If you'd like to try some extra credit, get back on the roller again, drop your head and hands toward the floor and roll your pelvis diagonally on the floor rather than straight up.

- Press with the right foot to roll your pelvis up and to the left. Press with your left foot to roll your pelvis up and to the right.

- Add in a Wishbone movement of lifting one foot if you would like to. Try this at different segments along your back. Reassess your contact with the floor again.

Brief discussion – Differentiated Back Bends

This lesson starts with a global torso flexion movement, lifting your pelvis and head off the floor at the same time. By directing our student to lift sequentially along the spine in each direction, we are asking for even distribution of movement into flexion. By directing the student to lower each end sequentially, we are asking for lumbar and cervical flexion with thoracic extension. Get out a model of a spine and try this out.

Round the whole thing into a full round and place the middle of the spine on the floor with the two ends lifted. Then press the two ends toward the floor and notice the thoracic spine move into extension relative to a starting position. This movement alone, when performed accurately, is a great one for our half arch folks. Combined with the roller or other toy, it is the strategy of choice for mobilizing the thoracic spine/chest/ribcage into extension while protecting the low back and neck.

The basic principle has already been introduced. Look back to Sitting Circles II and Pelvic Tilts. Place a roller, towel or ball under the thoracic spine or just laterally along the posterior ribs while lying supine. Gravity is assisting in mobilizing the thorax into extension while the legs work to roll the pelvis into posterior tilt. This creates the ever-so-elusive nonhabitual differentiated pattern of thoracic extension and lumbar flexion. By lowering the head to the floor with the chin tucked and the back of the neck pushing towards the floor, this also encourages that other ever-so-elusive nonhabitual differentiated pattern of thoracic extension and cervical flexion.

A word of caution to this tale – use your legs or you will fail

There is a very important detail to this technique: you have to be very clear about Using the Legs to roll the pelvis into posterior tilt. Many people will try to roll the pelvis with the abdominals, but this defeats the purpose. The idea is to get upper belly and anterior intercostal inhibition so the thorax can extend. They must be inhibited for this to work! Train your students well in pushing the pelvis upward with the legs without the toy first.

Palpate or have them palpate just below the bottom of the sternum to make sure the abdominals are not kicking in. Develop an eye for seeing the subtle lowering of the chest, the raising of the shoulders and the turtling of the neck that accompanies the use of the belly. Try this deliberate error yourself several times while on the roller, and then be clear about using your legs to move your pelvis. Compare and contrast the results.

Many subvariations of this basic technique are possible. Placement of the toy asymmetrically, rolling the pelvis diagonally, or side-bending the head/neck/upper back to the right or left on the toy creates multiplanar differentiations. A larger toy gives more generalized movement, and a smaller toy can be more specific to individual vertebrae. Sitting on a stool or backward on a chair with your back against a wall and placing a ball or roller between wall and mid back is a positional variation of the same basic movement. Use hands behind your head as in supine. Be sure to use your legs to push the pelvis back on the seat into posterior tilt.

Although this belly-up technique is great for mobilizing the mid back into extension, we also need ways to strengthen the mid back extensors without going into lumbar extension. This basic technique has also been described earlier – we called it the hamstring constraint. This belly-down technique involves bending over from a variety of positions far enough to significantly flex one or both hip joints. By moving to the end-range of hip extension we are using the hamstrings, gluteals and short and stubbies to constrain further movement of the pelvis into anterior tilt (Box 6.14).

We then lift the upper body and head in the contexts of orientation, manipulation or transitions to direct spinal extension to the mid back. Positional possibilities include bending over from a sit-kneeling position, side-sitting, long sitting, sitting on a low stool, chair sitting, half-kneeling, split stance, horse stance or modified plantigrade. Be creative and make up diagonal variations; focus on right or left thoracic extensors and posterior intercostals.

Create rotational differentiations with the corkscrew movements of the pelvis in TA Leg Lifts. Keep your lower back against the floor to constrain lumbar rotation and to funnel that movement up to the lumbothoracic junction and thoracic spine. Modify the Dead Bug Roll, or look ahead to Heel to Toe by drawing the lifted leg toward your chest instead of toward the ceiling. Roll your chest and shoulders back to rotate

---

Box 6.14 Differentiated Back Bends

Using toys to mobilize thoracic spine into extension – Using the Legs to push the lumbar spine into flexion

Rotational and side-bending variations – unilateral thoracic extension

Using the hamstring constraint to strengthen the thoracic extensors without lumbar extension

Moving toy to low back for the rare half round differentiation

through your mid torso, but keep pressing the bottom leg out and down into hip extension and abduction to posteriorly rotate your pelvis and flexion-lock your lumbar spine to prevent rotation from happening there.

Look ahead to Horsing Around and Rolling the Foot and use supine and standing/leaning back against a wall to provide a constraint and a reference point for your pelvis and lower back. Use triangle arms or imagined beach ball. Roll ball or tilt triangle left and right, but use legs to posteriorly tilt pelvis and to stabilize pelvis and lower back on the floor or wall to funnel rotational movement to thoracic spine.

The rare nonhabitual differentiation

There is another differentiated spinal pattern besides the half arch: the half round. Although this is much more rare than its mirror image, you will probably see some folks with this organization in your office occasionally. I tend to work more with global torso extension patterns (with differentiated hip flexion), but will occasionally use the toy technique in a slightly different way.

Instead of placing the toy at the mid back to encourage thoracic extension and lumbar flexion, place it in the low back and encourage thoracic flexion by placing head and hands together and lifting the head to look toward the feet. The ball creates lumbar extension and constrains lumbar flexion; combined with lifting head and shoulders, we get a nonhabitual differentiated pattern.

Movement model for treating low back pain

How do we treat our students with lower back pain? We use exercise, electrical modalities, massage, mobilization, orthotics, manipulation, acupuncture, heating pads, strain/counterstrain, myofascial release, biofeedback, injections, desensitization, meditation, mechanical traction devices, guided imagery, drugs, braces, visceral manipulation, ice, nutritional supplements, magnets, mental health counseling, taping, surgery and desperate appeals to a higher power.

We might hold to a structural model, a medical model (disease or injury), an energetic model, a muscle imbalance model, a chemical/nutritional model or a metaphysical/emotional model. Everywhere you go, there are chiropractors and physical therapists, massage practitioners, physicians, acupuncturists, mystics and just plain old quacks who are busy and prosperous working with people with lower back pain. It is endemic in our society. Products that are touted as cures for back pain include beds, topical crèmes, chairs, TENS units, braces, arch supports, shoes and an assortment of magic pills.

Why is so much time and money spent on solutions to low back pain? Because it afflicts so very many people and because the causes and solutions are not very clear-cut. Back pain isn't like malaria, with a proscribed set of symptoms, an identifiable bug, a specific drug regimen and you are good to go. With back pain, most people are looking for the magic bullet, the one thing that can stop their pain. This is the medical model of the malaria example.

Looking for the fix – or putting the ball in their court

One leg is longer than the other; I need a heel lift or orthotic. A vertebra is out of place; I need a spinal adjustment. My disc is blown; I need surgery. My ligaments are irritated; I need an anti-inflammatory. My energy meridians are clogged; I need acupuncture. My cartilage is deteriorating; I need chondroitin. My muscles are weak; I need to lift weights. My posture is bad; I need tape. My attitude is poor; I need a vacation. All of these solutions have worked for some people, even if only anecdotally. On the other hand, none of these solutions has worked for everyone.

Many people come to see us about their lower back pain. Many of them make statements to the effect that they would do anything to feel better and to be able to do the things they want to again. What they often mean is that they will spend the money, put in the time, take the pill religiously, wear the device, buy the product or come to your office five times a week. What doesn't often cross their minds is that we would ask them to begin to pay attention to how they move and how they hold themselves, and to pay attention to how are they misusing their equipment and to learn new ways of doing familiar tasks. We don't always ask them to both take responsibility for their pain and take credit for their improvement.

Whether your framework for thinking about back pain is medical, structural or energetic, movement education can be a valuable adjunct. Because we are dealing with pain from musculoskeletal tissues and because the role of the musculoskeletal system is movement, it makes sense to have a well thought-out and flexible movement education program as part of your treatment regimen. It is not enough to say you need strong stomach muscles to protect your back. When and how you apply that strength, and recognition of functional context and categories of stressors, is needed as well.

It is not enough to give someone a knee-to-chest exercise because lumbar flexion feels good. This global movement pattern is not as applicable to real life. It is not enough to train someone in intersegmental stabilization if their pelvis is sloshing about on top of their legs. There is unlikely to be arthokinematic stability of the vertebrae in the absence of stability of the pelvis. It is not enough to instruct someone to sit with their hips and knees at 90°. Supporting the vertical position of the pelvis from the legs rather than from the torso is much more important than geometrical tidiness.

It is not enough to tell someone to lift with their legs. What does that feel like and what part of my legs do I use? It is not enough to tell someone to stand with one foot up on a stool. If they are not pushing with that foot, their pelvis can and probably will still fall forward into anterior tilt. It is not enough to demonstrate or show a picture of proper posture or movement.

They have to experience it and judge for themselves whether it feels better. There is no one magic muscle that, if stronger, guarantees success in stabilization. Stabilization of the back is a motor skill requiring both a new set of physical skills and a more attentive and educated proprioceptive system.

Our role is to facilitate self-awareness and motor skills

We need to give our students access to skills and information. Pattern and effort recognition skills. Recognition of stressors. Principles of distribution of movement and use of the legs to control the pelvis. Help them find a new and improved spinal neutral. Train them in different functional categories. Help them to blend intersegmental stability and phasic mobility. Guide them toward physical activities consistent with nonhabitual patterns of movement for them. Be specific and picky with your exercises.

Educate them on a movement model of pain and the central role the student plays in the process. Help them with examples of how to preplan movements with recognition of categories of stressors. Emphasize the use of one or both upper extremities for weightbearing assistance, to add a stabilizing third or fourth point of contact, and to greatly widen the base of support for lifting, bending or leaning functions.

Although needles, manipulation and massage are things we do to people to help them feel better, we also need something we can do with people to help them to help themselves. We need to encourage them to take responsibility for their own comfort. With responsibility comes an enhanced feeling of control and a reduction in the feeling of powerlessness these folks may have. We also need to encourage them to find movements or get into positions that feel good for their back. They need to be able to experience pleasurable sensations from their back!

The main problems we run into when treating people with back pain are their inability to focus amidst the chaos of the rest of their lives and their unwillingness to look or feel different. The inertia of the CNS is such that, for the most part, people go about their daily lives in a proprioceptive fog. The nature of movement and postural patterns are such that, once established, awareness of them tends to fade into the background. People are not aware, even when you have shown them what they are doing multiple times in your office, that they are doing something they know is damaging.

It's not how you feel – it's how you look

They are simply not aware enough in the course of their busy day to recognize stressful behavior. How do you get someone to focus on what they are doing when there is not an immediate pain associated with it? Train them in pattern recognition, categories of stressors for that individual, and give them homework to find particular stressors in those categories. Lead your horse to water; it is then up to them to drink.

How do you get someone to accept looking differently? With any kind of low back instability, we are probably going to work towards a recalibration of neutral spine and towards different movement solutions to everyday functions. By definition, they will look different. One issue is looking different from how they usually move: postures will feel exaggerated and

wrong and movements will feel choreographed – 'That's just not me.' Another issue is looking different from everyone else.

The guy standing at the water cooler during break would rather suffer backache than to squat. The prim lady bending over to cut a rose would rather hurt than stick out her pelvis. What would people think if I stood with a low horse stance while washing my dishes or unloading my grocery cart? Won't people think me brazen if I let my pelvis move as I walk? Won't everyone stare at me if I stand in line at the cinema in a split stance? Would management kick me out if I were half-kneeling in their restaurant?

I want to feel better, I know the way I move contributes to my pain, but I want to look and move like everyone else (80% of whom also have back pain). I don't want to draw attention to myself by acting differently. What do you say to that? Assure them that most people are in such a kinesthetic fog that they don't notice what you are doing anyway? Model flamboyant movement in your office to let them know they aren't the only ones?

Assure them that they shouldn't care what other people think of them? Tell them to move differently only when there is no one else around? Send them to a psychotherapist to work through their issues? Why aren't things as straightforward as they are in school, books and continuing education classes? Why can't we just pretend we are working with organic machines? Why can't I just prescribe an exercise and have the muscle stay stronger or longer (Box 6.15)?

Why can't I correct a pelvic imbalance just once and have it stay? Why does she keep slouching every time I see her after I told her not to do so? Although machines would be a lot more predictable and easier to work with, people are far more interesting and require a far greater range of skills on the part of the practitioner. Embrace and enjoy the challenge!

Home program – the low back kata

In many styles of martial arts, practitioners learn and practice a prescribed series of movements called a form or kata. These kata put several movements together in a sequence and serve to prod the practitioner to further improve basic skills of stance, weight-shift, one-legged balance, integration of arms with pelvis and torso and so on. The movements simulate kicks, punches and blocks.

The lessons in this chapter provide a wealth of information and dozens of different movements. If we have our students continue to do everything we teach them, they will need to quit their day job and hire a housekeeper. We don't want to overwhelm them, but we don't want them to forget what they

---

Box 6.15 Low back kata

Compilation of summary movements from various lessons – not every movement is for everyone

Continuation on a home exercise program – keeping the student involved long term

Reinforce importance of frequent nonhabitual movement – and provide an exercise routine that does just that

have learned either. As you go through a series of lessons with your students, have them practice all or most of each lesson that you do, then pick one or two movements from that lesson to continue with even as you progress to the next lessons in the series.

A possible compilation of those summary movements is described in the following low back kata. All these movements are great for extension instabilities. Most of them work for multidirectional instabilities: just go slower and smaller and avoid side-sit twisted positions. Most of them work with flexion instabilities too, but with some modifications on use of legs as previously described. This is not a one-size-fits-all kata; use your clinical judgment.

Low back kata

Variations

A. Lie on your back with your legs down long and take a moment to do a quick scan of your contact against the floor.

- Feel the shape of your back and the balance of your pelvis from side to side. Take a couple of minutes to just feel before moving.

- Take a few minutes to direct movements of the breath and pelvic floor to reaccess your intersegmental stabilizers.

- Find your transverse abdominis and keep that as you breathe independently. Continue to hold this thread throughout the kata, except when resting.

B. Bend up your knees and roll your pelvis up and down on the floor.

- Roll up and down 8–12 times and take a couple of minutes to do it slowly. Try to roll from your legs. Emphasize your direction of comfort (Fig. 6.69).

C. Still on your back with both knees bent.

- Lift your left foot to reach your left knee up and out toward your left arm on the floor.

- Do this five times to this side, five times to the other side, and five times alternately from side to side (Fig. 6.70).

- Keep some part of your lower back pressed against the floor, but do let your pelvis roll from side to side on the floor.

D. Still on your back with both knees bent or up to lean back on elbows.

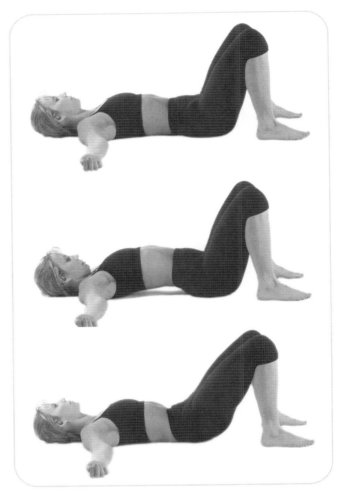

Fig. 6.69 Alternating rolling pelvis downward then upward on the floor.

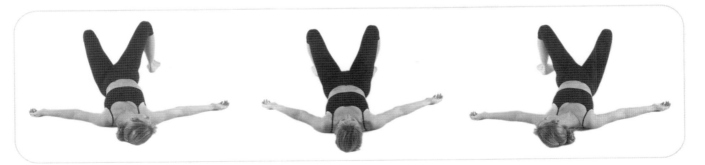

Fig. 6.70 Press one foot and lift the other – keep one side of lower back against the floor.

- Continue to lift one leg up and out, but now enlarge the movement to straighten your leg down long (Fig. 6.71).

- Straighten your knee and almost put your leg down long, but keep it lifted. Keep pressing with the other leg; keep some part of low back on the floor.

- Do this five to eight times on the left, then do the same thing to the right.

E. Lie on your back and lift both feet off the floor, one at a time. Reach both hands toward the ceiling, like a dead bug.

- Separate your arms and legs; open them like the covers on a book to slowly roll to your left side (Fig. 6.72).

- Roll your torso like a log and control the fall to your sides. Alternate rolling from left side to right side five to eight times in each direction.

F. Lie on your left side and hold on to your right knee with your right hand.

- Still holding your knee, roll yourself backward and pull your right knee toward your chest (Fig. 6.73).

- Roll forward and extend your right knee down and forward toward your left foot.

- Alternate back and forth between these two movements several times, then extend the movement of rolling forward and reaching your right knee toward your left foot to come up to sit.

- Do five times lying on left side and five times on right.

G. Hold your knee to roll yourself up to left side-sit, right foot behind.

- Place your hands in front of your left knee and slide first the right hand three to four times forward and back, then both hands forward and back (Fig. 6.74).

- Find a place where your back is neither round nor arched and keep it that same shape as you push up to sit.

- From sitting, lean back over again to place your hands or elbows on the floor. Keep your back neutral and control movement from left leg.

- Do the same thing to the other side. Do five to eight each side (Fig. 6.75).

H. From side-sitting position.

- Place the palms of your hands on the front of your thighs near your knees and keep them there.

- Alternate from left side-sit to right side-sit. Do this five times each side (Fig. 6.76).

- Continue the same movement, but straighten your legs down away from your pelvis as you round way back through the middle.

I. Come up to half-kneeling.

- Alternately slide right hand and left up and down the pole. Keep back neutral and bend and turn around your hips (Fig. 6.77).

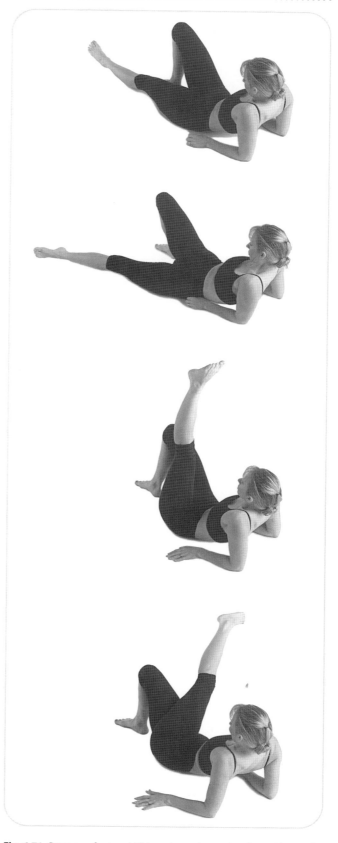

Fig. 6.71 Press one foot and lift long leg – then swing from side to side.

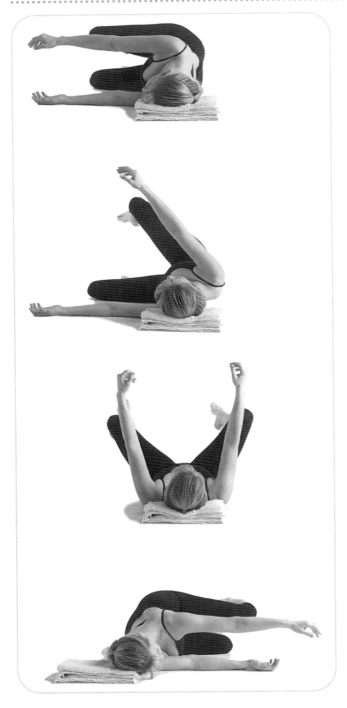

Fig. 6.72 Log rolling from side to side.

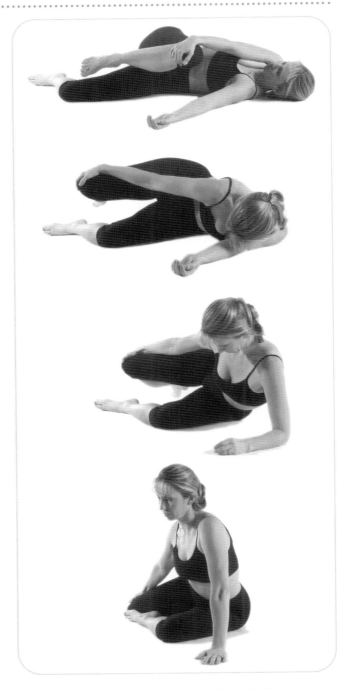

Fig. 6.73 Hold knee to transition from side-lie to side-sit.

- Do the same thing to the other side. Alternate five to eight times each, each side.

J. Come up to split stance.

- Alternately slide right hand and left up and down the pole. Keep back neutral and bend and turn around your hips (Fig. 6.78).

- Do the same thing to the other side. Alternate five to eight times each, each side.

K. Stand on telephone book or low stair.

- With your left foot on the riser, reach and slide your right foot back on the floor. Let yourself lean forward and turn to the left.

- Come back upright again and lift your right knee high toward your right shoulder. Or slide your right foot up the outside of your pole.

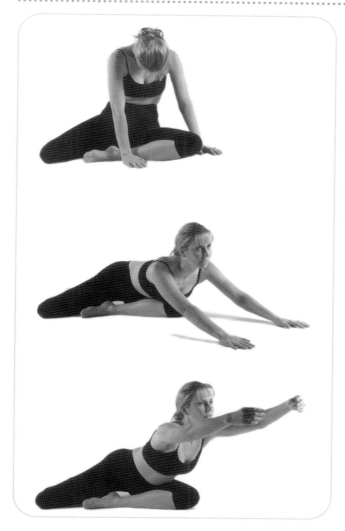

Fig. 6.74 Sliding one or both hands together forward and back – lift one or both for extra credit.

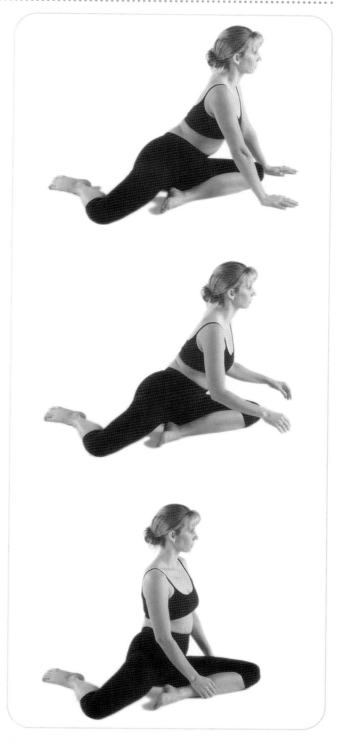

Fig. 6.75 Finding a neutral spine, then staying neutral while bending and coming upright.

- Do the same thing to the other side. Eight to 12 times to each side (Fig. 6.79).

L. Stand in a horse stance. Feet wide and parallel with knees slightly bent.

- Bend over to let your head and arms dangle toward the floor and press your feet outward from this position. Does your pelvis posteriorly rotate?

- Push outward to tuck your tail then progress by rolling up one vertebrae at a time to standing, making sure to keep your knees slightly bent.

- Roll your pelvis underneath and tuck your tail as you approach standing. Repeat three to six times (Fig. 6.80).

M. Stand in a horse stance. Feet wide and parallel with knees slightly bent.

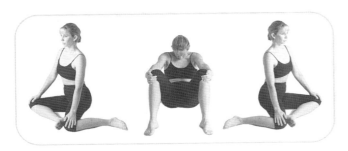

Fig. 6.76 Transition from right to left side-sitting without using hands.

- Keep your knees wide out over your feet as you shift your weight from side to side. Turn your pelvis and shoulders as a unit but rotate your pelvis around your legs.

- Continue the same basic movement, but now bend forward as you come through the middle, then push taller as you come to each side. Be sure to keep your feet tripods and knees out over feet (Fig. 6.81).

N. Stand in a short split stance; left foot back and right foot a little in front.

- Shift your weight back on to your left foot and turn your pelvis and chest to the left as you slide both

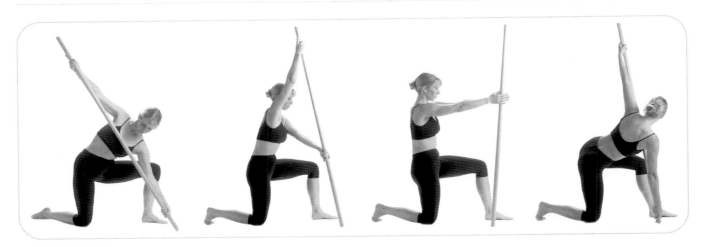

Fig. 6.77 Alternately slide one hand then the other toward the ground – keep back neutral.

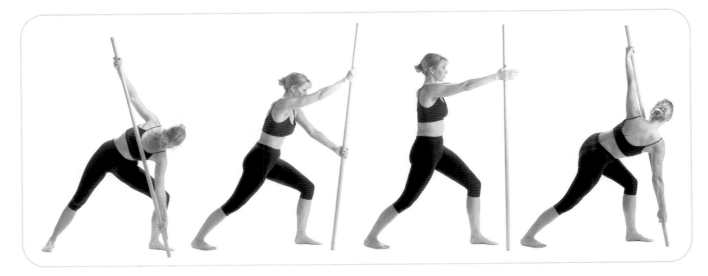

Fig. 6.78 Lengthening the hamstrings by turning and bending toward the front leg – keep back neutral.

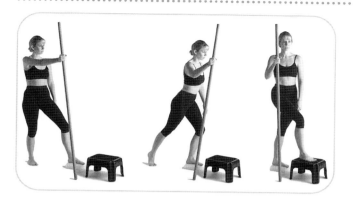

Fig. 6.79 Alternating steps to half standing – turn twice both coming forward and moving back.

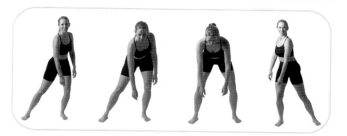

Fig. 6.81 Bending forward and swooping lower in the middle and pushing taller to each side – keep knees out over tripod feet.

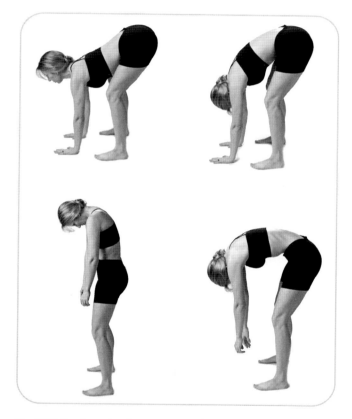

Fig. 6.80 Bend over in a horse stance and press outward – can you feel the top of your pelvis roll back? Progress by rolling up one vertebra at a time.

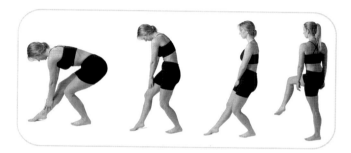

Fig. 6.82 Bending from a split stance position – the front leg is empty. Progress by lifting the empty leg.

6.82). Lower your foot back down, slide hands down leg, and repeat to push taller and lift front foot.

- Do four to eight times on each side; switch which foot is forward and which leg you put weight on.

Establish a budget for your lower back

Use the analogy of a budget when discussing strategies for better living with your low back pain patients. There are two factors involved in a budget: how much you spend and how much you earn. For every time you twist up out of the car without engaging your intersegmental stabilizers, deduct $5. For the bag of groceries you picked up without stabilizing your pelvis, deduct $10. For every minute of one-legged flop standing with lumbar hyperlordosis, deduct 50 cents. For every hour of sitting slumped at a computer, deduct $15. For the 150 pound landscaping rock you just awkwardly caught as it toppled out of the back of your pickup, better refinance your mortgage.

This is a question of recognition of stressors. This is a question of finding creative solutions to avoid those stressors. This is a question of motor preplanning and stabilizing yourself in the presence of those stressors you can't avoid. There is also the question of what you can do to replenish your account. What movements or positions feel good for your back?

For every 10 minutes spent supine with legs up on the wall or a couch, deposit $12. For every repetition of Half-kneel Bending into full posterior tilt and full hip flexor length,

hands down the front of your right thigh and shin. Keep your back neutral.

- Slide both hands back up your leg and continue to straighten your hip and knee while keeping your pelvis vertical, then –
- Lift your right foot slightly away from the floor several times as you come up to push taller (Fig.

293

deposit $2. For every repetition of Side-sit Bending with the front leg straight and full hamstring length, deposit $3. Find ways to incorporate stretches or nonhabitual differentiated movements into every day life. Substitute half-kneeling for sitting some of the time. Do the dishes while in a split stance. Push the vacuum with a horse stance. Empty the clothes dryer with a homolateral bending stance. Read the newspaper in side-sitting. Stand by leaning against a wall and pushing your feet into the floor. Be creative and find ways to accumulate wealth during the course of your daily activities. Be faithful and do your personalized low back kata.

Try recommending yoga for your gluteal-biased folks: this discipline tends to emphasize global spinal extension with ham-string and adductor length. Try recommending tai chi for your iliopsoas-biased folks: this discipline tends to emphasize a vertical pelvis and a straight thoracic spine with hip flexor and adductor length and gluteal/short and stubby strength. Both disciplines might be a bit much for your more acute low back pain sufferers initially. Use movement lessons to work toward needed physical skills and to assess readiness for more challenging activities such as yoga, tai chi or other martial art, or just to return to the local gym and get back on the gerbil machines, but now with an awareness of how to recognize and control their particular stressors.

References

1. Kahle W, Leonhardt H, Platzer W. Color atlas/text of human anatomy. Vol. 1 The locomotor system. New York: Thieme; 1992.
2. Hides JA, Stokes MJ, Saide M, Jull GA, Cooper DH. Evidence of lumbar multifidus muscle wasting ipsilateral to symptoms in patients with acute/subacute low back pain. Spine 1994;19:165–77.
3. Hides JA, Richardson CA, Jull GA. Magnetic resonance imaging and ultrasonography of the lumbar multifidus muscle: comparison of two different modalities. Spine 1995;20:54–8.
4. Hides JA, Richardson CA, Jull GA. Multifidus recovery is not automatic following resolution of acute first episode low back pain. Spine 1996;20:2763–9.
5. Hodges PW, Cresswell AF, Thorstensson A. Preparatory trunk motion precedes movement of the upper limb. Experimental Brain Research 1998;124:69–79.
6. Hodges PW. Changes in motor planning of feedforward postural responses of the trunk muscles in low back pain. Experimental Brain Research 2001;141:261–6.
7. Hodges PW, Richardson CA. Contraction of the abdominal muscles associated with movement of the lower limb. Physical Therapy 1997;77:132–44.
8. Hodges PW, Richardson CA. Feedforward contraction of transversus abdominis is not influenced by the direction of arm movement. Experimental Brain Research 1997;114:362–70.
9. Hodges PW, Richardson CA. Delayed postural contraction of transverses abdominis associated with movement of the lower limb. Journal of Spinal Disorders 1998;11:46–56.
10. Hodges PW, Cresswell AF, Thorstensson A. Preparatory trunk motion accompanies rapid upper limb movement. Experimental Brain Research 1999;124:69–79.
11. Hodges PW, Richardson CA. Altered trunk muscle recruitment in people with low back pain with upper limb movement at different speeds. Archives of Physical Medicine and Rehabilitation 1999;80:1005–12.
12. Hodges PW. Is there a role for transverses abdominis in lumbo-pelvic stability? Manual Therapy 1999;4:74–86.
13. Hodges PW, Cresswell AF, Daggfeldt K, Thorstensson A. Three dimensional preparatory trunk motion recedes asymmetrical upper limb movement. Gait and Posture 2000;11:92–101
14. Richardson CA, Toppenberg R, Jull G. An initial evaluation of eight abdominal exercises for their ability to provide stabilization for the lumbar spine. Australian Journal of Physiotherapy 1990;36:6–11.
15. Richardson CA, Jull GA. Muscle control–pain control. What exercises would you prescribe? Manual Therapy 1995;1:2–10.
16. Wohlfahrt DA, Jull GA, Richardson CA. An initial investigation into the relationship between dynamic and static function of the abdominal muscles. Australian Journal of Physiotherapy 1993;39:9–13.
17. Gallagher S, Kryzanowska R. The Pilates method of body conditioning. Philadelphia, PA: Bainbridge Books; 1999.
18. Johnson J. The multifidus back pain solution. Oakland, CA: New Harbinger Publications; 2002.

CHAPTER SEVEN

A leg to stand on

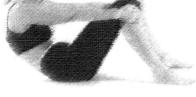

Chapter outline

Lower extremity stressors

- Application of overwhelming force – blows and falls.
- Inability to control lateral or rotational stresses – ligament strains and cartilage tears.
- Miscalibration of medial/lateral balance – bones aren't aligned (pronation, valgus knees). Repetitive stress injuries.
- Violations of the good housekeeping rule – uneven distribution of movement and disproportionate contributions from synergists. Another repetitive stress injury.

Balancing the foot

- Organizing principle is the way the foot interacts with the ground.
- Facilitating balanced movement and antagonists in three dimensions.
- General motor learning strategy of focusing on areas of disproportionately high representation in the CNS. Foot, hand, tongue, lips, eyes.

The three dimensions of the foot

1. Abduction/Adduction balance – whether toes point in or out.
   - Global patterns – hip external rotation with toe-out and hip internal rotation with toe in.
   - Differentiated patterns – hip internal rotation and tibial/knee external rotation creating toe out and hip external rotation with tibial/knee internal rotation creating toe in.
2. Pronation/supination balance – how the feet are rolled in or out.
   - Choices in rolling foot inward/pronating – hip adductors/internal rotators, popliteus/medial hamstring, peroneus longus and extensor digitorum longus.
   - Choices in rolling foot outward/supinating – hip abductors, hip external rotators, posterior tibialis, anterior tibialis, flexor hallucis longus, abductor hallucis, lateral hamstrings and the windlass effect created by big toe dorsiflexion/extensor hallucis longus.
   - Kinematic linkages – cascading sequence of bony movements. Foot controlled on the floor by the hips – head controlled in space by the pelvis – hand controlled in space from shoulder girdle and thorax.
   - Differences in medial/lateral balance of the right and left foot – may be attributed to habitual rotation of the pelvis right or left or imbalanced pelvic force couples.
3. Dorsiflexion/plantarflexion balance – how the weight is distributed front to back.
   - Dorsiflexor bias tends to accompany gluteal bias – differentiated pattern.
   - Plantarflexor bias tends to accompany iliopsoas bias – differentiated pattern.

- Modified ski jumper pose – hard to tell where weight falls (forward with pelvis or back with chest?).

Foot abduction/adduction balance

1. Lesson 1 – *Slip and Slide*. Use of slippery board to facilitate knee internal and external rotation control and balance.

   - External knee rotation driven by biceps femoris – constrained by semimembranosus, semitendinosus and popliteus.

   - Internal knee rotation driven by semimembranosus, semitendinosus and popliteus – constrained by biceps femoris.

   - For training control of excessive knee rotation – plant foot and pivot while protecting MCL and ACL.

   - For training control of miscalibrated left/right postural and movement balance – reducing repetitive stress.

   - Blended with training left/right ankle/foot control. Facilitates peroneus longus/posterior tibialis balance and integration. Sprained ankles – withdrawal and stabilization strategies.

   - Use of slippery board helps train hamstrings to extend hips – de-emphasizing use of quads. Press foot to floor by straightening hip rather than straightening knee – proportionality principle in action.

Pronation/supination balance

2. Manual technique of pressing medially and laterally against distal tibia, resulting in rolling of the foot in and out.

   - Allowing a rolling in and out of the foot on the floor – facilitating inhibition of peroneals/toe extensors and of anterior and posterior tibialis.

   - Preventing rolling in and out of the foot – facilitating stabilization of foot through peroneals and posterior tibialis.

   - Ankle eversion – calcaneal valgus – relative forefoot varus – pronation.

   - Ankle inversion – calcaneal varus – relative forefoot valgus – supination.

3. Blame, consequences and amelioration of pronation pattern.

   - Surrender to gravity and tight hip adductors as prime suspect for blame. Accomplices are peroneus longus and extensor digitorum longus. Excessive hip external rotation with marked toe out another possibility.

   - Hip and knee joint degeneration, patellar tracking dysfunction, ITB syndrome, plantar fasciitis, Achilles tendinitis are victims.

   - Hip abductors/external rotators prescribe the antidote, assisted by the posterior tibialis.

   - Associate subtalar neutral/vertical heel with equal weight between first and fifth metatarsal heads, creating the tripod.

- Differentiated pattern of calcaneal varus and forefoot valgus requires both motor control (coordinating hip abductors/external rotators or posterior tibialis with peroneals) and reduction of articular stiffness.

- Description of self-mobilization of the foot.

4. Lesson 2 – *Rolling the Foot*.

   - Rolling by tilting knee – use to find vertical thigh.

   - Rolling by lifting – anterior tibialis rolls outward and extensor digitorum longus rolls inward.

   - Rolling by pressing – posterior tibialis rolls outward and peroneus longus rolls inward.

   - Rolling by knee rotation/medial and lateral hamstrings – party trick.

   - Rolling by pushing/pulling hips – adductors roll in and abductors roll out.

   - Coordinating the adductors and posterior tibialis – stabilizing the foot in the presence of pulling to stop or pulling to move laterally movements. Use also with bow-legged or over-supinated/pes equinus.

   - Coordinating the abductors and peroneus longus – stabilizing the foot in the presence of pushing to stop or pushing to move laterally movements. Use with knock-kneed or over-pronated/pes planus.

   - Pushing to stop or to go with the abductors a preferable strategy to pulling to stop or to go with the adductors.

5. Lesson 3 – *Horsing Around*. Continuation of Rolling the Foot. Emphasis on pushing outward and stabilizing the foot.

   - Review of pushing out simultaneously to roll the pelvis posteriorly and alternately rolling the pelvis from side to side in supine.

   - Changes of venue – doing same movements while leaning on wall, standing with variable positions of feet and knees, side-lie with feet on wall and top leg lifted.

   - Variations to lengthen the hip flexors.

Front-to-back balance

1. Lesson 4 – *Heel to Toe*.

   - Coordinating and differentiating ankle and toes.

   - Coordinating torso, hips and pelvis with ankles, feet and toes.

2. Lesson 5 – *Toeing Off*. Standing version of Heel to Toe.

3. Lesson 6 – *Starting Blocks*.

   - Hands and knees mobilization of knees, ankles and feet.

   - Facilitating a vertical, skeletal weightbearing foot.

   - Facilitating roll along the foot.

4. Lesson 7 – *Squat Pivots*.

   - Adductor and hamstring length.

   - Facilitating a vertical, skeletal weightbearing foot.

- Pivoting – facilitating rotational stability of foot, ankle and knee.

Change of direction and rotational stability

1. Lesson 8 – *Peerless Pivots*.
    - Summary lesson for the section.
    - Open, closed and reverse T-stances.
    - Lots of step/pivot variations and drills.

Common lower extremity stressors

We started the Tyrannosaurus section of the book with explorations of the use of the legs in general. We learned how to teach more efficient use of the legs in balance, orientation and transitions, and became acquainted with concepts of iliopsoas/gluteal biases and pelvic force couples. We then built on this foundation by managing with movement education a particular clinical problem: lumbopelvic instability.

We created a focus around which everything else revolved: intersegmental stabilization. We can now blend that intersegmental stabilization piece with any of the previous lessons in the tyrannosaurus section (Chapter 5), as we did with the lessons from the just-completed stabilization chapter or as we could do from the current chapter focusing on the legs.

We could continue with a proprioceptive focus on intersegmental stability as the organizing principle of the lessons in this chapter, but although we will not be doing so here, feel free to experiment and create your own. This chapter on the legs could even be thought of as a continuation of the last chapter: use the lessons for more advanced lumbar stabilization. This is particularly true for lateral and rotational stability.

The way the feet interact with the floor, the way the knees balance over the feet, the way the pelvis balances over the legs and the way the lower spine balances over the pelvis are all manifestations of the same basic thing: lower body stability. This means that lumbar stabilization requires knee, ankle and foot stability, as well as multifidus/TA and pelvic control.

Our organizing principle in this chapter will be the foot and how it interacts with the ground. Instead of focusing on the hip/pelvis/lower back relationships of the stabilization chapter, we will be focusing in this chapter on hip/knee/foot relationships. Note that the hips are the common denominator for both. We will discuss kinematic linkages from hip to foot and explore medial/lateral biases. We will mirror the stabilization chapter somewhat by discussing front-to-back and lateral stresses as they relate to lower extremity function and health.

Lower extremity stresses and the problems they create

Let's start with a list of the more common lower extremity orthopedic problems we encounter. The list could include the following:

- Trochanteric bursitis
- Joint degenerative disease or hip joint replacement
- Hip flexor, hamstring or adductor strain
- Iliotibial band syndrome
- Anterior knee pain/chondromalacia/patellar tracking dysfunction
- Medial and lateral collateral ligament strains/tears
- Anterior and posterior cruciate ligament strains/tears
- Torn medial or lateral meniscus
- Total knee replacement
- Calf strain or Achilles tendinitis
- Anterior or posterior shin splints
- Medial or lateral ankle sprains
- Peroneus longus and posterior tibialis tendinitis
- Plantar fasciitis and bunions
- Tibial/fibular/femoral/tarsal fractures
- Postoperative repair or reconstruction of knee ligaments or cartilage, ankle ligaments or tendons, Achilles tendon or various foot surgeries.

Note that some of these injuries are traumatic, whereas others are self-induced/repetitive stress injuries. With traumatic injuries, we have pathology creating a deterioration of movement. We will want to restore normal mobility, stability and muscular control over the affected part and the synergistic whole. With repetitive stress injuries, we have inefficient movement creating pathology.

With repetitive stress injuries, we will want to train our students in proprioceptive awareness of their movement and postural patterns, how this contributes to their problem and how to develop the self-awareness and physical skills needed to control those stresses. This is much like the movement model for lower back pain as outlined in the previous chapter.

What are the main categories of stressor for the legs?

- There are the various violations of the good housekeeping rule.
- There is a miscalibration of medial/lateral balance in straight forward movements.
- There is an inability to control lateral or rotational forces.
- There is an overwhelming application of external traumatic forces.

Traumatic injuries

Let's start with the obvious one first. External traumatic forces could include blows, falls or scalpels. If a steel beam lands on your thigh, you might break a femur. If you fall from 30 feet, a fibula might snap. If a speeding 260-pound linebacker hits your knee from the side, you might tear a medial collateral ligament. If you are in a car accident and jam your knee into the dashboard, you might get a tibial plateau fracture or a posterior cruciate tear.

If you kick your car in frustration, you might sprain your first metatarsophalangeal joint. Surgery might also fall into this category. What this category doesn't include are traumatic bone breaks, ligament tears or meniscal damage from movement stresses not related to blows or falls.

Our second category is an inability to control lateral or rotational stresses. An example of catastrophic tissue failure because of your inability to control your own actions might be making a sharp cut to elude a tackler and tearing your anterior cruciate ligament (ACL). You could be planting your foot to take the wide-open jump shot and roll your ankle over. These are examples of an inability on the part of the CNS to control lateral or rotational forces. Inversion ankle sprains, distal fibular fractures and lateral collateral ligament sprains/tears are consequences of not controlling lateral forces.

Eversion ankle sprains, medial collateral ligament sprains/tears and adductor strains/tears are consequences of not controlling medial forces. Anterior cruciate ligament, medial and lateral meniscus tears and ankle sprains are consequences of not controlling rotational forces. Our first two stressors result in traumatic injury; the next two are of the self-inflicted variety.

Self-inflicted wounds

The third major category of lower extremity stressor is when there is a miscalibration of medial/lateral balance in forward-oriented movements or postures. This means that when standing and orienting forward, or when walking or running straight forward (or skipping, hopping or cycling for that matter), your bones are not aligned efficiently.

These arthrokinematic inefficiencies lead to asymmetrical tissue strains and to repetitive stress injuries. There may be an internal or external rotation bias at the hips, a varus or valgus bias at the knee, or a pronation or supination bias at the feet. These medial/lateral imbalances may be contributing factors in trochanteric bursitis, patellar tracking dysfunction, iliotibial band syndrome, shin splints, Achilles tendinitis, plantar fasciitis or bunions.[1–14] James,[1] in his book on adolescent patellar pain, described the 'miserable malalignment' of femoral internal rotation, relative to knee external rotation and foot pronation. This is the most common and most deadly of the medial/lateral imbalances possible in the legs and is the pattern we will want to have multiple teaching strategies to influence.

The fourth category of stressor consists of the various ways in which you can violate the good housekeeping rule and the proportionality principle. Not enough movement at a joint, or invariant weightbearing stresses on cartilage can lead to hip or knee joint degenerative problems and eventual replacements. Insufficient movement of the hip joints into extension can create knee hyperextension stresses and might contribute to posterior ligament or capsular strain or to patellar tracking problems.[15,16]

Insufficient movement of the hip joint into extension may make the hamstring work unnecessarily hard against a tight hip flexor and contribute to hamstring pulls. Tight hamstrings necessitate more work from the quadriceps and increased patellar stress.[17–20] Insufficient movement of the ankle into dorsiflexion creates a pronation stress on the foot and may overstretch and irritate the plantar fascia.[21–24]

Box 7.1 Lower extremity stresses
The various violations of the good housekeeping rule
A miscalibration of medial/lateral balance in straight forward movements
An inability to control lateral or rotational forces
An overwhelming application of external traumatic forces

Disproportionate use of the calf muscles in push-off because larger synergist inaction of the hamstrings and gluteals might contribute to Achilles tendinitis or eventual rupture, or to posterior shin splints.[25,26] Constant contractions of the anterior compartment muscles leading to shin splints might be linked to insufficient iliopsoas use and not enough hip flexion to clear a plantarflexed ankle.

The four categories of stressors are not mutually exclusive. You might get mildly tackled by a linebacker and fail to control the attendant medial stresses at your knee. You might have a biomechanical fault leading to surgery and have to work with both motor restoration (full motion/full function) and motor reorganization (reduction of underlying biomechanical fault).

In Achilles tendinitis, you might be combining medial/lateral imbalance stresses with good housekeeping stresses. Try not to get too hung up on the various categories and specific diagnoses. By continuing our theme of reciprocating multidirectional movements, you will be doing pretty much the same thing with all of them. What will change from diagnosis to diagnosis is pace, intensity, and how to emphasize different proprioceptive foci and different nonhabitual directions (Box 7.1).

This is a pretty big list of stuff to cover in one short chapter. My intention here is not to give the complete story of the etiology, histology, evaluation and treatment options for each problem, but to give you a motor control perspective on common lower extremity problems and common motor mistakes people make, to assist you in developing yet another tool in your bag, another color for your palette. We will be focusing on the motor control aspect of lower extremity dysfunction or injury recovery within the framework of lower extremity stressors outlined above.

For the freak accident/external traumatic factor sort of injury, what we will emphasize is the use of motor control techniques to facilitate a full return to efficient locomotion, lateral and rotational stability and biomechanical efficiency (accurate medial/lateral skeletal balance, even distribution of movement and use of proportionally stronger muscles to do the bulk of the work). For the biomechanical faults, we will explore strategies for facilitating more balanced and efficient movement and postural patterns. For injuries with biomechanical inefficiencies as a contributing factor, we will work with both tracks.

Balancing the foot – the three dimensions

The organizing principle for lumbar stabilization was intersegmental muscle control. The organizing principle when working with cervical dysfunction will be eye or tongue position and movements. The organizing principle for upper extremity dysfunction and injury will be the organization of the hand. The organizing principle for this chapter will be the way the foot interacts with the ground. The hands, especially the thumb, and the eyes are among the most generously wired parts of our bodies.

For their relatively small size, they account for a relatively very large amount of incoming and outgoing signals from the brain: they have a disproportionate representation in the CNS.[27] Each motor nerve ending might control tens of muscle fibers rather than hundreds or thousands. Each patch of skin, ligament, muscle spindle and joint capsule is swamped with sensory nerves. This both allows for finer discrimination in sensation and finer variations of motor response. The foot is similarly richly equipped with dense motor and sensory nerves.

Whereas the hand is the intersection between outer world and inner self in manipulation functions, the foot is the intersection between outer world (floor/ground) and inner self in locomotion and in standing balance/posture. The eyes are our window on the world in orientation. The lips and tongue are also highly innervated and will provide focus in the vegetative chapter.

Part of the benefit in linking functional context to exercise is that it takes advantage of this disproportionate CNS representation of the feet, hands, eyes and mouth by making these areas a focal point for sensation and intension. In this chapter, we will explore the relationship of the foot to the floor and how the foot fits with various synergistic patterns of movement and posture.

We will look at feet and their relationship to the floor in three dimensions. One dimension is the question of where the toes point: are the feet parallel to each other, turned inward to point toward each other or turned outward to point away from each other? Another dimension is weight distribution across the sole of the foot: is there more weight toward the inside or the outside edge of the foot?

The third dimension is the question of weight distribution forward and back: is there more weight forward on the toes or back on the heels? Let's take each dimension in turn and begin describing global and differentiated patterns, synergistic relationships and possible clinical consequence of particular movement or postural errors, then design some lessons around facilitating balance, biomechanical efficiency and motor control of these three aspects of the feet.

Foot abduction/adduction balance

Why would someone stand with their toes pointed out away from each other or in towards each other? Let's examine our choices. In toeing-out, there could be excessive external rotation at the hip joints and the femur, tibia and foot all angle

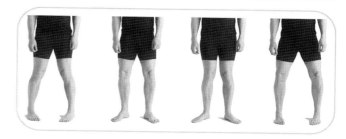

Fig. 7.1 Global internal and eternal rotation patterns – valgus and varus differentiations.

Box 7.2 Foot abduction/adduction balance

Global internal and external rotation patterns – hips responsible for direction toes point

Differentiated patterns – rotation at knee controls direction toes point

---

outward as a reflection of femoral external rotation. Although some people might have retroverted hips and have a bony abnormality reason to point the toes out, your garden-variety students who toe-out are doing so as a result of hip internal and external rotator muscle imbalance.

The intrinsic hip external rotators, along with the gluteus maximus, are firing and the tensor fascia latae is inhibited/weak. The feet are angled out, but so are the knees. If you visualize this organization in line with the orientation of the foot, the knee, foot and toes all line up more or less vertically. This is a lower extremity global external rotation pattern (Fig. 7.1). It tends to correspond to gluteal-biased pelvic patterns, but remember to take all generalizations with a grain of salt.

When toeing-in, there could be an excessive amount of internal rotation at the hip joints, owing to either anteverted hips or, more commonly, a hip muscle imbalance. The intrinsic hip external rotators will be weak and the TFL, anterior gluteus medius and gluteus minimus will dominate. With hip, knee, foot and toes lining up more or less vertically still, this would be a lower extremity global internal rotation pattern (Fig. 7.1). This pattern tends to correspond to iliopsoas-biased pelvic patterns (Box 7.2).

Of course, where there are global patterns there are also differentiated ones. It often happens that someone is biased toward rotating her hips inward and then compensating with an external rotation movement at the knee. This combination of relative femoral internal rotation (and/or adduction) and knee external rotation is quite common (the miserable malalignment described by James) and contributes to numerous lower extremity movement impairments. This is a differentiated external rotation pattern commonly known as knock-kneed or genu valgus (Fig. 7.1).

Although it is less common, you will occasionally see the mirror image of this. Sometimes, when femoral external rotation is compensated for at the knee through tibial/knee internal rotation, you will see a differentiated internal rotation pattern commonly known as bow-legged or genu varus (Fig. 7.1). Whereas in the global patterns the rotational asymmetry at the foot comes from the hips, in differentiated patterns the apparent toe-in/out of the foot comes more from the knees.

Choices in Rolling the Foot outward on the floor

What is someone doing when they stand with their weight perched more toward the outside edges of their feet or collapsed into the inside edges? What are their choices in rolling their feet in and out (Fig. 7.2)? If the feet are rolled outward on the floor, it could be coming from the lower legs or the hips. The anterior tibialis could work to hoist up the arch and roll the foot outward, the posterior tibialis could roll the foot outward by pressing the fifth metatarsal head into the floor, or the flexor hallucis longus could press the great toe into the floor, resulting in a roll outward.

Somewhere down in party trick status, the abductor hallucis has some capabilities. Also, try the following experiment. Sit on the floor with your right knee bent up and your right foot flat on the ground. Use your fingers to pull the right big toe slowly into dorsiflexion. This should result in shortening and lifting your arch and rolling your foot outward on the floor. Using the extensor hallucis longus to supinate the foot might just be another party trick, but the passive 'windlass' effect of great toe dorsiflexion is one that may have an important roll in re-supinating the foot in push-off, when the toes dorsiflex and differentiate from the plantarflexing ankle.[28]

The posterior tibialis and flexor hallucis are very important to lower extremity health and efficiency, but using such relatively small muscles to support the entire weight of your body would be a gross violation of the good housekeeping rule. Let's go a little further up the chain to search for other possibilities in rolling the feet outward.

Sit on the floor again with your right knee bent up and your right foot on the floor. Grasp the top of your tibia with both hands and gently begin to guide it in an alternating internal and external rotation movement. Although this can be performed passively, the idea is just to suggest a direction of movement that your CNS can then recognize and control muscularly. This tibial or knee external rotation is driven by the lateral hamstrings and results in a rolling outward of the foot on the floor.

This is yet another party trick. We won't want to train someone to roll the foot outward with his or her biceps femoris. This muscle is usually going to be associated with valgus knees and pronating feet. Moving further up the chain, we get to the real power behind the throne. It is the relative balance of the hip musculature that determines the medial/lateral balance of the foot on the floor.

Rolling the feet outward can also be a result of hip external rotation, abduction, or even hip internal rotation. Stand up for a moment and organize your feet so they are oriented straight ahead and parallel to each other. Contract your gluteus maximus and hip external rotators: pinch your cheeks together as if denying access to the nurse with the thermometer. As the femurs externally rotate, they grab the tibiae and externally rotate them (though the knees are internally rotating). The externally rotating tibiae then grab the talar bones, which in

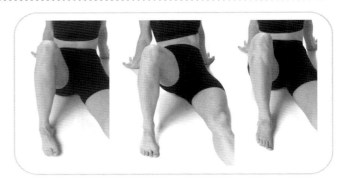

Fig. 7.2 Supination – about neutral – pronation.

Box 7.3 Feet rolling outward
Anterior tibialis – hoist up the medial foot
Posterior tibialis – press the fifth metatarsal head
Flexor hallucis longus – press the big toe
Windlass effect – dorsiflex the big toe
Biceps femoris – don't train this one
Hip abductors and external rotators

turn roll the calcaneus and navicular bones and the rest of the merry band of foot bones outward on the floor (Fig. 7.3).

This cascading effect of sequentially externally rotating bones is called a *kinematic linkage*. Kinematics is a term used to describe a body in motion regardless of the forces that produce that motion. Kinematic linkages are sequential movements of linked bodies (bones): one bone moves, which moves the next, which moves the next and so on. We are interested both in how the linked bones move relative to each other and in why or how they move. The examination of these forces acting on the body (inertia, gravity, ground reaction forces) and their effects on the body is the study of *kinetics*.[29–31]

Just as action of the muscles around the hip joints had domino effects on the organization of the pelvis and therefore on the spine and on the head and neck, the muscles of the hips have a profound effect on the organization of the knees and feet. The neck and arms start at the hip joints, and so does the foot. As the muscles and bones of the spinal system start with large bones and muscles (pelvis and hip musculature) and taper to smaller bones and muscles (atlas and axis and suboccipital muscles), so does the lower extremity system.

The larger bones and muscles (pelvis/femur and hip joint musculature) initiate and provide the bulk of power for movements, whereas the smaller bones and muscles (tarsals and intrinsic foot musculature) provide fine-tuning movements and continuous proprioceptive feedback. The proportionality principle applies to the lower extremities as well as to the spine. Get your big muscles involved in re-educating the foot: use the gluteus maximus and short and stubbies to create a cascading external rotation pattern, or the lateral gluteals and TFL to create a varus movement (Box 7.3).

Rolling the feet outward in a kinematic linkage can also be a result of hip abduction. Stand again with feet parallel and contract your TFL, gluteus minimus and medius and upper gluteus maximus. Push your feet away from each other as if intending to rip apart the carpet between your feet. The kine-

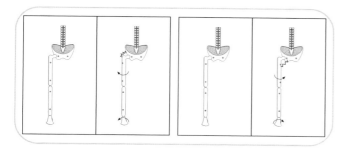

Fig. 7.3 Kinematic linkage in lower extremity external/internal rotational patterns.

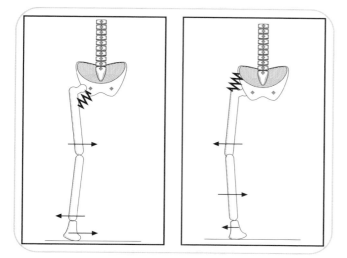

Fig. 7.4 Kinematic linkage in lower extremity adduction/abduction patterns.

matic linkage here is one of pushing bones out laterally. The femur abducts, which pushes the proximal tibia laterally (varus movement at the knee), pushes the talus, calcaneus, etc. laterally, and rolls your weight on to your outside edge (Fig. 7.4). If this rolling outward on to the outer edges of your feet is not happening, why not? What could you be doing to prevent the free rolling of your foot outward on the floor?

Rolling the feet out can go along with hip internal rotation bias in standing. Stand again and point your toes in toward each other. Straighten or even lock your knees and observe what happens at your feet. Exaggerate this by having your feet close together. Perhaps because of the abduction component of the internally rotating TFL and small gluteals, or perhaps because of more passive external rotation or abduction kinematic linkage, the feet roll on to their outside edges (unless you do something at your foot or ankle to counter this). Make it more obvious by pushing your feet outward while in this toe-in position.

Choices in rolling the feet inward

What action might be responsible for rolling your weight inward on your feet; who is the culprit in pronation? At the foot and

Box 7.4 Feet rolling inward

Extensor digitorum longus – lift the lateral foot and toes
Peroneus longus – press the first metatarsal head
Medial hamstrings and popliteus – party trick only
Hip adductors and internal rotators

ankle, there will probably be an imbalance between the medial and lateral lower leg musculature. The posterior tibialis will probably be the weaker partner in its pairing with the peroneals. Does this mean that if we stretch the peroneals and strengthen the posterior tibialis that the foot won't pronate as much?

Dream on: finer and more tertiary muscles, being designed for fine-tuning and proprioceptive acuity, are not well suited for long periods of tonic support of the whole weight of the body. What we need to figure out is what the hips are doing that drives or contributes to pronation, and what the hips are not doing that could be Rolling the Foot outward.

Probably the most common action at the hip that contributes to foot pronation is adduction. Stand up with your feet parallel and your knees straight and make a movement of pulling your feet in toward each other. Imagine squeezing a ball between your knees or sliding your feet toward each other as if bunching up the carpet between your feet, and observe proprioceptively how this rolls your feet inward.

This over-stimulation of the adductors in weightbearing and push-off functions is a major contributor to repetitive stress injuries of the lower extremities. The adductors are often not well differentiated from the hamstrings and over-contribute to movements that call for hip extension. Another version of the adductor-driven pronation is with knee external rotation patterns. As the hips adduct and internally rotate, the tibia compensates by rotating outward from the knee.

This toe-out orientation of the foot, especially along with excessive adductor tone, collapses the feet inward. Try this yourself. Stand and point your toes outward at 20–30° and pull your knees in toward each other as if protecting your genitals from attack. Observe this common pattern – this miserable malalignment – with your students; notice if their knees are closer together than their feet and where their toes point.

Another common pattern that manifests in foot pronation is excessive hip external rotation. This might fly in the face of logic, because you just felt proprioceptively a few paragraphs back how, if you stand and externally rotate at your hips, you roll on to your outer edges. However, this is only true if you start from a parallel or even an internally rotated position.

If you start with your hips significantly externally rotated and your feet pointed out, what usually happens is a collapse of the foot inward as the weight of the body falls forward and in. Try externally rotating more from this toe-out position to try and roll toward your outside edges. What makes this so hard is that you are already so externally rotated that there isn't much more room available in that direction. These folks are usually very short/tight in their short and stubbies, hamstrings and gluteals (Box 7.4).

They also tend to engage their posterior long adductors, often being undifferentiated from the tight hamstrings. Try this in standing: point your feet away from each other, squeeze your cheeks to deny thermometer access, and pull your heels in toward each other. The whole effect is one of guarding the posterior pelvic floor and collapsing the feet inward.

Other contributing factors to pronation include weakness or tightness of selected lower extremity muscles. Pronation has been linked to tightness of the hamstrings, gastrocnemius, soleus, iliotibial band (ITB), hip rotators and hip flexors and to weakness of the ankle inverters, hip rotators and gluteus medius, as well as to leg length discrepancies.[32]

Excessive foot pronation is a common clinical presentation and is associated with a wide variety of lower extremity repetitive stress injuries. Pronation has been linked to anterior knee pain and patellar tracking problems.[33–37] Pronation has been linked to plantar fasciitis,[38,39] Achilles tendinitis[40,41] and shin splints.[42,43] The savvy practitioner would do well to have a variety of ways to address this problem: perhaps a little motor skill facilitation could be tried before resorting immediately to the orthotics?

Imbalance of pelvis affecting medial/lateral balance of feet

To make things even more complex, there are often differences in the amount of roll-in and roll-out and in the amount of toe-in or toe-out, between the left and right feet. Stand again with feet parallel and turn yourself alternately from side to side; rotate your pelvis and torso together slowly left and right. Notice what happens at your feet. As the pelvis turns to the left, the left hip initially internally rotates, then the hip runs out of room to rotate and the left femur is pulled into external rotation.

This external rotation movement of the femur internally rotates the left knee, and then externally rotates the tibia and fibula. This in turn moves the talus, the calcaneus and the whole merry band of foot bones outward. At the same time as the pelvis turns to the left and the left foot rolls outward, the right hip joint is initially externally rotating, then pulling the right femur into internal rotation. This creates an external rotation movement at the right knee joint, internal rotation of lower leg and pronation of the right foot. The kinematic linkage got a bit longer by now involving the pelvis.

But what moved the pelvis in the first place? It was the left pelvic force couple musculature: right gluteals and short and stubbies and the left iliopsoas and adductors (perhaps the TFL?). Logic could tempt us to suspect the side with the stronger short and stubbies and abductors would coincide with the less pronated foot. This is often not the case because of this phenomenon of kinematic linkages. In this scenario, the gluteal-dominant side is both pushing the pelvis away and turning the pelvis away from that leg.

This can result in the pronation of the pushing foot and the supination of the pulling or iliopsoas-dominant side because of the turn of the pelvis away from the gluteal side. Similarly, we could be tempted to suspect more knee external rotation on the iliopsoas-dominant side because of the concurrent dominance of the adductors on that side. This is again sometimes not the case, and the toe-out-from-tibial-rotation might be greater on the side of the dominant push-off leg.

When assessing orientation of the feet on the floor and differences between the two sides, you'll need to keep in mind

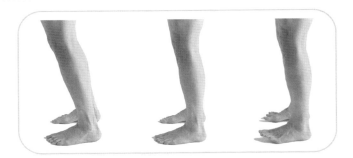

Fig. 7.5 Weight distributed way forward on foot – about neutral – and way back.

the varying amounts of rotation at the knee/hip/pelvis and mentally juggle the sometimes complicated compensation movements among the different parts to come to a satisfactory understanding of the situation. Or you could just cut the Gordian knot by training your student in principles of well organized movement.

Heel-to-toe balance

The last dimension of the foot we will discuss, in addition to the orientation of the toes in or out and the distribution of weight across the foot from inside to outside, is the distribution of weight along the foot from front to back (Fig. 7.5). As in previous dimensions, balance of the foot from front to back is a blend of antagonist balance of both lower leg and hip musculature. Lie supine for a moment and notice how your ankles are bent. Are they dorsiflexed or plantarflexed?

What are we going to call neutral or ideal here, and how do we define at what angle of the ankle we change from being neutral to being dorsiflexed, or at what angle we change from being neutral to being plantarflexed? This assessment is about as subjective as it gets: there is no ideal angle. If the ankles are approaching a 90° angle we could say they are dorsiflexing and would suspect gastrosoleus weakness and anterior tibialis/peroneal/toe dorsiflexor bias.

If the ankle is approaching 180°, we could say it is plantarflexing and would suspect anterior tibialis/peroneal/toe dorsiflexor weakness and gastrosoleus bias. Figuring out the nuances around the 115–165° range is a matter of repeated observation and judgment.

In looking at synergistic lower extremity patterns, we might expect a global relationship between all of the stepping muscles and all of the push-off muscles. If our student is gluteal biased we might expect strong and/or tight gluteals, hamstrings and gastrosoleus. Everything along the back of the leg contracts to assist in pushing off in gait. If our student is iliopsoas biased we might expect strong and/or tight iliopsoas, rectus femoris and the ankle and toe dorsiflexors.

Everything along the front of the leg contracts to assist in stepping. In reality, what we often see are differentiated relationships among the ostensible synergists. Plantarflexed ankles and gastrosoleus that dominate the anterior compartment muscles will often go with an iliopsoas bias. Dorsiflexed ankles and dominating anterior compartment muscles often go with

Box 7.5 Heel to Toe balance

Dorsiflexor/plantarflexor balance

Correlation to pelvic bias

a gluteal bias. To better understand this, come back up to standing.

Stand with your feet apart and parallel to each other. Anteriorly rotate your pelvis – let your pubic bone fall toward the floor and let your tailbone lift. Is one of the effects of this movement to shift your center of mass forward? If not, do this deliberately anyway. As your center of mass shifts forward, you have to adjust by contracting your ankle (and perhaps toe) plantarflexors to not fall forward. Therefore, most people with iliopsoas tightness and gluteal weakness tend to have more weight forward on their toes, necessitating gastrosoleus contraction and differentiation of the ankle from the hip musculature (Box 7.5).

This tendency toward antagonist imbalance in the direction of the plantarflexors is exacerbated in gait, where the relatively inhibited gluteals and hamstrings are not doing enough in push-off and the plantarflexors have to compensate by doing more. Additionally in gait, the iliopsoas-biased person tends to walk by falling forward. The pelvis is falling forward on the legs and the weight is distributed more forward on the foot, again necessitating constant plantarflexor effort. Think back to the Tinkerbell pose and imagine the heels she is wearing and how she would look walking – get up and walk like Tinkerbell to feel what she feels.

Does this mean that the gluteal-biased person will organize her weight more toward her heels? Sometimes that is the case. Movement of the pelvis backward in space and backward on the legs simulates a falling-backward movement (or should – there are many people who don't know how to posteriorly rotate their pelvis in a falling reaction in this position). Gluteal-biased people with posterior pelvic rotation (a reaction to falling back) are sometimes rocked back on their heels. This results in constant anterior compartment contraction, plantarflexor weakness and ankles that are stiff into plantarflexion.

Can you simulate this movement in standing? Stand up with your feet parallel and rock your weight back toward your heels. When do your toes start to lift and your toe and ankle dorsiflexors start to kick in? Do you have sufficient pelvic anterior/posterior balance to allow for posterior pelvic tilt in this position? Are your iliopsoas long enough? Are your gluteals active enough? What does it feel like to walk while rocked back on your heels?

To make things just a bit more complex, a gluteal-biased person is not always back on her heels: sometimes she will throw her pelvis forward over her toes to hang on her anterior hip ligaments. When doing this, she has two choices of what to do with her torso. She could straighten her back and angle it in a continuation of the angle of her legs and pelvis. This is a ski jumper pose, requires tremendous plantarflexor effort and is not often seen.

More commonly, she will compensate for this forward movement of her pelvis by sinking and collapsing her chest backward. This results in the short and compressed lumbar lordosis and long thoracic kyphosis we discussed in previous chap-

ters. With regard to the weight distribution along the feet from front to back, this organization can be tricky to assess. Whereas the legs will be angled forward and the pelvis will clearly be more forward over the toes than back on the heels, if the chest falls back far enough she may still be able to have more weight back on her heels. There is a choice within this configuration.

Where there will not be a choice for this person is in further rocking back. If while rocking back she is not able to extend her thoracic spine and push her head taller to move the center of mass of her chest forward, she will quickly reach her limits in that direction and will topple backward. Use this movement in your initial assessment of both lower back and lower extremity problems. We want to find out what sort of biases people have and what sort of postural adjustments they can make when slowly and gently pushed forward and back on their feet. Can they posteriorly rotate? Can they extend their thoracic spine? Can you? Get up on your feet and try it out!

Are all the various dimensions of the feet independent of each other? Of course not. How the feet are arranged on the floor, how the weight is distributed along and across the feet, how weight is distributed between the two feet, and differences in orientation and weight distribution along and across the two feet are a multiplanar mixture that defies hard and fast rules.

There are too many variables in standing to be able to boil things down to a couple of clear-cut categories. Watch for commonly occurring patterns (foot pronation and hip adduction, femoral internal rotation and knee external rotation, global lower extremity external rotation and foot pronation, etc.) and use reciprocating, pattern-specific and functionally relevant movements to train efficiency and balance of the whole pelvis/lower extremity complex – cut the Gordian knot, rather than trying to unravel the thing!

Foot adduction/ abduction balance

Let's get experiential now and do a series of lessons relating to lower extremity function and health. As in previous chapters, we will be breaking down these lessons for their muscular and functional relevance and will be discussing why and when to use them clinically. In our first lesson, we will be exploring the orientation of the feet inside and out and will be refining some previously introduced bridging movements: gaining more accuracy in pushing the foot into the floor from a supine position.

Slip and Slide

Variations

A. Stand for a moment in your bare feet. Let your arms hang at your sides, feet around shoulder width apart and look straight ahead.

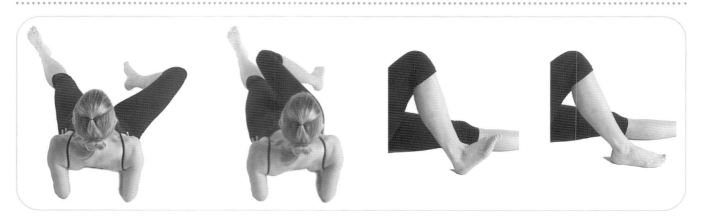

Fig. 7.6 Tilt knees out and in to find center – lift and lower your forefoot.

- Notice your feet against the floor. What direction do your toes point?

- Do you have more weight forward on your toes or back on your heels?

- Are your feet rolled in to flatten your arches, or are you rolled on to the outside edges of your feet?

- Walk around a bit and feel for movement of your ankles or toes. Does your ankle bend and straighten? How clearly can you feel your toes? Which toes do you use to push off of?

- Get a general sense of the springiness of your legs and how you are propelling yourself forward. How are your legs moving your pelvis in space?

B. Sit on the floor and lean back on your hands or elbows behind you. Rest your left leg down long on the floor with your knee straight. Bend up your right leg so the sole of your right foot is flat on the floor.

- Notice first the direction that the toes on your right foot point. Do they angle in? Out? Straight ahead?

- Notice if your right knee is pointed straight to the ceiling or whether it tends to angle in or out a little. Feel proprioceptively, then confirm visually.

- Tilt your right knee alternately inside and out to establish a place where your knee is pointed straight toward the ceiling (Fig. 7.6). Stay there.

- Keeping your right heel on the floor, lift and lower the front of your right foot several times (Fig. 7.6). Your toes and the balls of your foot will lift away from the floor then lower back down again. How smooth is this?

- Continue to lift and lower your right forefoot, but instead of putting it straight down each time, alternate diagonal movements.

- Reach toward the floor to your left with your right little toe several times.

- Then reach toward the floor to your right with your right big toe. These movements twist your ankle from

side to side. Can you also feel anything happening in your right knee (Fig. 7.7)?

C. Sit on the floor again, leaning back on your elbows or hands. Have your left leg down and long again and your right leg bent up. Place a smooth board (clipboard, ziplock bag, plastic cutting board; anything that is a bit slippery) under the sole of your bare right foot. Make sure the flooring surface is a carpet or smooth blanket so the board can slide easily across the floor.

- With your right knee still pointed to the ceiling, make a movement with your right foot to spin the front of the board alternately right and left (Fig. 7.8). The toes of your right foot will alternately point inward then outward.

- Confirm this visually by peeking at your right big toe as it slides into view inside your right thigh, then by peeking at your little toe as it slides into view to the outside of your thigh. Can you feel a movement at your knee?

- After sliding the front of the board right and left several times, use this movement to help you to establish that place where the toes of your right foot are pointed straight forward.

- From this place, push your right foot back into the board and lift your right hip away from the floor (Fig. 7.9). Your pelvis rolls back and to the left and the left side of your lower back pushes out and rounds.

- Return your right hip to the floor then repeat; push your foot, lift your right hip, then lower it back down again. Let your chest twist and roll your head opposite your pelvis.

- Experiment with pushing your foot and lifting your hip with the front of the board angled to the right (Fig. 7.9). How does it feel to push your foot into the floor when your toes are pointed outward?

- Angle the board to the left and lift and lower your hip several times. How does it feel to push with your toes angled inward (Fig. 7.9)?

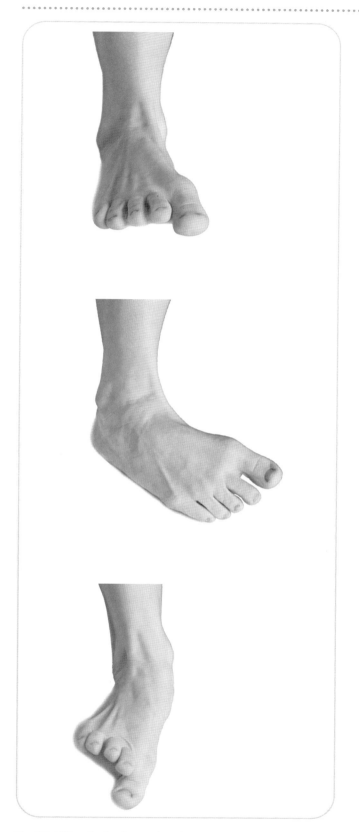

Fig. 7.7 Lifting the forefoot and reaching toward the floor inside – and outside.

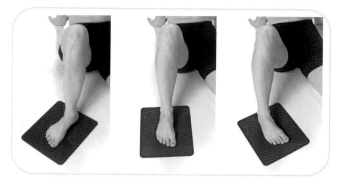

Fig. 7.8 Sliding the front of the board inside and out – knee internal and external rotation.

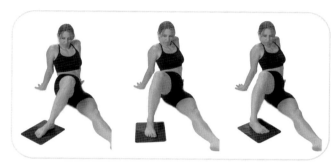

Fig. 7.9 Pushing foot and lifting hip with foot centered – with toe out – with toe in.

- Find center and lift your hip several times here. Which of the three variations feels most stable at your ankle? Knee?

- Can you lift your right hip and keep it lifted as you slide the front of the board alternately from side to side?

D. Come up to sit again. This time, have both knees bent and both feet on the floor. Put your right foot on the slippery board again.

- Center your foot; toes point straight forward. Point your knee to the ceiling.

- Keep your knee pointed to the ceiling and slide the whole board alternately right and left (Fig. 7.10). Your right knee will move alternately from side to side along with your sliding foot. Your right knee stays over your foot.

- As you do this sliding movement, notice whether there is an effect on your pelvis. Does your pelvis stay where it is, or does it roll on the floor from side to side?

- Continue this same movement but modify it a bit by leading the movement in each direction with your heel (Fig. 7.10).

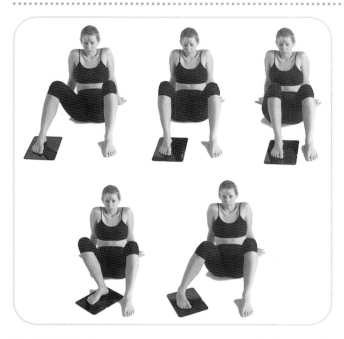

Fig. 7.10 Sliding board keeping knee over foot – then leading with the heel.

- As you slide the board out, your heel moves to the right and your toes point in. As you slide the board in, your heel moves in to the left and your toes point out.

- Repeat this movement many times. Is anything happening at your pelvis? Can you let it move? Try allowing your pelvis to roll to the left as you slide the board to the right and to the right as you slide the board to the left.

- Center your foot and board again and press your right foot into the board again to lift your right hip (Fig. 7.9). Feel how pushing your foot into the slippery board requires you to use the back of your thigh both to push your foot and to keep the board from sliding.

- Add in lifting your left foot from the floor and reaching your left knee up and out. Think about bringing your left knee in the direction of your left arm or elbow.

- Take the board out from under your right foot. Push your foot into the floor, lift your right hip and then lift your left foot from the floor. How stable/grounded does this feel?

- Go back to the movement of lifting your right forefoot from the floor and reaching with your big toe to the right and your little toe to the left. How does this movement feel in comparison to when we started?

E. Come up to sit again, this time with your right leg long and your left foot on the ground.

- Repeat movements as in B. Notice the direction of your toes, lift and lower your forefoot and reach from side to side with big and little toes. How does this side compare?

- Repeat movements as in C. Slide the front of the board left and right. Push your foot and lift your hip with toes pointed out, in and centered. Lift your hip and keep it up while turning the board left and right.

F. Come to sit again, but with both legs bent.

- Repeat movements as in D to this side. Slide the whole board from side to side so your knee stays over your foot. Add in leading the movement with your heel; your toes point in the opposite direction of where the board slides.

- Push your foot into the board to lift your left hip and add in lifting your right foot.

- Take the board out and push your left foot into the ground. How stable does it feel? Reach with your big and little toes from side to side. How smooth and complete is this now? Can you more clearly sense movement at your knee?

G. Lie on your back with both knees bent and both feet on the floor.

- Repeat the same sequence of board sliding movements with your right foot as in sitting.

- Slide the front of the board right and left to point your toes in and out.

- Push your foot into the board and lift your right hip with your toes pointed in, out and center. Lift your hip and keep it lifted while you slide the front of the board from side to side.

- Slide the whole board from side to side.

- Continue, but lead with your heel and allow full pelvic movement.

- Press your foot, lift your hip, and then lift your opposite foot from the floor.

H. Lie on your back with both knees bent and both feet on the floor.

- Repeat as G to the opposite side. Put the board under your left foot and slide it around. Lift left hip and right foot. Compare your two sides.

- Take the board out from under your foot – have both knees bent, both feet flat on the floor and the toes of both feet pointed straight forward. Press both feet into the floor and lift both hips and assess your legs for control/stability/power.

I. Stand up again.

- Notice your feet against the floor. What direction do your toes point?

- Do you have more weight forward on your toes or back on your heels?

- Are your feet rolled in to flatten your arch, or are you rolled on to the outside edges of your feet?

- Walk around a bit and feel for movement of your ankles or toes. Does your ankle bend and straighten? How clearly can you feel your toes? Which toes do you use to push off of?

- Get a general sense of the springiness of your legs and how you are propelling yourself forward. What do your hamstrings feel like? How are your legs moving your pelvis in space now?

Baselines – Slip and Slide

For our initial baseline, stand in your bare feet. Notice the orientation of your feet and how your weight is distributed along and across your feet. This initial static baseline asks questions about the three dimensions of the feet to provide an initial point of reference. We will revisit these questions in subsequent lessons, each with a slightly different emphasis. The initial dynamic baseline in this lesson involves walking and attending to the sensations created by the feet. The three points of focus were the amount, balance and smoothness of ankle plantar- and dorsiflexion, how the toes move relative to the foot and which metatarsal heads you push off from.

These are questions about how anterior and posterior lower leg muscles are balanced, how the push-off and stepping function is balanced at the ankle, whether your toes move globally with or differentiated from your ankle and whether you are able to organize your foot vertically for maximum skeletal weight-bearing effect in push-off. We will discuss more on each of these topics later. The question about springiness in your step is a general question about quality, ease, efficiency and liveliness, whereas the question about how your pelvis moves in space is that old question about pelvic force couple use and balance.

Tapping your toes

Our first exploratory movement in this lesson is one of abducting and adducting the foot. In variation B, sit on the floor and lean back on your hands behind you. Rest your left leg down on the floor long, with your knee straight. Bend up your right leg so the sole of your right foot is flat on the floor. The question about whether your toes point in or out in this position is a question of tibial/knee joint rotation and abduction or adduction of the foot.

The second question is about hip musculature bias. A knee that tilts in probably has dominant adductors and a knee that tilts out probably has dominant abductors/external rotators. You then tilt your knee from side to side to establish vertical, that place where your knee is pointed to the ceiling and your knee is over your foot. It is this ability to keep your knee over your foot that will be a recurring theme in treating both knee and foot/ankle injury and biomechanical faults.

The next movement variation in this section is to dorsiflex your ankle and lift your forefoot from the floor. We could observe for medial/lateral balance here. Does the forefoot lift straight up, or does it angle off to the outside or to the inside? The former would indicate a peroneal and toe dorsiflexor bias and the latter an anterior tibialis bias. These dorsiflexion imbal-ances may be accompanied by knee rotation. Observe for a spinning movement of the tibia medially or laterally.

The next movement is to deliberately reach your big toe to the outside and your little toe to the inside to create an alternating dorsiflexion eversion and dorsiflexion inversion movement. This reciprocating movement assists in balancing and coordinating the peroneals/extensor digitorum longus and anterior tibialis/posterior tibialis and can be a next step up from gentle isometrics when working with someone with an acute ankle sprain or other foot injury.

Getting the sole of the foot back on the ground as soon as possible after injury is very important for people with sprained ankles. This position of sitting up and bending up one leg allows for negligible weightbearing while still stimulating the proprioceptors on the sole of the foot (modify by leaning farther back, holding on with your hands behind your thigh, or lying supine and putting your foot up on the wall).

The floor provides for both a reference point and a destination for movement while also providing a constraint for too much movement of the ankle into plantarflexion. This initial active movement into dorsiflexion is the preferred direction at this stage, whereas the orientation to gravity allows the dorsiflexors (anterior tibialis and extensor digitorum longus) to do both shortening and controlled lengthening contractions.

This movement is also designed to assess range/balance of movement and degree of motor control over your tibial rotators. The movement of reaching the big toe laterally not only triggers ankle dorsiflexion and eversion, but also a movement of tibial or knee joint external rotation. This movement is performed through contractions of the lateral hamstrings: the biceps femoris.[7]

The movement of reaching the little toe to the inside not only triggers ankle dorsiflexion and inversion, but also a movement of knee internal rotation. This movement is performed through the semimembranosus, the semitendinosus and the popliteus.[8] It is the balance and coordination between medial and lateral hamstrings that plays a pivotal role in orientation of the foot in a medial/lateral direction and in stabilizing the knee in the presence of rotational stressors.[9]

This combination of ankle dorsiflexion and eversion with foot abduction (driven through knee external rotation) is regionally global. The foot, ankle and knee are moving synergistically with each other, though usually differentiated from the hip. Usually, this pattern is seen with adduction and/or internal rotation biases at the hips. The whole pattern is a nice one initially after ankle sprains, as this simulates a withdrawal function of the foot away from the floor.

Spraining your ankle

Ankle sprains usually happen for one of two reasons: you have stepped on an irregular surface, or you couldn't control lateral or rotational stresses with your foot on a flat surface. If you unexpectedly step in a hole, on rock or root, or come down from a rebound to land on someone else's foot, you could be in trouble. If unexpected enough, or if the surface you landed on is sufficiently skewed from the horizontal, you could be rolled over on your ankle before you have much of a chance to react.

At that point, it doesn't matter how strong your peroneals are: they have no chance of stopping your ankle from rolling into inversion and plantarflexion. Your only chance at that point is to get your weight off that foot. You need to withdraw your foot from the floor. This involves not just the ankle dorsiflexors but also the hip flexors on the same side and the hip extensors on the opposite side, which have to push that foot into the floor and quickly take additional weight. You will want to very quickly inhibit the hip extensors, quadriceps and calf muscles on the affected side to get weight off the unstable foot.

This linkage of the iliopsoas into the ankle and foot movement can be facilitated by lightening the heel away from the floor just a bit as you dorsiflex and evert. Try linking this to our various incarnations of the Wishbone movements where you press one foot while lifting the other. Initially, just do in the withdrawal direction for the affected side, but then progress to lifting the opposite foot and pressing the affected foot into the floor as your student becomes able to begin simulating push-off functions. The pelvic force couple rears again its massive head.

If your foot is flat on the ground and your ankle sprains, you are not controlling lateral or rotational stresses as your body moves in space on top of your foot. It is usually the peroneals we especially want to work again, but in a different way and for a different reason. Instead of using the peroneals to evert the ankle as part of a withdrawal from the floor function, we want them to work while on the ground as part of a stabilizing function.

This movement of lifting the foot and moving it left and right by reaching with the toes is useful initially to train resistance to lateral and rotational stresses through peroneal contraction, but needs to be refined further to be translated into foot and ankle stability with the foot on the floor. At some point we are going to want to differentiate peroneal support of the foot on the floor from synergistic lateral hamstring contractions and knee external rotation.

People who have sprained their ankle walk with their foot pointed out already. This minimizes the necessity to move into end-range of dorsiflexion and to engage the gastrosoleus in push-off. Let's not perpetuate the tendency to point the toes outward, let's not reinforce a compensatory movement by overemphasizing the use of elastic bands or tubing and resistance into eversion and dorsiflexion. Be aware that you are also probably getting knee external rotation that we will eventually want to extinguish. Keep this in mind early on in rehabilitation by training them early with reciprocating movements. Allow them to move some amount into ankle inversion with foot adduction and knee internal rotation, as we are doing in this variation.

Other contexts in which control over tibial internal and external rotation movement is useful are for plantar fasciitis and patellar tracking dysfunction. The external knee rotation pattern tends to shift weight medially and collapse and over-stretch the arch. This may contribute to plantar fasciitis.[38,39] When the tibia is rotated externally, it drags the patellar tendon and the patella laterally along with it, increasing the Q angle and contributing to patellar tracking problems.[44–46]

In addition, having control over rotational movements of the tibia through medial and lateral hamstring balance and competence is necessary for controlling rotational stresses at the knee during rehabilitation from (or avoidance of) collateral and cruciate ligament and knee meniscal damage or post surgical repair.[47–49] We could use both this initial movement and subsequent movements in this lesson with all of the scenarios listed above.

The initial lesson in this lower extremity chapter is concerned primarily with the abduction/adduction balance of the foot on the floor, peroneus longus/posterior tibialis balance, and the control of lateral and medial rotation movements of the knee. Subsequent variations of this lesson are designed to enhance balance, smoothness and competence in these movements. How did this movement compare at the end to what it was like to begin?

Controlling knee rotation

In variation C you begin to explore these knee internal and external rotation movements with your foot on a slippery board. The directions to slide the front of the board alternately inward and outward again stimulates the medial and lateral tibial rotators to work cooperatively in turning the tibia and the foot inside and out. The biceps femoris rotates the tibia laterally and the semimembranosus, semitendinosus and popliteus rotate it medially.[50–52] As a corollary, the biceps femoris stabilizes the knee from rotating too much into internal rotation and the medial hamstrings and popliteus stabilize the knee from rotating into too much external rotation.

As was the case in previous examples, we are using this reciprocating movement to facilitate an ability to move equally easily in each direction and to assist in establishing a truer neutral position of the foot on the floor and of the tibia underneath the femur. Once having found that neutral place, you then press your foot into the board to lift your hip away from the ground. Here we are functionalizing this new position by bearing increased weight through your foot, ankle and knee. We then play Goldilocks again by pressing your foot and lifting your hip with your toes pointed out, then in, then neutral again. Where is your subjective sense of stability, skeletal weightbearing and easy effort at its best? How do you know unless you've tried? How do you distinguish ideal from familiar?

As a final variation in this section, press your foot to lift your hip then stay there as you turn the front of the slippery board left and right. This variation ups the ante for the tibial rotators, as they now have to control knee rotation with increased weight. The contraction of the hamstrings to lift the hip also adds an element of complexity to the movement. Both medial and lateral hamstrings need to work to keep the hip up, but then have to also reciprocally lengthen and shorten to rotate the tibia. Enhance control by introducing errors and applying constraints.

The slippery board constraint – pressing the floor with hip extension

The slippery board serves several purposes here. One, it provides a nice reference point by having it as the focus of your intentional movement. Two, it helps in breaking up our more primitive regional global pattern. Instead of ankle eversion with knee external rotation and ankle inversion with knee internal rotation, the ankle stays more neutral, with the sole of the foot staying flat on the board while the tibia rotates in a more differentiated way. Three, the slippery board is an excellent adjunct in training hamstring competency in push-off functions.

Placing a slippery board under your foot with your lower leg angled the way it is will tend to make the board slide out or away from your pelvis on the floor. To prevent this, the hamstrings need to contract to keep the knee from straightening and the board from sliding away. This alone tends to stimulate the hamstring to contract more fully to push the foot and lift the hip. Add to this the constraint you have now placed on the quadriceps.

If you use your quadriceps and straighten your knee to push your foot into the ground, the board will go slip sliding away. One of the main benefits from using this slippery board is to encourage more competent use of the hamstrings and gluteals. Under what circumstances might we want to teach this strategy of pressing the foot into the floor with the hamstrings?

What we are facilitating here is an ability to press the foot primarily through hip extension rather than with knee extension or back extension. This is very useful in cases of lower back pain and/or instability because of extension stressors. Start with this slippery board lesson with these types of people to get them used to pushing with their hamstrings and gluteals. Then link that particular piece in with the supine and floor sitting rocking movements in Pelvic Tilts, standing and leaning with your pelvis against the wall described variations of Side-sit Bending, or pushing the foot into the floor while lifting the other foot movements in Wishbone. Link to pressing the feet to roll the pelvis in sitting and in the linebacker position in Sit to Stand, pressing the foot to stabilize the pelvis movements in TA Diagnals and TA Leg Lifts, and pressing the foot to control forward bending extension stressors and pushing the pelvis back to full vertical in Half-kneel Bending and Split Stance Bending. Link to pressing the foot to propel forward in Steppin' Out. This work is very modular: pick a piece then blend it into a number of different places.

Other circumstances in which we might want to encourage pressing the foot into the floor through hip extension rather than knee extension include working with people with chronic hip flexor strains, ACL strains or reconstruction, for hamstring strains or tears, for patellar tracking problems and for Achilles tendinitis. Recurrent hip flexor strains may be an indication of an iliopsoas bias. The strong iliopsoas is overpowering the weaker hip extensors, and forward movement is more through stepping out than pushing off.

Level off the hip flexor/extensor imbalance with the same basic progression as in the low back pain scenario. Perhaps emphasizing pushing the pelvis to vertical movements in Sit to Stand, Half-kneel Bending, Steppin' Out and Split Stance Bending to fully lengthen/require the inhibition of the hip flexors.

With anterior cruciate ligament sprains or reconstructive surgeries, we will want to de-emphasize the push-off function of the quadriceps because of the anterior shear movement of the tibia on the femur that they create.[53,54] By emphasizing the hamstrings in push-off, we are both reducing potential quadriceps-created drawer strain at the knee and training the rota-tional stabilizers of the knee to be balanced and available for push-off.

If the hamstring strain or tear of the person you are working with is partially because of quadriceps and hip flexor tightness that requires the hamstrings to work harder, especially at end-range of hip extension, where the resistance from the anterior muscles are more pronounced, then the slippery board might be a nice tool. If the hamstring strain is partially because of weakness of the hamstrings and their inability to hold up under repetitive or sudden acceleration impacts, they also need to learn to facilitate a more accurate and powerful hip extension and could use the board.

Patellar pain

In addition to possible knee rotation or foot pronation and to probable medial/lateral quadriceps imbalance[55–58] as contributors to patellar tracking problems, you may have noticed that people who are prone to this problem tend to do things in a very knee-intensive way. Have them stand and put one foot up on a chair seat, then ask them to press that foot into the seat. What they will most often do is to fire the quadriceps and straighten the knee. Watch for a straightening movement at the knee and for a tendency of the pelvis and torso to rock backward in space.

If performed from the hip extensors and hamstrings, this movement will not straighten the knee at all but will extend the hip and posteriorly rotate the pelvis instead. Do a variation of this test movement standing and leaning against a wall with the feet spread apart and placed a fair bit away from the wall. The knees are bent and hands are on the knees like a football linebacker. Ask them to roll their pelvis up the wall and watch to see if they roll their pelvis and keep their knees bent, or whether they either roll or slide their pelvis and straighten their knees.

Is their strategy knee or hip intensive? Try this while sitting in a chair and leaning with your elbows on your knees as in Sit to Stand. Watch for a subtle almost-sliding of the feet forward. These movements are clues to how they organize themselves for walking, going up and down stairs, running, bending over or squatting down, or getting up from Sit to Stand.

Think back to some of our basic principles of movement: even distribution of movement and proportional effort. The whole lower extremity is an integrated system just like the spine. Like the spine, we would like to organize the lower extremity system to move from proximal to distal. In the spine, that meant starting movements of the spine at the pelvis, where the biggest bones and strongest muscles are, then tapering off intensity of muscular effort as you got to the neck, where the smallest bones and most delicate muscles are.

In the lower extremity, this means initiating movements of the legs and providing the bulk of the power for a movement of the legs from the all-powerful muscles of the hip joints, then using progressively less effort as you move distally through the knee, ankle and toes. People who are knee intensive in their movements are in violation of the good housekeeping rule and need to learn to associate an intention to press the foot into the floor with primary activation of the hip extensors rather than of the quadriceps.

Whereas left/right malalignment is a primary ingredient in patellar pain, the other prime ingredient is patellar contact pressure. Contact pressure is increased (and compressed cartilage is put at risk) through hyperflexion of the knee or through resistance against extension.[59–62] In other words, the harder the quadriceps has to work, the more compressive force is placed on the patellofemoral cartilage. Reduce quadriceps overuse by training the hip extensors to push the feet into the ground.

The vastus medialis

I realize that de-emphasizing the quadriceps seems to contradict conventional wisdom and its emphasis on the strengthening of the vastus medialis, though I do not believe a conflict actually exists. This approach emphasizes more medial/lateral balance of the knee in space controlled from the hip joint, the abduction/adduction balance of the foot on the floor controlled through the balance of the medial and lateral hamstrings and popliteus, and pressing the foot functions primarily being performed from the more powerful hip extensors when working with people with patellar tracking problems. That doesn't mean we should ignore the vastus medialis.

Think of medial/lateral quadriceps imbalance as an outgrowth of adductor/abductor or internal rotator/external rotator bias at the hips. People who are adductor or internal rotator biased tend to have medial knee collapse and vastus medialis insufficiency. By addressing hip muscular imbalance, keeping the foot centered on the floor and keeping the knee above the foot in this and subsequent lessons in this chapter, we can reactivate the vastus medialis and achieve better medial/lateral quadriceps balance.

Strengthen the vastus medialis by funneling movement constraints down to a place where it has to work functionally with the foot or leg on the floor. Progress by getting into various standing and kneeling postures and shifting weight backward. These falling-back movements are excellent functional contexts for strengthening and balancing the quadriceps. More on this later.

This is why the slippery board is of such benefit for people with patellar tracking problems. It helps to reduce knee external rotation, foot abduction and pronation. It emphasizes hip extension and hamstring contraction, and it relegates the quadriceps to its proper secondary role. By pressing the foot and lifting the hip in this position, you are requiring hip abduction and external rotation and are inhibiting the probably overactive adductors and hip internal rotators. Use lessons and variations as described above for extension-related back pain, but with more proprioceptive focus on the foot on the floor and the subjective feeling of stability at the knee.

Other places to work with patellar tracking problems besides the lessons listed above include pressing the leg to control bending and return to vertical movements in Side-sit Bending or its described variations, the hip abduction movements in Side-lie Transitions and Dead Bug Roll, the pelvic force couple balancing movements in Wishbone, Side-lie Transitions, Cat/Camel and Side-sit Transitions and the walking simulation movements of Steppin' Out.

Are the hip extensors your Achilles heel?

Another example of when we would want to facilitate an ability to press the foot into the floor, emphasizing hip extension rather than ankle extension, is in Achilles tendinitis. Irritation of the Achilles tendon may be related to a violation of the good housekeeping rule. The tertiary muscles of the calf are carrying too much of the load and are breaking down their tendon. The stronger hip extensors need to shoulder a greater proportion of the responsibility. Use progressions and relate to previous lessons as outlined above for back and knee.

This illustrates again how the same basic movement imbalance can manifest itself in a number of different sites of tissue irritation, and how the same basic exercise approach can work with a number of different diagnoses. What you are really doing is teaching basic movement skills, then varying your language and varying how you direct your student's proprioceptive attention to be specific to each particular person's problem.

Coordinating medial/lateral hip, knee and foot balance

In variation D you are asked to balance your foot in a medial/lateral or abduction/adduction direction and then to slide the whole board from side to side on the floor. In the initial movement of this variation, the toes maintain their forward orientation and the knee stays above the foot. This movement is an abduction/adduction movement of the hip or a hybrid of adduction/abduction and horizontal adduction/abduction.

Note the synergistic relationships of hip and foot. As the hip abductors contract to slide the board outward on the floor, you will need to make an adjustment to prevent your foot from rolling outward on the floor. The peroneus longus needs to contract. As the hip adductors contract to slide the board inward, you will need to make an adjustment to prevent your foot from rolling inward on the board.

The anterior or posterior tibialis needs to contract; we will want to cue the posterior tibialis. We will be seeing these synergistic connections between hip abductors and peroneus longus and between hip adductors and posterior tibialis again later in this chapter.

A common mistake people make when doing this variation is in sliding the board outward on the floor with hip internal rotation rather than hip abduction. They might also slide the board inward with hip external rotation rather than adduction. Cue the sliding board through hip horizontal adduction and abduction; keep the knee over the foot!

What would be the benefit of doing this movement? It allows for a cooperative reciprocation between the adductors and abductors. The way this antagonist pair is balanced affects the position of the distal femur in space; it determines medial/lateral balance at the knee joint and is a major factor in determining the amount of pronation and supination of the foot.

We will continue to explore adductor/abductor balance and function more specifically in the next lesson and will discuss then some of the implications of adductor/abductor imbalance in injury prevention or recovery, in the treatment of biomechanical faults and in enhancing athletic performance. This variation of sliding the whole board from side to side is introduced in this lesson in anticipation of going on to the next lesson, and makes for a good starting place for working on adductor/abductor balance and competence. It is closed kinetic chain but partial weightbearing – a functional but safe place to begin learning.

Can you think through, visualize or feel proprioceptively what adjustments have to be made at the knee to keep the toes pointed straight forward regardless of whether the femur is adducted or abducted? These are differentiated patterns of hip abduction with knee internal rotation and hip adduction with knee external rotation. Which movement is a common enemy of the patella and which movement is its rescuer?

Can you feel or imagine the adjustments your ankles need to make as you slide the board from side to side? This movement is also a good place to start working with ankle inversion/eversion control and to balance and improve competence of the posterior tibialis/peroneus longus antagonist pair. As an alternative, try centering your foot on the board or the floor – then tilting your knee in and out without allowing your foot to roll in or out with your tilting knee. This movement also requires competence and control from our foot/ankle medial and lateral stabilizers.

Exaggerate the hip/knee differentiation – lead with the heel

In the next movement of this section you continue to slide the whole board left and right on the floor, but lead the movement in each direction with your heel. When sliding the board to the outside and engaging your abductors, you now are directed to deliberately rotate your tibia internally to engage your medial hamstrings and popliteus. This is a more exaggerated differentiated pattern, very different from the hip abduction, knee external rotation, ankle eversion movements we teach with elastic tubing or bands. In particular, this is the differentiated pattern that would be so beneficial to so many people with biomechanical faults of the knees or feet.

A very common movement imbalance that many folks with genu valgus and pronation have is an adductor bias. They angle their femurs inward by pulling with the adductors. The knee needs to compensate by angling or rotating the tibia outward (see Fig. 7.1). This is the hip adduction with knee external rotation pattern we see in the other half of the movement: sliding the board inward and leading with the heel. This common pattern may manifest itself in the many lower extremity problems listed previously.

These reciprocating differentiated movements – hip adduction with knee external rotation and hip abduction with knee internal rotation – help in balancing not just local antagonist muscle pairs but also regional differentiated pattern pairs. In the case of the commonly seen hip adduction and knee external rotation patterns, emphasize the nonhabitual direction of hip abduction and knee internal rotation. For those somewhat rarer folks who habitually bow their legs into hip abduction and knee internal rotation, emphasize their nonhabitual direction as well.

Box 7.6 Slippery board

Use of toy constraint to facilitate medial/lateral hamstring balance – stabilizing the knee with rotational stresses and postural balancing

Use of toy constraint to facilitate awareness of pushing foot into the floor through hip extension rather than knee extension

Coordinating hips, knees and feet in habitual and nonhabitual differentiated patterns

Description of alternative toy – the hard foam roller

The last subvariation of this section is to feel for, then to direct, movement of the pelvis as a consequence of sliding the board and contracting the adductors and abductors. Recall how the gluteal group of muscles pushed the pelvis away from and how the iliopsoas group of muscles pulled the pelvis toward that leg. The adductors and abductors work similarly. The abductors act to push the pelvis away from, and the adductors act to pull the pelvis toward that leg.

If your right foot is on the board and you slide the board outward to the right, your pelvis will roll on the ground to the left if you allow it to do so. Whereas anatomy books describe a moving insertion bone and a fixed origin bone, in reality a muscle contraction will move both bones toward each other. If your pelvis did not roll on the floor to the left as you slid the board to the right with your right foot, you were doing something else to stabilize or otherwise prevent your pelvis from moving as a consequence of your abductor contraction (Box 7.6).

If your pelvis did not roll to the right as you slid the board inward with your right foot, you were doing something to keep your pelvis from responding. Try to learn to allow your pelvis to move; give yourself an opportunity to experience that particular choice. With the foot sliding, the movement is not very large. In the next lesson, we will enlarge on this idea but use the friction of the floor to create larger and more powerful movements of the pelvis directed from the adductors and abductors.

Comparing baselines

The last movement variation in this section is to return to center, press your foot and lift your hip. After having made exploratory movements to find where your toes point forward and where your thigh is neither adducted nor abducted, you now return to this dynamic baseline of pressing your foot, then adding in lifting your opposite foot to complete the pelvic force couple movement.

How is this by-now-familiar movement organized at this time, and what did you learn from having your foot on a slippery board while you did it? Remove the board and press your foot into true ground. How does it feel now? Return to your initial dynamic baseline and lift your forefoot to reach big and little toes laterally and medially to the floor. Is your ankle moving any more smoothly, or are you any more aware of how to create, control and balance the knee rotation movement from your hamstrings?

Variations E and F are just mirror images of variations B–D and variations G and H are change of venue variations of the same movements. Lying supine while doing these movements is a degree of difficulty progression both because it tends to accentuate the tendency of the board to slide away and the hamstrings to work and because you now can't see what you are doing with your foot. This requires greater refinement of your proprioceptive listening skills. On the other hand, many people are not very comfortable sitting up and leaning back on their hands. Often, you will just skip straight to doing this whole lesson supine.

Describing variations

Positional variations for this lesson include doing it while sitting on the floor and leaning back on your forearms, or lying on your back with your feet up on the wall. With your feet on the wall, you could still use a board if it will slide without damaging your wall covering. Use a small patch of carpeted wall for both feet-on-the-wall and leaning-against-a-wall lessons.

Alternately, you could just have people slide their forefoot left and right on the wall like windshield wipers, or do it this way with the feet back on the ground again. Progress sliding board or windshield wiper movements by changing venue to chair sitting (perched near the front edge and feet out in front of you), to half-kneeling, to leaning on a wall with feet out in front, or to a long split stance position.

We could also use touch/pressure as a reference point for the knee rotation movements. Many people have difficulty in accessing this movement, and many more have difficulty in differentiating the movement of the knee from the movement of the ankle and the effort of the lower leg musculature. Try lying on your side with your hips and knees bent at about 90° and with your knees and feet together.

Keeping your first metatarsal heads in contact with each other, lift your top heel and lower it back down again. This is a movement of knee internal rotation performed through the medial hamstrings and popliteus, both eccentrically and concentrically. Then keep your heels in contact as you lift your forefoot and toes. This is a movement of knee external rotation. Palpate your lateral hamstring tendons to verify activity. Alternate lifting heel and toes to facilitate medial/lateral hamstring balance. Do this in prone and hogtied positions as well. Lie on your belly, bend up your knees to 90°, place knees and feet together and move heels or toes away from each other.

Try lying on your belly with one knee bent at 90°. Could you hold the board horizontally with your foot in this position? Imagine holding a water glass with the board! How do you find horizontal in eversion and inversion directions, dorsiflexor and plantarflexor directions, and all the diagonal directions in between? By moving. Design a lesson around reciprocating ankle dorsiflexion and plantarflexion movements to find neutral (Fig. 7.11).

Continue with eversion and inversion movements, again reciprocating to establish center. Try turning the front of the board left and right while keeping it horizontal. Can you differentiate knee rotation from the ankle movements that will tend to spill your board and its imaginary water glass? Try bending and straightening your knee and making dorsiflexion

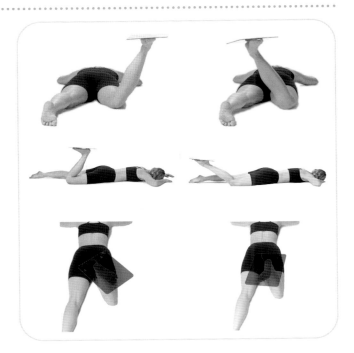

Fig. 7.11 Working with foot-to-knee relationships in prone – ankle eversion and inversion – ankle dorsiflexion and plantarflexion – knee internal and external rotation.

and plantarflexion adjustments to keep your board horizontal (Fig. 7.11).

Try tilting your lower leg alternately left and right through hip joint internal and external rotation and making ankle eversion and inversion adjustments to keep the board horizontal (Fig. 7.11). Make a circle with your lower leg in space and make multiplanar adjustments at your ankle. Lower your foot almost back to the floor and make your hamstrings and calves work synergistically. Are you able to allow your pelvis to posteriorly rotate and your lower back to flatten as a consequence of your hamstring contractions? Can you differentiate hip and lumbar extensors in this position?

Try lying on your back with both knees bent. Lift your right foot towards the ceiling and place your board on the sole of that foot. Do ankle movements as in prone to find horizontal balance in both planes and in circles. Raise your right foot toward the ceiling. This rolls your pelvis to the left by engaging your left adductors, as in TA Leg Lifts. Lower your right knee towards the floor to your right. This rolls your pelvis to the right, as in Wishbone and TA Leg Lifts by engaging your left hip extensors and abductors.

Alternate these movements to associate with pelvic force couple movements, but with added complexity of ankle/foot adjustments in keeping the board horizontal (more or less) (Fig. 7.12). Segue into a movement of rolling through your side and back to your belly while keeping the board on your foot to link up with prone variations. This latter suggestion is extra-extra credit.

Another prone facilitation of knee rotation control can be performed with both legs bent up to 90° while lying on your

and feet together, lower legs vertical, with legs tilted together as if hogtied to one side, then the other. Vary the position of your arms and the orientation of your head to preview some strategies for thoracic and ribcage mobility facilitation that we will be doing in the section on shoulder girdles.

A new toy

As an alternative toy to the slippery board, 3–6-inch hard foam (or cardboard or wood) rollers work well in helping your student to recalibrate knee rotation neutral. Sitting on the floor or lying supine with one leg bent up, place the sole of that foot lengthwise on the roller so that the middle of your heel and that spot between the first and second metatarsal heads is on the top of the roller. Angle the roller on the floor parallel to the midline of the torso. Create a constraint that requires the foot to be straight to start by artificially redefining neutral.

Roll the roller a little bit from side to side to train ankle eversion and inversion balance and competence, and to find middle. Press your foot into the roller to lift your hip. If you press with an adductor bias, your knee will tilt in and your roller will want to roll out. If you press with an abductor bias, your knee will tilt out and your roller will want to roll in. Using the roller lengthwise is a constraint that rewards the ability to keep the knee over the foot (Fig. 7.13). Use the same principle while supine with rollers on the wall, sitting with rollers on the floor, standing and leaning back against the wall with rollers on the floor and, for the thrill seekers among you, standing away from the wall with rollers on the floor.

Try placing the roller perpendicular to your foot and to where you just had it. Roll the roller toward and away from you to find the middle of your foot. Press your foot and lift your hip. If your weight is toward the back of your foot, you will have to engage your ankle dorsiflexors to prevent your ankle from plantarflexing. If your weight is toward the front of your foot, you will have to engage your calf muscles to prevent your ankle from moving into dorsiflexion. Directing awareness to the change in effort of the lower leg muscles leads to directing awareness to the balance and minimization of effort of the lower leg muscles when the foot is centered front to back (Fig. 7.14).

Taking this a step further, try standing up and rocking forward and back on your feet. Feel the effort in your calf as you rock forward on to your forefoot and feel the effort in your anterior compartments as you rock back on to your heel. Use awareness of effort to find center. Leaning forward from a chair and linebacker positions are other good places to experiment with forward/back weight distribution and to play with standing crosswise on rollers.

Placement of the roller crosswise also fulfills another function of the slippery board: it tends to roll away from your pelvis and requires the hamstrings to kick in. Using the roller crosswise is a constraint that rewards an ability to press your front-to-back-centered foot into the ground with your hip extensors. Try this with your feet on rollers and up on the wall.

Think back to previous lessons where one or both feet have been on the floor and think of how you could add further refinement, variety and complexity to those lessons by adding in either the slippery board or the crosswise and lengthwise

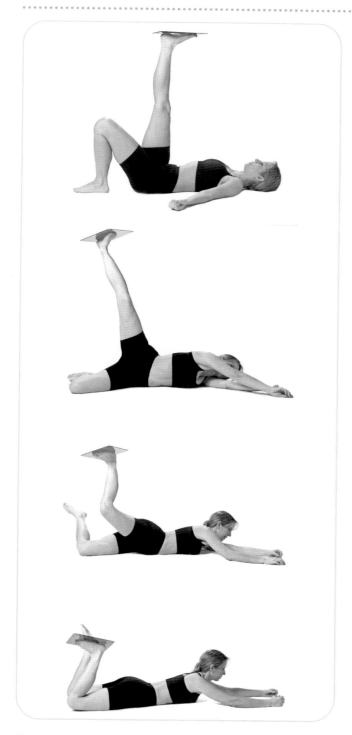

Fig. 7.12 Working with foot-to-knee-to-hip relationships in supine – segue into transitional movement to roll across the floor.

belly and placing your feet and knees together; no board this time. Design a lesson around moving one heel away from the other, then reverse, then move both heels away from each other at the same time. Move one metatarsal head away from the other, then reverse, then simultaneously. Do this with knees

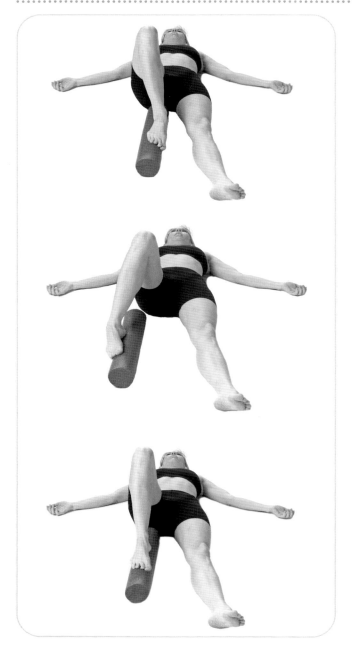

Fig. 7.13 Using a 3-inch roller lengthwise along the foot – facilitating peroneal/tibialis posterior balance and heightening an awareness of a neutral or skeletal weightbearing foot in a medial/lateral plane.

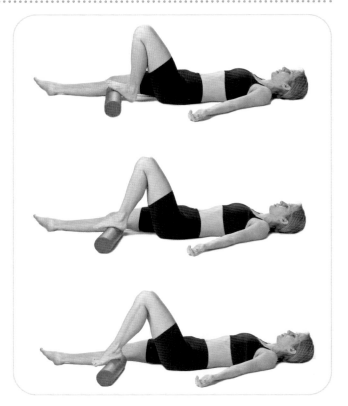

Fig. 7.14 Using a 3-inch roller crosswise across the foot – facilitating anterior tibialis/extensor digitorum longus to gastrosoleus balance and heightening an awareness of neutral or skeletal weightbearing foot in an anterior/posterior plane.

Medial/lateral foot balance

We will go on to our next lesson now to explore ways of further improving medial/lateral balance and stability of the lower extremities. After having facilitated a more neutral foot on the floor in an abduction/adduction direction, we will turn our attention to facilitating a more neutral foot on the floor in a medial/lateral direction.

Before doing this lesson with people, use a manual technique to help them to experience what you mean when you ask them to roll their foot inside and outside on the floor and then to stabilize their foot on the floor. Ask them to either sit or lie supine on the table or the floor and bend up one knee to place the sole of that foot flat on the floor, with the foot neither adducted nor abducted. Place one hand on their knee and ask them to give you the weight of their leg while you place your other hand on the medial aspect of the distal lower leg, a few inches above the ankle.

Allowing and controlling the rolling foot – manual facilitation

Gently and slowly press with your bottom hand to push the distal end of the lower leg laterally. This movement of the lower

rollers. Mix and match the two toys – put the foot on top of the board and board on top of the roller. Don't forget alternatives in which you have a knee rather than a foot on a roller. Be creative, adjust your language to fit the intention and the specific problem, and have fun!

Don't forget to use toys with neurologic and medical folk as well. Use boards and rollers to apply movement and stabilization constraints and to refocus kinesthetic awareness on affected side.

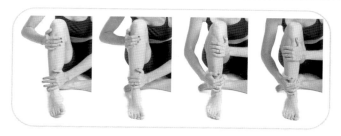

Fig. 7.15 Push out to roll out – then stabilize. Push in to roll in – then stabilize.

Box 7.7 Pronation/supination balance

Pronation is differentiated relationship of hindfoot valgus and forefoot varus

Supination is differentiated relationship of hindfoot varus and forefoot valgus

Coordinate hip abductors or external rotators with peroneus longus to stabilize and balance the foot

leg laterally drags the foot along with it and the ankle rolls into inversion, outward on to its outer edge. Do this movement of pressing laterally against their lower leg then letting it go to allow the foot to roll back inward again several times until your students are aware of the connection between pushing their lower leg out and rolling their ankle outward into inversion. They will need to learn to inhibit their peroneals and toe dorsiflexors to allow their foot to roll. Change the position of your hands and put your bottom hand on the lateral aspect of the lower leg. Push the distal tibia medially; this rolls the ankle inward into eversion (Fig. 7.15).

Notice that as the ankle everts, the calcaneus rolls inward. This is a *valgus* position for the heel. The forefoot however, can't follow the heel fully into valgus because it runs into the floor. As the heel rolls inward, it drags the midtarsal bones inward along with it, but because the floor is in the way, the forefoot can't just continue to roll inward with the calcaneus. The resultant twisting of the forefoot into varus relative to the calcaneus flattens and lengthens (overstretches) the medial longitudinal arch and presses the first ray into the floor. This creates a *varus* position of the forefoot relative to the rear foot; here is yet another differentiated pattern. We call this differentiated position of rear foot valgus and relative forefoot varus *pronation*.[63–65]

Notice that as the ankle inverts, the calcaneus rolls outward. This is a varus position for the heel. As the heel rolls outward, it drags the midtarsal bones outward along with it. Because the floor is no longer in the way, the forefoot can roll outward along with the heel. This results in lifting the whole medial edge of the foot away from the floor and loss of contact of the head of the first metatarsal. This is not a stable foot: think of a two-legged stool!

For the foot to be stable left and right, both the first and the fifth metatarsal heads need to be on the ground (preferably in good balance). When Rolling the Foot outward, then, the forefoot needs to differentiate from the rear foot and move into relative valgus. We call this differentiated position of rear foot varus and forefoot valgus *supination*.[63]

Assess this skill yourself. Push your distal tibia laterally to roll your heel outward then see if you can reach the head of your first metatarsal back to the floor without rolling your heel back inward (Fig. 7.15). This results in shortening the distance between first metatarsal head and heel and creates a high medial longitudinal arch. The farther you can roll your heel outward without the first metatarsal head leaving the floor, the higher

and shorter the arch becomes. Which is your habitual way of differentiating your foot?

After having established an ability on the part of your student to recognize how to allow the foot and ankle to move as a result of these applied medial and lateral stresses, we now want her to be able to counteract these stresses and stabilize her foot on the floor. Going back to pushing the distal tibia laterally again, direct your student to gently press the bottom of her first metatarsal head into the floor (Box 7.7).

This activation of the peroneus longus now resists the rolling outward movement of the foot on the floor and prevents you from pushing her lower leg farther laterally. This peroneus longus activation is not automatic: often people will substitute by contracting the toe dorsiflexors rather than plantarflexing the head of the first metatarsal. This is an extremely valuable skill to have for people with a wide variety of conditions.

Application of skill – stabilizing the foot

Consider the person with an inversion-style sprained ankle. We want her to be able to protect her ankle from rolling out again and straining the distal fibular ligaments and related lateral ankle tissues. The peroneals are just the muscles for the job. How do we train her to use the peroneals accurately and at the right time? How do we get her to recognize lateral movement stressors? How are we going to cue her to kick in her peroneals? What can her functional intention be?

By manually pushing her lower leg laterally, we are helping her to recognize the effects of lateral stresses on her foot and ankle proprioceptively. We do it here first under hothouse conditions, then progress it to where she can do it with her own effort, then gradually increase weightbearing loads and simulate lateral movement stresses with more advanced lessons.

We cue her to stabilize her foot on the floor by asking her to press her first metatarsal head into the ground. The intention to press the big ball of the foot into the floor is a much more functionally relevant way of engaging peroneus longus contraction and control than eversion isometrics or moving the ankle against rubber tubing resistance. Although these strategies may be appropriate initially after injury, we need to progress our students with sprained ankles past this regionally global, more primitive and open kinetic chain exercise.

We don't want to continue to associate peroneal contraction with lateral hamstring contraction and knee external rotation. We don't want to continue to associate peroneal contraction with ankle dorsiflexion and eversion. We don't want to continue to associate peroneal contraction with lifting the forefoot off the floor.

We do want her to associate peroneal contraction with preventing the foot rolling to its outside edge. We do want to associate peroneal contraction with a closed kinetic chain position. We do want to associate peroneal contraction with proprioceptive recognition of lateral stresses acting on the ankle.

When stepping unexpectedly on an irregular surface, sudden withdrawal of the foot from the floor through the simultaneous activation of peroneals, the common toe dorsiflexors and the hip flexors is appropriate. To prevent the right ankle from rolling over when planting that foot and changing directions or cutting, another strategy is needed. We want her intention to be one of pressing the first metatarsal into the floor instead of everting the ankle against resistance. This is pattern-specific exercise, making exercise look something like the activity we are trying to influence. The following lesson will give you an opportunity to explore this movement proprioceptively in more depth.

Blame, amelioration and consequences of pronation

Who else besides those with ankle sprains might benefit from this skill of pressing the first metatarsal head into the ground with the peroneus longus? Paradoxically, people who pronate could benefit greatly from learning this and related movement skills. In pronation, the ankle everts, the calcaneus comes to a valgus position and the forefoot collapses inward but inverts, or comes to a varus position relative to the heel. The medial aspect of the ankle overstretches and the lateral aspect compresses. If the peroneals are shortened here, why would we want to train people who pronate to contract them more?

The peroneals are not going to roll the heel outward on the floor – that job goes to others. What the peroneals do is to control the forefoot's relationship to the floor and to differentiate it from the rear foot. It is responsible for the necessary forefoot valgus as the heel and midtarsals are rolled outward. We could use a number of different strategies to roll the heel outward (hip abduction or external rotation, knee external rotation, posterior tibialis, anterior tibialis or flexor hallucis longus). All are possibilities, though all are not necessarily created equal. Each possibility requires the ability to make a differentiated movement of the foot, the ability to press the first metatarsal head back to the floor, and the ability to organize a stable foot to stand on, propel forward on and change direction on.

Hip and knee relationships to pronation

Let's journey further up the chain of command from the foot and ask about what the rest of the leg musculature is doing to contribute to pronation. Hip adduction is a prime suspect: high adductor tone may be pulling the foot inward on the floor. Hip internal rotation bias, along with adductor bias, can contribute to compensatory knee external rotation and to the collapse of body weight inward on the feet. Stand for a moment with feet apart and pull them inward with adductor contractions. Feel your feet roll into pronation. Stand and rotate your femurs inward. There are a couple of ways of interpreting this. Some

will roll their hips inward by doing a hybrid adduction movement and contracting the adductors; the knees collapse toward each other and the feet roll inward.

Others contract the tensor fascia latae and gluteus minimus to effect a truer internal rotation movement. This may very well lead to a rolling-outward movement of the foot as the abduction component of those muscles counteracts the rolling inward of the foot. Let's stay with the adductors as prime suspects. Along with this, we might anticipate a collapse of the lateral ankle and shortening of the peroneus longus and extensor digitorum longus, the unwitting accomplices, possibly along with biceps femoris, if there is a knee external rotation component.

To counteract the adductors, the hip abductors and/or the external rotators need to be trained to push or roll the foot outward on the floor. When the abductors contract in a closed kinetic chain situation, they move the distal end of the femur laterally and create a varus movement at the knee and an inversion movement of the ankle, Rolling the Foot outward on the floor.

Combined with the peroneus longus as it stabilizes the forefoot on the ground, this movement skill can ameliorate a number of postural and movement stresses through the hips and legs that are associated with pronation of the foot. As the distal end of the femur pulls the proximal end of the tibia laterally, this brings both the femur and the tibia toward a more vertical orientation. This seats the knee joint surfaces differently relative to each other as the legs change their configuration to bear weight more skeletally.

Knee valgus/external rotation consequences

When the adductors are pulling the femur inward and creating a valgus position at the knee, the lateral joint surfaces will become relatively more compressed and the medial joint surfaces will gap. This uneven distribution of weightbearing is detrimental to articular surfaces both medially and laterally: healthy cartilage requires intermittent compression and decompression. One of the consequences of a valgus knee on tissue health is that this arthrokinematically imbalanced joint may be prone to developing meniscal stresses or osteoarthritis.[66]

Another possible consequence of a valgus knee is patellar tracking dysfunction. The shallow V-shaped angle of the femur and tibia in a valgus knee creates lateral movement stresses on the patellofemoral complex and imbalances the arthrokinematic functioning of that joint as well. In a valgus knee, the medial collateral ligaments and medial capsule are overstretched whereas the lateral collateral ligaments are slack. Can you appreciate how the medial support tissues might be susceptible to postural stresses and resultant chronic conditions as well as medial or external rotational movement stresses and resultant recurring strains?

We can turn this question around and ask what we really want to do with people who are recovering from medial collateral ligament sprains or surgical repair. How much do we want to emphasize adductor strengthening? Wouldn't these folks be better served by proprioceptively recognizing medial knee stressors and by learning to control those stressors through the hip abductors and their side-kicks, the peroneals?

Another possible consequence of a valgus knee is iliotibial band syndrome. This may seem paradoxical, because we might think a tight distal iliotibial band would go with tight or dominant hip abductors.[67,68] Shouldn't this syndrome go along with a varus knee and hip abduction bias? Although this is sometimes the case, sometimes the pattern will be reversed. These people will have an adductor bias and valgus knees. This combination lengthens the ITB at the hip but shortens it at the knee.

With the femur and tibia fitted together in a shallow V, the distal ITB and other lateral knee tissues become shortened as the lateral knee surfaces become compressed. We might then get adaptive shortening of the lateral connective tissue and that dense and stringy feel we see with iliotibial band syndrome. Irritation and possible inflammation of that area is then precipitated by repetitive flexion and extension movements of the knee in a biomechanically imbalanced movement, as in running.

Although adductor bias and valgus knees contribute to foot pronation, so does knee external rotation. This resultant twisting or external rotation movement at the knee, usually as a compensation for adduction/internal rotation at the hip joints, is another example of imbalanced joint arthrokinematics with similar articular cartilage and meniscal consequences to a valgus knee, perhaps even magnified by the compressive effect of the cruciate ligaments as they are stretched by the twisting knee.

The medial collateral ligament and surrounding capsular tissues are again put at risk in this scenario, to both postural stresses and movement stresses (pivoting, cutting, change of direction). With the lateral movement of the tibial tuberosity pulling the patellar tendon and hence the patella laterally along with it, this hip internal rotation/knee external rotation pattern also alters normal patellofemoral joint arthokinematics and contributes to patellar tracking syndromes/chondromalacia.

In this schematic it is the hip external rotators that play a starring role in recovery. As they contract, they pull the femur into external rotation. This turns the knee internally toward a neutral position, then turns the tibia outward and rolls the calcaneus toward varus. The forefoot then needs to be differentiated from the rear foot through the peroneus longus.

In reality, the adductor bias/valgus knee and hip internal rotation/knee external rotation patterns are very close relatives, even interbreeding and spawning hybrids. We could say that both of these patterns are probably manifestations of a more general iliopsoas bias. The muscles that pull the pelvis toward the leg (iliopsoas and adductor groups) dominate the muscles that push the pelvis away from the leg (hip extensors, abductors and short and stubbies/hip external rotators).

Short and stubbies to the rescue – creating the tripod

We could say that both of these patterns could benefit from some of the gluteal/iliopsoas balancing lessons that have preceded this chapter, and that they could especially benefit from pelvic force couple balancing lessons with an emphasis on the pushing or gluteal component. Comb back through the Tyrannosaurus chapters for movements within lessons that empha-

---

Box 7.8 The tripod
Even distribution of weight front to back – ankle dorsiflexor/plantarflexor and hip flexor/extensor balance
Even distribution of weight between first and fifth metatarsal heads – peroneus longus/posterior tibialis and hip adductor/abductor balance
Subtalar joint in neutral – bearing weight skeletally on vertical calcaneus

size abductor and short and stubby strengthening. What does hip abductor/external rotator strengthening for various knee conditions have to do with using the peroneals to control foot pronation (Box 7.8)?

We left off our description of the kinematic linkages in the abduction scenario at the point where the distal femur pushed laterally, bringing the proximal tibia along with it, and the knee moved into varus. From here, the continued use of the hip abductors pushes the distal end of the tibia laterally and rolls the calcaneus outward on the floor. This is where the ability to stabilize the foot on the floor with the peroneals comes in handy. For a number of lower extremity injuries and repetitive stress syndromes, we want to have stronger/more competent hip abductors and external rotators.

For these muscles to be effective, they need to be synergistically matched with the peroneals. For the person who pronates, pushing or rotating outward from the hips would be a very beneficial direction of movement. We want to train people who pronate to control that medial postural stress with their large and in-charge hip muscles in a kinematic linkage, rather than having to rely on the much smaller foot intrinsic and lower leg musculature to prevent the collapse of the arch against gravity and full body weight.

How far outward should the foot roll as a consequence of abductor/external rotator contractions? To the middle! *Subtalar neutral* (palpate for subtalar neutral in yourself or others if you know what to feel for). Subtalar neutral has been described as a place where all vertical bones are vertical and all horizontal bones are horizontal. Subtalar neutral has also been described as a place at the mid point of 20° inversion and 10° eversion of the calcaneus.[69–72]

Proprioceptively, roll the foot to the middle of the heel, then make adjustments so the first and fifth metatarsals are bearing weight equally. Think of a well-balanced tripod: equal weight distributed between the heel and forefoot and equal weight between the first and fifth metatarsal heads.[s]

If the abductors are unchecked, the foot will roll into complete inversion and the medial aspect of the foot will lift completely from the floor unless an adjustment is made. This rolling-outward movement is arrested by pressing the first metatarsal head into the ground. Make the varus movement of the heel from the hip and the valgus movement of the forefoot with the peroneus longus.

The peroneus longus needs to contract to stabilize the foot on the floor in response to hip abductor contractions, just as it did when we manually pushed the distal tibia laterally. This is why learning this peroneal stabilization skill is so important for control of both movement stresses (lateral acceleration and

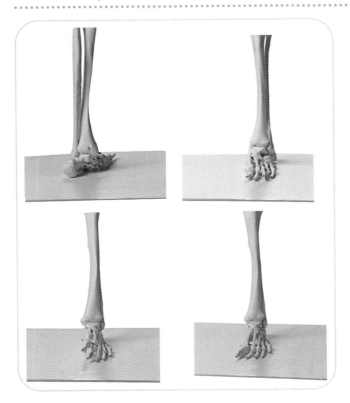

Fig. 7.16 Bare bones representation of hindfoot valgus and forefoot varus differentiation – of the same differentiated pattern in subtalar neutral – and the opposite differentiated pattern of hindfoot varus and forefoot valgus.

deceleration movements or stabilizing against lateral forces) and postural stresses (the foot loses its skeletal weightbearing property as it collapses inward into pronation). This forefoot varus/hindfoot valgus is a very common one clinically (Fig. 7.16).

What we would often like to train is a nonhabitual differentiated movement into rear foot varus and forefoot valgus. How do we go about teaching this motor control skill? We could train the posterior tibialis, the hip external rotators or the hip abductors to roll the calcaneus outward on the floor. Because the forefoot is used to being in a varus configuration relative to the heel, the habitual pronator will roll the forefoot outward as well and the whole first ray/big toe will lift from the ground (Fig. 7.16).

To prevent this, it again requires the peroneus longus to work to keep the first metatarsal head on the floor (Fig. 7.16). This differentiated pattern of calcaneal varus and forefoot valgus requires both motor control (coordinating hip abductors/external rotators or posterior tibialis with peroneals) and often additional mobility in the foot articulations (reduction of joint and fascial stiffness). Use your favorite manual technique, use squatting lessons introduced later in the chapter, or teach a self-mobilization technique to your more flexible students.

Self-mobilization of the foot

Side-sit with your right foot in front of you. Reach underneath your right heel with your right hand to lift the heel away from the floor. This moves the calcaneus into varus/inversion. Then use the heel of your left hand against the bottom of your first metatarsal head to press the top of the first metatarsal head into the floor. This moves the forefoot into varus as well. Use the heel of your left hand to press the dorsal aspects of the first through fifth metatarsal heads into the floor and to work along the bottom of the metatarsal shafts to press the dorsum of the midfoot into the floor. This is a regionally global pattern of forefoot and rear foot varus.

Now press again the dorsal surface of the first/second metatarsal heads and midshafts into the floor as you reverse the position of your right hand. Put the heel of your right hand against the medial aspect of your right heel and gently press the lateral side of your right foot towards the floor. This mobilizes the foot into a differentiated pattern of rear foot valgus and forefoot varus, needed by some but overdone by many. Use with very high arches/pes equinus/over-supinated foot. Play with variations of where to press and what to press with. Use with pronators to provide awareness and proprioceptive contrast.

Now, to create the opposite differentiated pattern, continue to press your right heel into the floor, this time with your left hand, as you reach underneath the outside of your right foot with your right hand. Grasp the heads and distal shafts of the fourth and fifth metatarsal heads with the second through fourth fingers of your right hand. Place the pad of your right thumb on the dorsal surface of your right first metatarsal head.

Use the fingers of your right hand to pull your right foot into ankle dorsiflexion and forefoot valgus/eversion, and the right thumb to push the head of the first metatarsal in a plantar direction. The whole effect is to use the right hand to twist the forefoot into eversion/valgus.

At the same time, you are using your left hand to press the right heel into the floor. Although this is initially a movement of the heel in the direction of valgus, at some point the floor constrains more movement. It is then possible to continue the movement of the forefoot into a valgus position relative to the more neutral and stabilized calcaneus. Use with low arches/pes planus/over-pronated foot. We are using the floor as an extra pair of hands to facilitate an ability to mobilize the foot into differentiated patterns.

See if you can spend 10 or 12 minutes in this side-sitting position, explore how to use your hands, how to allow your bones to be moved and how to turn off chronically working muscles of the foot and lower leg. Explore all three variations with some curiosity. Be creative, but be careful. Don't push too hard to protect both the foot and knee. You might notice that these are good self-mobilization techniques for knee internal and external rotation as well! Get up and walk around a bit after doing one side and feel for differences between left and right sides. Then get back down again to play with the other foot.

When integrated with hip abductor/external rotator control, we can train peroneus longus control with people who have plantar fasciitis, sprained ankles and patellar tracking dys-

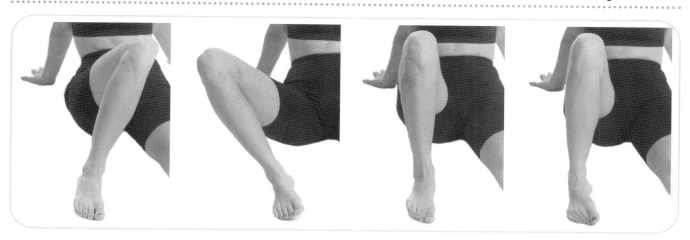

Fig. 7.17 Rolling the Foot in and out by tilting knee, then by using lower leg muscles.

function, medial collateral ligament strain, iliotibial band syndrome and knee osteoarthritis. This skill is very useful for people recovering from various hip, knee and ankle surgeries or joint replacements. Don't let the inevitable withdrawal function dominate, perpetuate and set the stage for future sloppy biomechanics.

Let's get on the ground and experiment with both pushing out and stabilizing the foot (abductors/peroneals) pattern and its reciprocal pair: pulling in and stabilizing the foot (adductors/tibialis posterior) pattern.

Rolling the Foot

Variations

A. Stand for a moment in your bare feet. Let your arms hang at your sides, feet around shoulder width apart, and look straight ahead.

- Notice your feet against the floor. What direction do your toes point?

- Are your feet rolled in to flatten your arch or are you rolled on to the outside edges of your feet?

- Do you have more weight forward on your toes or back on your heels?

- How is your weight distributed between the big ball (first metatarsal head), the small ball (fifth metatarsal head) and the middle of your heel? Does your foot feel like a well-supported tripod?

- Walk around a bit and feel for movement of your ankles or toes. Does your ankle bend and straighten? How clearly can you feel your toes? Which toes do you use to push off with?

- Get a general sense of the springiness of your legs and how you are propelling yourself forward. How are your legs moving your pelvis in space?

B. Sit on the floor and lean back on your hands behind you. Rest your left leg down on the floor long, with your knee straight. Bend up your right leg so the sole of your right foot is flat on the floor.

- Notice first the direction that the toes on your right foot point. Do they angle in? Out? Straight ahead?

- Lift and lower your right forefoot a few times, then alternate between reaching towards the floor to the left with your right little toe and reaching towards the floor to the right with your right big toe.

- Use this movement to help you establish center, that placement of your foot on the floor where your toes point straight forward.

- Notice how your weight is distributed across your foot from inside to outside edge. Is there more weight toward your big toe side or your little toe side? How high is your arch?

C. There are several ways of rolling left to right across the sole of your foot.

- The first way is to simply tilt your right knee alternately right and left. Do this movement several times and notice how, as you tilt your right knee outward to the right, your weight shifts toward the outside edge of your foot.

- When tilting your knee inward, your weight shifts toward the inside edge. Alternate back and forth a few times, then come to stop where your knee is angled neither in nor out but where your knee points toward the ceiling (Fig. 7.17). Now you should have your toes pointed straight forward and your knee pointed straight at the ceiling.

- The second way of rolling your foot in and out is to use the muscles of your lower leg (Fig. 7.17). Try rolling your foot toward its outside edge without allowing your knee to tilt out. Can you feel an effort at the front of your ankle or up along your shinbone?

- Observe visually for a large bulging tendon on the front/inside of your right ankle (this is the anterior tibialis). This is a way of Rolling the Foot outward that relies on lifting the inside edge of the foot.

- The third way of Rolling the Foot outward is to press the ball of the little toe (the head of the fifth metatarsal) into the ground. This strategy of pressing the fifth ball into the floor to roll outward is one we will be emphasizing. Try this pressing-to-roll movement many times.

- Now try rolling your foot towards its inside edge without allowing your knee to tilt inward. There are several choices here as well.

  ○ The first way of Rolling the Foot inward relies on lifting the outer edge of the foot. Can you feel effort across the top of your foot or up along the outside of your lower leg? Observe visually for lifting your toes and bulging of several smaller tendons along the top of your foot and outer ankle (these are the toe dorsiflexors).

  ○ The second way of Rolling the Foot inward is to press the ball of the big toe (the head of the first metatarsal) into the floor. This is again a strategy of pressing the ground to roll that we will emphasize. Alternate rolling your foot in and out using these lower leg muscles several times. Press the outer/small ball into the floor to roll out and the inner/big ball to roll in (Fig. 7.17). Can you make this movement without using the muscles on the front of your leg and the top of your foot? Can you press the first ball without lifting the four outer toes, and without pressing the pad of the big toe?

- Alternately roll your foot by alternately pressing inner and outer balls. Use this movement to find a tripod. Find that place where your weight is in the middle of your heel and where there is equal weight between the first and fifth metatarsal heads.

  ○ You could try finding this tripod arrangement by simultaneously pressing first and fifth balls into the ground.

  ○ You could find this arrangement by Rolling the Foot outward. Do this by pressing the fifth ball, letting the big toe and big ball lift initially, then pressing the big ball of your foot gently back toward the ground without allowing your whole foot and ankle to roll back inward.

  ○ This is a subtle movement of pressing the first metatarsal back toward the ground and shortening the distance between big ball and heel. Your arch will lift!

- Find your tripod and stay there.

  ○ Press your right foot into the floor and lift your right hip (Fig. 7.18). Roll your pelvis on the ground to the left as you keep your knee pointed to the ceiling and your foot centered.

  ○ Repeat several times to appreciate quality of movement and accuracy of skeletal alignment.

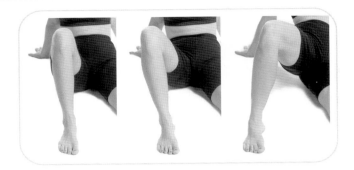

Fig. 7.18 Rolling the Foot inside and outside edges to find center, then pressing the tripod foot into the floor to lift the hip.

G. Come up to sit and lean back on your hands. Put your right leg down long and bend up your left leg.

  - Repeat instructions as in B–F to the opposite side.

H. Lie on your back.

  - Bend your right leg up and straighten your left leg down long. Roll your right foot in and out without tilting your knee. Press little ball to roll out and big ball to roll in. Find your tripod and stay there as you press your right foot into the floor and lift your right hip several times (Fig. 7.19).

  - Bend up your left leg and straighten your right leg down long. Repeat as above with the left foot. Find the tripod and press the foot to lift the left hip.

I. Lie on your back with both legs bent up. Arrange your feet reasonably close to parallel and point both knees toward the ceiling.

  - Roll both feet in and out by pressing first and fifth balls. Find the center and stay there.

  - Now make a movement of pressing outward with both feet at the same time. Imagine you are trying to stretch or tear apart the carpet between your feet. Press outward from your hips, but keep your tripods stable on the floor. To do this, you will need to press the first balls into the ground.

  - Try a few times of pressing outward, as if to tear the carpet between your feet and letting your feet roll to their outside edges. Instead of stabilizing your feet on the floor, can you allow them to roll outward as a consequence of the pushing-outward movement you are initiating from your hips?

  - Go back to pressing outward and stabilizing your feet. Don't let them roll to their outer edges. Do this slowly and gently so you can feel how you counteract the rolling-out movement by pressing the first balls into the ground.

J. Lie on your back with both legs bent up. Arrange your feet reasonably close to parallel and point both knees toward the ceiling.

  - Roll both feet in and out by pressing first and fifth balls. Find the center and stay there.

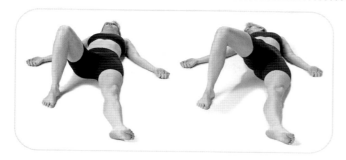

Fig. 7.19 Finding the tripod again while lying on your back and pressing foot to lift hip.

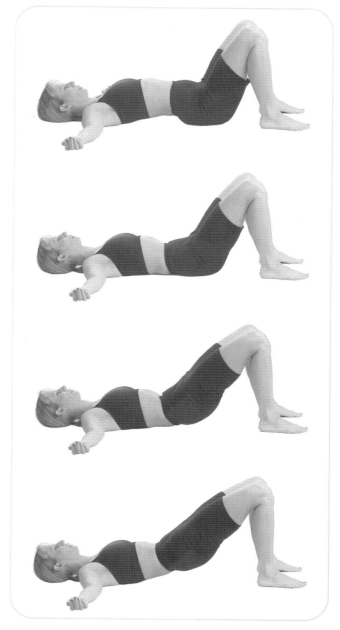

Fig. 7.20 Pressing both feet outward, then pressing both feet into the floor to roll your pelvis upward – then lift pelvis from floor.

- Now make a movement of pulling inward with both feet at the same time. Imagine you are trying to bunch up the carpet between your feet. Pull inward from your hips, but keep your feet stable on the floor. To do this, you will need to press the fifth balls into the ground.

- Try a few times of pulling inward, as if to bunch up the carpet between your feet, and letting your feet roll to their inside edges. Instead of stabilizing your feet on the floor, can you allow them to roll inward as a consequence of the pulling-inward movement you are initiating from your hips?

- Alternately push out and pull in, both stabilizing your feet on the floor and allowing them to roll in and out.

K. Lie on your back with both legs bent up. Establish where the toes of both feet are pointed straight forward and where both knees are pointed toward the ceiling.

- Press outward from your hips to roll your feet outward, just to the middle of your heels. Press the first balls into the floor to stabilize your feet in this position. This is another way of establishing a tripod. Keep pressing outward from both hips – keep your tripods centered.

- Then press both feet into the floor to roll your pelvis upward on the ground. Your tailbone will lift and your lower back will press back into the floor. Do this movement of simultaneously pushing outward (tearing carpet) and pushing backward (pressing tripods into the ground) to lift your tailbone several times (Fig. 7.20).

- Lift your tailbone and stay in this position for a while. Can you maintain your ability to push your feet outward from your hips and your ability to stabilize by pressing the first balls of your feet?

- Continue with the same movement but enlarge it: lift your tailbone, then pelvis, then lower back and so on up your spine. How far can you lift your pelvis without engaging the extensor muscles of your lower back? Keep tripods.

L. Lie on your back with both legs bent up. Establish where the toes of both feet are pointed straight forward and where both knees are pointed toward the ceiling.

- Press your feet outward; stabilize your centered tripods by pressing the first metatarsal heads.

- Keep your feet centered as you roll your pelvis alternately from side to side on the floor. Press outward more with your right foot to roll your pelvis to the left (Fig. 7.21).

- Press out more with the left foot to roll your pelvis to the right. Alternate from side to side.

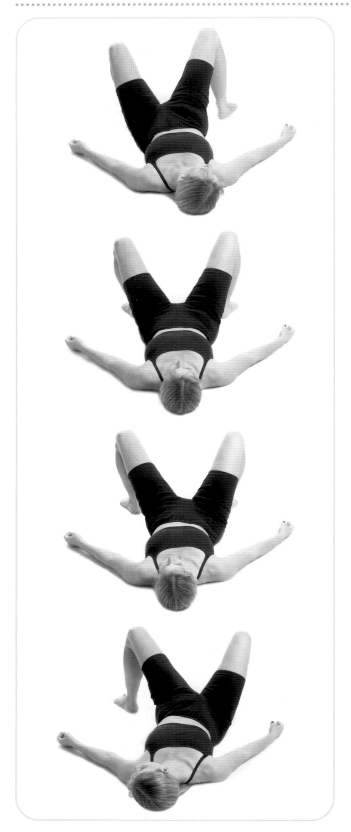

Fig. 7.21 Pushing the pelvis from side to side – first and fifth metatarsals continually planted.

- Add in lifting one foot and then the other. March in place while keeping the pushing foot centered (Fig. 7.22).
- Try swinging a long lifted leg left and right both down low to the ground and pointed toward the ceiling. Try this flat on your back or propped up on your forearms (Fig. 7.23).

M. Stand for a moment in your bare feet. Let your arms hang at your sides, feet around shoulder width apart, and look straight ahead.

- Notice your feet against the floor. What direction do your toes point?
- Are your feet rolled in to flatten your arch, or are you rolled on to the outside edges of your feet?
- Do you have more weight forward on your toes or back on your heels?
- How is your weight distributed between the big ball (first metatarsal head), the small ball (fifth metatarsal head) and the middle of your heel? Does your foot feel like a well-supported tripod?
- Walk around a bit and feel for movement of your ankles or toes. Does your ankle bend and straighten? How clearly can you feel your toes? Which toes do you use to push off from?
- Get a general sense of the springiness of your legs and how you are propelling yourself forward. How are your legs moving your pelvis in space?

Baselines – Rolling the Foot

After our initial assessment of the three dimensions of the foot in variations A and B, we come back to sitting on the floor with one leg long and one leg bent up in our first movement variations. We start here by making a link to our previous lesson. Do the toes of the standing foot point inward, outward or straight ahead? We revisit the initial exploratory movements of the previous lesson by lifting and lowering the forefoot and reaching big and little toes inward and outward. After re-establishing a truer neutral in a foot abduction/adduction dimension, it's on to the main event.

The primary focus of this lesson is the balance of the foot on the floor in pronation/supination. Is the foot rolled inward or outward on the floor? The initial inquiries and the initial exploratory movements in this lesson are then concerned with whether your foot is rolled in or out to start with, and how it is possible to roll the foot in and out by various means.

Choices in Rolling the Foot

The first and perhaps most obvious way of Rolling the Foot in and out is by tilting the knee inward and outward. If the knee is tilting inward, either here in supine or in a standing position, the foot will roll toward its inside edge. If the knee is tilting outward, the foot will roll toward its outside edge. We can use these reciprocating movements to begin to train our student in recognizing the relationship of the knee to the foot and the

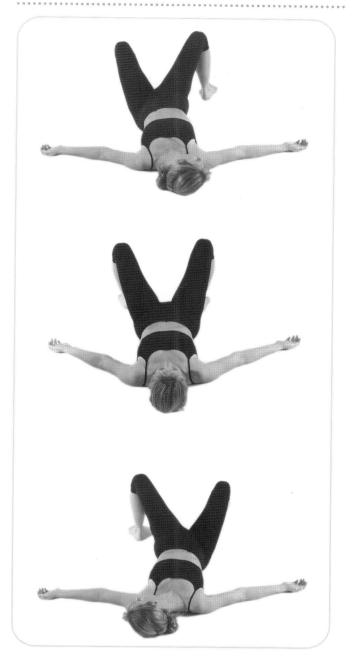

Fig. 7.22 Press one foot down and out while you lift the other – marching.

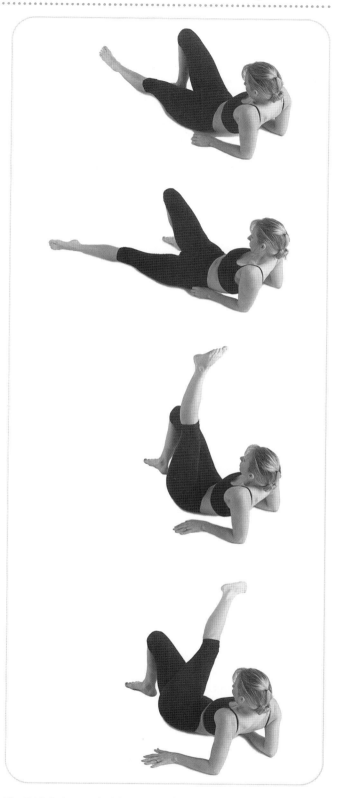

Fig. 7.23 Swinging the lifted leg from side to side – what do you have to do to keep your standing foot stable on the floor?

importance of finding and maintaining that place where the knee is organized vertically over the foot.

The second way of Rolling the Foot in and out is by moving the ankle and foot through local muscular effort. The peroneus longus can press the first metatarsal into the floor, or the extensor digitorum longus can lift the lateral forefoot from the floor to roll the foot inward. There is a choice. The posterior tibialis can press the fifth metatarsal into the floor, or the anterior tibialis can lift the first metatarsal away from the floor to roll the foot inward. There is a choice again. Which choice do we want to emphasize with most of our students?

We'll probably want to train peroneus longus/posterior tibialis access and balance, using a pressing the foot against the floor context to roll medially and laterally or to prevent the foot from rolling on the floor. The anterior tibialis/common toe extensor strategy is the Peter Pan choice: all lifting into the air and very short on grounding. This pair will emerge later, however, and have more of a starring role in front/back foot balance. What we will want to see in our students is an ability to press the fifth metatarsal and to roll the foot outward on the floor without anterior tibialis effort. Are you able to make the differentiation?

We also want to see an ability to press the first metatarsal head into the floor without toe dorsiflexion. Can you differentiate the peroneus longus from the extensor digitorum? Because what we are really talking about here when assessing medial/lateral foot balance is the ability to prevent the foot from rolling in or out on the floor; the pressing into the floor option becomes increasingly attractive. There is also an intrinsic choice in Rolling the Foot outward. You could press the pad of your big toe into the floor and use the flexor hallucis longus to assist in supination.

Doing the movement of Rolling the Foot alternately inward and outward on the floor by alternately pressing the first and fifth metatarsal heads is our classic reciprocating movement designed to help balance the antagonists and to find a truer neutral. Could we just stop right here, train peroneal/posterior tibialis balance, throw on some weights and call it good? No, using these small muscles to control the foot on the floor in full body weightbearing is asking way too much from the wee lads. This would be an egregious violation of the good housekeeping rule.

Why are we introducing this as a way of Rolling the Foot then? In the case of Rolling the Foot by lifting one side, we want our students to also be able to feel what not to do or how not to do it. This introduction of deliberate error is a variation of the Goldilocks principle. In the case of the Rolling the Foot by pressing one metatarsal head, we do want to use them to stabilize the foot on the floor in the presence of medial, lateral or rotational stressors.

Think of these as analogous to the intersegmental stabilizers of the lumbopelvic area. In the lower extremity, as in the lower back, we can think of having several layers of stability. How do we mobilize or stabilize the pelvis on top of the legs? How do we move or stabilize the femur on top of the tibia? The tibia on the foot? The foot on the floor? Rather than acting as primary supporters of the foot, we can think of medial/lateral balance (equally competent posterior tibialis and peroneus longus) as being an outgrowth of hip and pelvic balance (or an indication of bias/imbalances of the more proximal musculature).

Gaining better motor control and balance over the intrinsic foot and lower leg musculature can reflexly enhance balance and control over associated musculature further up the chain, whereas gaining better hip musculature control and balance necessitates a change in distal muscle balance and competence. Work the system from both ends to enhance efficiency at both ends.

What we are often looking for is that reduction of pronation is associated not with posterior tibialis activation alone, but with peroneal activation within the pattern of a hip abduction or external rotation-initiated kinematic linkage that results in an outward rolling of the heel on the floor. The peroneals act as a brake to prevent the heel from rolling too far into varus and to differentiate the forefoot into valgus. In this scenario, the flexor hallucis can be synergistic with the peroneus longus as both the first toe and the first metatarsal head can press into the floor to assist with reducing foot pronation and its accompanying physical ailments.

The instruction to press the first and the fifth metatarsal heads simultaneously into the floor is about creating a dynamic placement of the foot on the floor in a way that distributes weight evenly between the medial and lateral columns and suggests to the CNS to reproduce that balance through proximal control. The idea of the foot as a tripod can be a very powerful proprioceptive cue: equal weight front and back and equal weight left and right. Facilitate this ability to press simultaneously the first and fifth metatarsal heads by turning your hand away from you and moving thumb and little finger tips toward each other while keeping your palm as broad as possible.

Use the more familiar neurologic connections to your hand to provide a template for action at your foot. Try lifting the middle three toes away from the floor while pressing the outer two. Try small wedges; place them under the medial column to facilitate posterior tibialis control and under the lateral column to facilitate peroneus longus control. There are, of course, exceptions to the rule of proximal initiation and control of the foot. In the presence of a very unstable knee, initiating movements from the hips could be detrimental. In this instance, the posterior tibialis and flexor hallucis are going to have to be prime movers in Rolling the Foot outward.

A third way of Rolling the Foot in and out on the floor in this position that we didn't explore in the lesson is through rotational movements at the knee: tibial internal and external rotation. As you sit or lie in this half hook-lying position, a contraction of the lateral hamstring and its resultant knee external rotation could roll the foot outward if you inhibit the peroneals sufficiently to allow this to happen. Medial hamstring and popliteus activation rotates the tibia inwardly and rolls the foot inward.

Despite having potential as a great party trick, this is not something we will teach much; it is not pattern specific. By Rolling the Foot this way, we are linking pronation with knee internal rotation and supination with knee external rotation. Most commonly, we will want to favor an internal rotation (reduction of external rotation) movement at the knee joint associated with a supination movement of the foot on the floor. To achieve this, we will need to go a little higher up in the kinematic chain; let's get the hip joint involved.

Connecting the stabilizers of the foot to the hip abductors and adductors

The remainder of the lesson explores the relationship between the adductor/abductor balance of the hip and the position of the foot on the floor, on the relationships between the hip abductors and the peroneus longus, and between the hip adductors and the posterior tibialis in stabilizing the foot on the floor.

In the next section, we start by re-establishing an ability to roll the foot in and out by pressing the first and fifth metatarsal heads and establishing a centered tripod. From there, press this tripod into the floor to lift one hip. If you keep your foot centered, the hip needs to adjust by abducting, extending and externally rotating. If your hip abductors and external rotators are active, the peroneus longus also needs to hop to it if the foot is to stay stable on the floor.

Try adding in an intention to press the foot outward with the hip abductors (as we did in the slippery board lesson when sliding the board outward). Experiment with allowing your foot to roll outward (inhibiting the peroneals) and stabilizing it (in a subtalar neutral position) by pressing the first metatarsal head into the floor.

Reverse to roll your foot inward on the floor using your adductors, again allowing this to happen by inhibiting the posterior tibialis or stabilizing (in subtalar neutral) by pressing the fifth metatarsal head. These unilateral movements echo the bilateral movements we make in the next section of this lesson. Try allowing your pelvis to roll from side to side. Push out and stabilize your right foot, allow your pelvis to roll to the left. Pull in and stabilize your right foot, allow your pelvis to roll to the right.

Rolling the feet from the hips

In variations I and J bend up both legs, establish your tripods, and intentionally press the feet outward as if tearing the carpet between your feet or pulling the feet inward as if bunching up your carpet. Initially, the instruction is allow your feet to roll freely in and out. This can help our students in early recognition of medial and lateral stresses and how they act on the foot and ankle.

We then took the next step. After having focused on the ability to allow the foot to roll in and out, we now want to develop an ability to use that rolling movement to find a more accurate neutral position of the foot on the floor, then finally on an ability to keep that proprioceptively redetermined neutral or centered position even in the presence of medial and lateral stresses. We trained our students in stabilizing the foot on the floor.

The outward pushing of the foot on the floor from the hip abductors results in Rolling the Foot laterally on the floor until the peroneals are activated through an intention to press the first metatarsal into the floor. Confirm this connection visually or by palpation both with yourself and with students. This peroneal contraction stops the rolling movement of the foot; it resists lateral movement of the foot on the floor. This associative connection between the hip abductors or external rotators and the peroneals is a very important one in change-of-direction activities.

For a basketball or tennis player moving laterally and then stopping to change direction, or for an ice skater coming to a stop, the same basic thing has to occur. The hip abductors on the side toward which they are moving have to do a lengthening contraction to keep the hip from adducting and the pelvis and torso from succumbing to their lateral inertia and falling over in the direction they were moving. This abductor contraction stabilizes the lateral knee, which would tend to snap the knee in the direction of varus and protects the lateral collateral ligament through the ITB.

The peroneals then have to contract to keep the ankle from inverting/rolling outward and spraining the lateral ankle ligaments. In either case, with lateral collateral ligament protection at the knee or with lateral ankle ligament protection, our proprioceptive focus should be on the ability to initiate movements of the foot from the hip and to stabilize the foot laterally through an intentional pressing of the first metatarsal into the floor, not on laterally lifting an open kinetic chain leg in sidelying to quantitatively strengthen the abductors, and not on everting and dorsiflexing the ankle against resistive elastic bands or tubing.

A similar mechanism is at work in controlling rotational stresses. Stand up for a moment with your feet just a bit wider than your hips and with your feet turned in toward each other at 30 or 40°. Turn your whole body to the left: turn your pelvis, torso, shoulders and head. As you do this, notice how your left foot tends to roll outward on the floor. Initially, allow this to happen. After having established a proprioceptive awareness of the relationship between rotational movements of the pelvis and torso and the position of the left foot on the floor, stabilize that left foot now by gently pressing your first metatarsal head into the floor.

Feel how this prevents your foot from rolling farther toward its outside edge. Here, the peroneals are connected to the left hip short and stubbies. As you turn to the left, as if swinging a baseball bat or a golf club, the left hip rotators do a lengthening contraction to decelerate the ballistic turn of the pelvis to the left and to keep you from bouncing off your posterior hip ligaments or from falling down. Turning the pelvis to the left drags the left femur along with it and the femur externally rotates. This creates an internal rotation stress at the knee that could result in cruciate ligament strains or tears or knee meniscal damage. What controls this rotational stress at the knee? The lateral hamstrings.

We started exploring medial/lateral hamstring balance and competence in controlling knee rotation in the previous lesson, and will explore this in more detail in subsequent lessons. For now, we will continue to focus on hip-to-foot relationships. After the left femur has externally rotated and the knee has internally rotated, the tibia externally rotates and in turn rolls the left foot outward on the floor, necessitating again a peroneal contraction to stabilize the foot on the floor. This is the peroneals-to-hip-short-and-stubby connection.

The inward pulling of the foot on the floor from the hip adductors results in Rolling the Foot medially or a pronation movement of the foot on the floor until the posterior tibialis is activated through an intention to press the fifth metatarsal into the floor. Confirm this connection visually or through palpation with yourself and students. This posterior tibialis contraction stops the rolling movement of the foot inward: it resists medial movement of the foot on the floor and eversion ankle sprains.

Pushing or pulling to go or to stop – the secondary force couple

This associative connection between the hip adductors or internal rotators and the posterior tibialis is also an important one. Think again of the movement of the basketball or tennis player coming to a stop from moving laterally. If the player is moving to the left, for instance, she could stop herself with the left leg and use the abductor/peroneal connection established in the first movement, or she could stop herself with the right leg and use an adductor/posterior tibialis strategy.

The right adductor would fire to prevent the inertia of the pelvis and the torso from continuing to the left and toppling over, and to prevent the right hip joint from moving into too much abduction with a resultant strain or tearing the right adductors. Here again we find ourselves with choices. Do I engage my leading leg and the abductors on that side in a pushing-to-stop movement, or do I employ my trailing leg and the adductors on that opposite side in a pulling-to-stop movement? Or, do I engage them both simultaneously to create a synergistic relationship of opposite-side hip adductors and abductors, a sort of *secondary pelvic force couple* relationship?

We have been looking at strategies to come to a stop from moving laterally and have described choices. What happens when accelerating laterally from a stop position? What are our choices? Essentially the same as in coming to a stop, but reversed. When moving to the left from a standing position, for instance, the pelvis could be pulled to the left by the leading or left leg adductors, or it could be pushed to the left by the trailing or right leg abductors. Whereas the secondary pelvic force couple organization in the decelerate-to-stop-lateral-movement scenario was eccentric or lengthening, in the accelerate-to-move-laterally scenario the secondary force couple organization is concentric or shortening. Potential stresses on knee and ankle joints and supporting tissues are identical.

Moving down the kinematic chain, the right distal femur is dragged medially and a valgus strain is applied to the knee, putting the right medial collateral ligament at risk. This is true with decelerating lateral movements to the left and with accelerating lateral movements to the right. What stabilizes the knee here? The sartorius, gracilis and semitendinosus cross the medial knee joint and provide some stability, but not as much as is supplied laterally through the massive ITB and the big guns up in the posterior and lateral hip. Do you find that as curious as I do? Why is the medial knee not as well protected muscularly? Why do we tend to see more medial collateral injuries than we do lateral collateral injuries? Why do we see more groin pulls than gluteus medius pulls?

Could it be that we are better equipped to control stresses on the lower extremities resulting from movements from side to side on the floor primarily through the hip abductors rather than from the adductors? The short lever arm, stocky physique and close proximity to the joint of the hip abductors gives them the power advantage over the long lever arm and rail-thin build of the adductors.

The ITB provides passive lateral stability and allows the hip muscles to assist in lateral knee stability, whereas most of the adductors fall short of even crossing the knee joint. The instances of medial thigh and knee injuries are higher than for lateral thigh and knee injuries.[75] Although it is important to train our students in both choices and to employ the two simultaneously to create a third, the secondary force couple, emphasize more the abductors as a primary means of moving or decelerating laterally.

How can the medial collateral ligament be protected by the hip abductors? Let's start with the stopping-while-moving-left movement. The right medial collateral ligament is at risk, especially if your strategy is to use that right leg in a pulling-to-stop movement. The right adductors contract to pull the distal thigh medially while the right posterior tibialis fires to plant the fifth metatarsal head and stabilize the foot on the ground.

That leaves the sartorius and gracilis to counteract the valgus stress on the knee created by the much more powerful adductors. They are quickly overwhelmed, and the passive structures of the medial knee are then left defenseless. This situation could have been avoided by switching to a pushing-to-stop strategy: use the left hip abductors and left peroneals to stop the pelvis in space and stabilize the foot on the floor.

What about the accelerating-to-move-right movement? The right medial collateral is again at risk if your strategy is to use that right leg in a pulling-to-go movement. The right adductors again contract to pull the distal thigh medially, while the right posterior tibialis again works to stabilize the foot on the ground. The consequence is the same and the solution is the same. Use the left abductors as primary movers in a push-to-go movement to the right.

Use the abductors to protect the medial knee and groin

What about getting hit in the knee from the outside? If my student has been tackled from the right and has had her right knee knocked medially or leftward in space, she would be at risk of spraining her right medial collateral ligament. What prevents this movement of the distal end of the femur too far medially? The right hip abductors.

The same rationale can be used when discussing groin pulls. The abductors can protect the adductors from being overstretched. The left abductors protect the right adductors by stopping the pelvis from moving to far leftward in space in stopping-lateral-movement-leftward scenarios. The abductors can protect the adductors from being overcontracted. The left abductors initiate and power lateral-movement-to-the-right instead of making the right adductors do it.

Might a violation of the good housekeeping rule – disproportional distribution of effort – be common with groin strains? As we go through this and subsequent lessons in this chapter, we will be primarily emphasizing the abductors and their starring role in the stability of the foot on the ground, the stability of the knee over the foot, the stability of the pelvis on top of the legs and the stability of the lower back on top of the pelvis.

We could use this lesson to help someone to recover from an injury – or to prevent one – resulting from an inability to recognize and control lateral or rotational stressors. We could also use this lesson with someone with a repetitive stress lower extremity injury resulting from a miscalibration of medial/lateral balance. Rather than use the lesson to control

Box 7.9 Rolling the Foot

Manual facilitation – learning to allow the foot to roll freely on the floor and how to stabilize

Exploring possibilities in rolling the feet in and out on the floor – distal and proximal choices

Coordinating hip adductors with posterior tibialis – coordinating hip abductors with peroneus longus

Creating a secondary pelvic force couple – coordinating opposite adductors and abductors to control lateral weight shift

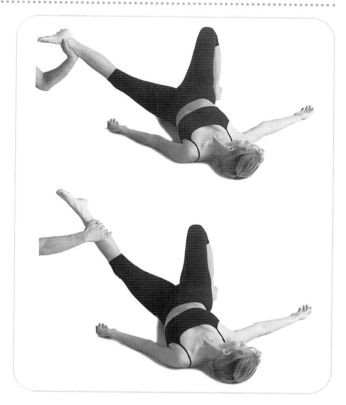

Fig. 7.24 Resisting the swinging leg to challenge tripod stability of the standing leg.

medial/lateral movement stresses, we could use it to help recalibrate medial/lateral postural imbalances (Box 7.9).

Where is your foot centered in a rolling-in/rolling-out dimension? Use this lesson to influence control over the amount of foot pronation and the detrimental effects it has on the plantar fascia, bunions or the Achilles tendon. Where is your knee in neither valgus nor varus? Use this lesson to influence control over the amount of knee valgus or knee joint external rotation and the detrimental effects it has on patellar tracking, distal ITB irritation, knee joint cartilage tears or ligamentous strains.

Where is your hip neither adducted nor abducted? Use this lesson to help in balancing the pelvis on top of the legs and reducing asymmetrical hip strains resulting in trochanteric bursitis or hip joint degeneration. Use this lesson to help in mobilizing and centering the pelvis on top of the legs and reducing lateral hypermobility stresses and asymmetrical stresses on the SI joints and lumbar spine.

Playing both ends against the middle – pelvic tilt and left/right balance

In variation K you push outward with the abductors to find subtalar neutral, then differentiate the forefoot and stabilize the foot on the floor with the peroneus longus. Find your tripod. Continue to press outward to effect a posterior rotation movement of the pelvis. This is a very important, but elusive, motor skill in lumbar stabilization and one that we will return to in the next lesson. The ability to posteriorly rotate the pelvis in standing from the hip abductors is a nice alternative to gluteus maximus or abdominal contractions.

Variation L features rolling the pelvis from side to side on the floor with alternate abductor contractions. One variation has you pressing outward with both abductors and playing them against each other in a game of tug-of-war. One hip abductor provides resistance for the other to work against. The abductors are antagonists in rolling the pelvis left and right and synergists in rolling the pelvis posteriorly.

Another variation is our familiar marching movement: lifting the leg in the classic Wishbone or pelvic force couple movement, but with intention/attention on pushing outward with the hip abductors. Blend primary and secondary pelvic force couples to create an irresistible force.

A final variation asks you to swing the lifted leg from side to side as a trigger to roll your pelvis from side to side. This coordinates the antagonistic adductors (rolling the pelvis toward the standing leg) and abductors (rolling the pelvis away from the standing leg) of the standing leg. It also coordinates the antagonistic rollers and stabilizers of the foot of the standing leg (peroneus longus and posterior tibialis). Try resisting this movement manually or with pulleys/elastics (Fig. 7.24).

Variations

As a possible subvariation of this rolling the pelvis movement, deliberately combine pushing out with one foot and pulling in with the other, both while allowing the feet to roll in and out on the floor and while stabilizing the feet on the floor. Alternately rolling the pelvis from side to side with this simultaneous pushing/pulling secondary pelvis force couple organization and with stable feet could be another cumulative movement of this lesson, and lends itself well as a focal point for home exercise.

Are there some positional variations to this lesson? Positional variations include lying supine with feet on a wall and progressing from farther away to closer to the floor. This can be particularly entertaining when your feet are close to the floor, your knees are nearly straight and your pelvis is in posterior rotation with your lower back pressed back into the ground. Sitting in a chair can work, though it tends to constrain the movement of the pelvis from side to side compared to doing it supine.

Side-lie with feet against wall, then slide your top foot upward and stay there by pressing out with abductors in both directions. Press out with your top foot as if to roll upward on the wall but stabilize foot with peroneus longus. Then move your top knee alternately forward and back (rolling pelvis and shoulders in log roll) to simulate rolling pelvis from side to side on the floor. Progress farther and farther away from the wall to work more in hip extension. Other variations follow in the next lesson. Horsing Around is a companion lesson and a progression from rolling the foot.

In addition to applying this lesson and these motor skills to orthopedic problems, try parts or variations of this lesson with your neurologic students, enhance lateral stability and balance in posture and change of direction activities. Provide conditions in which they will have to stabilize the affected foot on the floor. Use this lesson with amputees: direct their attention to the way their new foot interacts with the ground, and how to control it with the hips.

This next lesson picks up where we left off. Horsing Around is an extension of Rolling the Foot.

Horsing Around

Variations

A. Stand in your bare feet on a carpeted surface.

- Notice your feet against the floor. What direction do your toes point?

- Are your feet rolled in to flatten your arch or are you rolled on to the outside edges of your feet?

- Do you have more weight forward on your toes or back on your heels?

- How is your weight distributed between the big ball (first metatarsal head), the small ball (fifth metatarsal head) and the middle of your heel? Does your foot feel like a well-supported tripod?

- Begin to make a movement as if you were going to sit down in a chair or stool behind you. Use a chair if one is handy.

- Notice if there is a change in how your weight is distributed across your foot. Do your feet roll in or out?

- Notice if there is a change in the distance between your knees. Do they move toward or away from each other? Could you sit on a horse?

B. Lie on your back on the floor and bend up both knees; both feet are flat on the floor with your toes pointed straight forward and with both knees pointed toward the ceiling.

- Pick up here where we left off in the last lesson. Push out with both feet at the same time. Your right foot pushes out to the right, and you plant your right big ball as you do the same thing with your left foot. This simultaneous pushing out of both legs will cancel each other out in terms of side-to-side movement.

- Do this a few times and notice if there is a rolling of your pelvis up or down on the floor. Try letting your tailbone make a small lifting movement and letting your lower back flatten toward the floor (Fig. 7.25).

- After doing this simultaneous pushing out and releasing a few times, push out and hold it. Can you sustain this pressing outward from your hips along with pressing the big balls of your feet to stay centered on your tripod?

- Hold for 30–60 seconds, release, and repeat a few times. Adjust weight forward and back on your tripods as appropriate. Pause for a moment.

- Then push your feet back into the floor and roll your pelvis upward on the floor. Continue to enlarge this movement to lift your pelvis and lower back away from the floor (Fig. 7.25).

- In this position, now press your feet away from each other and plant your first metatarsals to center your tripods. Hold this for a bit, lower down slowly and repeat. Pause for a moment and rest with your pelvis on the floor and both knees still bent.

- Push out with both legs again to slightly lift your tailbone, and then hold that for a moment. Now keep pushing out with both legs but roll your pelvis from side to side on the floor (Fig. 7.26).

- One leg pushes a little harder as the other side lightens up, but both legs are pushing out and both feet are centered by maintaining pressure with your metatarsal heads. Your legs are playing a game of catch with your pelvis, tossing it from side to side.

- Roll from side to side several times in this cooperative tug-of-war. Don't let your knees tilt inward at all. Keep them out over your feet.

C. Stand up and lean back against a wall. Place your feet a bit wider than shoulder width on the floor out away from the wall. Let both knees bend (to about 135°).

- Arrange your toes straight forward, so your feet are parallel. Imagine you are straddling a horse.

- Move your knees toward and away from each other several times. Feel how this rolls your feet in and out.

- Use this movement to establish where your knees are over your feet; your knees point straight forward rather than angling in or out (Fig. 7.27).

- With your feet parallel and your knees over your feet, roll your ankles in and out using effort from your lower legs; alternately press the big and little balls of your feet. Find that well centered tripod and stay there.

- Push both feet out away from each other, as if tearing the carpet apart, and press your first metatarsals into the floor as you were doing while lying on the floor. Does this roll your pelvis up the wall a bit or round your lower back toward the wall?

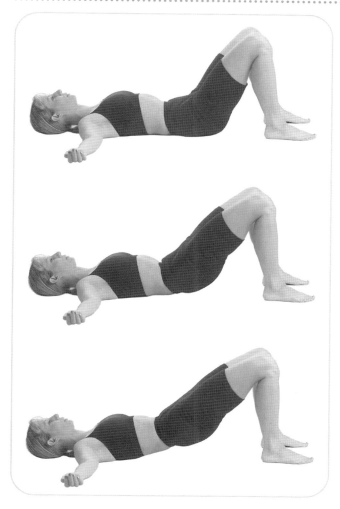

Fig. 7.25 Pressing feet outward to lift tailbone – add in lifting pelvis while maintaining outward press.

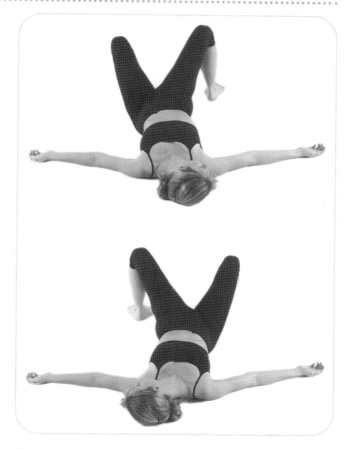

Fig. 7.26 Pressing feet outward and rolling hips from side to side – legs play catch with the pelvis.

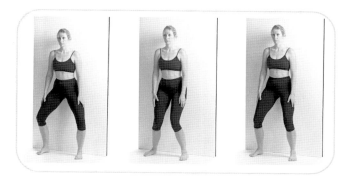

Fig. 7.27 Push knees away – pull knees in – horse stance with knees over feet and centered on the floor.

- Push both feet out to neutral, stabilize your feet by pressing the first metatarsal heads, and maintain that pressure with both feet as you roll your pelvis from side to side on the wall (Fig. 7.28).

- Let your chest and shoulders roll from side to side along with your pelvis. Think of rolling from side to side like a log. Notice how you shift your weight in the direction of your turn.

- What adjustments do you have to make in your hips and feet to keep your knees from moving in or out, or to keep your feet from rolling toward their inside or outside edges? Repeat several times.

D. Stand up away from the wall.

- Put your heels together so they touch and angle your toes outward at about 45° each (Fig. 7.29). Rock your weight toward your heels, bend your knees a bit

and tuck your tail in or point your tailbone towards the ground.

- From here, push your feet outward on the floor and plant your first metatarsals to stabilize your tripod. In this position, your knees should be over your toes.

329

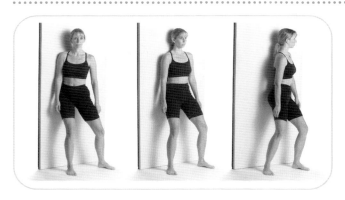

Fig. 7.28 Pressing feet out and rolling pelvis while standing with your back on a wall – keep tripods centered.

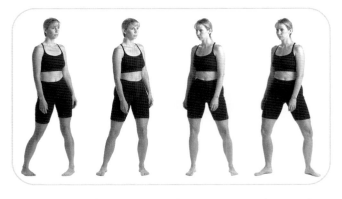

Fig. 7.30 Toe-in – horse stance – and toe-out versions of turning the pelvis – keep the tripods.

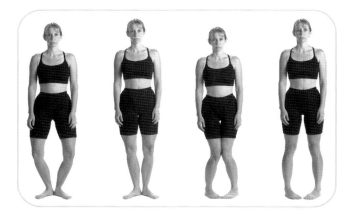

Fig. 7.29 Push taller and sink lower in toe-out and toe-in pose – feel how your gluteals work with each.

Your kneecaps are pointing out away from each other at 45°.

- Keeping your knees balanced out over your tripod feet, slowly and gently bend further and then straighten your knees (Fig. 7.29). Be sure to keep your knees out and your feet centered the whole time. Let your tailbone lift and move backward a bit as you bend your knees, lean your torso forward a bit and get shorter.

- Then push your pubic bone forward and tuck your tail as you straighten your knees to get taller. Do this several times, making sure to keep your feet centered and your knees pointed out at the same angle as your feet, then pause in normal standing for a moment. Your gluteals should be working very hard to do this and you may not be able to fully straighten your knees.

E. Stand up.

- Put your big toes together so they touch and angle your heels outward at about 45° each. Push out and

find your tripod feet, and bend and straighten your knees several times in this position. Does this movement seem easier in this position or with your toes pointed outward (Fig. 7.29)?

- Feel what happens at your ankles and feet as you straighten your knees. Try allowing your feet to roll outward a few times. Then resist this rolling movement by planting your first metatarsals.

F. Stand.

- Arrange your toes straight forward, so your feet are parallel. Soften your knees and sit back toward your heels a bit; point your tailbone toward the ground.

- Move your knees toward and away from each other several times. Feel how this rolls your feet in and out. Use this movement to establish where your knees are over your feet, where your knees point straight forward rather than angling in or out.

- Maintaining this position, push both feet out away from each other and press your first metatarsals into the floor, as you were doing while lying on the floor. Does this roll your pelvis more toward vertical? Rest for a moment.

- Push both feet out and maintain that pressure with both feet as you turn your pelvis from side to side and shift your weight from right to left foot. Your legs play catch with your pelvis (Fig. 7.30).

- Be sure to maintain a vertical pelvis and centered tripods. What do you have to do in your right hip to keep your right knee from drifting inward as you turn your pelvis to the left and shift your weight toward your left foot?

G. Stand.

- Push both feet out and turn your pelvis from side to side but with your feet at varying widths. Try this with your feet nearly touching; how stable is this?

- Try it with your feet very wide apart; how mobile is this? Try it at varying widths and assess for a good compromise between mobility and stability.

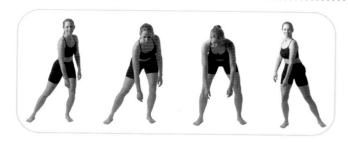

Fig. 7.31 Bending forward and swooping lower in the middle – pushing taller to each side. Keep knees out over tripod feet.

- This is a horse stance: feet a bit wider than hips, knees bent, back straight with tailbone pointed to the floor, and feet parallel with weight centered between inside and outside edges (Fig. 7.30).
- Turn your toes inward with your feet at wider-than-shoulders distance and try the same pushing out and tossing your pelvis from side to side (Fig. 7.30).
- What sort of hip movement is needed to keep your knees over your feet? What sort of ankle and foot adjustments are necessary to keep your feet from rolling completely to your outside edges?
- Turn your toes outward and do the same thing. What sorts of hip, foot and ankle adjustment are needed here (Fig. 7.30)?
- Shift your weight from side to side, but now bend forward as you come through the middle and then push taller as you come to each side. Let your head and shoulders move in a U-shaped curve. Be sure to keep your feet tripods and knees out over feet (Fig. 7.31).
- Walk around and feel your feet, ankles, knees and hips as you walk. How do they feel?

Baselines – Horsing Around

After assessing standing and walking organization again in variation A, we start our movement explorations in variation B by reviewing one of the last variations from the last lesson. Lie supine and roll your pelvis from side to side on the floor by coordinating opposite abductors in a tug-of-war. After refamiliarizing your student with this review movement, we press on by now pressing out with both feet at the same time as if ripping apart the carpet between your feet.

The opposite-side abductors/short and stubbies seem to be doing an isometric contraction. They are working against each other in a way that allows no lateral movement of the pelvis on the floor. That doesn't mean that movement of some kind won't happen. If you simultaneously push out from the hips and stabilize with the feet on the floor in this position or in subsequent changes of venue in this lesson, your pelvis

will roll into posterior tilt and your back will move toward flexion.

Pushing out to tilt pelvis posteriorly

This can be subtle for many people, especially once fully in standing with the knees straight. It may be difficult for some to differentiate the lumbar extensors from the hip abductors/external rotators, and posterior pelvic tilt may not occur for some. It is still a very valuable movement to learn, to have in your personal movement arsenal and to teach your students.

For the low back pain sufferer, the ability to push out simultaneously with the abductors is a way to press the feet into the floor and to push the pelvis to vertical. This relieves postural extension stresses on the low back. Although posterior pelvic tilt can be performed from the abdominals, this has drawbacks in terms of reduced power in comparison to the hip musculature and in terms of negative consequences on breathing, on thoracic mobility and on the shoulder girdles and neck.

Posterior pelvic tilt can also be performed from the lower gluteals. Pinch your cheeks together to deny thermometer access. This may have drawbacks in terms of having to lock down the pelvis on top of the legs and in terms of the associative havoc it may trigger in the lower digestive tract. Try walking like this and try not to giggle.

Our most elegant solution in standing is then one of pressing the feet away from each other and activating the TFL, gluteus minimus and medius, and the upper gluteus maximus. Stand as you did in the final sections of this lesson, press your feet out away from each other and palpate along the inferior aspect of the iliac crest for contractions of these muscles. Palpate for ability to differentiate/inhibit the lower gluteus maximus and appreciate the possibility of standing with a relaxed distal digestive portal.

Putting down roots

The back pain sufferer also benefits from learning this simultaneous pushing-out movement through an enhanced ability to control lateral stresses acting on the pelvis, especially when those stresses are intermittent and from random directions. Think of standing in a concert crowd and getting jostled from all directions, or standing on a boat in choppy water or swell, or trying to survive a rollercoaster ride or a ride in a car with a teenager. If you are pulling or pushing laterally but suspect the object you are moving might suddenly slip, protect yourself by pushing out some in both directions and cover all your bets.

Athletes who need to control lateral stresses coming from unexpected directions could benefit from learning this. The football lineman grappling with the behemoth in front of him might utilize some element of pressing outward to help protect his knees and ankles from blows from the sides and unexpected lateral movement stresses. Ditto for the wrestler clawing for a hold, the power forward trying to stake a claim to piece of floor under a contested basket, the hockey goalie trying to maintain his place in front of the net while still being able to move laterally in either direction, the surfer trying to maintain a grip on her board, the hiker when fording the calf-deep river when the bridge washes out, or the flight attendant on a turbulent flight.

This stance reeks of stability, of putting down roots, of grounding into the earth and refusing to be moved by forces human or elemental. Sadly, with the advent of paved walkways, cars and sedentary lifestyles, competence in lateral stability is sorely lacking in people of more technologically advanced societies. This movement of pushing out to stabilize is unfamiliar for most people, with predictable results concerning hip abductor/short and stubby weakness and adductor bias.

Practitioners of the martial arts have known this about this 'grounding' ability for centuries, but have never put things into Latin terms and applied it to western medicine. On the other hand, scientists know the lingo but probably lack the juice (proprioceptive acuity and personal movement experience). Each discipline has things to learn from the others' perspective, and there is a common ground. Quality of movement is where objective science and subjective art can meet.

Other variations in this section include pushing out in both directions and holding it: tonic postural muscles should be able to hold a submaximal contraction for long periods of time. How many minutes did you go? We then combined pressing outward with the feet against the floor with pressing the feet back into the floor with the hip extensors, as we did previously in Pelvic Tilts by coordinating posterior and lateral hip musculature to posteriorly tilt and lift the pelvis in a bridging movement.

Then press out with both feet and maintain some abductor effort with both sides as you roll your pelvis from side to side. One side works a little harder while the other side gives a little to allow lateral movement. In this variation, the legs are playing another version of controlled catch with the pelvis. Use this to simulate pushing laterally against resistance. Have your student put her palms together with both arms reaching toward the ceiling and manually resist lateral movement of the straight arms, initiated from the legs. Recall the described variation of this drill holding a vertical pole in the lumbar lateral stability section. Prepare proprioceptively for a standing version of the same movement. Relate upward to low back stability or down to knee and foot stability and balance.

Changing venue – leaning on the wall

In variation C we have a change of venue but are doing the same basic thing while standing and leaning the pelvis and torso back against a wall. This position is a degree of difficulty progression, with more weight going down through the legs and into the feet. We did much the same here as we did in previous variations.

We find parallel feet and find centered feet by tilting the knees, rolling the ankles from the lower leg musculature, and by pushing out and pulling in from the hips. Pushing out both feet and stabilizing the feet through peroneal activation in this position may be similar in terms of its effect on the pelvis and lower back, as it was in supine. Did your pelvis roll up the wall into posterior tilt as you did this? If not, why not?

Having the wall is handy in terms of being able to use a reference point to feel for movement of the pelvis into posterior

tilt, and handy because the hip joints are not yet at end-range extension, taking tight hip flexors out of the equation and making this movement easier to do than our next variation in full standing. Having a wall also provides a nice reference point and measuring stick for your ability to push your pelvis from side to side, to turn your pelvis left and right while keeping your feet centered on the floor.

How do you move your pelvis from side to side and what do you have to do to keep your feet centered with your knees over your feet? To roll your pelvis to the left on the wall, you could push the pelvis with the right hip abductors and external rotators or you could pull your pelvis with your left hip adductors and internal rotators. To keep your back knee over your back foot, the hip on that side needs to do some serious external rotation. This is a great context for training knee-over-foot concepts.

You'll have to watch very carefully here: it's very easy to let that back foot roll inward on the floor and for the back knee to collapse inward. A very small inaccuracy here makes a huge difference. Be very picky with this movement and insist that your student go only as far as she can go accurately. In this lesson you are asked to roll from side to side using the abductors/external rotators against resistance provided from the opposite abductors/external rotators. This is a lengthening contraction of the left and a shortening contraction of the right.

Your feet will tend to roll on the floor unless otherwise stabilized. The left foot will roll outward into supination and the right foot will roll inward into pronation. Movement of the left foot too far outward into supination can be arrested with the left peroneals. Movement of the right foot into pronation needs to be arrested by the right posterior tibialis, but where most people make their mistake in this movement is by allowing the right knee to drift too far inward to overpower the little tyke.

They are not allowing for (adductors tight) or fully contracting into (short and stubbies, gluteus maximus) right hip extension/abduction. The right hip external rotators in particular have to be very active to keep the right knee from drifting too far inward and dragging the foot inward on the floor along with it.

This ability to turn the pelvis away from the trailing leg in cutting movements is central to protecting the cutting knee and ankle from medial rotational stresses. This twisting movement of the knee into external rotation would tend to strain the right medial collateral ligament, the medial meniscus and the anterior cruciate ligament.[23] It is again the hip abductors and external rotators that protect the knee from these stresses. The adductors and internal rotators need to be sufficiently long to allow full hip external rotation and abduction, and the abductors and external rotators need to be sufficiently strong to keep the distal thigh stable in space over the foot.

We will be exploring cutting/change of direction movements in more depth in the last lesson of this Tyrannosaurus section, Peerless Pivots. In that lesson, we'll be looking a bit more into strategies to facilitate better knee rotational stability through hamstring/popliteus activation, through controlling the position of the knee in space from the hip joints, and by recognizing rotational stressors acting on the leg though proprioceptive awareness of the foot on the floor.

The Goldilocks gambit

In our next change of venue variations D and E you are fully standing without wall support. Placing either toes or heels together and angling feet at 45° each, you again tilt both knees towards and away from each other to establish where the knee is over the foot. In variation D your heels are together and your toes are pointed outward at 90° to each other. Is it easier to move the knees inward or outward in this position?

Although it's pretty easy for most of us to allow our knees to fall inward from this position, it's also pretty difficult for most of us to push our knees outward far enough in this position to roll to our outer edges. The hip external rotators need to get busy! Use this as part of a progression designed to wake up the short and stubbies and assign them to various functional chores: lateral stabilization of the lumbar spine, protection of the medial collateral/anterior cruciate/medial meniscus complex from medial stresses on the knee, and assistance in organizing the bones of the lower extremity to bear weight more efficiently, reducing external knee/knee rotation and foot pronation.

The movement of tilting your knees inward from this position can give you an exaggerated perspective on what it feels like to valgus. This common pattern of hip internal rotation, knee/knee external rotation and foot pronation is mimicked when you point your toes away from each other and pull your knees inward. Try walking like this, bend over to pick something up off the floor, or get up and down from a chair. Exaggerate the pattern to exaggerate the tissue strain on feet/ankles, knees, hips and low back and exaggerate the pattern to enhance proprioceptive self-awareness.

In variation E your toes are together and your heels are pointed outward at 90° (more or less) to each other. What is particularly interesting about tilting the knees in and out in this position is what happens when moving the knees outward. Push the knees outward and the external rotation of the lower extremities quickly starts rolling the feet toward their outer edges. This is therefore a great place to work with peroneal control of rotational stresses in a fully weightbearing position.

Initially, as when we started this process supine in Rolling the Foot, let your feet roll to their outer edges and feel what it is like to allow your foot to move. Then add in the intention to press the first metatarsal heads to stabilize the feet. Use this as part of an ankle sprain progression. Use this as part of an anti-pronation campaign. Use this to create a unique sensation: foot supination with tibial/knee internal rotation with hip external rotation. For people who valgus, this nonhabitual differentiated pattern of movement is the antidote to their self-inflicted poison. Do be judicious in the use of this particular medicine. It is fairly easy to over-rotate at the knee, so keep it mild.

Pushing taller and sinking shorter

We added in a new movement in variations D and E: bending and straightening the knees. The description of the movement included directions on leaning forward a little and lifting your tail as you bent your knees, then straightening up and tucking your tail as you straightened your knees. This is really just another version of a variation we did back in Sit to Stand.

In that lesson, you were standing with your hands on your thighs near your knees and were lowering and raising yourself in much the same way as in this lesson. You straightened your knees, tucked your tail and rounded your back, then bent your knees, lifted your tail and arched your back. Review that movement if the toe-in/toe-out versions are unclear (Sit to Stand variation F, Fig. 5.75). The movement in this lesson is different from the movement in Sit to Stand in how the feet are oriented. The constraints which may be created might be useful in helping someone learn to use their legs more efficiently.

By having the toes pointed outward and requiring that the feet stay centered, we are providing a constraint in which the hip external rotators have to be very active. By bending the knees and leaning over to get shorter, we are loading a series of springs. The ankle, knee and hip are all flexing. As the ankle moves into dorsiflexion, the temptation for most people is to start letting their knees fall inward. With foot pronation and knee external rotation being a substitute for ankle dorsiflexion, this is the path of least resistance for many. By adding the constraint of keeping the foot centered, however, we eliminate pronation as a choice and require the ankle to dorsiflex along a more neutral pathway.

Although we will be covering heel-to-toe connections and ankle dorsiflexion and plantarflexion in more detail in the next section, we could still introduce this movement in this position as an Achilles and soleus stretch. We could also use it for patellar tracking problems. Keeping the feet centered means keeping the knee over the foot and then training the quadriceps, especially the vastus medialis, to work functionally in lowering your center of mass.

By straightening the knees and hips together while keeping the feet centered, we are releasing the springs. The ankles, knees and hips are all extending. By keeping the feet centered, we are creating a constraint that disallows movement of the hips into internal rotation as they extend. The pelvis might tilt more posteriorly; this is what will happen 'naturally' if you let it. Stand for a moment and come back to this movement.

As you straighten your knees, just let your feet roll where they will. Do they tend to roll inward a bit? Can you feel how you have to keep pushing outward to straighten the knees with the feet centered? We are linking quadriceps, and especially vastus medialis, with the hip external rotators/abductors as they work in pushing you away from the ground. Add weights now that a specific pattern is established, or use plyometric concepts. Continue the movement if you like by coming up on the toes, add in the calf to the push-off function, and link to jumping efficiency.

By requiring that the tail tuck when straightening the knees, we are linking the hip extensors with the knee extensors. The proportionality principle maintains that the largest muscles do the bulk of the work. Could you feel your gluteals contract hard? Or did you mostly just straighten your knees and let the quadriceps take over a primary role? By requiring that the tail tuck when straightening the knees, we are providing another constraint.

The tendency with most iliopsoas-biased folks when doing this movement is to let their pelvis roll into anterior tilt as they near full knee extension – their hip flexors get in the way. By disallowing anterior tilt, we are requiring a differentiated pattern of hip extension and lumbar flexion. We are requiring the hip extensors and external rotators/abductors to work very strenuously. We are requiring the iliopsoas and its kin to lengthen. For the vast majority of people, straightening the knees fully with these constraints is impossible, but in attempting to do the impossible many valuable physical skills can be learned, practiced, refined and blended in with functional activities.

Try standing with your feet a bit wider apart, but with the toes still pointing outward at 45°. Keep your toes pointed outward and slowly slide your left heel toward your right heel. Maintain posterior pelvic tilt and experiment with more or less knee bend. Feel the gluteals, hamstrings and adductors work to do this! This is a great drill off this lesson; it provides a nifty constraint that facilitates an ability of the weightbearing leg to pull the weight of the body toward itself. Think of the requirements on the adductors and hamstrings of a hockey player. Switch weightbearing and sliding legs and compare sides. Try at wider distances. Try with feet in different orientations (toes in, toes out and toes parallel). Try this with a slippery board, using deliberate movements of the board as constraint and functional context.

Try a one-legged version of this movement. Stand with the left foot up on a chair seat, knee bent, while the right foot is on the floor with the knee straight initially. Bend the right knee and let the pelvis fall back into posterior tilt. It will be easier in a position where both hip flexors are on slack. Keep the pelvis in posterior tilt as you slowly straighten your right knee, and make sure your right knee stays out over a centered right foot.

Go only as far as you are able while still maintaining a posterior pelvic tilt. For people who can 'get' this, it is a great iliopsoas stretch. Try pressing down with the left foot into the chair seat to assist in pushing the pelvis into posterior tilt. Use the left hamstrings to stretch the right iliopsoas! Doing this movement of bending and straightening the knees in a toe-in position can be useful as another progression in teaching peroneal control and lateral/rotation stability of the foot on the floor.

Straightening the knees and hips from this toe-in position tends to roll the feet outward on the floor. Cue pressing the metatarsal heads to arrest outward roll. Cue to push out a little to create hip external rotation, tibial/knee internal rotation, foot supination, and link skeletal weightbearing sensations of joints in this position with bending/straightening of knees and recalibration of quadriceps/vastus medialis.

A horse of a different shape

In variations F and G we continue with the basic movements of pushing out with both feet or pushing out and turning the pelvis and torso from side to side. After having performed movements with toes pointed away from and toes pointed toward each other, we might get a more accurate sense of where the feet are parallel. In variation F you find parallel, push out and turn left and right. This is progression of what we did on the floor and while leaning against a wall.

Box 7.10 Horsing Around

Companion lesson to Rolling the Foot – picking up where we left off

Exploring possibilities in rolling the feet in and out on the floor – distal and proximal choices

Coordinating hip adductors with posterior tibialis – coordinating hip abductors with peroneus longus

Creating a secondary pelvic force couple – coordinating opposite adductors and abductors to control lateral weight shift

Subsequent movements in variation G are both Goldilocks explorations and specific constraints. Using Goldilocksian principles, you did these same movements of pushing out and turning side to side with feet very wide apart, very close together and just right. Trying to turn from side to side with feet very wide apart constrains mobility. The adductors tend to get in the way. This provides us with an opportunity to reset the muscle spindle length of the adductors.

Think of a progression of hands and knees with knees wide apart, plantigrade with feet wide apart, leaning back on a wall with feet wide apart and standing with feet wide. Weight-shifting and turning the pelvis in all these positions challenges the adductors. Try a few of each and see if you can recognize the pattern and how it morphs from hip horizontal adduction/abduction, through various hybrids, to hip internal rotation/external rotation (Box 7.10).

Turning from side to side with the feet very close together challenges stability. It is very easy to move your center of mass outside your base of support. Think of a progression from hands and knees with knees and feet very close, to plantigrade, to leaning on a wall, to standing. We might use this to help someone identify the disadvantages in keeping their knees perpetually locked together. Use the two extremes to help establish a width between the feet that provides the best compromise between stability and mobility.

The last instruction of the lesson is to add a bending and straightening movement of the torso to the weight-shifting movements. This variation links lateral stability with bending movements and is a great cumulative movement to continue in a home program. Try doing this movement while pushing out laterally in each direction; use one leg to resist the other in this weight-shifting movement. The abductors are pushing against each other but in a cooperative way that allows the smooth movement of the pelvis from side to side.

Use the subvariations of turning and weight-shifting in toe-in (closed horse stance) and toe-out (open horse stance) positions with feet at the compromise width to provide specific constraints. Toeing in requires short and stubby length and toeing out requires adductor length and short and stubby strength. Doing the two versions back to back again helps in establishing a truer neutral, that place where the feet are parallel and centered – a true horse stance.

Variations

Use manual resistance techniques for lateral stability of the knees and feet, as described in the lumbar stabilization chapter. Change the emphasis of proprioceptive awareness from an

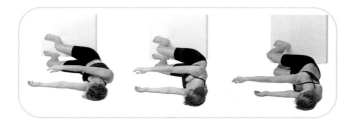

Fig. 7.32 Side-lie with feet on wall and log roll forward and back – requiring the abductors to work – link to tripod feet and posterior tilt of pelvis. Progress by moving further away from the wall.

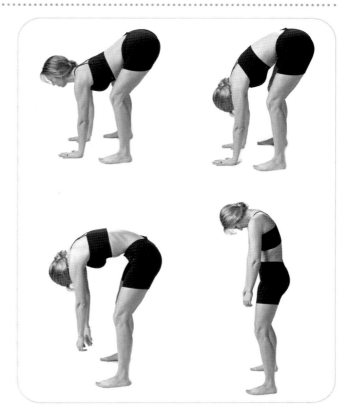

Fig. 7.33 Bend over in a horse stance and press outward – can you feel your pelvis move towards posterior tilt? Progress by rolling up to stand one vertebra at a time.

ability to coordinate intersegmental stability with pelvic stability to an ability to keep the knees over the feet and the feet centered and stable on the floor.

Use a variation of this lesson while lying down (Fig. 7.32). Lie on your side with your feet against a wall, hips and knees bent at about 90°. Slide the top foot up the wall. As you know from the Side-lie Transitions and Dead Bug Roll, the act of lifting the top leg engages the hip abductors from both sides. This mimics the simultaneous pushing-out movement we did in supine and standing. Does your pelvis posteriorly tilt as you slide your foot up the wall? Press out with both feet deliberately and plant your first metatarsal heads.

Keep pressing out and bias toward mild posterior tilt as you move your top knee alternately forward and back; keep your feet centered and your knees over your feet as before. This movement is similar to the log rolling forward and back we did in Dead Bug Roll, but with the feet on the wall. The rolling forward and back mimics the rolling of the pelvis from side to side on the floor or wall, or turning the pelvis left and right in standing. Visualize it as a three-dimensional pattern.

Progress the lesson by moving farther away from the wall, culminating in a position where your hips and knees are very close to straight. From here, use the top leg to push and pull the top side of your pelvis forward and back. The movement of the top hip forward mimics push-off. Progress by moving farther away from the wall. Culminate in having both hips and knees as close as possible to straight while still being able to maintain outward pressure with both legs. It will look increasingly like standing and walking.

This lesson variation is a great one – one of my personal favorites – but can be elusive. You will have to experiment and be creative. Use the few clues I have given to design a whole lesson. What will be your static and dynamic baselines? How will you describe the movements? What are the proprioceptive clues you want your student to focus on? Watch for subtle imperfections.

Are the toes pointed out and the knee externally rotated? Are the knees closer together than the feet or hips? Is the back arching when rolling forward? Is the top knee lifting toward the ceiling when rolling back, or dropping toward the floor when rolling forward? Are the feet staying centered? What does each of these imperfections mean, and how do they relate to your student's complaint?

Try standing in a horse stance, bending over to let your head and arms dangle toward the floor and pressing outward from

this position. Does your pelvis posteriorly rotate? Progress by rolling up one vertebrae at a time to standing, making sure to keep your knees slightly bent to fully appreciate the ability of the hip abductors and extensors to push your pelvis to vertical (Fig. 7.33).

We have now looked at two of the three dimensions of the foot. We have explored ways of influencing the degree of foot abduction and adduction in Slip and Slide. We explored ways of influencing the degree of foot pronation and supination, and ways of protecting the ankles and knees from rotational and lateral stresses in Rolling the Foot and Horsing Around. After having explored lateral and rotational movements of the lower extremities in these three lessons, we will now direct our attention to straight-ahead movements and front-to-back balance of the foot on the floor.

Front to back balance

Why did we leave the question of front-to-back balance of the foot and how to influence straight-ahead movements for the end? Why didn't we start with straight forward movements, as walking and running forward are much more common than cutting and turning?

Walking and straight forward locomotion is much more firmly ingrained with habitual muscle imbalances and movement asymmetries. They are more difficult movements to influence because they are more fully under the influence of the automatic pilot. We might want to work first with the legs in lateral and rotational movements. More unfamiliar movements require more attentive proprioceptive listening and can bring medial/lateral imbalances to the attention of your student.

Much of what we are working to correct in walking is medial/lateral imbalance. Is the foot pronated or supinated too much in push-off? Is the knee in too much valgus or varus? Is the hip too internally or externally rotated? Are there imbalances or inefficiencies in the pelvic force couples? How much does your student's medial/lateral imbalance in gait manifest itself in a repetitive stress injury at their feet, knees, hips or back? We might want to work first on ways of addressing medial/lateral lower extremity imbalances so that we can blend those newly learned skills into a recalibrated gait.

These next lessons involve ankle dorsiflexion and plantarflexion, and how movements of the ankle are coordinated with movements of the hip and knee in gait. We will be exploring ways of both reducing medial/lateral imbalances in gait and reducing good housekeeping violations, facilitating proportional distribution of movement and effort. The first lesson is a mostly open kinetic chain lesson that we can use early on after injury, or as an initial way of facilitating appropriate foot/ankle/knee/hip/pelvis relationships in gait. Subsequent lessons blend these patterns or Legos into closed chain situations.

In search of the perfect step

Let's take a moment to analyze an 'ideal' step. We can use a movement of stepping up on a stool as a microcosm for walking. How does the stepping leg act, how does the push-off leg act, and how are the pelvis/torso/shoulders organized? Recall the gait variations described in Chapter 6 relating to pelvic movement and lumbar stability. Four basic types were described: the doll body walk, the swish walk, the waddle walk and the force couple walk.

We could assess gait by observing the real deal; get your student on a treadmill or walk them out in the hall. Videotape if you have the equipment; high-speed film would be great! Sometimes, though, too many things are happening too fast to get a sense of what is happening in gait. What is the orientation of the feet? Are the knees biased into valgus or external rotation? What are the force couples doing? Is the pelvis turning on the legs?

Perhaps we can slow things down a bit and get a sense of basic movement and postural tendencies by breaking walking down to one step. Ask your student to stand and slowly put one foot up on a stool (Fig. 7.34). Observe for turn of the pelvis in space, where the knee ends up relative to the hip, where the knee ends up relative to the foot, and the direction the toes point. After observing the initial stepping movement several times, have your student step up slowly on to the stool. Watch for collapse of the knee and foot inward, whether the

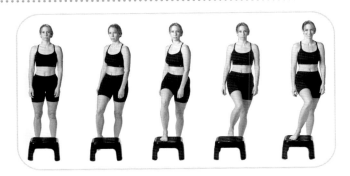

Fig. 7.34 Assessing stepping movement on low stool – watch for turn of pelvis, relationship of knee to hip and relationship of knee to foot. Watch for knee extensor/hip extensor balance.

pelvis turns, and whether the torso stays upright or bends over to engage the hip muscles.

Adduction and internal rotation on the hip of the stepping leg is very common and results in a poor relationship between hip, knee and foot. This organization contributes to medial knee strain, patellar tracking problems and foot pronation stresses through the lower legs. When assessing your students, watch for the placement of the knee relative to the hip: is the knee in narrower than the hip? Watch for placement of the knee in space relative to the foot. Is the adducted thigh pronating the foot? Is the knee externally rotating as a compensation for the adducting thigh?

Watch for knee wobble or collapse inward when stepping up on to a stool or telephone book. Watch for the same tendencies when watching your student getting up from sitting on a chair to standing. Do the knees come toward each other? Do the feet roll inward? Watch for the same tendencies when watching your student bend down to pick something up off the floor from a standing position. Watch again for knee collapse and foot pronation. This tendency of many people to organize the hip/knee/foot relationships this way over a number of different functional contexts (locomotion, transitions and manipulation) illustrates again the complex and interwoven nature of habitual motor patterns and emphasizes the importance of training the same motor corrections with multiple changes of venue.

When a person with a doll body walks (little or no rotational or lateral movement of the pelvis, minimal forward bending of the torso) or steps up on a stool, the hips are not generally the primary mode of stepping up. There will be little or no rotation of the pelvis on the legs as neither the hip flexors nor the extensors are showing sufficient signs of life. The torso will stay relatively vertical, as she won't flex and horizontally adduct the hip to load her hip extensor springs. These folks tend to do press-the-foot movements in a knee-intensive way, emphasizing the quadriceps and increasing contact pressure on the patella.

When a person with a waddling gait steps up, we might see a turn of the pelvis in the direction of the push-off leg. If she is stepping up on to a stool with the right foot, the pelvis may turn to the left. This often results in movement of the right knee medially in space and an arrangement of the knee in space consistent with valgus postures (Fig. 7.34). Watch here for knee external rotation bias. Pushing the right foot into the stool to step up without having the benefit of aligning the knee over the foot in a skeletal weightbearing organization results in imbalanced stresses on knee joint, patellar complex, ankle and foot. Stepping tends to be knee intensive: hip extension is not a waddler's forte. Assess differences between the two sides and correlate to the side of symptoms.

When a person with a force couple gait steps up, there is a turning of the pelvis in the direction of the stepping leg. This tends to align the knee more accurately with the hip. Try this yourself. Step up on a stool with your right foot and turn your pelvis to the left; notice whether your knee ends up medial to your hip. This is a very common tendency, but it doesn't have to be if the adductors on that side lengthen and allow the thigh to differentiate from the pelvis.

Now step up on the stool while turning your pelvis to the right; notice whether your knee ends up more laterally or more in line with your hip. In fact, by turning the pelvis in the direction of the stepping leg, we are applying a short and stubby constraint that prevents hip movement farther into horizontal adduction/internal rotation. Try moving your right knee inward with your pelvis turned to the right.

Next, step up on the stool with your pelvis turned first to the left, then to the right. When turned to the left, the right knee tends to collapse farther inward and the foot collapses into pronation. Now step up with your pelvis turned to the right. Notice how the turn of the pelvis helps keep the knee out over the foot. Correlate to what you learned about gait in Steppin' Out.

For your last experiment, try stepping up on to the stool by keeping your torso very erect, then by leaning forward a little bit toward the forward/stepping/right leg. Feel how, by keeping your torso upright, you are emphasizing pressing the foot with the quadriceps. Feel how, by allowing your torso to bend over (the deeper the bend the fuller you get into your hip) in the direction of the stepping leg, you are able to better recruit your hip muscles and can propel yourself forward with proximal initiation (Box 7.11). Watch for similar styles of disproportional lower extremity muscle use with Sit to Stand and bending from standing.

This stepping assessment can give us valuable clues about shock absorption and push-off competence, force couple balance and habitual lower extremity differentiated patterns. Make your observations here then take your student out into the hall or up on a treadmill, and notice whether there are correlations. Be prepared to be hopelessly confused sometimes.

Box 7.11 Stepping assessment

Assessing turn of pelvis on initial step – how does this bias the alignment of hips, knees and feet?

Assessing stability of knee and foot in push-off to step up – is there a collapse of knee and foot inward?

Assessing distribution of effort in step up – is it quadriceps or gluteal intensive?

Heel to Toe

Variations

A. Stand in your bare feet on a carpeted surface.

- Notice your feet against the floor. What direction do your toes point?
- Are you rolling your feet inward to flatten your arches or rolling out on to the outside edges of your feet?
- Do you have more weight forward on your toes or back on your heels?
- How is your weight distributed between the big ball (first metatarsal head), the small ball (fifth metatarsal head) and the middle of your heel? Does your foot feel like a well-supported tripod?
- Change your standing position to a split stance, left foot well in front of the right and both feet still about shoulder width apart (Fig. 7.35).
- From here, shift your weight forward on to your left foot and lift your right heel. Come on to the balls of your right foot (Fig. 7.35). Is your weight more towards the big or the little toe of your push-off foot?
- Shift your weight back on to your right foot and lift your left forefoot, still keeping your left heel on the ground (Fig. 7.35). Does your left forefoot lift straight up, or does it veer off to the right or left?
- Alternate shifting your weight forward and back, lifting right heel and left forefoot. Assess quality, balance and coordination.
- Change into the opposite split stance, right foot now forward and left foot back. Do the same movement to this side. How does it compare?

B. Lie on your back with your left leg long and your right leg bent up. Bring your right heel as close to your pelvis as is comfortable.

- Alternately lift your right forefoot to rest your weight on your right heel then lift your right heel to come

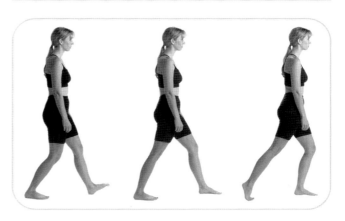

Fig. 7.35 Shifting weight forward and back from a split stance.

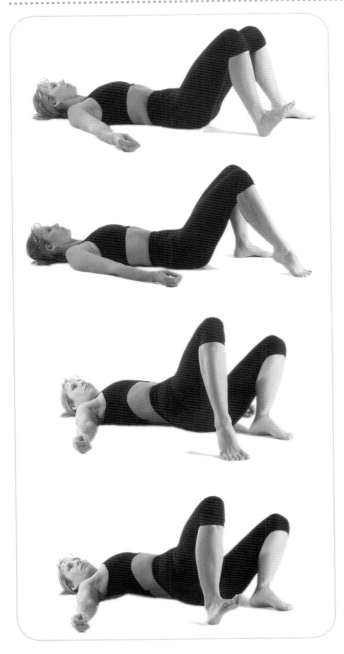

Fig. 7.36 Heel to Toe – then lifting the hip.

up on to your toes (actually the balls of the feet – the metatarsal heads) (Fig. 7.36). Do this alternating movement several times.

- Then lift your heel, support your weight mostly on the first and second balls of your right foot, and stay there. From there, push your foot into the floor and lift your right hip (Fig. 7.36). How stable does this feel?

- Lift your forefoot and stay there. Press your heel into the floor and raise your right hip (Fig. 7.36). How stable does this feel?

- Alternate back and forth between pressing your heel and pressing your metatarsal heads into the floor to raise your hip. Then leave both heel and toes on the floor and press your whole foot into the floor several times.

- How is your weight distributed along your foot from Heel to Toe? Can you find the place that splits the difference? Where is that sweet spot?

C. Lie on your back with your left leg bent up and your right lower leg crossed over your left thigh.

- Start to flex and extend your right ankle. Do it slowly and gently to start with – don't do a full movement. How smooth is this movement? What do your toes do when you flex your ankle up (dorsiflexion)?

- Do they also flex up? Are they not moving relative to your foot? What do your toes do when you extend your ankle downward (plantarflexion)? Do they curl?

- Deliberately curl your toes as you extend your ankle downward and flex up your toes as you flex up your ankle (Fig. 7.37). Do this several times.

- Then go back to just flexing and extending your ankle gently and see if you can make the movement at your ankle without moving your toes relative to your foot.

- Flex and extend your ankle, but deliberately move your toes in the opposite direction. Curl your toes when you flex your ankle up and flex your toes as you extend your ankle downward (Fig. 7.37).

- Alternate many times to coordinate this ankle/toe differentiation.

D. Lie on your left side with your hips and knees bent up to about 90°. Place your left upper arm on the floor above your shoulder but bend your elbow a bit more than 90° to rest your head on your left hand and upright left forearm.

- Lift your right heel away from your left but keep your toes in contact with each other (Fig. 7.38). Return and repeat several times.

- Lift your right toes away from your left but keep your heels together (Fig. 7.38). Repeat.

- Alternate lifting toes and heel. What happens to the shape of your ankle? Can you feel anything happening in your right knee? Pause for a moment.

- Then lift your whole right thigh, knee and foot away from your left so that your thigh and lower leg are parallel to the floor.

- Lift alternately heel and toe in this lifted position (Fig. 7.38). Is this easier here or more difficult? Use this movement to find neutral: where is it that neither heel nor toe is closer to the floor and where your whole foot is parallel to the floor?

- Stay in this place while you alternately flex and extend your right ankle, differentiating your toes to move

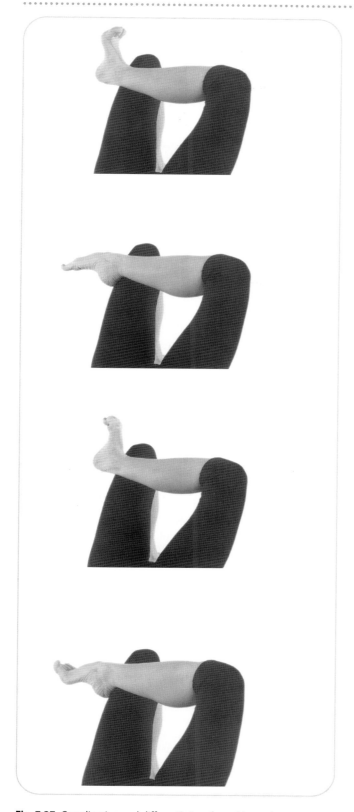

Fig. 7.37 Coordinating and differentiating the ankles and toes.

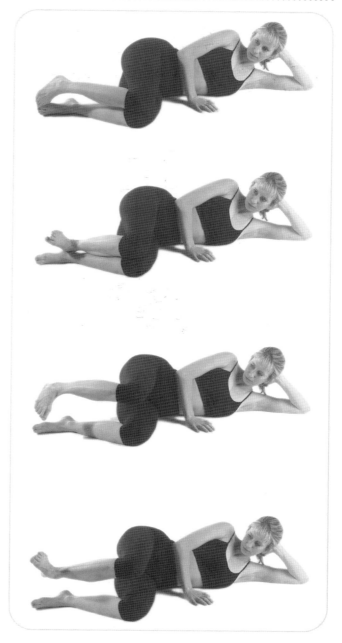

Fig. 7.38 Lift heel – then toes – find neutral. Can you sense movement in your knees? Then do with lifted leg.

them in the opposite direction (Fig. 7.37). Do this several times, then rest on your side for a bit.

- Lift your right leg again so foot, lower leg and thigh are parallel to the floor. Continue the movement of flexing up your right ankle and curling your toes as you now add in drawing your right knee up toward your chest.

- Allow your pelvis, chest and shoulders to roll backward. You might come close to touching your head to the floor (Fig. 7.39). Repeat this several times.

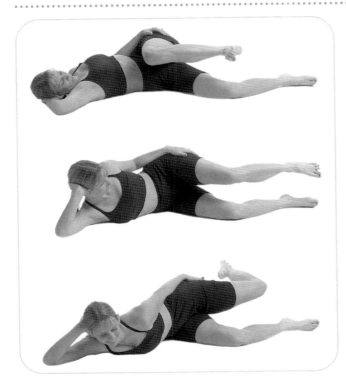

Fig. 7.39 Coordinating stepping movement with ankle/toe differentiation.

- Then move in the opposite direction. Extend your leg down and back as you extend your ankle and flex your toes. This will roll you forward, perhaps even letting you touch the floor with your head in this direction (Fig. 7.39).
- Alternate many times between these two movements.
- Roll back on to your back and bend up your right leg again. Alternately lift your right heel and forefoot and press your foot in each of these positions. Do you feel any more stable pressing through your foot while up on your toes now?

E. Lie on your back and repeat instructions B and C to the opposite side, with the left foot.

F. Sit up to lean back on your elbows and forearms. Lift your feet off the floor to bring your knees up over your belly.

- Alternate rolling from side to side, transitioning from one elbow to the other through your back. Keep both legs lifted and stay on one or both elbows the whole time (Fig. 7.40).
- Straighten the top leg down and back while you bend the bottom leg up. Add in differentiation of toes and ankles and add foot movements into larger movements of torso and hips.
- Straighten your ankle and bend up your toes as you extend the top leg down and back.
- Bend your ankles and curl your toes as you draw the top leg up toward your chest. Coordinate feet and

toes of both bottom and top leg simultaneously for extra credit.

G. Lie on your back.

- Bend up both legs and lift both heels from the floor to come up on to your toes. Press both feet into the floor to lift both hips from the floor. Lift sequentially along your spine; lift and lower one vertebra at a time. Repeat several times.
- Then keep your pelvis on the ground, but roll it from side to side by pressing first with one foot then the other.
- Now have both heels and toes on the floor and lift sequentially a few times. How stable do your knees, ankles and feet feel? Roll your pelvis a few times from side to side and feel for your ability to keep your knees over your feet and your weight centered on your first and second metatarsal heads.
- Repeat these same instructions but with your heels off the ground. Come up on to your metatarsal heads and press one foot then the other into the ground to roll pelvis from side to side.
- Press both feet into the ground to lift/bridge up sequentially. How stable is the foot now with the heel off the floor in comparison to when you began?

H. Stand up.

- Notice your feet against the floor. What direction do your toes point?
- Are you rolling your feet inward to flatten your arches or rolling out on to the outside edges of your feet?
- Do you have more weight forward on your toes or back on your heels?
- How is your weight distributed between the big ball (first metatarsal head), the small ball (fifth metatarsal head) and the middle of your heel? Does your foot feel like a well-supported tripod?
- Change your standing position to a split stance: left foot well in front of the right and both feet still about shoulder width apart (Fig. 7.35).
- From here shift your weight forward on to your left foot and lift your right heel. Come on to the balls of your right foot. Is your weight more toward the big or the little toe?
- Shift your weight back on to your right foot and lift your left forefoot, still keeping your left heel on the ground. Does your left forefoot lift straight up, or does it veer off to the right or left? Alternate shifting your weight forward and back, lifting right heel and left forefoot. Assess quality, balance and coordination.
- Change into the opposite split stance: right foot now forward and left foot back. Do the same movement to this side. How does it compare?
- Walk around the room and feel how your weight goes through your feet from Heel to Toe, which toes you use to push off, and any change in the shape of your ankles as you walk.

Baselines – Heel to Toe

After dispensing with the usual questions in variation A about how your feet are organized on the floor in the three dimensions, we introduce a new dynamic baseline. Standing in a split stance, you are directed to first shift your weight forward on to the front foot while lifting the back heel, then to shift your weight back on to the back foot while lifting the front forefoot. The questions asked during this initial proprioceptive scan concern the movements of the ankle and the way the foot is organized at the moment of push-off. There are also questions about movements of the pelvis on the legs.

The sweet spot – between first and second metatarsal heads

When shifting your weight forward from a split stance, the first question has to do with how you come on to the balls of your push-off foot. Is your weight concentrated more towards the little toes or towards the big toes? Where should it be?

In keeping with our theme of bearing weight skeletally, where would your weight be centered if the foot were vertical? Stand up and get into a split stance with your right foot back. Shift your weight forward on to your left foot and lift your right heel. Which metatarsal heads do you put most of your weight on? Take a look over your left shoulder to confirm visually what you perceive proprioceptively.

Move your right heel from side to side and notice how this rolls your weight from first to fifth metatarsal heads. Proprioceptively find that place for your heel in space where your weight is centered around your second metatarsal head or just medially, in that space between the first and second metatarsal heads. Is your foot vertical in this position?

Find a partner where you can try the following experiment. Find that placement of your heel in space where your weight is around the second metatarsal head and have your partner push vertically through the back of your heel, through the mid and forefoot and into the metatarsal heads. Feel the stability of a vertical foot. Now roll your right heel outward to bring your weight on to your fourth or fifth metatarsal heads. Have your partner push vertically through the (inside) back of your heel in this position. What do you have to do to keep your ankle from inverting further?

Roll your heel inward to bear weight a bit to the inside of your first metatarsal. Have your accomplice push vertically through the (outside) back of your heel from here. What stabilizes your foot from going farther into eversion? Try each of the three versions several times, or make even finer distinctions. What is the proprioceptive difference between bearing weight on the inside of your second metatarsal and the outside of your second metatarsal? Switch roles and try this out on your partner, and do remember that you are pushing down through the foot to refine proprioceptive sensation, not engaging in a test of strength.

In terms of intension, that sweet spot between first and second metatarsal heads is a critical one. We can use a proprioceptive awareness of that spot and we can direct intentional movement with that spot as a focal point to improve both change of direction movements and push-off/propulsion

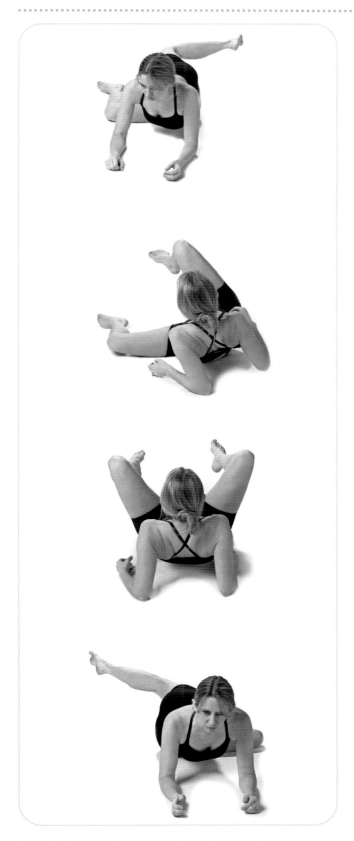

Fig. 7.40 Transitions from right to left side-lie scissor kicks – coming through both elbows in the middle.

efficiency. What happens if your weight is directed more medially in push-off, towards the inside of the first metatarsal head? Observe how this pushes the big toe medially or creates a hallux valgus; could a medial/lateral miscalibration contribute to bunions?

Note how a pelvic force couple gait, with a turn of the pelvis in the direction of the stepping leg, reduces the tendency of the heel to move medially and the tendency of the big toe to be pushed laterally. Note how a waddle gait, with a turn of the pelvis in the direction of the push-off leg, increases the tendency of the heel to move medially and the tendency of the big toe to be pushed laterally. Are weak gluteals/short and stubbies and tight adductors and hip flexors contributing to bunions?

We will be exploring change of direction or pivoting movements in the last lesson of this chapter, Peerless Pivots, where we will use the sweet spot as a pivot point. This current lesson and the next two lessons after this will be focusing on straight forward movements: how to engage that sweet spot in running, walking and jumping.

Assessing push-off and shock absorption competence

What is it that makes for an efficient push-off in gait? We would certainly like to see a powerful and well-balanced coordination of the pelvic force couples: an ability to allow the hips to flex and internally rotate/horizontally adduct in the heel-strike/shock absorption phase loads the spring for a powerful push-off. A well-used iliopsoas and a turn of the pelvis in the direction of the stepping leg set the stage for a more powerful hip extensor contraction.

Review lessons throughout the Tyrannosaurus section for ways of facilitating better performance and better balance of the pelvic force couples. Cat/Camel, Wishbone, Side-lie Transitions, Side-sit Transitions, Knee Walking and Steppin' Out all have pelvic force couples in starring roles. Can you find individual variations in each lesson that mimics gait?

We would like to see a hip joint that fully extends. Short hip flexors rob the hip extensors of power at end-range and shorten the stride. Review lessons throughout the Tyrannosaurus section for ways of facilitating longer hip flexor trip wires: Pelvic Tilts, Wishbone, Side-sit Transitions, Knee Walking, Steppin' Out and Half-kneel and Split Stance Bending. Which variations are belly-up lengthening contractions of the hip flexors? Which are initial movements of using gluteal contractions to create reciprocal inhibition of the hip flexors, and which are the more demanding movements of pushing the pelvis to vertical on a weightbearing leg to demand length of the hip flexors as they near end-range?

We would like to see hamstrings that work in push-off to extend the hip and to assist in straightening the knee, and would like to see the medial and lateral hamstrings balanced. Review lessons in the T. Rex section for ways of facilitating hamstring use in pushing the foot into the floor: slippery board, Pelvic Tilts, Wishbone, Split Stance Bending, Sit to Stand or variations of Side-sit Bending where you are leaning back against a wall and bending over straight, diagonally or in circles. Use toys with variations of each of these lessons: slippery board

or crosswise rollers. Do bridging movements with the feet high on a wall.

We also would like to see calf musculature contribute to push-off, and for the ankle joint to fully plantarflex. We then need the anterior compartment muscles of the shin to lengthen and the toes to be able to differentiate from the plantarflexion movement of the ankle to move into full dorsiflexion. These are the issues we will be focusing on in the next several lessons.

By cueing our students to direct their proprioceptive attention to pushing off from a vertical foot, by directing weight-bearing to the space between the first and second metatarsal heads, we are helping to make all of the above happen more efficiently. The propulsion forward off the metatarsal heads almost requires the calf musculature to engage and strongly encourages synergistic muscles along the chain to participate.

The hamstrings and gluteals tend to be much more active. The longer stride and fuller gluteal and hamstring contractions impose a demand on the hip joint to extend more fully, and help lengthen the hip flexors. Pushing off from the sweet spot rather than from the inside or outside of the forefoot helps to balance out the inner and outer hamstrings and helps in reducing knee rotation bias.

Ironically, what can muck up this whole beautifully orchestrated coordination of pelvis, hip, knee and ankle are the lowly and often neglected toes. If the toes can't move into adequate dorsiflexion, the whole push-off function is compromised. Use this and subsequent lessons to refine the way your whole lower extremity works in gait, from the engine for gait at the hips and pelvis, through the transmission for gait at the knees, to where the rubber meets the road at the feet.

Open chain foot and ankle movements

In variation B we establish some dynamic baselines while supine. How fully does the ankle plantarflex and dorsiflex? What part of your heel and how far toward the ends of your metatarsal heads can you get? How is your foot organized when pushing down through the middle of your foot. Where is there equal weight between the front and back of the foot?

The primary antagonist pair we are working with in this lesson is the gastrosoleus to anterior compartment relationship. Lifting the forefoot to press the heel into the floor requires the anterior tibialis and toe dorsiflexors to work. Lifting the heel and pressing the metatarsal heads into the floor requires the calf muscles to work. Which of these two movements seems most familiar – which seems more difficult? What is your bias? We could ask further questions about which of the five metatarsal heads receive more of the weight, or whether the dorsiflexing ankle has an inversion or eversion component, or we could wait for more variations in this series.

In variation C you now get the foot in question off the floor by crossing your lower leg over your opposite thigh. This variation explores the coordination of the ankle and toes in dorsiflexion/plantarflexion directions. There is an initial question about the spontaneous organization of your toes. Did they move globally with the ankle, differentiated from the ankle, or completely independent of the ankle?

You are then directed to explore the global and differentiated patterns. Most people will spontaneously move their toes and ankle in the same direction or globally, ankle dorsiflexion with toe dorsiflexion and vice versa. In this open kinetic chain position and without specific directions to do otherwise, this is a perfectly legitimate choice. It is just not pattern specific relative to gait.

In walking and running, ankle plantarflexion needs to be coordinated with toe dorsiflexion. The ankle and toes need to differentiate. The next instruction in this section is to move your ankles and toes in the opposite direction. Whereas some people will take to this like a duck to water, others might take to it like a cat to water. This will be very foreign to some and will require slow and patient attempts to develop any sort of smoothness and reproducibility. We will see this ankle plantarflexion/toe dorsiflexion pattern many times over the next several lessons.

Other subvariations we might teach in this section include plantarflexing and dorsiflexing the ankle without engaging the toe musculature at all, or doing diagonal movements. Completely separating the movements of the toes from movements of the ankles is just another way of training the CNS for more options and further refining motor control over an often neglected part of our bodies.

Moving in diagonals helps with medial/lateral balance at the foot and ankle. Try crossing your leg over your thigh and moving your ankle down and in (ankle plantarflexion and inversion) then up and out (ankle dorsiflexion and eversion). Do this several times to feel for coordination. Switch to move your ankle down and out (plantarflexion and eversion) then up and in (dorsiflexion and inversion). Closely observe yourself and your students in attempting straight plantarflexion/dorsiflexion movements, and feel for biases.

Do you dorsiflex more with the toe extensors (dorsiflexion and eversion) or more with the anterior tibialis (dorsiflexion and inversion)? Do you plantarflex more with the posterior tibialis (plantarflexion and inversion) or with the peroneals (plantarflexion with eversion)? Use diagonal movements to balance medial and lateral dorsiflexors and plantarflexors, or isolate and gain control over one of the antagonist pair.

Proximal/distal coordination – simulating stepping in side-lie

In variation D you now coordinate the ankle/toe differentiation patterns into a larger pattern that coordinates the foot and ankle with the knee, hip, pelvis and torso. The first thing you do in this left side-lying 'Cleopatra' position is to do a previously described variation: with the feet and knees together, you should alternately lift the right heel and toes. This movement of lifting the heel is an internal rotation movement of the right knee.

Lifting the toes stimulates an external rotation movement at the knee; palpate the lateral hamstring tendons to confirm. This movement previews the next instruction in this section, where you are asked to do the same knee internal/external rotation movements of the knee but with the right leg lifted. This both engages the hip abductors on both sides and takes away your contact reference: you can't play the feet off against each other to monitor your movements.

Getting the thigh, tibia and outside edge of the foot all parallel to the ground defines hip abductor/adductor, hip inter-

nal rotation/external rotation and knee internal rotation/external rotation neutral, and approximates the 'hip over the knee and the knee over the foot' organization we are looking for in standing and gait. Hip abduction/adduction balance defines whether the knee is valgus to, directly under or varus to the hip joint.

Hip internal/external rotation balance defines whether the lower leg will need to compensate into tibial external or internal rotation. Knee internal/external rotation balance defines whether the foot is adducted, neutral, or abducted relative to orientation. You are to then keep these parallel relationships as you add in foot/ankle/toe movements and rolling-forward and back movements of the pelvis and torso.

After a review of the ankle/toe differentiations you did in supine, you then add in the rolling-forward and back movement of the pelvis and torso. We saw variations of this movement in Side-lie Transitions and Dead Bug Roll. In this side-lying variation your head is propped up on a vertical forearm. Moving your head toward the floor in back and bringing your top knee towards your chest while keeping your elbow where it started on the floor is a constraint that links a stepping movement of the top leg with a turning/rotation of the pelvis and torso in the direction of the stepping leg.

This is another pelvic force couple movement. Moving your head toward the floor in front and bringing your top leg down and back is a constraint that links a push-off movement of the top leg with a turning/rotation movement of the pelvis and torso in the opposite direction of the push-off leg – another pelvic force couple.

We then link the stepping movement to the roll-back movement with ankle dorsiflexion/toe plantarflexion and the push-off movement to the roll-forward movement with ankle plantarflexion/toe dorsiflexion. It is the push-off with ankle plantarflexion/toe dorsiflexion differentiation combination that is of particular interest here. Although hip flexion and ankle dorsiflexion certainly go together in gait (and this part of the lesson could be particularly useful in working with foot drop), the toes don't necessarily have to plantarflex here.

The purpose of going in both directions here is to create a reciprocating movement and all that that implies in terms of helping to balance out the anterior and posterior lower leg musculature. This is a fairly complex movement. Watch yourself and your students carefully for subtle details.

Does your thigh stay horizontal; can you adjust the hip joint in horizontal adduction/abduction to keep the knee from dipping toward the floor when rolling forward and to keep the knee from lifting toward the ceiling when rolling back? Does your lower leg stay horizontal? Can you adjust the hip joint to internally and externally rotate relative to the pelvis so that the foot doesn't lift toward the ceiling or lower toward the floor? Does your foot stay horizontal; can you adjust the amount of internal/external rotation at the knee? Is your spine/ribcage sufficiently mobile to alternately arch/twist and round/twist?

Comparing baselines and doing a summary movement

The last variation of this section returns us to our supine dynamic baselines. How does the right ankle now dorsiflex and plantarflex? Where is the 'center' of your foot? How stable does it feel to push the toes into the floor? You might anticipate an improvement in all these parameters. Variation E is a mirror image of the first half of the lesson. This is one of those lessons where you do nearly every variation of the lesson to one side first, which heightens contrast and facilitates better proprioceptive listening skills.

Variation F is a summary movement that revisits our transitional movements from lying to side-sitting, but with a few variations. Rolling across from elbow to elbow gives you an opportunity to feel back-to-back pelvic force couples and to further coordinate them with knees and feet. Rolling across the elbows like this is also an excellent way to mobilize and balance the shoulder girdles and chest, but we're getting a bit ahead of ourselves.

In variation G you come back to your back again and bend both legs up. Lift both heels to come on to your metatarsal heads and stay there as you bridge; lift and lower pelvis and spine like a chain. Then roll the pelvis from side to side on the floor as you did in Wishbone and Horsing Around, but while up on your toes. Combine intentional movements of pushing outward to challenge the hip abductor/peroneal connections in this more vulnerable position. Learn to stabilize your foot without your heel on the ground. Challenge further by applying manual resistance at the knees or the distal lower legs.

Come back up to standing in variation H, and revisit our initial baselines. Pay particular attention to the movements in split stance of shifting weight forward and lifting the back foot in imitation of a push-off movement. Is your foot vertical? Do you use the various muscles along the push-off chain more forcefully? How is your pelvic force couple doing? Is your pelvis turning in the direction of the forward leg as you come forward?

How is the movement of shifting weight toward the back leg and lifting the front forefoot? Whereas we might anticipate a freer and better balanced ankle dorsiflexion and clearer choices in terms of how to organize the toes for this, perhaps another change may have occurred in the primary weightbearing leg. As you shift your weight back to the back (right) foot, that ankle needs to be able to dorsiflex. Does the ankle purely dorsiflex, or does it also pronate or abduct?

Pattern specificity – Achilles and psoas stretching – VMO strength

This tendency to pronate or abduct the foot is very common, and could be because adductor bias is pulling the knee in or because of tight Achilles/calf musculature. Reduce the tendency of the foot to collapse inward while shifting your weight backward by turning your pelvis and torso in the direction of the back leg. This creates a kinematic linkage that rotates the pelvis to the right, which internally rotates the hip, which grabs and externally rotates the right thigh.

This movement then externally rotates the lower leg and foot, Rolling the Foot outward towards supination (or to prevent movement of the foot into pronation). This is a great heel cord and soleus stretch if performed accurately, and is a must for pronation-related plantar fasciitis. It also dovetails nicely with the pelvic force couple. Recognize the pattern from homolateral bending, Knee Walking and Steppin' Out.

Stand up for a moment in this split stance position, left foot forward and right foot back. Shift weight forward and on to your left foot, turning pelvis and torso to the left. Then shift weight back and on to your right foot, turning your pelvis to the right. Feel how the right hip alternately flexes/internally rotates/horizontally adducts, then extends/externally rotates/horizontally abducts. This simulates what the hip does on initial shock absorption through push-off.

Shifting back makes a dandy context for stretching the deep hip rotators, soleus and Achilles of the back leg and for stretching the adductors of the forward leg. Shifting back is also a great context for strengthening the quadriceps, and in particular the vastus medialis. By keeping the knee out over the foot, you are arranging the arthrokinematics of the knee joint in such a way that is excitatory to the eccentrically contracting VMO. Try this yourself using visual, palpation or EMG feedback. Shift back and turn pelvis to ensure knee stays over the foot, then shift back and allow the knee to collapse inward and the foot to roll into pronation. Which way facilitates better VMO use (Box 7.12)?

Shifting forward provides a dandy context for stretching the gastrocnemius and hip flexors of the back leg. Delay lifting the back heel to encourage the gastrocnemius stretch and emphasize moving the pubic bone up and forward to encourage iliopsoas length. Shifting forward also helps strengthen the short and stubbies, gluteals, hamstrings and calves when doing the movement faster/more explosively, when resisting forward movement with your forward leg (another cooperative tug-of-war), or when manually or plyometrically resisting the movement. This is an important movement that we have already seen in Steppin' Out, and that we will see again in this chapter, but with a different proprioceptive focus.

Applications and variations

What sort of folks could benefit from this lesson? Trochanteric bursitis might respond to a recalibration of medial/lateral balance and by varying the use and length of the hip abductors and short and stubbies. Adductor strains might benefit from training the bottom leg abductors for pushing-to-go and pushing-to-stop movements, and from recalibrating the medial/lateral push-off function to de-emphasize the engagement of the posterior adductors. The knee rotation components of this lesson could be used for initial medial/lateral hamstring control in rehabilitation from knee ligament sprains or with patellar tracking problems. The ankle plantarflexion/dorsiflexion movements might be particularly useful as a beginning movement for someone with shin splints.

Box 7.12 Heel to Toe

Side-lie and open kinetic chain (for the top leg) facilitation of force couple gait pattern

Coordinate force couples with differentiated ankle/toe piece – time the movements appropriately

Clarifying hip over knee over foot relationships – keep all the bones parallel to the floor

Functionally, we could anticipate that someone with anterior shin splints might have habitual postural and movement patterns that would predispose her to this particular malady. In shin splints, there is an overuse irritation of the anterior compartment muscles and their attendant fasciae. Overuse of the anterior compartment might be linked with postures that roll the pelvis backward and shift weight back on the heels.

Tightness of the anterior compartment muscles mirrors weakness of its antagonist. The calf will not be adequately engaged in push-off movements. By linking ankle plantarflexion movements and weightbearing through a vertical foot to gait, we are reciprocally inhibiting the anterior compartment muscles and giving them a rest period when walking or running. The key to reducing anterior compartment strain is to train the gluteals, hamstrings and calf to all work synergistically in push-off. This scenario is again dependent on one small but important detail: the toes need to be able to dorsiflex adequately. Subsequent lessons further challenge this skill.

Use at face value for gait retraining in neurologic, geriatric and general medical applications. Work with foot drop by coordinating ankle dorsiflexors with hip flexors in the stepping or withdrawing the foot from the floor contexts.

Positional variations utilizing this same ankle/toe differentiation movement could be performed in a prone and hog-tied position. Think of balancing the board on the foot variation of Slip and Slide, but with both legs bent up (Fig. 7.41). Make the same basic alternating ankle dorsiflexion and plantarflexion movements, differentiate the toes, then coordinate to move both feet at the same time, switch to move one ankle one way and the other in the opposite direction. Or, do the same movements in long sitting. Move ankles opposite to each other and link to force couple movements at the hips and pelvis (Fig. 7.41).

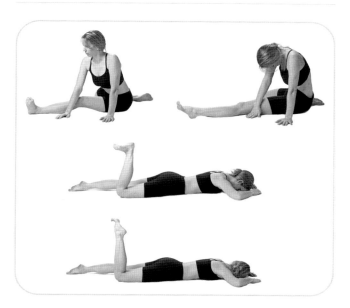

Fig. 7.41 Ankle/toe differentiations in other positions – long sitting and prone.

The next lesson picks up where we just left off, in standing, exploring weight-shifting movements from split stance. Toeing Off is really just a recycled and slightly modified version of Steppin' Out. It has nearly identical movements but with a different proprioceptive focus. In Toeing Off there are more cues to attend to the feet and toes and no reference to intersegmental stability. Because the lessons are fraternal twins, we will not be reanalyzing this lesson.

Go back to the Steppin' Out section of the last chapter and review analysis if desired, but think of the advantages of a force couple walk to the legs instead of the advantages to the back. Because Toeing Off is an extension of Heel to Toe, apply the same reasoning as to who might benefit from this lesson. I would suggest getting up on your feet and going through the lesson experientially again, but with a different proprioceptive focus. Either lose yourself in the glorious sensations of the lesson again, or do a condensed version with a quicker pace and fewer repetitions of each variation.

Toeing Off

Variations

A. Stand for a moment in your bare feet. Let your arms hang at your sides, feet around shoulder width apart and look straight ahead.

- Notice your feet against the floor. What direction do your toes point?

- Do you have more weight forward on your toes or back on your heels?

- Are your feet rolled in to flatten your arch or are you rolled on to the outside edges of your feet?

- Walk around a bit and feel for movement of your ankles or toes. Does your ankle bend and straighten? How clearly can you feel your toes?

- Pay particular attention to which toes you use to push off and how active are the backs of your legs, thighs and hips in propelling yourself forward.

B. Stand with your left foot on a half-roller and hold on to a long pole with your right hand (approximately 5–6-foot long half-inch dowel). Hold on to the pole with your right hand in front of you and out a bit to the right. Place your left foot on the half-roller (or tightly rolled blanket or towels) lengthwise so that the middle of your heel and the spot between the first and second balls of your left foot are on the top of the curve of the roller. Let your right leg dangle off the right edge of the roller (Fig. 7.42).

- In this position, make a few movements of tipping your pelvis forward and arching your lower back, then tucking your tail under and flattening your back. After doing this a few times, tuck your pelvis under you, flatten your lower back and point your tailbone down towards the ground. Now keep your back this same shape but let your pelvis and torso lean forward a little as you –

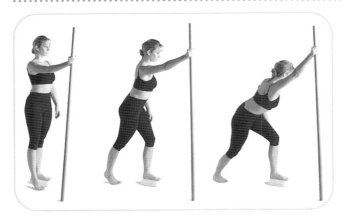

Fig. 7.42 Dangling your right foot – dropping it a little – then sliding it backward on the floor.

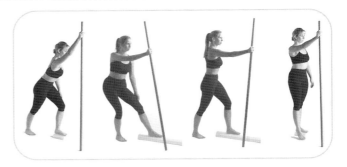

Fig. 7.43 Shift weight back to right foot – then power back forward again to dangle foot.

- Slowly lower your right foot toward the ground (Fig. 7.42). Make it a small movement and don't worry about touching the ground.
- Can you do this movement and keep your back from arching?
- Which direction do you turn your pelvis? Try turning deliberately to the right – to the left – stay in the middle. Which way seems smoothest?
- Add in sliding your right foot backward on the floor (Fig. 7.42).
- You will have to lean forward a bit to accommodate this movement of sliding your right foot behind you. Let your pelvis turn to the left, but keep holding on to the vertical pole with your right hand.
- Reverse to return; bring your torso back upright as you slide your right foot forward and twist pelvis and chest to the right to come back to where you started with your right foot dangling (Fig. 7.42).
- Reciprocate several times, and then lie on your back to rest. Compare your two sides, especially your legs, ankles and feet.

C. Stand this time with your right foot on the half-roller and your left foot dangling off the left edge. Hold on to the pole with your left hand.
- Repeat B as above to the opposite side.
- Compare strength, flexibility, familiarity and coordination between the two sides.

D. Stand again with your left foot lengthwise on the roller and with your right foot dangling; hold the pole with your right hand as before.
- Drop your right foot toward the floor, turn your pelvis and chest to the left, lean forward a bit and slide your right foot backward a little bit on the ground behind. Repeat this several times, then slide your leg about halfway back and stay there.
- From there, shift your weight back on to your right foot and turn your pelvis and chest to the right (Fig. 7.43). Lean forward a bit and stick your right hip out and to the right.
- Alternate. Shift your weight forward on to your left foot to come upright with your torso while tucking your tail and turning your pelvis to the left.
- Then shift your weight back on to your right foot while turning your pelvis and chest to the right. Stick out your right hip and lean forward a bit. Keep both heels down for now.
- What do you have to do to keep your knees over your feet? How do you prevent your feet from rolling in and out as your pelvis rotates right and left?
- Enlarge this shifting-forward movement to come up on to the balls of your right foot. Think of centering your vertical foot over that spot between the first and second balls of your foot.
- Reverse to drive your right heel back to the floor, then sit or sink yourself back and down to bend as completely as you can over your right ankle. Make sure your foot doesn't roll inward as you do this! Keep your right knee out over your right foot.
- Continue now to lift your right foot off the floor again to come to your starting position, balancing on one foot with the right foot dangling off the edge of the roller. Combine the two movements to again slide your right foot back, shift weight back on to it, shift back forward again to lift your right foot and return to the start.
- Focus your attention on the activity in your calf, pelvis and the back of your thigh as you push off in coming forward. Focus your attention on your ability to keep your right knee out over your right foot as you bend back fully over your right ankle. Pause for a moment and rest in this position.
- Resume this same basic movement, but this time as you shift your weight forward on to the left foot and turn your pelvis to the left, continue now to take a step up on to something (chair, stair, bench, table) with your right foot (Fig. 7.44).

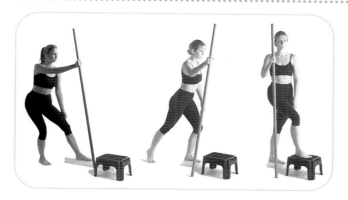

Fig. 7.44 Alternating steps to half-standing – turn twice both coming forward and coming backward.

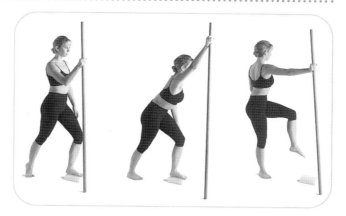

Fig. 7.45 Lifting the front leg – spilling your pelvis backward – and straightening standing knee to push taller.

- Place the sole of your right foot on the step so that your knee is directly over your foot. This is a half-standing position.
- Reverse this movement to slide your right foot back, shift your weight back on to and turn towards that right foot. Then reverse the movement again to come back forward to half-standing. Reciprocate several times.
- Try allowing your pelvis and chest to turn to the right as you come forward to half-stand in a counterpoint to the turning to the left of your pelvis and torso as you slide your foot back.

E. Stand this time with your right foot on the half-roller and your left foot dangling off the left edge.
- Repeat D as above to the opposite side.
- Compare and contrast the two sides.

F. Come back to place your left foot on the roller again with your right foot dangling off the edge.
- Drop and slide your right foot back on the floor about halfway and stay there.
- Shift your weight back on to the right foot and turn your pelvis and chest to the right. Sink yourself back on to your centered right foot and stay in this position as you alternately lift and lower your left foot slightly away from the roller several times (Fig. 7.45).
- As you lift your foot, tuck your tail again and let your pelvis fall back on your legs. Try pulling your ankle up and curling your toes as you do this!
- You are sitting back and putting all your weight into your right leg. Make sure your right knee is still above your foot. Repeat this several times, then rest.
- Enlarge this movement by straightening your right knee and pushing the top of your head toward the ceiling as you lift your foot away from the roller, then bending your right knee and sinking lower as you put your foot back down again (Fig. 7.45).
- Try letting your pelvis turn to the left as you lift your foot and to the right as you lower it back down. Tuck

your tail to get taller and lift it slightly to sink down/lean slightly forward.

G. Repeat instructions as above to opposite side.

H. Stand on both feet again, no pole.
- Feel how you are organized now in comparison to when you started.
- Take a step forward with your left foot – then step back – then forward – then back. Do the 'Charleston.'
- Do the same thing with your right foot.
- Walk around a bit and feel for movement of your ankles or toes. Does your ankle bend and straighten? How clearly can you feel your toes?
- Pay particular attention to which toes you use to push off and how active are the backs of your legs, thighs and hips in propelling yourself forward.

Brief remarks – Toeing Off

Toeing Off continues our theme of facilitating a differentiated pattern of ankle plantarflexion and toe dorsiflexion in a context of a push-off function. In this lesson, we added weightbearing and a change of venue to similar patterns of movement introduced earlier in Heel to Toe. Try keeping your heel off the ground even as you shift weight back on to the back leg. Can you maintain a vertical foot the whole time (Fig. 7.46)?

Expand on the described lesson by hopping forward, shift back on to the back leg, then come forward, turn and hop your front foot forward a foot or so. Repeat sequentially to hop across the floor, making sure to shift back and load your various springs before each leap (Fig. 7.46). Do several times on one side then walk around a bit to compare and contrast the two sides. Repeat hops and sequential hops to the other side (Box 7.13).

By shifting weight forward and pushing off a vertical foot we are again politely but more firmly asking for ankle plantarflexion/toe dorsiflexion differentiation and an ability to direct movement to that spot between the first and second

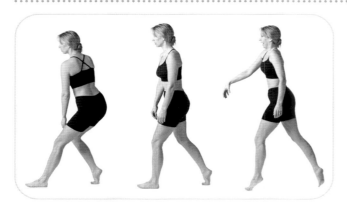

Fig. 7.46 Keep the foot vertical even as you sink your weight back on to it – and turn the whole movement into a forward hop.

Box 7.13 Toeing Off
Companion lesson to Heel to Toe – recycled version of Steppin' Out that focuses proprioceptively on hip to knee to foot relationships
Focus on orientation of knee and foot in stepping leg
Iliopsoas and soleus stretch context – work with knee hyperextension
Work with upper extremity facilitation of lower extremity function
Degree of difficulty progressions – heel on floor the whole time and hopping

metatarsal heads. What else can we teach that would ask the question even more rigorously? We can experiment with movements from various squatting positions. This next lesson is a bit on the rigorous side, so proceed with caution: it asks a lot of knees, ankles and toes.

One thing to note in this lesson concerning the organization of the stepping leg: foot placement and orientation matter. As the stepping leg swings through in a flexion and horizontal adduction movement of that hip the orientation of both the knee and the foot needs to be addressed. The student who habitually adducts her knee relative to her hip in swinging the stepping leg through needs to recalibrate the position of the knee relative to the hip towards a more horizontally abducted position. This can happily be facilitated by turning the pelvis in the direction of the stepping leg, with a subsequent constraint on the ability of the stepping leg to drift medially. This is one of the beauties of using a pelvic force couple organization with walking, running, hiking, stairs or biking.

The other orientation that needs to be addressed is that of the foot. When swinging through, we will want a balance between the medial and lateral hamstrings as they work to decelerate the straightening knee. Design a few variations of a lesson around placing the stepping foot on a stool or step and exploring knee-to-foot relationships. Try a few steps and attend to the orientation of your stepping foot. Is it abducted? Exaggerate the two extremes to recalibrate the middle.

Lift your leg to step with knee external rotation and foot abduction; point your toes way to the outside. Then lift your leg to step with knee internal rotation and foot adduction; point your toes inward, but still allow your pelvis to turn appropriate to your force couple. This skill emphasizes the ability to control the forward-swinging leg with the medial hamstrings.

Assess your ability to balance these two regionally opposite motor skills and use awareness to find middle. Try further variations with a slippery board on a stool or chair in standing; segue into the Charleston. For most, balancing this movement will require medial hamstring emphasis. Look back to slippery board for medial hamstring emphasis; find variations in Heel to Toe, Horsing Around or Rolling the Foot that do the same.

Play with upper extremity involvement in this lesson. Coordinate opposite leg and arm in push-off movement; emphasize pulling arm and shoulder back with latissimus to facilitate fuller opposite hip extension from the gluteals. Coordinate opposite leg and arm in stepping movement; emphasize reaching out with opposite arm and shoulder as if grabbing an imaginary something out in front of you to facilitate fuller opposite hip flexion. Use images of reaching out with your foot to grab the floor in front, then spit the floor back out behind you.

Work with knee hyperextension tendencies in this position. Knee hyperextension can be a compensation for a lack of hip extension or of ankle dorsiflexion. A common pattern features anterior pelvic tilt and knee hyperextension; extension-related low back pain and patellar tracking problems are possible manifestations of this laziness of the legs. The gluteals are allowing the pelvis to fall too far forward on the legs and the quadriceps abdicate all responsibility by hyperextending the knees and shifting weight forward.

Get up on your feet and check this out proprioceptively; note that as you posteriorly rotate your pelvis your knees unlock, and that as you shift your weight back toward your heels your quadriceps kick in. Get your students with weak quadriceps to spend more time with their weight rocked back toward their heels.

Use the push-off movement in this lesson with an emphasis on extending the hip and preventing the pelvis from rolling forward to retrain the CNS away from hyperextension tendencies in gait. Use the Horsing Around variations of pushing taller with posterior tilt to retrain the CNS away from knee hyperextension in standing. Use one-legged standing variations where you bend your knee to sink lower and maintain/exaggerate posterior pelvic tilt as you straighten your knee and push taller. All these variations emphasize powerful use of the gluteals and more complete hip extension.

Use the push-off movement in this lesson with an emphasis on extending the hip, keeping a centered heel on the floor behind and preventing the pelvis from rolling forward to lengthen the iliopsoas and the gastrocnemius. The temptations many people will succumb to here are to let their pelvis roll into anterior tilt, to bend the back knee, to let the back heel lift, to let the back heel slide inward on the floor or to roll the back foot into pronation. Get on your feet and try each of these cheats. Be accurate and feel for that deep and oh-so-satisfying stretch in the hip flexors and calf. Keep the front knee bent and push that foot into the floor. Cue the front leg hamstring to extend the front hip and create more posterior tilt of the pelvis.

Continue to push both front and back feet into the floor as you resume shifting weight forward and back. Resist the movement forward with the front leg and resist the movement backward with the back leg. Let your legs play a cooperative game of tug of war in this split stance position, analogous to what we did when shifting weight left and right and playing the hip abductors against each other in Horsing Around. Try a wider split stance and see if you can push simultaneously forward and back while adding in our previously learned movement of pushing outward bilaterally. Put down roots and stabilize yourself in 360 directions.

Steppin' down

So far we have discussed stepping forward and stepping up, but not stepping down. Where you will want to have teaching strategies for stepping down is in working with people who experience anterior knee pain when walking down slopes or stairs. Pain on going downhill is a very common complaint, and for those who love to hike, live at the top of a hill or work in a three-storey building with no elevator, this presents a problem.

People get their knees in a bunch going downhill because of medial/lateral imbalance problems and because of patellar compression problems. Observe your patellar students when they step down forward off a stool. Watch for a collapse of the back foot into abduction or pronation, and for a collapse of the back knee inward. Watch for how much of the function of lowering the center of gravity is done around the hips. What is the proportion of effort between the quadriceps and the gluteals/short and stubbies?

Start retraining efforts with a described variation of Steppin' Out (see Fig. 6.60). Place your left foot in front and your right foot back, then sink yourself back on to your right foot and lift just the heel of your left foot so only your left toes are on the ground and 80% of your weight is on your back/right foot. From here, slide both hands down your left leg toward your left foot. Be sure to keep your weight back on your right leg and your left toes just touching the floor.

Keep your back tripod stable and keep your knee out over your foot as you slide your hands repetitively up and down your left leg. This puts a premium on your right hip extensors and hip rotators and is great for teaching hip over knee over foot relationships, and for facilitating an active vastus medialis. Try both sides and compare range, strength and familiarity.

This bending-forward movement with weight on the back leg also simulates stepping down. Progress this movement by putting the back foot up on a thick book or 2–4 inch riser. Do the same basic movement, but focus on lowering the front foot to the floor in front with the same hip movement that previously resulted in a forward-bending movement.

Lean your torso forward a bit as you step down, let your pelvis turn in the direction of the back foot (!) and let the back/weightbearing hip flex, internally rotate and adduct. How much can you lower your front foot without bending your back knee? Be rigorous about not letting your foot or knee collapse inward; this will be assisted by letting your pelvis turn toward the weightbearing hip and allowing full ankle dorsiflexion.

Progress your student next to walking down inclines. Start with small steps and shallow inclines and emphasize dropping the center of mass with the omnipotent hip muscles. Gradually enlarge length of stride and steepness of incline to bring in some amount of knee flexion and some quadriceps activation. Cue balanced foot on the floor and balanced knee over foot to ensure balance of the medial and lateral quadriceps. Emphasize initial lowering movement from the hip to get the big guys involved and to improve medial/lateral balance of the knee joints and musculature.

As an alternative for going down stairs or taking a big step down on a hiking trail, try turning sideways and getting into a split stance. Find some stairs and stand with your left foot forward and your right foot back and on the same riser. Shift your weight forward and turn your pelvis to the left as you shift on to your left foot. Step down with the right foot to the riser below through left hip horizontal adduction, flexion and internal rotation. Keep the same split stance as you rock yourself forward and back to go down stairs. Apply to any large step down.

Starting Blocks

Variations

A. Stand for a moment in your bare feet. Let your arms hang at your sides, feet around shoulder width apart and look straight ahead.

- Notice your feet against the floor. What direction do your toes point?

- Do you have more weight forward on your toes or back on your heels?

- Are your feet rolled in to flatten your arch or are you rolled on to the outside edges of your feet?

- Walk around a bit and feel for movement of your ankles or toes. Does your ankle bend and straighten? How clearly can you feel your toes?

- Pay particular attention to which toes you push off from, and how active the backs of your legs, thighs and hips are in propelling yourself forward.

B. Come on to your hands and knees. Distribute your weight proportionally so there is a bit more weight back on your legs than forward on your hands. Hands and knees are under hips and shoulders and are around hip to shoulder width apart (Fig. 7.47).

- In this position, notice your feet.

- Are they closer together or farther apart than your knees? Are the fronts of your ankles close to or touching the floor? Or is there a space between them?

- Are your heels rolled out wider or rolled in narrower than your toes? Are there differences between the two sides?

- Bring your attention to your right foot. Roll your heel alternately inward and outward. Feel how this rolls the top of your forefoot and toes from side to side on the floor. What is the range of this movement? Does it roll more easily outward or inward?

- Does your pelvis move in space as you do this? Try shifting your pelvis in space to the left as you roll your

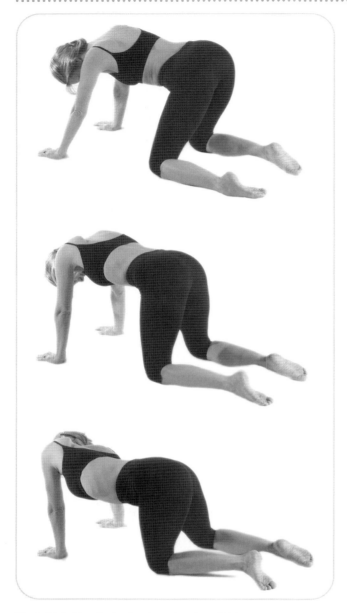

Fig. 7.47 Rolling the heel and moving the pelvis in opposite directions.

right heel to the right, and shift your pelvis to the right as you roll your heel to the left (Fig. 7.47).

- Do the same exploratory movements with the left foot; roll the left heel in and out, feel for any movement of your pelvis, then direct the pelvis and heel in opposite directions as above. Coordinate rolling both heels at the same time and move your pelvis!

C. Come back to your hands and knees again as before.

- Roll both your heels alternately in toward and out away from each other a few times. Use this movement to help establish where your foot is centered

with the heels rolled neither in nor out. Stop there once found.

- Then flex and extend your ankles (Fig. 7.48) Flex up your ankles to bring the bottoms of your toes or even the balls of your feet to touch the floor.

- Extend your ankles back down long again to bring the tops of your toes and the fronts of your ankles to flatten back toward the floor.

- Alternate several times. Which direction seems easier? How do you organize your hips and pelvis with this?

- Extend your ankles and toes down long and sit back toward your heels. Use your body weight to help in flattening the tops of your forefeet and the fronts of your ankles toward the floor.

- Which direction do your heels tend to roll? Do this several times, then flex your ankles up and your toes underneath to get into this starting-block position and sit yourself back to put more weight on your heels (Fig. 7.48).

- Which toes are supporting your weight? Which balls (metatarsal heads) are on the floor? Do this several times, then pause for a short rest.

- Still in hands and knees, extend your ankles long and sit back toward your left heel. Do this a few times, then stay there a moment with your pelvis resting on your heel. Move your pelvis alternately left and right to roll your heel from side to side (Fig. 7.49).

- Do this same movement to the other side; sit toward your right heel and roll it from side to side with your pelvis. Pause for a short rest again.

- Then flex up your right ankle to a starting block position and sit back to put weight on that heel if possible. Come back to hands and knees, then flex up your left ankle and sit back to put weight on that heel.

- Alternate from side to side, directing your weight on to the area of your foot between the first and second balls (metatarsal heads) (Fig. 7.49). This is a place where your foot is effectively vertical and you are bearing weight skeletally through your foot. Compare your ability to do this movement to each side.

D. Come to a right half-squatting position (first illustration of Fig. 7.53). The balls of your right foot are on the floor and your right heel is lifted. Most of your weight is on the right foot. Your left foot is flat and out in front of you a half step or more. Place your hands or knuckles on the floor in front of and to either side of your right knee and use them to assist with balance. Your right knee and thigh will be between your two arms.

- Rest your pelvis on your right heel and notice whether your weight is rolled inward to the inside of your right big toe or outward toward your right ring and little toes.

- Move your pelvis from side to side, moving your heel from side to side to shift weight across all five balls

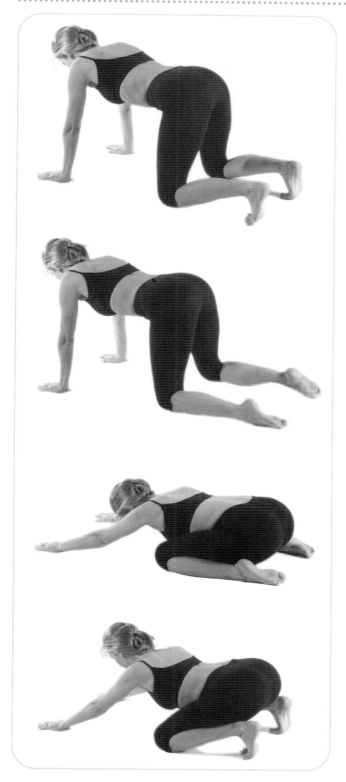

Fig. 7.48 Flex and extend your ankles – then sit back to put some weight on your heels in each position.

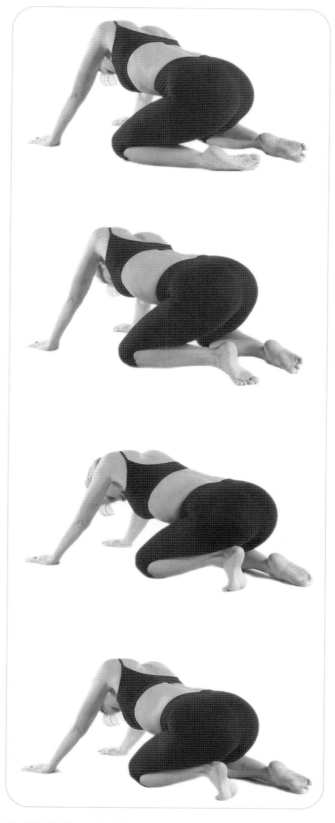

Fig. 7.49 Rolling the heel from side to side with the pelvis – two versions.

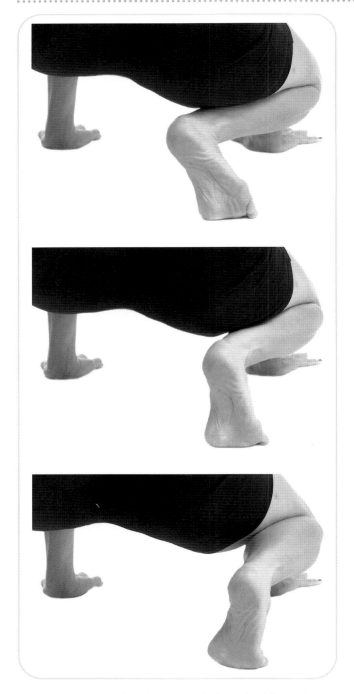

Fig. 7.50 Keep your pelvis where it is and roll your heel from side to side – scratching your tush with your heel.

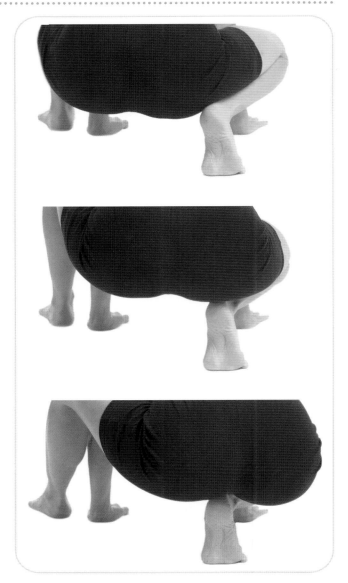

Fig. 7.51 Keep your foot vertical and move your pelvis from side to side – scratch your heel with your tush.

of your foot (Fig. 7.50). Go from side to side several times to establish kinesthetically where your foot is vertical and where you are bearing most of your weight between first and second balls.

• Stay here while you now move your pelvis from side to side, but keep your foot vertical and your weight between your first and second balls (Fig. 7.51).

• Think of scratching your heel with your pelvis. Find the place where your right sitting bone (ischial tuberosity) is resting on your right heel.

• From this place (sitting bone resting on a vertical foot), roll forward on the toes and balls to move your right knee toward the floor in front of you as if wanting to place your knee on the floor between and in front of your hands.

• Then roll backward on your metatarsals to move your right heel toward the ground behind you.

• Alternate back and forth between moving your right knee toward the ground in front and your right heel

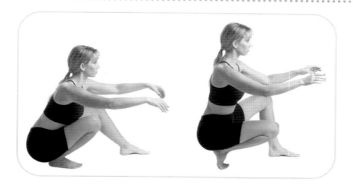

Fig. 7.52 Placing sitting bones on heel of vertical foot – then lifting and lowering heel.

toward the floor behind; roll along your foot, but stay between the first and second balls (Fig. 7.52).

- Do this several times, then stand up to rest for a moment and to feel for differences between your two feet as you stand and walk. You could also lie on your back and scan for differences in your feet, ankles, knees and hips.

E. Come to left half-squatting – rest your weight on your left heel and place your flat right foot on the floor in front.

- Repeat instructions as in D to the opposite side.
- Compare the movements on this side to the other.

F. Come to right half-squatting again.

- Rest your right sitting bone on your right heel with your right foot vertical and with your weight between your first and second metatarsal heads.

- Resume the previous movement of moving your right knee and right heel alternately toward the ground in front and in back. Do this a few times.

- Then, the next time you move your right knee forward slide your left hand forward on the ground a little past your left foot. While keeping both hands on the floor, lift your pelvis high toward the ceiling while driving your right heel back toward the ground behind (Fig. 7.53).

- This is a sequential movement that first brings your pelvis forward, then up toward the ceiling and back toward your heel. Reverse the trajectory to return to half-squatting.

- Repeat this movement several times and pay particular attention that you don't roll your weight on your right foot toward the inside of your big toe and that you don't allow your right heel to slide or move inward to the left. Keep your feet parallel and pointed straight forward.

- Get into that position, then push yourself all the way to standing; your right leg is still behind and your left knee stays slightly bent. Feel the work in the back of your left thigh as you do this.

- Rest for a moment, then try the following movements for extra credit if you are physically capable.

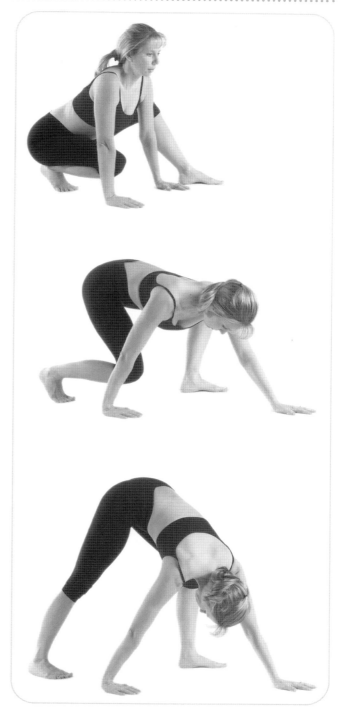

Fig. 7.53 Transition from half-squat to quadruped split stance – be reasonable!

- Come to right half-squatting but with both hands off the floor and both arms extended out in front of you at shoulder height. From this position, alternate back and forth between moving your right knee forward toward the floor and your right heel back toward the

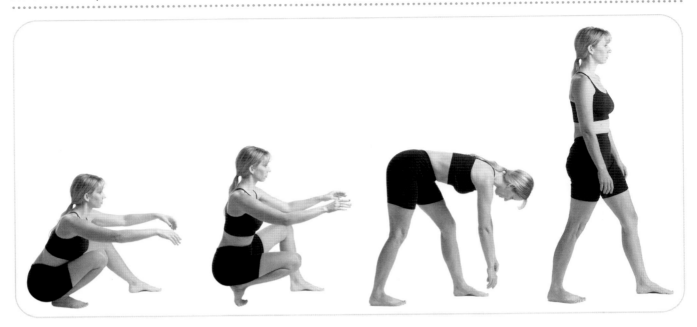

Fig. 7.54 Extra credit – half-squat to split stance with no hands. Keep feet centered.

floor (Fig. 7.54). This is the same movement as before, but without your hands to assist in balance and weightbearing.

- Now try extending this movement by driving yourself all the way up to a split stance from the half-squatting position (Fig. 7.53). Be mindful and respectful of your right knee; be reasonable! Can you return to right half-squatting from the right split stance? Is this movement reversible?

G. Come back to left half-squatting.

- Repeat instructions as in F to the other side.
- Compare and contrast the two sides.

H. Come back to your hands and knees again.

- Sit back toward your heels. Try this a few times with the feet long and the top of your feet and toes on the floor, then a few times coming back with your toes bent up in your starting block position.
- Sit back to your right heel a few times with each variation, then sit back toward your left heel.
- How are your ankles and toes bending and straightening now? Do you come on to your toes any more easily now?

I. Stand up.

- Notice your feet against the floor. What direction do your toes point?
- Do you have more weight forward on your toes or back on your heels?
- Are your feet rolled in to flatten your arch, or are you rolled on to the outside edges of your feet?

- Walk around a bit and feel for movement of your ankles or toes. Does your ankle bend and straighten? How clearly can you feel your toes?
- Pay particular attention to which toes you use to push off and how active the backs of your legs, thighs and hips are in propelling yourself forward. How does this compare to when you started?

Baselines – Starting Blocks

The questions in variation A are identical to the initial questions in Heel to Toe and Toeing Off: they pertain to straight forward locomotion. The questions in variation B, however, are different.

From your hands and knees, you are directed to notice the organization of your feet while in this position. Are your feet closer together or farther apart than your knees? This is a question of internal rotation/external rotation bias at the hips. Modify the lesson by sliding the feet right and left on the floor, exploring alternating internal and external rotation movements of the hips to establish a truer neutral.

Are the fronts of your ankles touching the floor? This is a question of calf/anterior compartment bias at the ankles. Are your heels rolled out wider than, or rolling in narrower than, your toes? This is a question of medial/lateral hamstring bias. Are there differences between the two sides? This is a question of force couple bias or injury avoidance/compensation.

Rolling the heels

The initial movements in this lesson are to roll the right heel in and out on the floor. This is a question of control and balance of tibial/knee internal and external rotation. We also explored the associations between this rolling movement of the heel and movements farther up the kinematic chain to the pelvis and torso.

Which way did you tend to move your pelvis when rolling the right heel in and out? If your pelvis moves in the same direction of the rolling heel (pelvis moves right when right heel rolls out), you are probably initiating your weight shift from your arms or torso and are moving them in the same/global direction to enlarge the range of movement of the heel. If your pelvis moves in the opposite direction to the rolling heel (pelvis moves left when right heel rolls out), you are probably engaging your legs more in your weight-shift.

By engaging the right hip abductors to push outward on the floor, they would drag the rolling right heel outward along with them, as in Rolling the Foot. Can you have the motor control necessary to both allow your heel to roll outward and to stabilize your heel in space when pushing off and have the awareness to know what you are doing differently? This differentiated movement of knee internal rotation with a push-to-move-left engagement of the right hip abductors/short and stubbies is just what many of your students with patellar tracking problems need.

The movement of rolling the right heel inward would then be linked to a pulling movement of the right adductors in a pulling-to-move-right strategy. Find the foot stabilizers here as similar to movements in Rolling the Foot. Rolling both feet at the same time either accelerates the secondary force couple movements (right abductors and left adductors working together to shift weight to left – right heel rolls out and left heel rolls in to move in same direction) or cancels them out (both abductors contract to roll both heels out, or both adductors contract to pull both heels in – heels roll in opposite directions and legs opposing each other).

Self-mobilizing feet, ankles and knees

In variation C you come back to hands and knees again to roll heels in and out. This time, use this reciprocating movement to find the middle and stay there. From this knee rotation neutral position, begin to flex and extend your ankles. Movements of the toes and ankles in this variation are global: the ankles and toes dorsiflex and plantarflex together. In this position, a vertical foot requires this global pattern, whereas our next movement in this sequence (sitting your pelvis back on to your heels to flatten the dorsal foot to the floor) requires a horizontal foot and another regionally global pattern, this time ankle and toe plantarflexion.

Use these vertical and horizontal positions of the foot and sitting your pelvis back on to your feet movements to stretch soleus/Achilles and the anterior compartment and to re-coordinate the antagonists associated with a brand new knee rotation neutral position. Use the sitting-back movements to encourage movements of the heels outward and to facilitate knee internal rotation.

What you will usually want to discourage is someone sitting back toward their heels with their knees farther inward than their feet (hips internally rotated) or with their toes pointed outward (knees externally rotated). This movement can be unsafe for the knees if the knees can't be out and the heels can't be out or neutral. Try it yourself if you have sturdy knees to appreciate proprioceptively the rotational strain it puts on your knees. Contrast with moving knees out, toes closer together and heels rolled out away from each other.

Sitting your weight back on to vertical feet can be just as challenging a feat for some as it is for others to sit back on to horizontal feet. Did you fit more neatly into one bias or the other, or was this an equal opportunity difficulty for you? This movement requires a lot of toe and ankle dorsiflexion and places even more weight on those bent-up little toes. Try developing a rhythm or coordination of simultaneously dorsiflexing the ankle and toes up to this starting block position while sitting your weight back.

Something about doing them together helps the CNS in placing the foot more vertically and more easily for many people. Something about sitting back and placing a significant amount of weight vertically through the foot also helps the CNS to figure out more accurately how to arrange the foot to bear weight closer to the second metatarsal. Be Goldilocks for a moment and deliberately sit back toward feet perched on their fifth metatarsal, or towards feet collapsed inward towards the medial aspect of the first metatarsal. Use trial and error to find a vertical foot and correlate with subjective feeling of stability and minimization of effort in the ankle and lower legs.

The next variation asks you to sit back on to one heel, in both vertical and horizontal orientations of the foot, and to use a side-to-side movement of your pelvis to roll the heel you are sitting on from side to side. While the foot is horizontal with the top of the foot flattened to the floor, the passive rolling of the heel is to improve ankle mobility into plantarflexion, inversion and eversion, and to improve knee mobility into internal and external rotation.

While the foot is vertical with the weight on your metatarsal heads, the passive rolling of the heel with the pelvis is to shift weight across the five metatarsals. This experience helps the CNS to identify and differentiate in sensation the different parts of the forefoot and helps in identifying a vertical foot. Roll across the metatarsal heads to find that sweet spot between the first and second balls of the foot.

A possible variation in this section would be to sit back on to one horizontal or vertical heel again and to roll the heel from side to side, but to keep the pelvis where it is. This is performed both vertically and horizontally to gain motor control/balance over knee internal and external rotation through the medial/lateral hamstrings and popliteus. Use it vertically again to establish through movement a vertical foot with weight between first and second metatarsal heads. Another possible variation is to continue this sitting-back movement by lifting the knee of the heel you are sitting on off the floor. This moves you farther back and completes a transitional movement from hands and knees to half-kneeling.

Half-squats and full weightbearing on tiny base of support

In variation D we explore new territory. Squatting positions are great for working with dynamic lumbar stability and for working with knee-to-foot-to-toe relationships. Sadly, many people from western cultures have difficulty with this position and its variations, so be reasonable with yourself and your students. The first position is right half-squatting. The balls of your right foot are on the floor and your right heel is lifted; most of your weight is on the right foot. Your left foot is flat on the floor and out in front of you about a half step.

Lean on your hands in front for support and move your right heel from side to side by moving your pelvis from side to side. This is a link to a previous variation performed in hands and knees. This again helps in finding a vertical foot and in experiencing the disadvantages of bearing weight too far out on the fifth or too far in on the first metatarsal head.

Once found, you now keep your weight between the first and second metatarsal and keep your foot vertical as you continue to move your pelvis from side to side. This skill of keeping the foot centered on the floor while the skeleton gyrates from side to side is valuable in terms of foot and ankle health. Figure out the knee internal rotation/external rotation and the hip rotational movements that need to be made to accomplish this.

Once you have found that place where the foot is vertical, the weight is between the first and second balls and the ischial tuberosity is sitting on or is vertically over the heel, stay there. This again defines the hip over the knee over the foot relationship we have been facilitating in other lessons. From here, we add in the plantarflexion and dorsiflexion movements again.

By rolling forward on to the right toes and metatarsal heads and moving the right knee towards the floor, we are asking for the always-in-popular-demand ankle plantarflexion and toe dorsiflexion differentiated pattern. This movement ups the ante on the ability of the toes to dorsiflex. Feel free to fold at any time during the game.

By rolling back toward the right heel and lifting the knee away from the ground, we are asking for ankle dorsiflexion and a movement of the toes into relative plantarflexion. This reciprocating differentiated movement in this position again reviews and refines a previously introduced movement. Do the same basic movement in a number of positions, functional contexts and weightbearing demands to provide for a progressive learning experience.

By directing the movement through the middle of the foot from sweet spot in front to middle of the heel in back, we are tracking the foot along a line we will want to establish for walking and running. Avoid the temptation to move the heel in or out to compensate for a tight big toe into dorsiflexion or a tight ankle/heel cord into dorsiflexion. Use squatting movements to further challenge and refine posterior tibialis/peroneus longus balance and competence. Cue awareness of forward foot. Maintain first metatarsal contact with the floor to facilitate peroneus longus and a high arch.

Use squatting movements and variations to work on improving toe dorsiflexion range of motion and control. Coming forward and reaching the knee toward the floor requires an eccentric contraction of the flexor hallucis longus, whereas coming back again requires the same muscle to work concentrically. These various squatting and split stance positions are great for functionally strengthening the flexor hallucis longus. This muscle may contribute to stabilizing the medial arch and to alleviating plantar fasciitis.

Transition – half-squat to split stance

In variation F, come to right half-squat again. Sit your right ischial tuberosity on your right vertical foot with your left foot flat on the floor a half step in front of you. Lean with your hands on the floor and overlap the last movements of the last variation; roll front to back along your foot. Add in sliding your left hand forward on the ground and lifting your pelvis high towards the ceiling while driving your right heel back towards the floor. This variation adds another functional context to the Rolling the Foot to balance movements we were exploring in half-squatting. This variation begins our transitional movement from half-squatting to a split stance.

Besides providing for an excellent gastrosoleus/heel cord stretch for the back leg and an excellent hamstring stretch for both front and back legs, this is another position to facilitate a precise hip over knee over foot relationship. Watch out that your back foot stays parallel to your line of movement. Most people will want to allow the heel to move inward to reduce the necessity to truly dorsiflex over a neutral foot and ankle.

Try unlisted variations from this position. Keep your feet where they are and centered, then lift your right hand toward the ceiling. Let your pelvis and torso rotate to the right as you do this, but keep your feet centered on the floor and keep your knees over your feet. Then reach your right elbow toward the ground. Let your pelvis and torso rotate to the left, but again keep knees and feet centered.

Try getting into this position then rolling the back foot inward and outward through pressing the first and fifth metatarsal heads. Use this movement to check for accuracy in making sure you are not compensating for heel cord shortness by pronating that foot. Do you feel an enhanced calf/heel cord stretch when rolling outward/pressing with the posterior tibialis?

After having raised and lowered your pelvis several times, now complete the transition by pushing yourself all the way to a right split stance position. Concentrate on keeping your front (left) knee slightly bent as you do this to provide a constraint that de-emphasizes pushing the foot into the floor with the quadriceps. Feel the strong use of the left hamstring as you raise yourself up to split stance, then lower your hands back towards the floor.

Review similarities to bending movements in Side-sit Bending, Half-kneel Bending and Split Stance Bending. This bending movement is a great way of getting hamstring and short and stubby length and strength, and is a great way to retrain accurate hip-over-knee-over-foot relationships. Cue to press both first and fifth metatarsals and enhance the sling effect through the foot.

Reverse the movement to come back to right half-squatting and put the whole thing together several times, moving from right half-squat to right split stance and back again. Try it faster, or set yourself a goal for the number of times you are going to do this. Working quickly, powerfully and even aerobically is another change of venue that both solidifies learning and develops physical skills.

The last variation of this section is an extreme continuation of the shifting weight back and forward movements we did in Toeing Off. Whereas in that lesson we stayed upright when

Box 7.14 Starting Blocks

Hands and knees facilitation of foot, ankle and knee – mobility, stability and accurate left/right balance

Half-squatting and rolling along the foot – define weightbearing trajectory front to back

Clarifying the sweet spot – bearing weight vertically through first and second metatarsal heads

Degree of difficulty regressions – chair, lean on wall, pull on bars in front or sit on balls of various sizes

sinking weight back on to the back foot, in this lesson we continue the movement to sink all the way back to sit on the back heel. I expect very few of those who do this lesson to actually do this movement, so why put it in?

I put it in to illustrate the modular aspect of this kind of exercise approach. Seemingly separate lessons suddenly have a connection via this variation. And if you are working with a high-level athlete, you will need to be able to figure out ways of imposing further demands within the framework of a particular function or particular movement pattern. Could we make this movement even more challenging (Box 7.14)?

Widen the distance between your feet; add in the hopping movement you did at the end of Toeing Off. Conversely, you will want to have an understanding of basic movement patterns sufficient to make movements easier for those of your students who struggle proprioceptively, lack the physical prowess to do the full movement, or are in too much pain.

Baselines and variations

In variation H we come back to hands and knees to reassess our initial dynamic baseline. Are the heels rolling more easily or more evenly from side to side? Do your toes bend more? Can you flatten your ankle to the floor more fully when you sit your weight back on it?

In variation I, we come back to standing and walking to reassess our initial dynamic baseline. Walk around a bit and feel for movement of your ankles or toes. How does your ankle bend and straighten now? How clearly can you feel your toes? Pay particular attention to which toes you push off from, and how active the backs of your legs, thighs and hips are in propelling yourself forward. How does this compare to when you started? Try going back to some of the last variations of the Toeing Off lesson and notice whether you have learned anything new.

One variation is to do the lesson sitting in a chair instead of squatting on the floor (Fig. 7.55). Sit in a firm chair without armrests and scoot yourself all the way to the right so that your right ischial tuberosity is off the edge of the seat. Start with an awareness of how the right leg now needs to press into the floor to keep from toppling over to the right. Lift and lower your right ischial tuberosity a few times. Move your right knee/right ischial tuberosity forward and back a few times.

Connect the dots and make a circle with the right side of your pelvis in space. Rest, then come back off the edge of the chair. This time place the balls of your right foot back on the floor so that your right foot is vertical and your right heel is

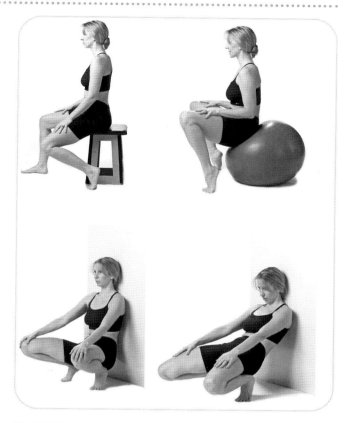

Fig. 7.55 Finding a vertical foot from a chair – on a ball – or leaning on a wall.

underneath your right ischium. Roll your heel from side to side to define vertical and center the vertical foot over the sweet spot. Do dorsiflexion and plantarflexion movements to track a parallel line along the foot from front to back.

Guide toward sit-to-stand movements; emphasize pushing off with back leg and turning a bit to the left. Cue to maintain sweet spot if working with legs; cue to maintain intersegmental stabilization and independent breath if working with low back instability. Modify this idea further by sitting on balls of various sizes. Reduce weightbearing stresses on the toes, metatarsals and knees while still training the same movements. Start with larger and progress to smaller balls and less support for the pelvis (Fig. 7.55).

Leaning back against a wall can be a great position to start working with metatarsal squatting skills: balance requirements are fewer and you don't need as much toe dorsiflexion as you do during the lesson. It's easier to get both the heels and the knees to the ground, and some of your weight is supported by the wall (Fig. 7.55). Design a lesson incorporating both squatting and half-squatting positions leaning against a wall. Include rolling the heel variations to challenge peroneus longus and posterior tibialis balance and competence, to mobilize the foot, ankle and toes, and to train for proprioceptive awareness of a vertical or skeletal weightbearing foot.

Standing up and placing one foot up on a high bench, table, counter or chair seat is another place to work on getting a

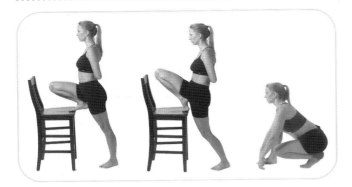

Fig. 7.56 Finding a vertical foot in standing with one leg up – upping the ante by placing a ball between heel and ischial tuberosity.

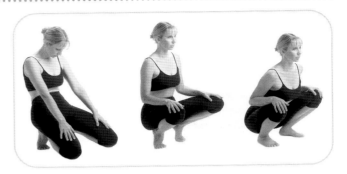

Fig. 7.57 Squatting – move knees then heels toward floor – round and arch back to find neutral.

vertical foot centered between first and second metatarsal heads. Roll left and right to find the sweet spot and move heel then knee towards the floor (Fig. 7.56).

Up the ante on any of these variations by placing a small ball between the ischial tuberosity and the heel of the vertical foot (Fig. 7.56). This challenges the ability of the peroneus longus and the posterior tibialis to stabilize the foot, and assists in defining a vertical relationship between the heel and the ischial tuberosity that we would like to see carried over in standing and walking.

Squatting is such an important function, for both lumbar stability and lower extremity health, that I'm going to throw in another squatting lesson here. This lesson might logically precede the last one, as it starts in bilateral squatting and moves toward half-squatting. Or it might logically follow the preceding one, as it introduces some pivoting movements that we will explore in the last lesson of the chapter. Either way, enjoy your Squat Pivots.

Squat Pivots

Variations

A. Squat down and balance there with your hands off the floor. Stabilize your intersegmentals and breathe independently throughout this lesson.

- How well balanced are you?
- How is your weight distributed between your two feet?
- Are your heels on or off the floor?

B. Squat with your hands off the floor.

- Begin to move both knees a little bit toward the floor in front of you. What do you need to do with your pelvis and back to stay balanced? Do this movement a few times.
- Then move both heels a little bit toward the floor behind you. What do you need to do with your pelvis

and back to stay balanced while moving in this direction?

- Alternate back and forth (Fig. 7.57). Try rounding your back and tucking your tail as you move your knees forward.
- Arch your back and lift your tail as you move your heels toward the floor. Gradually enlarge the movement in each direction.

C. Squat again, but place both hands on the floor in front of your feet so your arms are between your knees.

- Shift your weight to your left foot and take a step forward and to the right with your right foot (Fig. 7.58). Place the whole sole of the right foot on the floor. Return to your squatting position and repeat a few times.
- Then shift your weight to your right foot and take a step forward and to the left with your left foot. Return to squat and repeat the movement on this side a few times. Alternate back and forth – squatting to half-squatting to each side (Fig. 7.58).
- Now place your right foot forward and to the right and stay there, but instead of coming back to squatting, shift your weight on to that right foot, come up on to the balls of that foot and flatten the sole of your left foot to the floor.
- You are making a transition from left to right half-squatting. Now go back balancing on the balls of your left foot again and flatten your right foot to the floor.
- Try gradually widening the space between your feet as you continue to make this transitional movement between left and right half-squatting. How wide can you be and still be in control?

D. Squat again, but this time with your hands off the floor again.

- Move your right knee toward or onto the floor. It's OK to allow your pelvis and torso to turn to the left and for your left knee to swing outward. Try this a few times.

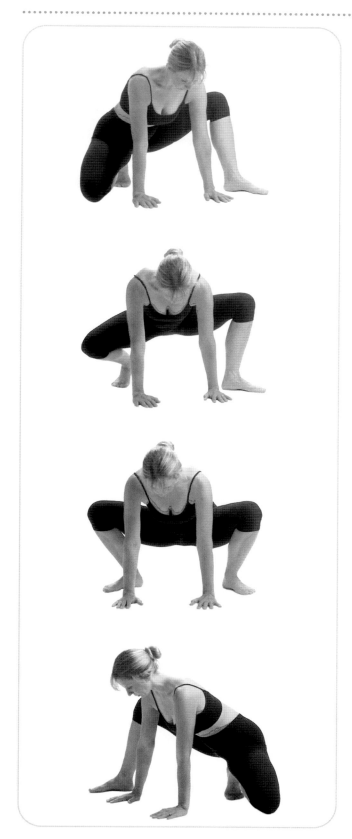

Fig. 7.58 Transition from right to left half-squatting.

Box 7.15 Squat Pivots

Transitions between various squatting and kneeling incarnations
Challenging the adductors to lengthen
Half-squatting and rolling along the foot – define weightbearing trajectory front to back
Clarifying the sweet spot – bearing weight vertically through first and second metatarsal heads

- Then move your left knee to the floor and let yourself turn to the right. How does this side compare?
- Alternate from side to side. This is a half-squat kneeling position (Fig. 7.59).

E. Squat with your hands off the floor.

- Move your right knee to the floor; turn to the left and let your left knee swing outward. Stay there.
- Now come off of the balls of your right foot and flatten the top of your right foot to the floor. Sit on your right foot so that the top of your foot and toes and the front of your ankle is pressing into the ground. This will also let the heel of your left foot touch the floor (Fig. 7.60).
- From here, shift your weight forward on to your left foot and come up on to the sole of your left foot. Keep the top of your right foot on the floor still.
- Alternate back and forth between coming up and forward on to the sole of your left foot, then sink back and down again on to the flattened right foot (Fig. 7.60).
- Do the same movement to the other side. This is a half-sit kneeling position.

F. Squat with your hands off the floor.

- Squat for a moment and feel your balance/stability.
- Go back to our original movement: alternately move both heels toward the floor, then both knees. How does this movement compare to when you started?
- Sit on both feet with the tops of the feet and the tops of the toes long on the floor. How stable does this feel?
- Stand up and walk around. How do your feet, ankles, knees and hips feel as you walk?

Brief remarks – Squat Pivots

This lesson starts in a squatting position with directions to alternately move heels and knees towards the floor. We could link these movements with an awareness of the movements of the pelvis and back. Finding spinal neutral and maintaining intersegmental stability, we could use this lesson with someone with low back pain. We could also link these movements to an awareness of the movements of the toes and ankles, and could direct intentional movement to roll on to the sweet spot between first and second metatarsal heads (Box 7.15).

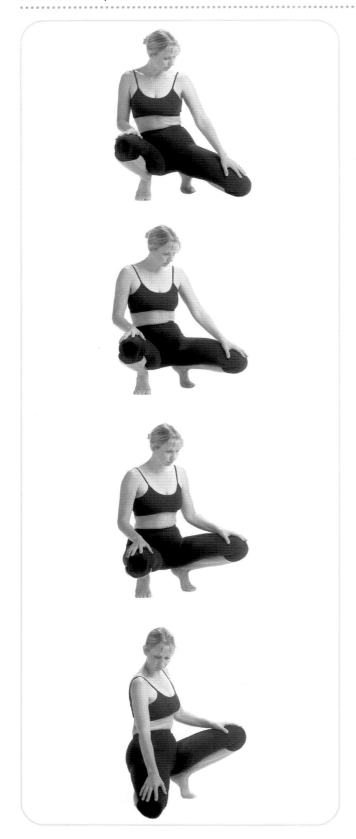

Fig. 7.59 Alternating left and right half-squat kneeling.

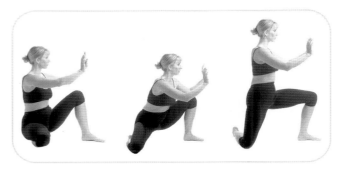

Fig. 7.60 Transition from half-sit kneeling to half-kneel.

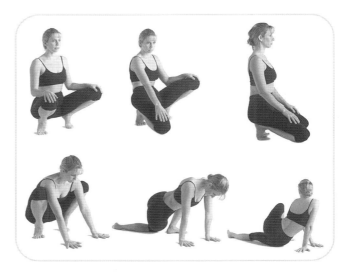

Fig. 7.61 Squatting to half-squat kneeling – to full squat kneeling – spiraling to sit from squatting.

Making a transition from squatting to half-squatting enhances stability for the lumbar patient who wants to move or lift something. Making transitions from right to left half-squatting introduces pivoting movements. Direct your attention to pivoting around the sweet spot. Transitions from squatting toward half-squat kneeling challenge the toes to dorsiflex and the quadriceps to lengthen.

Accentuate this quadriceps stretch by posteriorly tilting your pelvis and rounding your back as you move your knee toward the floor. When doing this, did you move into right torso flexion to create a diagonal? How does the opposite diagonal work, left knee toward floor and left torso flexion?

Transitions from half-sit kneeling (weight on the top of the foot rather than on the metatarsal heads) to half-kneeling complete the lesson. This variation could be modified to come up to sit on the heel of the front foot to a squatting rather than a kneeling position. Make up your own variations from here. How many transitions can you make from the various kneeling and squatting positions, either down to the floor or up to your feet (Fig. 7.61)? Use as described before for heel/toe balancing and straight forward gait, or as described before for lumbar stabilization.

Use balls to sit on as before, especially in the movement from half-sit kneeling to half-squatting. Use ball or roller between heel and ischial tuberosity to challenge foot stability and to clarify hip-to-foot relationship. Use low horizontal (or vertical) bars to hold on to while doing all squatting variations. This makes movements backward to bring heels toward the ground easier, and allows the arms to assist in pulling back forward to come on to toes. Can you move from right half heel squatting, though right half metatarsal squatting to stand without using hands for support? If not, use bars or rope/strap to assist in pulling forward or prevent from falling back.

Changing directions – rotational stability

So far in this chapter we have worked toward facilitating a foot balanced on the floor in three dimensions and have worked with push-off and shock absorption movements in front/back and left/right directions. This next lesson will have elements within it that reinforce and expand upon these earlier themes. It will also expand upon the pivoting movements we started in the last lesson. Peerless Pivots is a nice integrative lesson for much of what we have performed in the last two chapters. Include this lesson in your lumbar stabilization protocol with proprioceptive cues directed towards finding and maintaining a neutral spine and intersegmental stabilization.

Include this lesson in your return to function protocols for ankle or knee fractures or ligament or cartilage tears. Direct proprioceptive cues to a stable foot on the floor and establish a powerful and balanced pelvic force couple system. Include this lesson in your recalibration of neutral series for your students with biomechanical faults leading to lower extremity repetitive stress injuries. Direct awareness to hip over knee over foot organization and proportional effort initiated from the hip.

Include this lesson with athletes, dancers or other physically accomplished students to train for prevention of injuries and for performance enhancement. Improve the most basic building blocks of running, cutting and jumping. We will be working with pivoting movements in this lesson, exploring various combinations of weight-shift and turning movements. Sometimes you will be pivoting around the sweet spot, whereas at other times you will pivot on your heel. This lesson is derived in part from a classic Feldenkrais lesson and in part from what little I know about the martial art of tai chi.

Martial arts have much to offer us as medical professionals. These movement disciplines have been developed and refined over centuries, as has another movement discipline, yoga. Both precede the exercise model we have today. They emphasize whole-body integrated movements, self-awareness and movement toward an intentional functional goal.

The skills taught in these movement disciplines can be broken down into their muscular and functional components and correlated to the various medical or performance enhancement puzzles we come across, similar to what I have attempted

to do with the Feldenkrais Method in this book. We have actually already used some martial arts stances and movements in Horsing Around and Split Stance Bending.

As medical professionals begin to reconcile what they know about motor control theory with how they are going to teach exercise and movement skills, these movement disciplines, along with Feldenkrais and the Alexander Technique, can be a great resource. As we learn more about how people actually move and learn, we can start to replace our more antiquated systems of exercise with one derived from these various movement methods. Let's bring exercise into the information age!

Peerless Pivots

Variations

A. Stand for a moment. For this lesson you may want socks or even shoes, as you will be creating some friction on the skin of your feet when pivoting. Let your arms hang at your sides, feet around shoulder width apart and look straight ahead.

- Notice your feet against the floor. What direction do your toes point?
- Are your feet rolled in to flatten your arch or are you rolled on to the outside edges of your feet?
- Do you have more weight forward on your toes or back on your heels?
- How is your weight distributed between the big ball (first metatarsal head), the small ball (fifth metatarsal head) and the middle of your heel? Does your foot feel like a well-supported tripod?
- Take a few steps forward, then rapidly reverse your direction and walk a few steps in the opposite direction. Pace back and forth within a 10-foot span and notice how you change your direction.
- Do you round it off and walk in a tight circle to change direction? Or do you pivot on your feet to change direction?
- Which direction do you turn? Which foot is the forward one when you turn? What part of your foot are you pivoting on?

B. Stand with your feet a bit more than shoulder width apart. Bend your knees a bit, rock yourself back slightly toward your heels and drop your tailbone toward the floor; get into a horse stance (Fig. 7.62). If you use a pole for balance, hold it in your left hand.

- Slowly shift your weight to your left foot as you pick up the toes and the front of your right foot from the floor. Keep your right heel on the ground.
- Pivot around your right heel to turn the toes of your right foot inward to the left (Fig. 7.62). How close can your right foot come to pointing at the middle of your left foot?

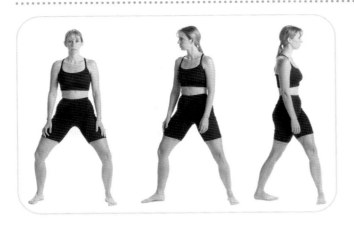

Fig. 7.62 Heel pivoting from a horse stance.

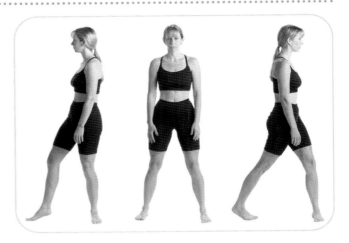

Fig. 7.63 Metatarsal pivoting from a horse stance.

- Reverse the movement to return to horse stance and repeat. Notice how your pelvis turns to the left around your left hip.
- Make sure your left foot tripod stays solidly on the ground. Keep your knee over your foot and don't let your weight roll in or out on your left foot. Pause for a moment in horse stance.
- Then shift your weight to your left foot again and pick up the front of your right foot but turn your toes this time outside to the right (Fig. 7.62).
- Feel how your pelvis turns to the right around your left hip. Make sure you don't allow your left foot to roll inward, even bias yourself a little to rolling to your outside edge, then plant your first metatarsal. Repeat this movement several times.
- Then alternate pivoting on your right heel to turn your toes in toward your left foot then out away from your left foot. Which direction of turn is the easiest?
- Add in shifting your weight on to your right foot as you turn your toes out and on to your left foot as you turn your toes in.
- Emphasize the turn to the right and explosively shifting your weight on to your right foot. This simulates a cutting movement to your right.
- Walk around a bit and compare sensations in your two hips, legs and feet.

C. Stand in your horse stance.
- Repeat instructions B as above to the opposite side.
- Compare and contrast abilities to pivot around left and right hips.

D. Stand in your horse stance.
- Alternate between turning your right toes out and turning your left toes out. Shift weight from side to side and shift your weight in the opposite direction of your direction of turn.
- Do this more quickly, but still be accurate in terms of keeping your weightbearing foot centered.

- Alternate between turning your right toes in and turning your left toes in. Shift weight from side to side and in the same direction as your direction of turn. Which of the two heel pivots feels easier?

E. Stand in your horse stance.
- Imagine a small pebble on the ground underneath your right foot, centered in that spot between the first and second balls (first and second metatarsal heads). This is the point you will be pivoting your foot around. Keep that sweet spot on the pebble.
- Lift your right heel a bit from the floor as you shift your weight toward your left leg. Turn your right heel outside to the right (Fig. 7.63). This will turn your pelvis and torso to the left, and you will pivot around the pebble. Return to horse stance and repeat the sequence again. Pause.
- Lift your right heel and turn it to the left. Your pelvis and torso will turn to the right as you shift your weight back on to your left foot (Fig. 7.63). Repeat several times.
- Alternate pivoting your sweet spot around your imaginary pebble as you turn your right heel alternately in and out. Remember to keep your left foot centered: don't let it roll in or out. Pause for a moment.
- Continue to alternate this pivoting movement, but now add in getting taller and shorter (Fig. 7.64). You can let your right toes drag in toward your other foot a little bit as you get taller.
- As you turn your right heel inward, straighten your right knee and push the top of your head and your eyes taller.
- If you push your pelvis to vertical, point your tail to the ground and keep your left knee well out over your left foot as your pelvis turns to the right, you might feel a very powerful contraction of your left gluteal muscles.

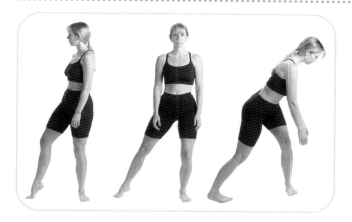

Fig. 7.64 Spiraling shorter and taller – moving pelvis around the left hip.

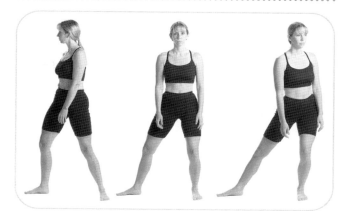

Fig. 7.65 Shifting weight in an open T-stance.

- As you turn your right heel outward, bend your left knee and lean your torso out and over your left leg as if reaching down toward the ground or as if ducking under something.

F. Stand in your horse stance.
- Repeat instructions E to the opposite side; pivot around your right hip.
- Compare and contrast the two sides.

G. Stand in your horse stance.
- Alternate lifting your right heel and turning it inward and lifting your left heel and turning it inward; spiral taller.
- Alternate lifting your right heel and turning it outward and lifting your left heel and turning it outward; spiral shorter.
- Which direction of metatarsal pivoting seems easiest?

H. Stand in your horse stance.
- Shift your weight to the left, lift your right forefoot and turn your toes out to the right. Stay there.
- Then shift your weight forward on to your right foot and lower your right forefoot and toes to the ground.
- Then, shift your weight back to your left foot and lift your right forefoot. Alternate shifting your weight between right and left foot while in this left open T-stance (Fig. 7.65).
- Pay particular attention to keep your knees out over your feet even as you let your pelvis turn slightly to the right when shifting right and to the left when shifting left.
- Think of this movement as a spring. Sink yourself back on to your left foot and hip, getting shorter, then exploding forward and up to the right. Try this movement of shifting forward on to your right foot quickly several times.

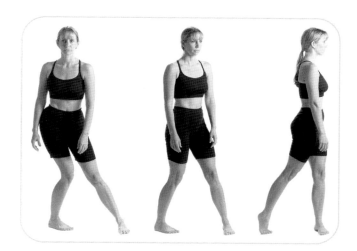

Fig. 7.66 Shifting weight in a closed T-stance – lifting the back heel to complete push-off.

- Do the same thing to the other side: shift your weight right, lift your left forefoot and turn your toes out to the left in the opposite right open T-stance.
- Shift back and forth while still keeping both feet centered. Load your spring and explode forward, up and to the left.

I. Stand in your horse stance.
- Shift your weight to the left, lift your right heel and turn your right heel outward to the right. Stay there.
- Then, shift your weight back on to your right foot and drive your right heel back toward the floor. Adjust your initial foot width to be able to accomplish this. This is a right closed T-stance.
- Shift your weight back to your right foot then forward on to your left again (Fig. 7.66). Enlarge the movement by exaggerating your spring.

- Sink back and down on to your right foot and hip, then explode forward and up on to your left foot. Do this quickly several times.

- Then enlarge this movement by lifting your right heel from the floor and coming on to the balls of your right foot (Fig. 7.66). Check visually and kinesthetically that your right foot is vertical and you are on your sweet spot (between first and second metatarsal heads).

- Do this movement quickly and explosively and emphasize the completion of the push-off with your calf. Try this with a constant vertical foot for extra credit: keep your right heel off the floor even as you shift back on to your right foot.

- Now do the same thing to the other side. From a left closed T-stance, shift weight from foot to foot, turn your pelvis and torso left and right.

- Load your springs and get low, then explode forward and to the right. Complete with emphasis on your calf and the sweet spot on the balls of your left foot.

J. Stand normally again.

- Notice your feet against the floor. What direction do your toes point?

- Are your feet rolled in to flatten your arch or are you rolled on to the outside edges of your feet?

- Do you have more weight forward on your toes or back on your heels?

- How is your weight distributed between the big ball (first metatarsal head), the small ball (fifth metatarsal head) and the middle of your heel? Does your foot feel like a well-supported tripod?

- Take a few steps forward then rapidly reverse your direction and walk a few steps in the opposite direction. Pace back and forth within a ten-foot span and notice how you change your direction.

- Do you round it off and walk in a tight circle to change direction? Or do you pivot on your feet to change direction?

- Which direction do you turn? Which foot is the forward one when you turn? What part of your foot are you pivoting on?

- Try walking in a square and making crisp 90° turns. Vary your organization and direction so you pivot both left and right off both left and right feet.

Baselines – Peerless Pivots

In variation A we begin with a standard standing scan of the three dimensions of the feet then establish an initial dynamic baseline. Taking a few steps forward, then turning 180° to take a few steps in the opposite direction gives us an initial reference point for the change of direction theme we will work on during the rest of the lesson. Do you round it off and walk in a tight circle to change direction? Do you twist around your knee, or allow your foot to slop around on the floor? Or do you pivot on your feet to change direction?

Someone who pivots might be more confident in her ability to decelerate, absorbing shock with ankle, knee and hip. Someone who pivots might be more confident in her ability to keep her ankle from rolling over or her knee from twisting, stabilizing knee and ankle against rotational stresses. Someone who pivots might be more confident in her ability to push off: quickly turning and moving in the other direction with a strong push-off can't be performed nearly as effectively when rounding out the turn. Which direction did you turn? Which foot is the forward one when you turn?

Pivoting possibilities

If you had your right foot forward and made a left hand turn, you probably did an inward pivot off your right foot. Although having your right foot forward and turning to the right is possible, it is a bit trickier. The pelvis would have to travel in almost a full circle in space to get around the right leg and back in front again.

Alternatively, you could pivot off the back leg. Do an outward pivot off the right foot and make what amounts to a step back with your left foot, placing it behind you to become your new push-off leg. Stand up for a moment and do inward pivots off both feet and both versions of the outward pivots off both feet. Which is quicker, more powerful, easier? Isn't it great to have several choices in any one movement?

What part of your foot are you pivoting on? Whereas pivoting around your heel or spinning your whole foot on the floor so that both heel and forefoot are moving in space is possible, the forefoot will usually be the preferred pivot spot. Is that spot directly between the first and second metatarsal heads? If not, where is it? If toward the outer metatarsals, that is an ankle sprain waiting to happen. If toward the medial aspect of the first metatarsal, this might give us clues about likely push-off from the medial aspect of the great toe and the abduction stress it places on the first metatarsophalangeal joint.

What are we looking for is a well organized pivot, whether to turn 180° to go in the opposite direction, 90° to lay a perpendicular course, 45° to cut off at an angle, or any of the other 355 possible directions. We want the foot to slide or pivot relative to the floor, but we don't want the tibia and fibula to pivot or rotate relative to the foot. Stabilizing the foot on the floor is the responsibility of the peroneus longus when executing an inward pivot.

Take a few steps, place the right foot forward and turn leftward (inward) to pivot around the foot and face 180°. Feel proprioceptively, observe visually and palpate a student or partner for peroneal use in preventing the outward roll of the foot into a potential right ankle inversion sprain. Stabilizing the foot on the floor is the responsibility of the posterior tibialis when executing an outward pivot. Experience this proprioceptively as well to learn to control eversion sprains.

We want the tibia to turn along with the femur and the foot to pivot/slide on the floor. We don't want an unstable knee moving into too much rotation. When doing an inward pivot with the right foot forward, the pelvis turns to the left. This in turn externally rotates the right hip joint, which runs out of room and internally rotates the right femur. This will then create an external rotation movement at the right knee. This puts the medial collateral ligament, medial meniscus and anterior cruciate ligament in grave peril.

This is a common injury and a common mechanism of injury. Perhaps the foot/shoe got stuck and couldn't slide on the ground surface. Perhaps the hamstrings didn't fire to maintain dynamic rotational knee stability. Perhaps the right hip joint couldn't externally rotate sufficiently and dragged the right femur prematurely into internal rotation. To have a stable knee when pivoting, you have to have a stable ankle and an ability to slide the foot or shoe on the ground. There is a limit to how much traction you want through cleats or tread. You also have to be able to control and direct rotational movements at the knee through the hamstrings and popliteus.

Think back to initial movements we did in the slippery board lesson where we worked to initially germinate this stabilization skill. We continued to work on this skill through Heel to Toe (side-lie lift heel and toe), Starting Blocks (rolling vertical and horizontal heel passively and actively) and Toeing Off (sinking back on to back leg and turning in the direction of the back leg creates an internal rotation movement in that knee).

We want the pelvis to be able to turn freely around the femur. We want there to be sufficient range of movement so the femur doesn't have to twist prematurely or too much. We want there to be sufficient strength in the short and stubbies to both power the push-off movement and absorb the deceleration of a turn. We have been working on these skills from the first lesson in the Tyrannosaurus section and through all three chapters. Subsequent variations in this lesson bring the various stabilization and initiation movements learned earlier to a climactic boil.

Heel pivots to closed and open T-stances

In variation B you are directed to get into a horse stance, to shift your weight to the left foot and to turn the toes of your right foot inward; this is an inward heel pivot. This movement requires decent ankle dorsiflexion range and facilitates it by requiring the anterior shin compartment muscles to fire and provide for reciprocal inhibition of the calf. This movement strongly suggests a turning movement of the pelvis and torso to the left.

The pelvis pivots around the left hip, which moves into an internal rotation and horizontal adduction hybrid. The movement is initiated from the left TFL and perhaps the adductors and is decelerated by the left hip external rotators. The knee moves into internal rotation, which is prevented from creating ligament and cartilage damage by the lateral hamstrings.

The tibia moves into external rotation and wants to roll the left ankle outward along with it. This is checked by the peroneals. This direction of movement simulates shock absorption at the hip, enhances control of lateral rotational movements at the knee, and is used to train someone in the prevention of inversion ankle sprains. Note the heel cord and calf length needed if you are to slide the heel accurately. Be aware that many people can't keep the heel on the floor if there is any kind of width between the feet to start with. Remember to allow for approximations.

The next movement in this sequence is to again shift your weight to the left from a horse stance, but this time to turn the toes of your right foot outward. Although this movement doesn't provide the same necessity for ankle dorsiflexion that the inward heel pivot does, this outward heel pivot again acts to turn the pelvis in space around the hip joint, this time rotating the pelvis to the right and externally rotating/abducting the left hip.

This is more reminiscent of a push-off movement. This is an excellent opportunity to functionally strengthen the left hip short and stubbies and to work on knee-over-foot relationships. It is very easy to allow the left knee to drift inward and to allow the left foot to roll inward on the floor when doing this movement. Be scrupulous in demanding that the knee remain over a centered foot.

Following the kinematic chain, if you allow the left femur to turn inward, the left knee moves into relative external rotation and valgus; stabilize with medial hamstring and popliteus. Use this movement to rehabilitate and to prevent medial meniscus/collateral ligament/anterior cruciate damage and to recalibrate knee-to-foot relationships in patellar tracking and pronation problems.

Alternate pivoting on your right heel to turn your toes in toward your left foot, then out away from your left foot. Alternately pivot left and right around left hip to simulate alternate push-off and shock absorption or to simulate inward and outward pivots. Which direction of turn is the easiest for you? Add in shifting your weight on to your right foot as you turn your toes out and on to your left foot as you turn your toes in; emphasize the turn to the right and explosively shifting your weight on to your right foot.

This simulates a cutting movement to your right and adds in a weight shift in the direction of the turn when doing the inward pivot. We will do some serial inward pivots later during the discussion of variations. Repeat instructions to the other side in variation C: how do the two sides differ? Which externally rotates more completely? Which internally rotates easier? Which leg feels stronger? Which fatigues faster?

In variation D you alternate between the two sides. Alternately turn left then right toes outward, then inward. This alternates external rotation movements at each hip, then internal rotation movements at each hip. Use back-to-back comparisons to heighten proprioceptive awareness and to recalibrate truer neutral standing.

Pivoting on the sweet spot – to closed and open T-stances

In variation E we move on to an exploration of metatarsal pivoting. There is an initial description of imagining a pebble on that spot between first and second metatarsal heads and focusing your intention to slide your foot around that sweet spot. This links Peerless Pivots with the heel/toe series we did where much of the proprioceptive focus was on that spot. From your horse stance again, shift weight to your left foot, lift your right heel and turn that heel outward to the right.

This turns your pelvis to the left, with all that entails through the left hip, knee, ankle and foot. Then turn your right heel inward to the left. This turns your pelvis to the right, with all that entails through the left hip, knee, ankle and foot. Although this variation seems much like the heel pivots we did earlier, there are a couple of important differences. One, we are pivoting around the forefoot. This is a much more functional pivot and one that you'll want to encourage over heel pivoting for most of your students. Two, by making the heel move right and left in space, you have created another constraint.

Either you could shift your weight further right or left, or you could sink your weight down and raise it back up again. It is this latter strategy that we want to encourage. Turning the right heel outward turns your pelvis to the left and suggests a sinking around and a leaning or bending of your pelvis and torso over that left leg. This exaggerates the lengthening and strengthening demand on the left short and stubbies (see Fig. 7.64).

Turning the heel inward turns your pelvis to the right and suggests a rising around and a straightening or pushing to get taller movement of your pelvis and torso around your left hip. This exaggerates the lengthening requirements of the left adductors and hip flexors and the strength requirement of the left hip rotators and extensors.

In variation F you repeat these instructions to the opposite side. In variation G you make alternating movements analogous to what you were doing with the heel pivots. Whereas in outward heel pivots you shifted your weight in the opposite direction of your turn, in alternating metatarsal pivots you will tend to shift weight in the same direction as your turn. This again allows for back-to-back comparisons and helps in establishing a truer neutral standing posture.

In variations H and I, you get into first an open T-stance (toes pointed outward) and then a closed T-stance (toes pointed inward) and shift weight forward and back between the two feet. Turn your left toes outward into a right open T-stance and shift your weight back on to your right foot then forward on to your left foot while maintaining the open T-stance. The challenge here is to recruit enough right hip rotator and abductor juice to simultaneously push forward in a pushing-out-into-abduction/external rotation movement while keeping the right foot centered on the floor.

This is really the same critical proprioceptive and motor skill – keeping knee over foot – that we've been working toward throughout this and previous chapters in the T. Rex section. The left leg is a bit easier to keep centered in this position, though the adductors on that side need to be long enough to allow the left knee to stay out over the left foot when shifting your weight back and to the right.

Turn your right toes inward to get into a right closed T-stance. Shift your weight back on to your right foot and forward on to your left foot while maintaining your closed T-stance. The challenges here for the back leg are many:

- The right short and stubbies get a stretch when shifting back on to the right leg.

- The right hip extensors get to work in a pushing-into-extension movement and the right hip flexors need to lengthen.

- The calf and heel cord need to lengthen to keep the heel from sliding in or the foot from collapsing into pronation.

Enlarge the movement by lifting the heel and coming on to the sweet spot with a vertical foot or segue into a hop, but with the left foot always pointed over to the right. Check visually and proprioceptively that your right foot is vertical and you are on your sweet spot (between first and second metatarsal heads). Do this movement quickly and explosively and emphasize the completion of the push-off with your calf. Try this with a constant vertical foot for extra credit; keep your right heel off the floor even as you shift back on to your right foot.

The challenge to the front leg in this closed T-stance weight-shifting is to have sufficient left hip short and stubby length to allow for a full turn of the pelvis to the left, that shock-absorbing hybrid of hip flexion, internal rotation and horizontal adduction. The left ankle is also challenged to keep from rolling into inversion. Use this movement in sprained ankle rehabilitation.

T time – pivot variations

Come back to our original questions once again in variation K. How are the feet organized in their three dimensions? How do you organize your change of direction when pacing? How many other lessons throughout the T. Rex section could be part of a line of lessons leading to this one?

These shifts of weight from open and closed T-stances are real goldmines. First, try weight-shifting in open and closed T-stance movements while leaning against a wall (Fig. 7.67). Put your feet out away from the wall a bit and turn feet into open and closed T-stances; roll your pelvis along the wall. Use the wall as a reference point and as a guide to direct turning and weight-shifting coordination. Enlarge to lift the back heel as before.

Second, try putting a series of pivoting steps together. Shift into a left open T-stance, then lift and turn your right toes to the right. Shift your weight forward on to your right foot, then step across to put your left foot in front of your right. This 180° right-hand turn faces you in the opposite direction to where you started and puts you in a right closed T-stance (Fig. 7.68).

Return to where you started (left open T) and repeat. Turn your body around your stationary right leg several times. Progress this by now stepping across into the right closed T,

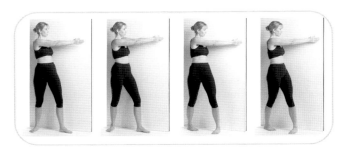

Fig. 7.67 Rotational movement of the pelvis around the hips while weight shifting in open and closed T-stances – using the wall as a reference point.

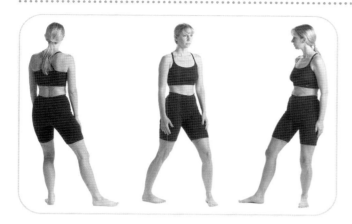

Fig. 7.68 Start from a left open T, step across into a right closed T – alternate back and forth. Then step into a closed T and pivot/snap around the front of the right foot to end up in a left open T.

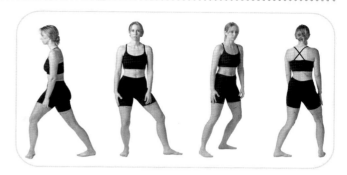

Fig. 7.69 Alternating right closed T-stances – stepping backward with the left foot then turning 180° by snapping the right heel outward. Follow pictures right to left.

shifting your weight forward on to your left leg and continuing your turn to the right by turning the right heel inward, to the right. This turns the toes of the right foot to point 180° from where they began and brings you into a right open T-stance (Fig. 7.68).

This transitional movement can make for a very snappy hip movement into extension, abduction and external rotation. The pivot happens around the toes of the right foot, which is nearly nonweightbearing. Making 180° pivots from open T to open T-stance allows the one standing leg the opportunity to do the same pushing-to-open-the-pelvis movement over and over. This is one strategy for learning.

Third, do alternating left and right open T-stances. Get into a right open T-stance, left toes pointed out to the left. Shift forward on to your left foot and step up to the back of your left heel with the inside of your right heel. Step out 90° with your right foot and shift weight forward now on to your right foot in a left open T-stance. Repeat by bringing the inside of your left heel to the back of your right heel, stepping out 90° to the left, shifting forward on to the left foot and so on. Slide heel inward and squeeze gluteals and posterior adductors. You make a zigzag across the floor.

Fourth, try making serial pivots from closed T-stance to closed T-stance. Shift into a left open T-stance; lift and turn your right toes to the right. Shift your weight forward on to your right foot, then step across to put your left foot in front of your right. This 180° right-hand turn faces you in the opposite direction to where you started and puts you in a right closed T-stance (Fig. 7.68). Return to where you started (left open T) and repeat; turn your body around your stationary right leg several times. This is similar to what you were doing a moment ago when making pivoting movements from left open T to left open T-stance; you are turning your body 180° around your right leg.

This time, alternate right closed T-stances. Step back into a left open T-stance, then turn your right heel 180° to the right (outside). This turns your whole body a half turn and brings you to a right closed T-stance (Fig. 7.69). Now shift your weight backward on to your right leg, step back with your left

Box 7.16 Peerless Pivots

Summary lesson for legs section – blends medial/lateral balance, rotational stability, shock absorption and push-off competence
Open, closed and reverse T-stances – and the transitions we love so well
Lots of step pivot variations and drills

foot into a left open T again, then turn your right heel outward to turn back to your right closed T (Fig. 7.69). Repeat this sequence slowly several times, then quicken the pace. Snap your hips a bit! Where the open T pivots were performed with forward stepping, the closed T pivots are performed with backward stepping. Be sure to experiment with both sides.

The actual pivoting the foot to turn movement can be very explosive. This simulates a push-off to move forward action, emphasizing turning in the direction of the stepping leg component of a powerful force couple movement. Much of the power from this turning movement comes from the left iliopsoas/internal rotators/adductors. Those muscles that pull the pelvis around them work to rotate the pelvis toward the standing leg.

This movement is central to swinging a baseball bat or a tennis racket, throwing a javelin or football, punching, and a number of other unilaterally performed athletic movements. Reciprocating these movements simulates walking, running and other straight forward locomotion movements. Might someone run faster or leap farther with enhanced force couple capabilities?

Fifth, and analogous to what we did previously with serial open T-stances, we could also do serial closed T-stances. Shift into a left closed T-stance – left heel out to the left and left toes pointed toward right foot. Slide your left toes forward to touch the inside of your right toes, then step out to the left with your left foot, leading with the outside edge. Pivot on the toes of your right foot to slide your right heel outward and point the toes of your right foot toward the inside of the left foot (Box 7.16).

This brings you into a right closed T-stance. Continue by bringing the right toes to touch inside of the left toes, then step out to the right with the right foot, leading with the outer edge and pivoting around the sweet spot on the left foot. Continue in zigzag fashion across the floor. Try both open and closed T serial pivots (zigzags) going backward.

Sixth, walk or run around in a square. Go counterclockwise and pivot 90° off the right foot; these are inward pivots around the forefoot. Go clockwise and pivot off the right foot; these are outward pivots around the forefoot. Change direction again and pivot off the left foot, then change direction again to complete inward and outward pivots around both left and right feet. Change directions again but go backward; pivot 90° both inward and outward and around both feet.

Seventh, try standing in a horse stance then shifting your weight toward your heels. Lift both forefeet slightly and slide both toes simultaneously to the right, then to the left. You end up turning somewhere between 45° and 75° to each side. Feel for stabilization strategies at ankles and knees. Switch your weight forward to your sweet spots and slide both heels right and left and pivot around the balls of your feet.

Feel for stability. Increase speed and put on some foot stompin'/butt-shakin' music. Where you did the Charleston before, now you do the Twist. Alternate these simultaneous heel and toe pivots. Turn your toes to the left, then slide your heels to the left, then toes, then heels and so on. This pivots you laterally across the floor. Do in both directions.

Eighth, up the ante by pivoting across the floor while staying up on your toes. Plantarflex your ankles as much as possible, come up as vertically as possible on to your metatarsal heads and pivot around that sweet spot around the second balls of your feet. Go slowly to start to appreciate the medial/lateral foot and ankle control necessary to do this and stay balanced. Extrapolate appreciation of peroneus longus and posterior tibialis competence and balance necessary to do this and stay balanced. This is the ultimate in foot ankle stability, proprioception and strength linked to pelvic force couple movements. Apply 'up on your toes' metatarsal balancing for any of the other pivoting drills. Vary speed, distance between feet and surface friction coefficient. Add throwing movements or plyometrics.

Ninth, do serial pivots on one foot. Stand and slide your right heel only to the right, then your right toes, then right heel and so on to somewhere short of the splits (Fig. 7.70).

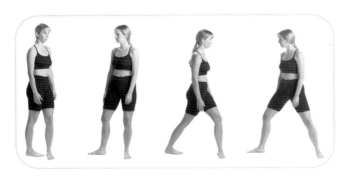

Fig. 7.70 Serial pivots. Keep alternating turning heel then toe outward – stop somewhere short of the splits. Return with serial pivots or by sliding the foot back in.

Return in the same way or by sliding the right foot back inward to train the adductors to assist in pulling the pelvis toward the standing leg (think roller skating, ice skating, certain types of cross-country skiing). Try this movement with the slippery board, or dispense with the serial pivots and just slide the board out to the side and back in again.

Having a strong and coordinated hip adductor/posterior tibialis synergy is important for foot, ankle and pelvic/low back stability in the presence of wide stances and wide lateral steps or jumps. The adductors are rarely used muscles for most people and are difficult to exercise in their closed kinetic chain functions. Some of the movements in Squat Pivots and some of these described pivot variations are excellent ways to strengthen and enhance control of these important but often neglected muscles.

Try experimenting with sliding the board out laterally with one foot. How much weight can you put on the board and still have it slide without catching the carpet? Can you feel how your tibialis posterior needs to be on its toes to do this in such a way that the whole sole of your foot stays on the board? Feel your ability to create a differentiated relationship of hip abduction and ankle inversion. Try experimenting with sliding the board back in again with the toes of your 'board foot' pointing out – this will put you in an open T-stance. Feel how this movement requires the gluteals and adductors of the standing leg to play nicely together.

Recall the same facilitation of the gluteal/adductor synergy in Rolling the Foot and some of its variations, especially lying on your back and tilting your long leg inward against resistance (see Fig. 7.24) Try sliding the board back inward again with the toes of your board foot pointed in – in a closed T-stance arrangement. What is the difference between pulling your weight towards your internally rotated standing leg rather than your externally rotated standing leg? Be sure to note the adductor/posterior tibialis synergy with the standing leg – don't allow your standing foot to collapse inward.

Since you're playing around with your board, try sliding it straight out in front of you and then sliding it back in again. Try two variations. If you slide the board forward with your right foot, reverse by turning your pelvis to the left and getting nearly all your weight back on your left leg. Slide the right foot and board back toward you again by cueing the left hip flexors to pull your weight in toward your internally rotated left hip. Alternately, slide the board forward with your right foot and shift your weight forward on to the board.

Keep as much weight on the right foot and into the board as possible. This gets the right hamstrings to work in a fashion similar to the original slippery board lesson. This also juices the left hip flexor to work in pulling your weight back in again. These movements can also be done without a slippery board: just slide your stocking feet on hardwood floor, your bare feet on rug, or your shod feet on concrete, grass, whatever. These are tai chi-based movements that help to wake up seldom-used hip muscles and muscle synergies.

Tenth, use a pole to facilitate the turning movements. Stand on your left foot and place your right foot on a pole held diagonally in front of you. Slide your right foot down the pole and out to the right while turning pelvis and torso to the left. Reverse this movement to slide your right foot up the pole and in toward midline while turning pelvis and torso to the right

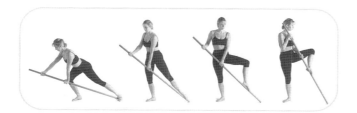

Fig. 7.71 Toy facilitation of pivoting – try this a few times quickly!

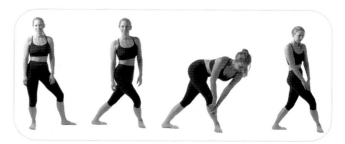

Fig. 7.72 Open T to reverse T – then bending and coming up from reverse T.

(Fig. 7.71). Which movements in Split Stance Bending or Toeing Off is this reciprocating movement reminiscent of?

Eleventh, try standing on your knees on the floor with your knees close together and your feet wider apart than knees. This internally rotates your hips. Turn to the right and lift your right knee off the floor to come to left half-kneeling. Turn back to center, lower your right knee to the floor near your left knee, then lift your left knee while turning to the left to come to right half-kneeling. Alternate from side to side and feel for similarities in movement patterns and sensations to some of the pivoting movements performed earlier in this lesson.

Twelfth, we've done open and closed T-stances, but there is a third T. Reverse T-stances. Shift into a right open T-stance, weight on right leg, toes of left foot pointing to the left and pelvis and torso turned to the left. Shift your weight forward on to your left foot and step forward with your right. Place your right foot on the floor in front of your left foot with the toes of your right foot pointed to the right. The toes of your left foot will point toward the outside of your right foot (Fig. 7.72).

Alternatively, stand in a horse stance and shift your weight to your left foot. Slide your right foot behind your left and continue to slide your right foot to the left while pointing your right toes toward the outside edge of your left foot. Whether getting into a reverse T-stance by stepping forward with the left foot or backward with the right, stay there for a moment. You will be in a right reverse T-stance; left foot forward and right toes pointed toward the outside of your left foot.

Place both hands on the inside of your left thigh and slide them down and across your left thigh to the outside of your left knee. Continue to slide hands down the outside of your left lower leg as you get the hang of this movement. Slide your hands back up the outside of your knee, then up and across to the inside of your left thigh again (Fig. 7.72). Twist and bend down and to the left in a spiraling movement as you slide your hands down, then spiral back up and to the right as you come back up.

Try alternating reverse T-stances. Start in standing, and then shift your weight to your left foot as you step forward with your right. Place your right foot on the floor in front of your left foot with the toes of your right foot pointed to the right: this is a reverse T-stance from stepping forward. Now keep your weight on your left leg as you sweep your right foot backward on the floor then leftward to slide behind your left heel. Slide your right foot to the left so the toes point toward your left foot: this is a reverse T-stance from stepping backward. Alternate these two movements several times, then switch legs and try the other side. Compare and contrast. Alternately, slide one leg in back of the other to get into a reverse T-stance, come back to where you started, then move into a reverse T-stance to the other side. Alternate from side to side, moving laterally on the floor. These are yet more variations in a long line of short and stubby-intensive movements that so many people need for such a wide variety of problems.

Thirteenth, progressions of the 90° and 180° pivots we did earlier can be done by coming as far up on to the metatarsal heads as possible before pivoting. The more ankle dorsiflexion and the closer the metatarsals are to vertical, the more demand pivoting places on ankle and foot stability. These pirouetting movements are the ultimate in foot stability and posterior tibialis/peroneus longus competence and balance.

Do pivots both inside (challenging the peroneus longus) and outside (challenging the posterior tibialis) at 90°, 180°, 270° and 360° while walking. Be sure to do these with both feet and compare/contrast for upper-level foot competence. Repeat a previously described variation but while high up on toes: stand in high horse stance, lift both heels high off the ground to come up on to metatarsal heads, and pivot both feet 60° left and right.

There are many other variations of pivoting and stepping movements possible. Making transitions between open and closed T-stances, reverse T-stances, open and closed horse stances and one-legged stances opens up nearly endless possibilities. Putting these various steps and stances together is the genius of tai chi. Check out the various tai chi styles and the various open hand and weapons forms that these styles have and marvel at the brilliant application of constraints that is tai chi.

Use change of direction movements with neuro, geriatric and general medical folk to improve balance, retrain lower extremity stability and competence and to reduce one side neglect.

Chapter applications and book considerations

Following are some motor control considerations and possible skill facilitation strategies for some common lower extremity orthopedic problems:

- **Bunions**. Watch for medial weightbearing and medial push-off tendencies. Watch for first metatarsophalangeal or ankle joint stiffness into dorsiflexion. Facilitate skills of vertical foot, directing movement over sweet spot. Facilitate force couple gait so back heel doesn't turn inward with turn of pelvis in the direction of push-off leg. Heel to Toe and Toeing Off, manual facilitation of nonhabitual foot differentiation, Peerless Pivots.

- **Plantar fasciitis**. Watch for pronation – medial weightbearing and medial push-off tendencies. Watch for short heel cord, valgus/externally rotated knees and adductor/internal rotation bias at hips. Facilitate skills of tripod foot in standing and vertical push-off from the sweet spot. Facilitate pelvic force couple gait. Slippery board, Rolling the Foot, Horsing Around, Heel to Toe, Toeing Off and Starting Blocks, manual facilitation of nonhabitual foot differentiation, Peerless Pivots.

- **Ankle sprains**. Early protection followed by gentle movements – slippery board and Heel to Toe. Partial weightbearing proprioceptive awareness and stability training – Rolling the Foot and its variations, Cat/Camel and beginning part of Sit to Stand with rollers. Progress to full weightbearing proprioceptive awareness and stability training – Split Stance Bending, Horsing Around, the rest of Sit to Stand and Peerless Pivots. Challenge peroneus longus/posterior tibialis balance and competence and redefine a vertical foot with squatting variations: start in a chair, progress to squatting against a wall, then to Starting Blocks and Squat Pivots. Recalibrate medial/lateral balance in gait – Toeing Off and Peerless Pivots. Ditto for foot joint sprains, tib/fib fractures, foot or ankle surgeries.

- **Peroneus longus tendinitis**. Watch for pronation bias and chronic shortening. Balance with antagonist/tibialis posterior and coordinate with hip abductors – slippery board, Rolling the Foot, Horsing Around, Peerless Pivots and Starting Blocks. Facilitate proportional push-off through lower extremity synergists – Wishbone, TA Leg Lifts, Half-kneel or Split Stance Bending, Knee Walking, Heel to Toe, Toeing Off.

- **Tibialis posterior tendinitis**. Watch for supination bias and chronic shortening or pronation bias and trying to use tibialis posterior to supinate rather than hip musculature. Balance with antagonist/peroneus longus and coordinate with hip adductors – slippery board, Rolling the Foot, Horsing Around, Peerless Pivots and Starting Blocks. Facilitate proportional push-off through lower extremity synergists – Wishbone, TA Leg Lifts, Half-kneel or Split Stance Bending, Knee Walking, Heel to Toe, Toeing Off.

- **Achilles problems**. Watch for pronation, tight heel cord, weight biased forward towards toes and disproportionate push-off. Facilitate medial/lateral balance of the foot and lengthen the heel cord – Wishbone and bridging variations with longitudinal rollers, slippery board, Heel to Toe, Toeing Off, Starting Blocks/Squat Pivots or some degree of difficulty regression. Cue hamstring juice with split stance or Half-kneel Bending. Facilitate anterior and posterior compartment balance with rollers crosswise; progress from supine to Sit to Stand.

- **Shin splints**. Watch for lack of full push-off and ankle plantarflexion – cue ankle plantarflexion and toe dorsiflexion differentiation. Heel to Toe and Toeing Off. Lengthen the anterior compartment and challenge push-off – Starting Blocks. Involve hip flexors more in lifting the stepping foot – Wishbone with cues to coordinate and differentiate from foot. Involve hamstrings more in push-off – slippery board and Split Stance Bending.

- **Patellar tracking**. Watch for hip adduction/internal rotation tendencies leading to knee valgus or external rotation tendencies leading to foot pronation and/or abduction. Watch for quadriceps-intensive pressing-the-foot functions. Facilitate foot abduction/adduction balance – slippery board, Sit to Stand with rollers under feet arbitrarily oriented parallel to each other and Horsing Around variations exploring different toe-in/toe-out arrangements. Facilitate hip over knee over foot relationships – slippery board/Wishbone variations, Horsing Around and Peerless Pivots. Facilitate a tripod foot – Rolling the Foot and Horsing Around. Facilitate a hip extensor strategy for pressing the floor – slippery board or crosswise rollers, Half kneel and Split Stance Bending, bridging supine with feet far away or up on a wall, standing and leaning back against the wall doing variations from Side-sit Bending. Facilitate balanced force couple gait to encourage knee to stay out over foot – applying the short and stubby constraint with Heel to Toe and Toeing Off.

- **Iliotibial band syndrome**. Watch for adductor/internal rotation bias at hips with valgus or externally rotating knee. Facilitate pushing out movements and activation of the abductors and external rotators – Side-lie Transitions and Heel to Toe. Creating differentiated patterns of hip abduction and external rotation with knee varus and internal rotation – slippery board, Rolling the Foot, Horsing Around and shifting back movements of Toeing Off. Hamstring and adductor lengthening – Squat Pivots, weight shift from plantigrade as described in Cat/Camel. Recalibration of medial/lateral balance in gait – Heel to Toe and Toeing Off.

- **Hamstring strains/tears**. Watch for tightness of hamstrings or hip flexors, weakness of gluteals. Facilitate hamstring length. Facilitate proportional use of lower extremity extensors – Wishbone, Side-sit Bending, Cat/Camel, Toeing Off. Facilitate hamstring awareness, control and strength – Wishbone, slippery board, Half-kneel and Split Stance Bending.

- **Adductor strains/tears**. Watch for adductor/internal rotation bias at the hips, pulling to stop or pulling to go strategies or over involvement of adductors in push-off. Facilitate adductor and hamstring length – Side-sit Bending, plantigrade variations of Cat/Camel, Starting Blocks or Squat Pivots. Facilitate lateral pushing to go or pushing to stop movements – Rolling the Foot, Horsing Around and Peerless Pivots. Facilitate reduction of adductor involvement in push-off – Wishbone, slippery board, Knee Walking and Toeing Off.

- **Hip flexor strains**. Watch for psoas bias and anterior pelvic tilt, incomplete hip extension in push-off. Facilitate hip flexor length – Wishbone, TA Leg Lifts, Half-kneel

Bending, Split Stance Bending and pushing taller variations of Horsing Around and Peerless Pivots. Facilitate hip extensors in push-off – Wishbone, Half-kneel and Split Stance Bending, peerless pivot variations of alternating closed T-stances – make it snappy!

- **Medial collateral ligament strain.** Extinguish avoidance and compensation behaviors – slippery board and Heel to Toe. Protect knee from medial movement and postural stresses – Rolling the Foot, Horsing Around and Peerless Pivots. Restore propulsive gait pattern and drill for return to activity – Toeing Off, Peerless Pivots, Starting Blocks and sequential pivoting drills described in Peerless Pivots.

- **Medial meniscus tear.** Extinguish avoidance and compensation behaviors: slippery board and Heel to Toe. Protect knee from medial movement and postural stresses – Rolling the Foot, Horsing Around and Peerless Pivots. Restore propulsive gait pattern and drill for return to activity – Toeing Off, Peerless Pivots, Starting Blocks and sequential pivoting drills described in Peerless Pivots.

- **Anterior cruciate ligament strain/tear/reconstruction.** Extinguish avoidance and compensation behaviors – slippery board and Heel to Toe. Protect knee from medial movement and postural stresses – Rolling the Foot, Horsing Around and Peerless Pivots. Protect knee from rotational movements – slippery board supine on floor or prone with board on foot, rolling the foot, Horsing Around, Toeing Off and Peerless Pivots. Emphasize pushing the foot with the hamstrings rather than with the quadriceps to reduce anterior shear stress – slippery board, Half-kneel Bending, Split Stance Bending and Toeing Off.

- **Total knee replacement.** Extinguish avoidance and compensation behaviors – slippery board and Heel to Toe. Protect knee from medial movement and postural stresses – Rolling the Foot, Horsing Around and Peerless Pivots. Protect knee from rotational movements – slippery board supine on floor or prone with board on foot, Rolling the Foot, Horsing Around, Toeing Off and Peerless Pivots. Emphasize pushing the foot with the hamstrings rather than with the quadriceps to reduce anterior shear stress – slippery board, Half-kneel Bending, Split Stance Bending and Toeing Off.

- **Total hip replacement.** Protect the hip from horizontal adduction strains: Dead Bug Roll, Rolling the Foot and Horsing Around. Restoring hip adductor and hamstring length – Wishbone, TA Leg Lifts, plantigrade variations of Cat/Camel, homolateral bending in half-kneel or Split Stance Bending. Restoring hip flexor length – Half-kneel or Split Stance Bending, TA Leg Lifts. Facilitating turns and change of direction – Peerless Pivots. Facilitating transitions; Side-lie Transitions and Sit to Stand.

- **Trochanteric bursitis.** Watch for adduction/internal rotation bias at hips, anterior tilt bias, weak abductors and short and stubbies and tight adductors. Work as with total hip replacement; may be able to get a bit more athletic. Work more in side-lie if pressure tolerable, works hip shorties length and strength.

- **Below-knee amputations with prosthesis.** Iron-clad knee rotational stability – slippery board, Horsing Around and Peerless Pivots. Facilitate force couple gait – Wishbone, Side-lie and Side-sit Transitions, Cat/Camel, Heel to Toe (forget the ankle/toe differentiation part), Toeing Off. Facilitate change of direction competence – Peerless Pivots.

The use of manual resistance, weight training or plyometrics concepts is complementary to a motor control approach, and vice versa. You could take some of the individual movements in these lessons and apply resistance through various means, dose the resistance intensity and repetitions, and still use the pattern-specific aspects of a movement to your advantage. The key is not to think of strengthening as having only qualitative properties, but to blend what you already know about the physiology of exercise with the art of a motor learning approach. Work on both qualitative and quantitative strengthening and stretching at the same time.

Selected muscles and how to influence them

We have progressed through this book looking at movement facilitation techniques and breaking movements down into their muscular components. We have been learning/teaching motor and proprioceptive skills and then discussing the effects of these movements on specific muscles. As physical therapists, however, we might be more familiar with evaluating our students and developing a treatment plan while thinking in terms of individual muscles, their strength, flexibility or imbalance. The following list is a cheat sheet for those of you who know they want to stretch the right quadratus lumborum or strengthen the flexor hallucis longus but can't remember all the possibilities enumerated throughout the book.

- **Flexor hallucis longus.** Work with stretching, strengthening, coordinating with and differentiating from ankle movements in Heel to Toe, Toeing Off and Peerless Pivots. Up the ante with Starting Blocks and Squat Pivots.

- **Peroneus longus.** Strengthen and coordinate with hip abductors or short and stubbies in slippery board, Rolling the Foot, Horsing Around and Peerless Pivots. Up the ante with Starting Blocks, Squat Pivots and pivoting and pirouetting drills at the end of Peerless Pivots (pivoting in the direction of heel sliding outward). Stretch with Horsing Around or Peerless Pivots or use sitting back on plantarflexed feet section of Starting Blocks, transitions from hands and knees to side-sit in Cat/Camel or transitions from side-sit to side-sit in Side-sit Transitions. Use longitudinal 3 inch rollers on floor or wall while in supine, using pushing movements in Pelvic Tilts, Wishbone or TA Leg Lifts. Progress by placing rollers under feet in Sit to Stand or Horsing Around.

- **Tibialis posterior.** Strengthen and coordinate with hip adductors in slippery board, Rolling the Foot, Horsing Around and Peerless Pivots. Up the ante with Starting Blocks, Squat Pivots and pivoting and pirouetting drills at the end of Peerless Pivots (pivoting in the direction of heel sliding inward). Stretching not usually an issue, but could use sitting back on plantarflexed feet section of Starting Blocks. Use longitudinal 3 inch rollers on floor or wall while in supine, using pushing movements in Pelvic Tilts, Wishbone or TA Leg Lifts. Progress by placing rollers under feet in Sit to Stand or Horsing Around.

- **Gastrosoleus**. Strengthen and differentiate from toe flexors in Heel to Toe, Toeing Off and Peerless Pivots. Up the ante with described variations from Toeing Off: shifting weight to back leg with that heel off the ground and turning the weight shift forward into a hop. The squatting twins and the pivoting and pirouetting drills from Peerless Pivots have some calf strength requirements. Stretch the calf with pattern specificity; don't allow foot pronation or abduction. Start with Heel to Toe and progress to Toeing Off and Peerless Pivots. Emphasize Achilles and soleus length in the sitting weight back and bending the back knee components of these lessons, and emphasize gastrocnemius length in the propelling weight forward, straightening the knee and driving the middle of your heel to the floor components of these lessons. Up the ante on the Achilles and soleus in Starting Blocks and Squat Pivots, and on the gastrocnemius while pushing your tush toward the ceiling with hands on the floor in Starting Blocks. Coordinate/balance with anterior tibialis by placing 3 inch roller crosswise on wall or floor under feet while supine in Pelvic Tilts, Wishbone or TA Leg Lifts. Progress to rollers crosswise under feet in Sit to Stand and Horsing Around. Use front-to-back weight shifts in Sit to Stand (sitting and during linebacker pose), standing variations of Horsing Around and one-leg standing variations of Steppin' Out or Peerless Pivots to focus proprioceptive awareness on balance of effort between anterior and posterior compartments.

- **Anterior tibialis and extensor digitorum longus**. Coordinate and differentiate from each other in Heel to Toe or described variations in side-sitting or standing and sliding a foot up and down a pole. Facilitate ankle dorsiflexion by engaging hip flexors and whole-body pattern of withdrawing the foot from the floor or stepping in Wishbone, TA Leg Lifts, slippery board or Steppin' Out. Stretch initially in Heel to Toe then progress to sitting back on plantarflexed feet in Starting Blocks. Emphasize full use of gluteal/hamstring/calf synergy in push-off to complete ankle plantarflexion and to lengthen the anterior compartment in Toeing Off and peerless pivot variations.

- **Popliteus, semimembranosus and semitendinosus**. Train ability to stabilize against tibial/knee external rotation stresses and ability to improve abduction bias of the foot and tracking balance of the patella in slippery board, side-lie variations of Heel to Toe, Horsing Around and Peerless Pivots (lesson and described pivoting and pirouetting drills).

- **Biceps femoris**. Train ability to stabilize against tibial/knee internal rotation stresses and ability to reduce adduction bias of foot in slippery board, side-lie variations of Heel to Toe, Horsing Around and Peerless Pivots (lesson and described pivoting and pirouetting drills).

- **Hamstrings**. Train contribution of hamstrings to hip extension. Strengthen hamstrings in supine with feet on wall or floor. Use slippery board or crosswise 3 inch roller under feet to emphasize hip extension/hamstring use over knee extension/quadriceps use. Use in slippery board, Pelvic Tilts, Wishbone, TA Leg Lifts. Place feet high up on wall or far away and on floor while supine and roll pelvis into posterior tilt. Stretch and strengthen the hamstrings by progressing to bending movements; use Side-sit Bending, Half-kneel Bending, Split Stance Bending and the final movement in Starting Blocks (pushing up to a split stance position from half-squatting). Use transitional movements from Sit to Stand, Cat/Camel and Side-lie Transitions to stretch and strengthen proximal hamstrings. Use belly-up orientations to activate the hip flexors and create reciprocal inhibition of hamstrings in Pelvic Tilts, Side-sit Transitions and leaning/falling back variations of Sit to Stand.

- **Quadriceps**. Train eccentric strength of quads in sitting weight back movements in Cat/Camel, Knee Walking and Half-kneel Bending. Progress on to feet to work with sitting back movements in Toeing Off and Peerless Pivots. Bias to shift weight back in Horsing Around stances and one-legged standing stances. Train medial/lateral quadriceps balance (usually activating the vastus medialis) with the same lesson variations. Cue to keep tripod foot, avoid foot pronation or abduction and to maintain knee-over-foot relationship in Toeing Off, Peerless Pivots and Horsing Around. Work with medial/lateral balance of hip and ankle musculature and reap the benefits at the knee. Stretch the rectus femoris in Knee Walking and Half-kneel Bending. Stretch the rest of the quadriceps in side-sit or sit kneeling. Tuck feet under hip(s) and lean back on hand(s), then alternate between anterior and posterior tilt. Progress to lean back on elbow(s). Contortionists may be able to lie back on their backs.

- **Hip adductors**. Train adductor/tibialis posterior coordination in slippery board, Rolling the Foot, Horsing Around and Peerless Pivots. Strengthen adductors by using a slippery board under nonweightbearing foot and doing serial pivots; alternate open and closed T-stances to get feet progressively wider, then pivot back to a narrower stance again. Vary by sliding the nonweightbearing foot out wide by leading with the heel (closed T-stance), then sliding foot back in closer by leading with the heel (open T-stance). This trains the adductors to control hip abduction and to pull the pelvis toward the weightbearing leg. Stretch the adductors in supine in Wishbone and TA Leg Lifts. Stretch in side-sitting with Side-lie Transitions and Side-sit Transitions. Stretch in hands and knees with feet wide and shifting weight to look over shoulder in Cat/Camel. Progress to described variations of Cat/Camel in plantigrade position. Use weight-shifting movements in Horsing Around and Peerless Pivots and close the deal with Squat Pivots.

- **Hip abductors**. Train abductor/peroneus longus coordination in slippery board, Rolling the Foot, Horsing Around and Peerless Pivots. Strengthen abductors in Side-lie Transitions, Dead Bug Roll and side-lie variations in Heel to Toe. Stretching the hip abductors and iliotibial band is a tough one; try variations of plantigrade movements off Cat/Camel, but instead of placing feet wide to challenge adductor length, cross one foot behind the other and shift weight. Try described variations of Peerless Pivots: get into a reverse T-stance and alternately bend and straighten.

- **Piriformis and other hip external rotators**. Train short and stubby/peroneus longus coordination in slippery board, Rolling the Foot, Horsing Around and Peerless Pivots.

Strengthen external rotators in Side-lie Transitions, Dead Bug Roll and side-lie variations in Heel to Toe. Progress to bending and pushing back upright movements in Half-kneel Bending, Split Stance Bending and Starting Blocks. Incorporate short and stubbies in gait push-off in Steppin' Out/Toeing Off and Knee Walking. Incorporate short and stubbies in change of direction functions in Horsing Around and Peerless Pivots (lesson, pole variations and drills). Stretch with Side-lie Transitions, Cat/Camel, Side-sit Transitions, Sit to Stand and all the bending movements (especially asymmetrical bending involving rotation of the pelvis and horizontal adduction of the hip joint). Link short and stubby length to shock absorption function in gait in Knee Walking, side-lie variations in Heel to Toe and Toeing Off.

- **Gluteus maximus**. Ditto as for deep hip rotators. Add in intention to 'pinch your cheek' or contract your gluteals at end-range hip extension in Pelvic Tilts (plus described bridging), Wishbone, TA Leg Lifts, Knee Walking, Half-kneel Bending, Split Stance Bending, Toeing Off (plus described variations of pushing taller and sinking lower in one legged standing), Horsing Around and Peerless Pivots.

- **Iliopsoas**. Train for function of pulling pelvis toward legs in belly-up orientations. Cue for upright sitting or as part of strong pelvic force couple that turns the pelvis in gait or throwing functions. Use Pelvic Tilts, Side-sit Transitions, Side-sit Spirals and lean/fall-back component of Sit to Stand and Sitting Circles III. Stretch with lengthening contractions in belly-up orientations; see previous lessons. Stretch by reciprocal inhibition; contract the hip extensors and allow the pelvis to posteriorly tilt and the lumbar spine to flex. Use pushing variations in Sitting Circles III, Pelvic Tilt, Wishbone, Cat/Camel and Sit to Stand. Progress to reciprocal inhibition/use of gluteals near end-range of hip extension. Use Knee Walking, Half-kneel Bending, Toeing Off, Split Stance Bending and Peerless Pivots. Use exaggerated posterior tilt with bent knees then pushing taller while maintaining posterior tilt in Horsing Around. Use one-legged version of same pushing taller with posterior tilt movement from Toeing Off or Peerless Pivots.

- **Lumbar paraspinals and quadratus lumborum**. Strengthen back muscles in gluteal-biased folks with London Bridges, Xs and Os, Cherry Turnover and Baby Rolls. Differentiate from hip extensors in Pelvic Tilts, Cat/Camel, Side-sit Transitions, Sit to Stand, Side-sit Bending and Split Stance Bending. Stretch with belly-up/falling back contexts. Use Be a Better Ball, Pelvic Tilts, Wishbone, TA Diagonals, Sitting Circles III and Sit to Stand. Stretch with belly down/push pelvis toward vertical movements in Side-sit Bending, Cat/Camel, Sit to Stand, variations of Half-kneel Bending and Split Stance Bending (instead of maintaining neutral spine the whole time, arch your back as you bend forward and round your back as you push back upright).

- **Thoracic extensors and posterior intercostals**. Strengthen globally with London Bridges, Xs and Os, Cherry Turnover and Baby Rolls. Differentiate from lumbar extensors with hamstring constraint; extend spine to orient or manipulate forward or upward from bent-over position. Use bending movements from Side-sit Bending, Half-kneel Bending, Split Stance Bending or Sit to Stand. Stretching

is less frequently required, but use falling/rolling-back movements in Be a Better Ball, Pelvic Tilts, Sit to Stand, Sitting Circles I and Side-sit Transitions. Progress by holding knees with hands variations of these lessons to emphasize shoulder girdle abduction and thoracic rounding.

- **Transverse abdominis and multifidi**. TA Facilitation, TA Diagonals and TA Leg Lifts explore coordination and differentiation of intersegmental stabilizers with pelvic floor, diaphragm and intercostals. The rest of the stabilization chapter blends intersegmental stability with pelvic mobility/stability and with thoracic mobility. Cue TA with slight falling-back movements in chair or floor sitting; remain upright and don't allow torso flexion as balance response. Cue multifidi with an analogous movement leaning/bending/falling forward.

- **Abdominal obliques, rectus abdominis and anterior intercostals**. Strengthen with falling-back movements in Be a Better Ball, Pelvic Tilts, Wishbone, TA Diagonals, Sitting Circles III, Side-sit Transitions and Sit to Stand. Train obliques for rotational stability of torso on pelvis with Dead Bug Roll and described variations lying supine with vertical pole or hand weight. Blend with wall pulleys for resistance but keep the pelvis moving. Stretch with belly breathing from TA stability series and with extension movements from London Bridges, Xs and Os, Cherry Turnover, Baby Rolls, Sitting Circles, Side-sit Spirals, Sit to Stand and the whole bending series. Emphasize upper abdominal and anterior intercostal length with Differentiated Back Bends. Facilitate lateral obliques/intercostal strength and flexibility and left/right torso balance with Be a Better Bow, Eskimo Roll and Side-sit Transitions.

Zen and the art of Using the Legs

This first volume of *A Manual Therapist's Guide to Movement* concerns movements of the worm and how it is controlled from the legs. This emphasis on the central role of the legs is not a new one. Even the Zen masters recognized what was important in life: when asked about the path to enlightenment, the answer was to 'chop wood and carry water.'

Chopping wood is an obvious reference to the ability to flex at the hips. The act of swinging the ax downward on to the wood is accompanied by bending the pelvis and torso forward on the legs in either a horse stance or a split stance. Picking up wood chunks from the ground is an even deeper bending from either horse or split stance, and additionally involves weight shift and rotation of the pelvis on the legs as you pick pieces off the ground from left to right. Chopping wood rewards long hamstrings and a strong back, the ability to allow the pelvis to fall forward on the legs, and the ability to access the hip shock absorption movement of flexion/internal rotation/horizontal adduction. Chopping wood is most easily done by the psoas-biased.

Carrying water is an obvious reference to the ability to extend the hips. The act of balancing a yoke of water buckets on your shoulders or an urn on top of your head requires an ability to push your bones close to vertical to create a column. The legs press into the ground to push the pelvis toward vertical and the thoracic extensors contract to verticalize that part of the column and push the head to a higher horizon. Carrying water rewards long hip flexors and a strong butt, the ability to push the pelvis backward on the legs and the ability to access the hip push-off movement of extension/external rotation/abduction. Carrying water is most easily done by the gluteal biased.

Enlightenment comes when you can chop wood or carry water with equal aplomb. Chopping wood and carrying water represent yet another dualism: dark and light, good and evil, yin and yang, gluteals and psoas, push-off and shock absorption. We could add another dualism: left and right force couple balance. The ability to use the legs in balanced way, both front to back and left to right, is critically important in treating lumbar instability, patellar tracking dysfunction and plantar fasciitis. The ability to use the legs in a balanced way is critically important in treating cerebrovascular accidents (CVA), cerebral palsy and multiple sclerosis. This ability is critically important in treating below-knee amputees and total hip replacements. And, as we will illustrate in the next volume of this saga, the ability to use the legs in a balanced way is critically important in treating cervical degenerative disc disease, glenohumeral impingements, tennis elbow and CVA-related upper extremity rehabilitation.

Wrapping it up

This completes the first volume of this book. The second volume on neck, shoulder girdles, arms and hands, vegetative and temporomandibular joint considerations and some simple manual facilitation techniques will follow in due course. I hope you enjoyed this tour of human movement. I hope you have a better understanding of what you want to teach and how you want to teach it. I hope you are as excited and as fascinated as I am about human movement and how to improve it.

I know this is a tough read; it's not easy going back and forth between reading and moving, between cognition and proprioceptive perception. I know it's not easy to learn movement from written words and a few pictures. I know that some of the concepts are new, confusing or even controversial. But I also know that this kind of approach can be both very beneficial to your students and deeply rewarding for you as a physical therapist.

It is my wish that this book be a catalyst for change in the way our profession and we as practitioners use movement and exercise. I would hope that the concepts of even distribution of movement, skeletal weightbearing, economy of effort and proportional use of synergists will be widely adopted. I would hope that proprioceptive awareness is emphasized more through the use of reference points and specific language cues. I would hope that we think about principles of pattern specificity and functional context before sending our students home with exercises. Change venues, reciprocate movements, apply constraints and introduce choice and problem solving to your exercises.

The way you learn to use these concepts and these exercises is to do them. Dive in and get your hands dirty. Get on the floor with your students and feel what they are feeling as they go through a lesson. Practice lesson parts or whole at home, and teach them to several people that day; notice how each responds. Build up movement experience by doing, teaching and observing. Develop language skills by describing movement: don't just read the texts of these lessons. Develop metaphors and tell stories that illustrate your point.

Teach your students about the concepts of ideal movement and provide proprioceptive examples. Break the lessons up into smaller chunks to spoonfeed to your students, or put chunks back together again in different ways to create a new lesson. Repeat the lessons again but much slower: each variation is a jewel in itself, and taking several minutes to do one repetition can help refine and improve your understanding movement. Just do it!

Neuroplasticity – stroke recovery or changing a 30-year motor habit

Whereas it used to be thought that movement and postural patterns were set in stone once developed, recent research indicates that even in adult nervous systems there is a certain amount of *neuroplasticity*.[75–87] Neuroplasticity is the ability of your nervous system to make morphological and functional changes as a result of injury (stroke, MS, Parkinson's disease) or changing environmental factors (musculoskeletal pain or injury). This capacity of the CNS to reroute familiar neural information over new neural pathways is critical to the recovery of function after stroke or other neurological insult. This capacity of the CNS to create new routes for unfamiliar neural information is critical to developing new and better motor patterns in the presence of musculoskeletal pain or dysfunction.

How much change can you expect from your students? If these movement and postural patterns and the vast quantity of interwoven subroutines have been present from early childhood, do we really stand a chance of changing their motor behavior? Yes, though it depends on how you define success. If you are thinking of absolute extinction of habitual patterns and total adoption of new and improved patterns, you will be disappointed. If you are thinking of success in terms of a reduction of harmful or inefficient patterns, increasing the amount of choice the CNS has when confronting a familiar movement problem and improving the amount of time a better motor solution is used in solving that problem, you will be happy.

We exercise our foot abduction students in parallel positions not because we expect them to suddenly adopt parallel feet in standing but to lessen the amount they abduct. We exaggerate a force couple gait not because we expect a longshoreman to walk like a runway model, but to help him recognize how to reduce to some degree the amount of rotation that happens around his lumbosacral junction. We are very specific with how we teach exercise, but are reasonable with the degree of change we expect. Allow approximations!

Donatelli wrote about recovery from an anterior cruciate ligament (ACL) injury: 'Motor learning is a primary goal of rehabilitation and entails the acquisition or reacquisition of skilled or coordinated movement. Coordination is defined as the process by which movement components are sequenced and organized temporally and their relative magnitudes determined to produce a functional movement pattern or synergy. A musculoskeletal system has the potential to move in multiple directions and use multiple muscles to produce a desired motion. Different neural pathways within the CNS influenced by vestibular, ocular or joint proprioceptive input may produce the same coordinated movements. Studies by Keshner demonstrated that different muscle recruitment patterns were induced with experimental manipulation of the environment that produced the same desired motion. To function with appropriate movement behaviors in a changing environment, the CNS must be able to identify and perceive sensory input under different conditions. Keshner suggests that therapeutic intervention provide different environmental circumstances that require multiple adaptive responses. She warns that overlearning a specific task can inhibit adaptation of motor responses; that she attempt to use that response when it interferes with generation of a more appropriate response. By progressively altering specific movement tasks and environments during closed kinetic chain training, altering overall afferent neural system input to the CNS and facilitating appropriate muscle recruitment and movement patterns, clinicians can improve the flexibility and variety of motor responses.'[88–92]

Hoo-Raa

In other words, movement education is the primary emphasis of rehabilitation professionals and movements are made up of patterns or synergies. There are literally too many choices in movement, and we have to reduce those choices by developing habitual patterns. Attending to and being self-aware of proprioceptive cues is key to coordinated movement. Exercise needs to be varied to avoid the circus bear phenomenon of situation-specific learning. Therapeutic intervention should include changing venues, applying constraints and widening choices, and should be pattern specific, functionally relevant and follow a progressive path. This, of course, is easier said than done.

Inertia is a powerful thing, and we as physical therapists have been looking at movement and exercise through a particular lens for a long time. But the era of isolated movements and compartmentalized exercises, of straight lines and cardinal planes and of mindless repetitions with strictly quantifiable goals needs to give way to a new exercise paradigm if we are to continue to grow as a profession.

Let us as physical therapists accept the challenges that go along with being movement teachers. Let us accept that we are working with motor behavior, and that strict objectivity cannot apply when we are seeking to influence that behavior. Let us accept that we cannot make someone change; that we are only facilitators for change for those willing to let us help them.

Let us expand our treatment goals beyond objective strength gains and goniometric measurements of range of motion to include goals of proprioceptive awareness, motor problem-solving abilities, integration of movement, accurate skeletal weightbearing, even distribution of movement, proportional use of synergistic muscles and economy of effort.

Let us prescribe exercise that is creative, adaptable and interest provoking. Let us scrutinize our favorite traditional exercises, inspecting them more closely under the light of pattern specificity and functional context, and being willing to make a change if there is a better alternative available. Let us embrace a new framework for exercise that is more specific, more complex, more functionally relevant, more cortical and admittedly more difficult to teach than our traditional approaches.

Let us rise to the challenge of upgrading our motor teaching skills, recognizing that pictures, demonstrations and putting in the repetitions alone are not enough. Let us hone our descriptive language skills and acquire a more critical eye for motor mistakes. Let us ask our students questions before dispensing advice, being willing to let them make motor mistakes and allowing approximate success within a progressive learning program.

Let us be the PhDs of experiential pathokinesiology!

References

1. James SL. Chondromalacia of the patella in the adolescent. In: Kennedy JC. The injured adolescent knee. Baltimore: Williams and Wilkins; 1979: 214–18.
2. Maquet P. Biomechanics of the knee. New York: Springer Verlag; 1984: 75–103.
3. Cyriax J. Textbook of orthopaedic medicine. Vol. 1. London: Tindall and Cassell; 1969.
4. Davies GJ, Larsen R. Examining the knee. Journal of Sports Medicine and Physical Fitness 1978;6:49.
5. Mayfield G. Popliteus tendon tenosynovitis. American Journal of Sports Medicine 1977;5:31.
6. Mangine R. Physical therapy of the knee, 2nd edn. New York: Churchill Livingstone; 1995: 34–41.
7. James SL, Bates BT, Ostring LR. Injuries to runners. American Journal of Sports Medicine 1978;6:40.
8. Clement DB. A survey of overuse running injuries. Physician Sports Med 1981;9:47.
9. Viitasale JT, Kvist M. Some biomechanical aspects of the foot and ankle in athletes with and without shin splints. American Journal of Sports Medicine 1983;11:125.
10. Lutter L. Injuries in the runner and jogger. Minnesota Medicine 1980;63:45.
11. Litletvedt J, Kreighbaum E, Phillips LR. Analysis of selected alignment of the lower extremity related to the shin splint syndrome. Journal of the American Podiatry Association 1969;69: 211.
12. Messier SP, Pittala KA. Etiological factors associated with selected running injuries. Medicine and Science in Sports and Exercise 1988;20:501.
13. Buchbinder MR, Napora NJ, Biggs EW. The relationship of abnormal pronation to chondromalacia of the patella in distance runners. Journal of the American Podiatry Association 1979; 69:159.
14. Mann RA, Baxter DE, Lutter LD. Running symposium. Foot Ankle 1981;1:190.
15. Scuderi G. The patella. New York: Springer Verlag; 1969.
16. Donatelli R. The biomechanics of the foot and ankle, 2nd edn. Philadelphia: FA Davis; 1996: 35.
17. Mangine R. Physical therapy of the knee, 2nd edn. New York: Churchill Livingstone; 1995: 90–1.

18. Cailliet R. Foot and ankle pain, 2nd edn. Philadelphia: FA Davis; 1983: 139.

19. Donatelli R. The biomechanics of the foot and ankle, 2nd edn. Philadelphia: FA Davis; 1996: 59.

20. Lutter LD. Running athletes in office practice. Foot Ankle 1982;3:153.

21. Clement DB, Taunton JE, Smart GW. Achilles tendinitis and peritendinitis: etiology and treatment. American Journal of Sports Medicine 1984;12:179.

22. Kibler WB, Goldberg C, Chandler TJ. Functional biomechanical deficits in running athletes with plantar fasciitis. American Journal of Sports Medicine 1991;19:66.

23. Donatelli R. The biomechanics of the foot and ankle, 2nd edn. Philadelphia: FA Davis; 1996: 198.

24. Mangine R. Physical therapy of the knee, 2nd edn. New York: Churchill Livingstone; 1995: 94.

25. Donatelli R. The biomechanics of the foot and ankle, 2nd edn. Philadelphia: FA Davis; 1996: 197.

26. Subotnick JI. The shin splints syndrome of the lower extremity. Journal of the American Podiatry Association 1976;66:43.

27. Juhan D. Job's body: a handbook for bodywork. Barrytown, NY: Station Hill Press; 1987: 42.

28. Donatelli R. The biomechanics of the foot and ankle, 2nd edn. Philadelphia: FA Davis; 1996: 210.

29. Norkin CC, Levangie PK. Joint structure and function: a comprehensive analysis. Philadelphia: FA Davis; 1989.

30. Deusinger RH. Biomechanics of clinical practice. Physical Therapy 1984;64:1860.

31. Rogers MM, Cavanagh PR. Glossary of biomechanical terms, concepts, and units. Physical Therapy 1984;64:1886.

32. Mangine R. Physical therapy of the knee, 2nd edn. New York: Churchill Livingstone; 1995: 94.

33. Cailliet R. Foot and ankle pain, 2nd edn. Philadelphia: FA Davis; 1983: 44.

34. Schilero J, Klein KK, Subotnick S. Letters to the editor-in-chief. Medicine and Science in Sports and Exercise 1981;13:ix.

35. Mangine R. Physical therapy of the knee, 2nd edn. New York: Churchill Livingstone; 1995: 94–5.

36. James SL. Chondromalacia of the patella in the adolescent. In: Kennedy JC. The injured adolescent knee. Baltimore: Williams & Wilkins; 1979: 214–18.

37. Buchbinder MR, Napora NJ, Biggs EW. The relationship of abnormal pronation to chondromalacia of the patella in distance runners. Journal of the American Podiatry Association 1979;69:159.

38. Lutter LD. Running athletes in office practice. Foot Ankle 1982;3:153.

39. Donatelli R. The biomechanics of the foot and ankle, 2nd edn. Philadelphia: FA Davis; 1996: 59, 210.

40. Clement DB, Taunton JE, Smart GW. Achilles tendonitis and peritendonitis: etiology and treatment. American Journal of Sports Medicine 1984;12:179.

41. Donatelli R. The biomechanics of the foot and ankle, 2nd edn. Philadelphia: FA Davis; 1996: 211.

42. Viitasale JT, Kvist M. Some biomechanical aspects of the foot and ankle in athletes with and without shin splints. American Journal of Sports Medicine 1983;11:125.

43. Donatelli R. The biomechanics of the foot and ankle, 2nd edn. Philadelphia: FA Davis; 1996: 213.

44. Ficat RP, Hungerford DS. Disorders of the patellofemoral joint. Baltimore: Williams & Wilkins; 1977.

45. Mangine R. Physical therapy of the knee, 2nd edn. New York: Churchill Livingstone; 1995: 40.

46. Scuderi G. The patella. New York: Springer Verlag; 1995: 69.

47. Mangine R. Physical therapy of the knee, 2nd edn. New York: Churchill Livingstone; 1995: 26.

48. Nissan M. Review of some basic assumptions in knee biomechanics. Journal of Biomechanics 1980;13:175.

49. Shoemaker SC, Markolf KL. In vivo rotary knee stability. Ligamentous and muscular contributions. Journal of Bone and Joint Surgery 1982;64A:208.

50. Mangine R. Physical therapy of the knee, 2nd edn. New York: Churchill Livingstone; 1995: 21.

51. Last RJ. The popliteus muscle and the lateral meniscus. Journal of Bone and Joint Surgery 1950;32B:93.

52. Barnett CH, Richardson A. The postural function of the popliteus muscle. Annals of Physical Medicine 1953;1:177.

53. Grood ES, Suntay WJ, Noyes FR, Butler DL. Biomechanics of the knee extension exercise. Journal of Bone and Joint Surgery 1984;66A:725.

54. Yack HJ, Riley LM, Whieldon TR. Anterior tibial translation during progressive loading of the ACL-deficient knee during weight bearing and non-weight bearing isometric exercise. Journal of Orthopedic and Sports Physical Therapy 1994;20:247–53.

55. Hungerford DS, Barry N. Biomechanics of the patellofemoral joint. Clinics in Orthopedics 1979;53A:1551–60.

56. Scuderi G. The patella. New York: Springer Verlag; 1995: 34–46.

57. Lieb FJ, Perry J. Quadriceps function. An anatomical and mechanical study using amputated limbs. Journal of Bone and Joint Surgery 1968;50A:1535.

58. Griffin L. Rehabilitation of the injured knee. St Louis: Mosby; 1995: 121, 126–30.

59. Ficat RP, Hungerford DS. Disorders of the patello-femoral joint. Baltimore: Williams & Wilkins; 1977.

60. Goodfellow J, Hungerford DS, Woods C. Patellofemoral joint mechanics and pathology: chondromalacia patellae. Journal of Bone and Joint Surgery 1976;58B:291–9.

61. Fox, J, Del Pizzo W. The patellofemoral joint. New York: McGraw-Hill; 1993: 54.

62. Radin EL. A rational approach to the treatment of patellofemoral pain. Clinics in Orthopedics 1979;144:107–9.

63. Donatelli R. The biomechanics of the foot and ankle, 2nd edn. Philadelphia: FA Davis; 1996: 130–s6.

64. Root ML, Orien WP, Weed JN. Clinical biomechanics, Vol. 2. Normal and abnormal function of the foot. Los Angeles, CA: Clinical Biomechanics; 1977.

65. Duckworth T. The hindfoot and its relation to rotational deformities of the forefoot. Clinics in Orthopedics 1983;177:39.

66. Maquet P. Biomechanics of the knee. New York: Springer Verlag; 1984: 75–103.

67. Noble CA. Iliotibial band friction syndrome in runners. American Journal of Sports Medicine 1980;8:232.

68. Kirk KL, Kuklo T, Klemme W. Iliotibial band friction syndrome. Orthopedics 2000;23:1209–15.

69. Schuster R. Podiatry and the foot of the athlete. Journal of the American Podiatry Association 1972;12:465.

70. Mangine R. Physical therapy of the knee, 2nd edn. New York: Churchill Livingstone; 1995: 88.

71. Root ML, Orien WP, Weed JN. Clinical biomechanics, Vol. 11. Normal and abnormal function of the foot. Los Angeles: Clinical Biomechanics; 1977.

72. Donatelli R. The biomechanics of the foot and ankle, 2nd edn. Philadelphia: FA Davis; 1996: 14–15.

73. Mangine R. Physical therapy of the knee, 2nd edn. New York: Churchill Livingstone; 1995: 88–90.

74. Mangine R. Physical therapy of the knee, 2nd edn. New York: Churchill Livingstone; 1995: 47.

75. Grimby G, Eriksson P, Nilsson M, Sjolund B. Neurobiology provides a scientific foundation for rehabilitation. Report from an international symposium. Lakartidningen. 2003;100:52–5.

76. Nielsen BG. Sequence learning in differentially activated dendrites. Network 2003;14:189–209.

77. Tjolsen A, Hole K. Pain regulation and plasticity. Tidsakuft for den Norske Laegeforening 1993;113:2921–4.

78. Bach-y-Rita P. Brain plasticity as a basis for recovery of function in humans. Neuropsychologia 1990;28:547–54.

79. Wilder-Smith OH, Tassonyi E, Arendt-Nielsen L. Preoperative back pain is associated with diverse manifestations of central neuroplasticity. Pain 2002;97:189–94.

80. Cheung ME, Broman SH. Adaptive learning: interventions for verbal and motor deficits. Neurorehabilitation and Neural Repair 2000;14:159–69.

81. Sanes JN, Donoghue JP. Plasticity and primary motor cortex. Annual Review of Neuroscience 2000;23:393–415.

82. Gispen WH. Neuronal plasticity and function. Clinical Neuropharmacology 1993;16(Suppl 1):S5–11.

83. Ren K, Dubner R. Central nervous system plasticity and persistent pain. Journal of Orofacial Pain 1999;13:155–63.

84. Bogerts B. Plasticity of brain structure and function as the neurobiological principle of psychotherapy. Zeitschrift fur klinische Psycologie, Psychiatrie und Psychotherapie 1996;44:243–52.

85. Taub E, Morris DM. Constraint-induced movement therapy to enhance recovery after stroke. Current Atherosclerosis Reports 2001;3:279–86.

86. Weiller C, Rijntjes M. Learning, plasticity, and recovery in the central nervous system. Experimental Brain Research 1999;128:134–8.

87. Van Praag H, Kempermann G, Gage FH. Neural consequences of environmental enrichment. Nature Reviews of Neuroscience 2000;1:191–8.

88. Donatelli R. The biomechanics of the foot and ankle, 2nd edn. Philadelphia: FA Davis; 1996: 338.

89. Scholz JP. Dynamic pattern theory – some implications for therapeutics. Physical Therapy 1990;70:844.

90. Keshner EA. Controlling stability of a complex movement system. Physical Therapy 1990;70:844.

91. Keshner EA, Woolacot MH, Deb B. Neck and trunk responses during postural perturbations in humans. Experimental Brain Research 1988;71:455.

92. Keggerreis S. The construction and implementation of a functional progression as a component of athletic rehabilitation. Journal of Orthopedic and Sports Physical Therapy 1983;4:14.

Index

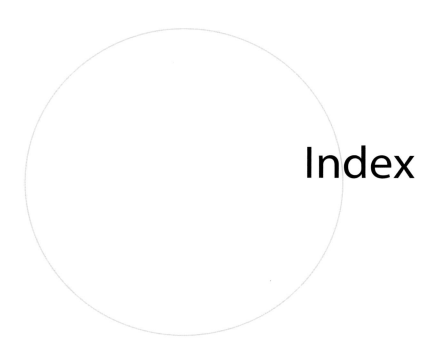
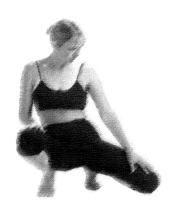